Diseases of the Swine

Diseases of the Swine

Edited by Anna Hunt

MURPHY & MOORE
www.murphy-moorepublishing.com

Published by Murphy & Moore Publishing,
1 Rockefeller Plaza,
New York City, NY 10020, USA
www.murphy-moorepublishing.com

Diseases of the Swine
Edited by Anna Hunt

International Standard Book Number: 978-1-63987-167-4 (Hardback)

Cataloging-in-Publication Data

Diseases of the swine / edited by Anna Hunt.
p. cm.
Includes bibliographical references and index.
ISBN 978-1-63987-167-4
1. Swine--Diseases. 2. Swine. 3. Veterinary medicine. I. Hunt, Anna.
SF971 .D57 2022
636.408 96--dc23

TABLE OF CONTENTS

PREFACE

The main aim of this book is to educate learners and enhance their research focus by presenting diverse topics covering this vast field. This is an advanced book which compiles significant studies by distinguished experts in the area of analysis. This book addresses successive solutions to the challenges arising in the area of application, along with it; the book provides scope for future developments.

Swine refers to the even-toed ungulates which are commercially bred for their meat, hair and leather. The health of swine is a significant area of research due to the possibility of zoonotic diseases. Pigs harbor an array of parasites such as taenia solium, brucellosis, trichinosis, cysticercosis, ascarid worms, etc. Pigs all suffer some diseases such as swine influenza, swine vesicular disease, foot-and-mouth disease, swine acute diarrhea syndrome coronavirus, etc. Swine influenza is characterized by fever, coughing, loss of appetite and difficulty in breathing. Vaccines are an effective way to prevent it. Swine vesicular disease is a viral disease cause by an enterovirus. The primary symptoms include vesicles with mouth ulcers and fever. Prevention measures include placing infected pigs in quarantine, maintaining high sanitation standards and hygiene management in the facility. This book provides comprehensive insights into the diseases of swine. It consists of contributions made by international experts. This book is appropriate for students seeking detailed information in this area as well as for experts.

It was a great honour to edit this book, though there were challenges, as it involved a lot of communication and networking between me and the editorial team. However, the end result was this all-inclusive book covering diverse themes in the field.

Finally, it is important to acknowledge the efforts of the contributors for their excellent chapters, through which a wide variety of issues have been addressed. I would also like to thank my colleagues for their valuable feedback during the making of this book.

Editor

1

African swine fever virus transmission cycles in Central Europe: Evaluation of wild boar-soft tick contacts through detection of antibodies against *Ornithodoros erraticus* saliva antigen

Jana Pietschmann[1†], Lina Mur[2†], Sandra Blome[1*], Martin Beer[1], Ricardo Pérez-Sánchez[3], Ana Oleaga[3] and José Manuel Sánchez-Vizcaíno[2]

Abstract

Background: African swine fever (ASF) is one of the most complex viral diseases affecting both domestic and wild pigs. It is caused by ASF virus (ASFV), the only DNA virus which can be efficiently transmitted by an arthropod vector, soft ticks of the genus *Ornithodoros*. These ticks can be part of ASFV-transmission cycles, and in Europe, *O. erraticus* was shown to be responsible for long-term maintenance of ASFV in Spain and Portugal. In 2014, the disease has been reintroduced into the European Union, affecting domestic pigs and, importantly, also the Eurasian wild boar population. In a first attempt to assess the risk of a tick-wild boar transmission cycle in Central Europe that would further complicate eradication of the disease, over 700 pre-existing serum samples from wild boar hunted in four representative German Federal States were investigated for the presence of antibodies directed against salivary antigen of *Ornithodoros erraticus* ticks using an indirect ELISA format.

Results: Out of these samples, 16 reacted with moderate to high optical densities that could be indicative of tick bites in sampled wild boar. However, these samples did not show a spatial clustering (they were collected from distant geographical regions) and were of bad quality (hemolysis/impurities). Furthermore, all positive samples came from areas with suboptimal climate for soft ticks. For this reason, false positive reactions are likely.

Conclusion: In conclusion, the study did not provide stringent evidence for soft tick-wild boar contact in the investigated German Federal States and thus, a relevant involvement in the epidemiology of ASF in German wild boar is unlikely. This fact would facilitate the eradication of ASF in the area, although other complex relations (wild boar biology and interactions with domestic pigs) need to be considered.

Keywords: African swine fever, Transmission cycles, Wild boar, *Ornithodoros erraticus*, Tick saliva antigen, ELISA

*Correspondence: sandra.blome@fli.bund.de
†Equal contributors
[1]Institute of Diagnostic Virology, Friedrich-Loeffler-Institut, Suedufer 10, 17493 Greifswald—Insel Riems, Germany
Full list of author information is available at the end of the article

Background

African swine fever (ASF) is one of the most important and complex notifiable diseases of both domestic and wild pigs. It is caused by the eponymous virus which belongs to the genus *Asfivirus* within the *Asfarviridae* family [1]. African swine fever virus (ASFV) is the only known DNA virus with an arthropod vector. The latter are soft ticks of the genus *Ornithodoros* [2]. In general, different transmission cycles are observed with ASFV: a sylvatic cycle, a soft tick-pig cycle, and a domestic cycle [3]. The former is of importance in Southern and Eastern Africa, where it involves warthogs and soft ticks of the *O. moubata* complex, while a similar sylvatic cycle in Europe, involving Eurasian wild boar and *O. erraticus* ticks has not been hitherto demonstrated [4]. The tick-pig cycle was up to now observed in Africa [5] and on the Iberian Peninsula [6], where it involved domestic pigs and *O. erraticus* ticks infesting the pig pens. This cycle can have a tremendous impact on transmission and long-term maintenance of ASF virus circulation [3] favoring endemic situations, especially in outdoor swine production [7]. However, once introduced into the domestic pig population, the virus does not rely on vector borne transmission, as both direct and indirect contacts are very efficient means of viral transmission [8].

The endophilous/ nidicolous ticks in the *O. erraticus* complex have been reported from the Iberian Peninsula, North and West Africa, and Western Asia [9–11]. On the Iberian Peninsula, *O. erraticus* ticks were found in close association with swine on free-range pig farms, hidden in holes, cracks and fissures inside and around pig-pens. They were also found in bird nests, in burrows of small mammals, under stones, or in the resting places of vertebrate host species, but always in the proximity of pig-pens [12]. So far, these soft ticks have never been reported from Central and Northern Europe [9, 11].

ASF was completely eradicated from Europe in the 1990's except from the Italian island of Sardinia, which has been affected since 1978 [9]. In 2007, the disease was introduced into Georgia. Subsequently, it spread to neighboring Trans-Caucasian countries, the Russian Federation, and more recently (2014), it re-entered into the European Union affecting Lithuania, Poland, Latvia, and Estonia (OIE WAHID, visited March 23rd 2015). In most of the affected European countries, the disease was detected in domestic pigs of all production sectors and in wild boar. The involvement of the latter is of special importance as the very high density of wild boar in Central Europe could favor the establishment of endemic situations that are most difficult to control. Although no evidences were found in the past that wild boar were parasitized by Ornithodoros ticks [13], the absence of this relationship has not been clearly demonstrated by scientific data. Considering that the presence and involvement of soft ticks would certainly further complicate ASF eradication in the area [14], the assessment of a possible tick-wild boar cycle is urgently needed and would be required in the framework of legal binding ASF control within the European Union (Council Directive 2002/60/EC and Commission Decision 2003/422/EC).

In order to assess the possible role of soft ticks in Central Europe, over 700 serum samples from German wild boar were screened for antibodies against tick saliva antigen using an indirect ELISA previously developed and largely employed to screen domestic pigs in Spain. This ELISA uses a salivary gland extract (SGE) as antigen and provides 100 % specificity and sensitivity with experimentally infested pigs, decreasing to 90 % in field conditions [15–17].

Methods

A total of 723 serum samples of hunted Eurasian wild boar from four different German Federal States, namely Rhineland-Palatinate (RP), North-Rhine Westphalia (NRW), Mecklenburg-Western Pomerania (MWP), and Brandenburg (BB), were investigated for antibodies against *O. erraticus* tick saliva antigen. The samples were obtained within the framework of an ongoing classical swine fever (CSF) surveillance program in the respective Federal States and were kindly provided by the competent regional veterinary laboratories (Rostock, Krefeld, Koblenz, and Frankfurt/Oder). The sampling areas were chosen to reflect the spatial extent of Germany (areas in the North-West, South-West, North-East, and East) and were taken from the sample collection at random.

The samples were transferred to the OIE-Reference Laboratory for ASF—Universidad Complutense de Madrid (UCM) to be tested in ELISA. All serum samples were analyzed against the SGE of *O. erraticus* and samples giving doubtful results were reanalyzed after deglycosylating the SGE with sodium metaperiodate to eliminate cross-reactivity by glyscosylated epitopes [Oleaga-Pérez et al. 1994]. The test shows an overall specificity of 100 % with experimental sera which drops to about 90 % under field conditions.

Sample results were normalized considering the controls of their plates (two positive controls and one negative control), and the sample to positive ratio (SP ratio, SP) was calculated for each sample. For the samples analyzed repeatedly in different plates, the maximum optical density (worst case scenario) was employed for the calculation of the final results.

Results

Based on the established sample to positive (SP)-categorization (see Table 1), a total of 595 samples (82.3 % of all serum samples) were placed into category 0 (negligible risk for tick presence), 112 samples (15.5 % of

Table 1 Classification matrix according to the sample to positive ratio (SP)

SP	Category	Definition
<10	0	Negligible probability of tick presence
1–30	+	Medium probability of tick presence
31–50	++	High probability of tick presence
>50	+++	Very high probability of tick presence

era) were assigned to category + (medium probability of ick presence) 9 (1.2 %) samples were categorized as ++ and seven samples (<1 %) were placed into the +++ category, which would mean, high and very high probability of tick presence, respectively. Of the seven samples in category +++, four samples originated from North-Rhine Westphalia (NRW), two from Mecklenburg-Western Pomerania (MWP), and one from Rhineland-Palatinate (RP). In category ++, samples were found from Brandenburg (BB; $n = 3$), MWP ($n = 3$), NRW ($n = 2$), and RP ($n = 1$). An overview of all SP results by region is presented in Fig. 1.

Follow-up of positive samples placed in categories ++ and +++ revealed that these samples did not show spatial clustering and showed low sample quality with high degree of hemolysis and impurities. None of the samples originated from areas where the climate would suggest tick presence.

Discussion

With the aim to assess the risk of a soft tick-wild boar transmission cycle of ASFV in Central Europe, and to explore the possible interest in direct tick sampling, more than 700 German wild boar sera available from an active classical swine fever surveillance were investigated by an indirect ELISA for the detection of antibodies against *Ornithodoros erraticus* tick saliva antigen. The results were categorized according to the SP ratio to indicate the possible presence of ticks in the region of origin.

From the total of 723 sera, 2.2 % were placed in categories that would indicate high and very high probability of tick presence. Given the fact that the ELISA has a specificity of 90 % under field conditions [15], these few

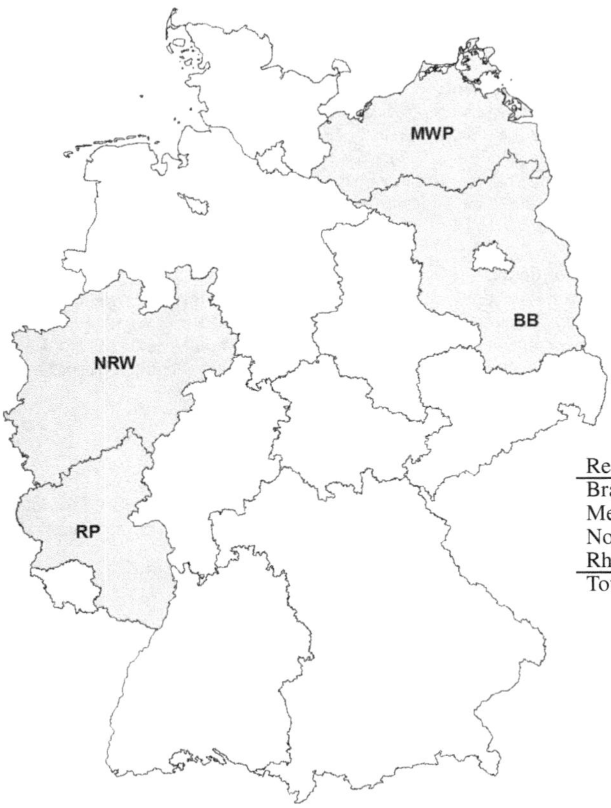

Region / federal state	0	+	++	+++	Total
Brandenburg	55	30	3	0	88
Mecklenburg-Western Pomerania	235	31	3	2	271
North Rhine-Westphalia	241	33	2	4	280
Rhineland-Palatinate	64	18	1	1	84
Total	595	112	9	7	723

Fig. 1 Origin of German wild boar sera analyzed utilizing the indirect antibody ELISA against salivary gland extract of O. erraticus ticks. Sampled areas are highlighted in grey and positive results are indicated by category in the adjacent table. Categorization of sera is done according to the sample to positive ratio (SP). The categories reflect the potential presence of Ornithodoros ticks in the respective regions from "negligible (0)" to "very likely (+++)" as defined in Table 1. NRW = North Rhine-Westphalia; RP = Rhineland-Palatinate; MWP = Mecklenburg-Western Pomarania; BB = Brandenburg.

high positive results could be within the false positive limits of the test system. This assumption is strengthened by the fact that these positive results were not spatially clustered, and were obtained from samples with low quality. Furthermore, these samples came from areas with suboptimal climate for tick maintenance, i.e., the respective soft ticks are highly resistant to high temperatures and dry conditions, but cold temperatures limit the development of their life cycle, which only starts when the external temperatures are in the range of 10–13 °C [18]. Therefore, the areas involved in the current study, presenting mean annual temperatures of 5 to 10 ° C, do not seem to be optimal for *Ornithodoros* presence. Based on these facts, false positive reactions are quite likely. Those reactions are known to occur quite frequently in serological tests with samples of bad quality. Some ELISA tests for the detection of antibodies against ASFV also presented this problem [19], specifically when raw antigens were employed instead of recombinant or more purified antigens [20]. These results enhance the importance of obtaining good quality samples for a correct diagnosis, what is not always possible when working with materials from wild animals.

Apart from the above mentioned high suspect samples, another 15.5 % were placed in the category with medium probability of tick presence. This rate would definitively surpass the expected range of false positives (roughly 10 % under field conditions) and thus, the possibility that these sera and those classified as ++ and +++ are true positives cannot be completely ruled out. Only direct sampling of places where positive wild boar were hunted could give certainty. This would mean a tremendous effort in a region that is considered suboptimal for soft ticks and was never shown to harbor those species [9]. However, sampling attempts are under discussion in representative areas. Apart from true positive reactions, cross reactions with hard ticks have to be considered. While Pérez-Sánchez et al. [17] discarded cross reaction between *O. erraticus* and the most usual species of hard ticks that also parasitize swine on free-range pig farms in Southwestern Spain (namely, *Dermacentor marginatus*, *Hyalomma lusitanicum*, *R. sanguineus* and *R. bursa*), these authors did not include *Ixodes ricinus* in their study since this species is rarely found, if ever, in the holm-oak savannah lands where these free-range pig farms localized [21]. In contrast, *I. ricinus* is by far the most common species of tick in Germany and wild boar are among the hosts [22]. Thus, cross reaction between *O. erraticus* and *I. ricinus* should not be discarded and this could account for the positive results obtained with these sera.

Conclusions

Based on the presented results, soft tick-wild boar contact and thus, a soft tick-wild boar transmission cycle of ASF in Germany seem unlikely. This conclusion has been previously suggested by other authors [13], but up to now, this is the first study supporting the previous hypothesis with field data.

These findings have an important impact on prevention and control strategies and should help to prioritize efforts and resources. Based on the presented data, the potential role of soft ticks in ASF persistence in German wild boar populations is mostly negligible and consequently, prevention measures should be focused on measures such as controlling artificial feeding and concentration points, analyzing home ranges and host interactions.

Further application of this serological test in other areas of Europe could help to understand and reveal the importance of ornithodoros ticks, and consequently assess its potential future implication in ASF epizootic cycles.

Competing interests

The authors declare that they do not have competing interests.

Authors' contribution

JP and LM carried out the ELISA, analyzed the results, and drafted the manuscript. SB, MB and JMSV designed and supervised the study and critically revised the manuscript, RPS and AO designed and validated the test system and critically revised the manuscript. All authors read and approved the final manuscript.

Acknowledgements

The authors would like to acknowledge the regional laboratories for providing the wild boar sera, Dr. Christoph Staubach for providing the shaded map of Germany, and Dr. Kerstin Wernike for critically reading the revised manuscript. This work has been funded by the European Research Project ASFORCE ("Targeted research effort on African swine fever", grant agreement 311931).

Author details

[1]Institute of Diagnostic Virology, Friedrich-Loeffler-Institut, Suedufer 10, 17493 Greifswald—Insel Riems, Germany. [2]VISAVET Center and Animal Health Department, Veterinary School, Universidad Complutense de Madrid, Avenida Puerta de Hierro s/n, 28040 Madrid, Spain. [3]Parasitología, IRNASA (CSIC), Cordel de Merinas, 40-52, 37008 Salamanca, Spain.

References

1. Takamatsu HD LK, Alonso C, Escribano JM, Martins C, Revilla Y, Salas ML. Asfarviridae. In: Virus Taxonomy. Volume Ninth Report of the ICTV. ednth ed. 2011. p. 153–62.
2. Penrith ML, Vosloo W. Review of African swine fever: transmission, spread and control. J S Afr Vet Assoc. 2009;80(2):58–62.
3. Costard S, Mur L, Lubroth J, Sanchez-Vizcaino JM, Pfeiffer DU. Epidemiology of African swine fever virus. Virus Res. 2013;173(1):191–7.
4. Thomson GR. The epidemiology of African swine fever: the role of free-living hosts in Africa. Onderstepoort J Vet Res. 1985;52(3):201–9.
5. Plowright W, Parker J, Pierce MA. The epidemiology of African swine fever in Africa. VetRec. 1969;85:668–74.
6. Sanchez-Bojita A. Reservorios del virus de la peste porcina Africana. Investigacion del virus de la P.P.A en los artropodos mediante la prueba de la hemoadsorcion. Bull Off Int Epizoot. 1963;60:895–9.
7. Sánchez-Vizcaíno JM, Arias M, Zimmermann J, Karriker L, Ramirez A, Schwartz K, et al. African swine fever. In: Diseases of swine. 10th ed. Ames: Blackwell Publishing Professional; 2012. p. 396–404.
8. Sanchez-Vizcaino JM, Mur L, Martinez-Lopez B. African swine fever: an epidemiological update. Transbound Emerg Dis. 2012;59 Suppl 1:27–35.

Vial L. Biological and ecological characteristics of soft ticks (Ixodida: Argasidae) and their impact for predicting tick and associated disease distribution. Parasite. 2009;16(3):191–202.

0. Trape JF, Diatta G, Arnathau C, Bitam I, Sarih M, Belghyti D, et al. The epidemiology and geographic distribution of relapsing fever borreliosis in West and North Africa, with a review of the Ornithodoros erraticus complex (Acari: Ixodida). PLoS One. 2013;8(11):e78473.

1. Boinas F, Ribeiro R, Madeira S, Palma M, de Carvalho I, Núncio S, et al. The medical and veterinary role of Ornithodoros erraticus complex ticks (Acari: Ixodida) on the Iberian Peninsula. J Vector Ecol. 2014;39(2):238–48.

2. Oleaga-Perez A, Perez-Sanchez R, Encinas-Grandes A. Distribution and biology of Ornithodoros erraticus in parts of Spain affected by African swine fever. Vet Rec. 1990;126(2):32–7.

3. Scientific Opinion on African Swine Fever, EFSA Journal. 2010; 8(3):1556 [149 pp.].http://www.efsa.europa.eu/en/efsajournal/pub/155.

4. Arias M, Sanchez-Vizcaino JM, Morilla A, Yoon KJ, Zimmerman JJ. African Swine Fever Eradication: The Spanish Model. In: Trends in Emerging Viral Infections of Swine. Volume 1. Ames: Iowa State Press; 2002. p. 133–9.

5. Oleaga-Perez A, Perez-Sanchez R, Astigarraga A, Encinas-Grandes A. Detection of pig farms with Ornithodoros erraticus by pig serology. Elimination of non-specific reactions by carbohydrate epitopes of salivary antigens. VetParasitol. 1994;52(1–2):97–111.

6. Canals A, Oleaga A, Perez R, Dominguez J, Encinas A, Sanchez-Vizcaino JM. Evaluation of an enzyme-linked immunosorbent assay to detect specific antibodies in pigs infested with the tick Ornithodoros erraticus (Argasidae). VetParasitol. 1990;37(2):145–53.

7. Pérez-Sánchez R, Oleaga-Pérez A, Encinas-Grandes A. Analysis of the specificity of the salivary antigens of Ornithodoros erraticus for the purpose of serological detection of swine farms harbouring the parasite. Parasite Immunol. 1992;14(2):201–16.

8. Scientific report submitted to EFSA prepared by Sánchez-Vizcaíno, J.M., Martínez-López, B., Martínez-Avilés, M., Martins, C., Boinas, F., Vial, L., Michaud, V., Jori, F., Etter, E., Albina, E. and Roger, F. on African Swine Fever. (2009), 1–141.

9. Gallardo C, Reis AL, Kalema-Zikusoka G, Malta J, Soler A, Blanco E, et al. Recombinant antigen targets for serodiagnosis of African swine fever. Clin Vaccine Immunol. 2009;16(7):1012–20.

0. Mur L, Boadella M, Martinez-Lopez B, Gallardo C, Gortazar C, Sanchez-Vizcaino JM. Monitoring of African swine fever in the wild boar population of the most recent endemic area of Spain. Transbound Emerg Dis. 2012;59(6):526–31.

1. Encinas Grandes A. Ticks of the province of Salamanca (Central/NW Spain). Prevalence and parasitization intensity in dogs and domestic ungulates. Ann Parasitol Hum Comp. 1986;61(1):95–107.

2. Schwarz A, Maier WA, Kistemann T, Kampen H. Analysis of the distribution of the tick Ixodes ricinus L. (Acari: Ixodidae) in a nature reserve of western Germany using Geographic Information Systems. Int J Hyg Environ Health. 2009;212(1):87–96.

African swine fever virus infection in Classical swine fever subclinically infected wild boars

Oscar Cabezón[1,2†], Sara Muñoz-González[1,3†], Andreu Colom-Cadena[2], Marta Pérez-Simó[1,3], Rosa Rosell[1,3,4], Santiago Lavín[2], Ignasi Marco[2], Lorenzo Fraile[5], Paloma Martínez de la Riva[6], Fernando Rodríguez[1], Javier Domínguez[6] and Llilianne Ganges[1,3*]

Abstract

Background: Recently moderate-virulence classical swine fever virus (CSFV) strains have been proven capable of generating postnatal persistent infection (PI), defined by the maintenance of viremia and the inability to generate CSFV-specific immune responses in animals. These animals also showed a type I interferon blockade in the absence of clinical signs. In this study, we assessed the infection generated in 7-week-old CSFV PI wild boars after infection with the African swine fever virus (ASFV). The wild boars were divided in two groups and were infected with ASFV. Group A comprised boars who were CSFV PI in a subclinical form and Group B comprised pestivirus-free wild boars. Some relevant parameters related to CSFV replication and the immune response of CSFV PI animals were studied. Additionally, serum soluble factors such as IFN-α, TNF-α, IL-6, IL-10, IFN-γ and sCD163 were analysed before and after ASFV infection to assess their role in disease progression.

Results: After ASFV infection, only the CSFV PI wild boars showed progressive acute haemorrhagic disease; however, the survival rates following ASFV infection was similar in both experimental groups. Notwithstanding, the CSFV RNA load of CSFV PI animals remained unaltered over the study; likewise, the ASFV DNA load detected after infection was similar between groups. Interestingly, systemic type I FN-α and IL-10 levels in sera were almost undetectable in CSFV PI animals, yet detectable in Group B, while detectable levels of IFN-γ were found in both groups. Finally, the flow cytometry analysis showed an increase in myelomonocytic cells ($CD172a^+$) and a decrease in $CD4^+$ T cells in the PBMCs from CSFV PI animals after ASFV infection.

Conclusions: Our results showed that the immune response plays a role in the progression of disease in CSFV subclinically infected wild boars after ASFV infection, and the immune response comprised the systemic type I interferon blockade. ASFV does not produce any interference with CSFV replication, or vice versa. ASFV infection could be a trigger factor for the disease progression in CSFV PI animals, as their survival after ASFV was similar to that of the pestivirus-free ASFV-infected group. This fact suggests a high resistance in CSFV PI animals even against a virus like ASFV; this may mean that there are relevant implications for CSF control in endemic countries. The diagnosis of ASFV and CSFV co-infection in endemic countries cannot be ruled out and need to be studied in greater depth.

Keywords: CSFV, CSF postnatal persistent infection, Subclinical CSF, ASFV, Wild boars, Viral load, Innate immune response, Adaptive immune response, Disease

* Correspondence: llilianne.ganges@irta.cat
†Equal contributors
[1]IRTA, Centre de Recerca en Sanitat Animal (CReSA, IRTA-UAB), Campus de la Universitat Autònoma de Barcelona, 08193 Bellaterra, Spain
[3]OIE Reference Laboratory for Classical Swine Fever, IRTA-CReSA, Campus de la Universitat Autònoma de Barcelona, 08193 Barcelona, Spain
Full list of author information is available at the end of the article

Background

African swine fever (ASF) and Classical swine fever (CSF) are highly contagious viral diseases of domestic pigs, wild boars and feral pigs [1, 2]. Because of their high socioeconomic impact, both diseases must be reported to the World Organisation for Animal Health (OIE).

ASF is caused by the large DNA virus African swine fever virus (ASFV), currently the only member of the *Asfarviridae* family [3]. ASFV encodes between 150 and 167 proteins, a number of which have been shown to modulate host immune responses [1, 4]. Since 2007, a highly virulent ASFV has spread from Sub-Saharan Africa to Eastern Europe being detected in Russia, Armenia, Azerbaijan, Estonia, Ukraine and Lithuania, among other places [5]. Direct contact between infected wild boars and domestic pigs has played a relevant role in the spread of the disease in the Caucasus region and the Russian Federation [5–8]. CSF remains endemic in areas of Asia, Europe, Central and South America and parts of Africa. The disease is caused by Classical swine fever virus (CSFV) which belongs to the Pestivirus genus within the *Flaviviridae* family [9]. CSFV is composed of a lipid envelope, a capsid and a single plus-strand RNA genome carrying a single, large open reading frame (ORF) flanked by two untranslated regions (UTRs) [10].

Both ASFV and CSFV share a tropism for immune system cells, mainly those that are derived from the monocyte-macrophage lineage, which are central in orchestrating innate and adaptive immune responses [1, 11, 12]. It is assumed that the infection of these cells plays an important role in virus replication and pathogenesis by exploiting their migratory ability, which promotes viral spread and persistence in the host for both ASFV and CSFV.

Type I IFN-α has beneficial effects for viral infections because it restricts viral dissemination, although it can promote immunopathological events when released at high levels over a longer duration [13]. CSFV induces a potent IFN-α response, which is detected in the serum of CSFV acute-infected pigs. This response has been hypothesised to be related to disease severity rather than to protective immune responses [13, 14]. Likewise, previous studies have demonstrated the increase in type I IFN-α response after infection with ASFV virulent strains ([15–17]). In addition, macrophages, the main target cells for ASFV replication, produce a range of inflammatory mediators, including chemokines that play an important role in the disease's progression [18]. Depending on many factors, including the nature of the viral strain and the age, breed and immune system of the host, varying degrees of disease severity can be observed, ranging from acute to subclinical or chronic forms in infections caused by both viruses [1, 4, 17, 19, 20]. In addition, the circulation of CSFV strains of low and/or moderate virulence has been associated with the maintenance of the virus in the field, generating unapparent forms of CSF [21–23].

Recently, it was proven that CSFV can generate postnatal persistence by infecting both newborn piglets and wild boars with either low- and/or moderate-virulence strains, respectively [24, 25]. During the 6 weeks after postnatal infection, most of the infected animals remained clinically healthy, despite persistently high virus titres in the blood, organs and body secretions. These animals were unable to mount any detectable CSFV-specific humoral or cellular immune responses [24, 25].

The superinfection exclusion (SIE) phenomenon is defined as the ability of a primary virus infection to interfere with a secondary infection caused by the same or a closely related virus [26–28]. In this regard, CSVF PI wild boars were protected from superinfection by the virulent CSFV Margarita strain, showing efficient suppression of superinfection in animals, especially in the absence of IFN-α, which might be associated with the lack of innate immune mechanisms [28]. Thus, considering the drastic effect of ASFV on the swine immune system, in the present study, we assessed the infection generated after African swine fever virus (ASFV) inoculation in CSFV PI wild boars. For this purpose, apparently healthy, CSFV postnatal PI wild boars (7-week-old) [24] were inoculated with a highly virulent ASFV strain. Some relevant parameters related to CSFV and ASFV replication and immune response were studied. Additionally, serum soluble factors including IFN-α, TNF-α, IL-6, IL-10, IFN-γ and sCD163 were analysed before and after ASFV infection to assess their role in the progression of disease in the CSFV PI animals. Additionally, virological and immunological parameters after ASFV infection in naive wild boars were also evaluated.

Methods

Cells and viruses

PK-15 cells (ATCC CCL 33) were cultured in Dulbecco's Modified Eagle Medium (DMEM), supplemented with 10% foetal bovine serum (FBS), pestivirus-free, at 37 °C in 5% CO_2. The cells were infected with CSFV 0.1 $TCID_{50}$/cell in 2% FBS, and the virus was harvested 48 h later. Peroxidase-linked assay (PLA) [29] was used for CSFV titration following the statistical methods described by Reed and Muench [30].

The CSFV Catalonia 01 (Cat01) strain used in this study was isolated from the Spanish CSF epizootic in 2000–2001 [31]. This isolate belongs to the CSFV 2.3 genogroup [22]. The course of infection from this strain was found to be mild [31, 32]. Finally, the moderately virulent E75 ASFV strain was used [33]. This strain was isolated in 1975 in Spain and propagated in pig leucocytes [17].

Experimental design

Two groups of three wild boars each (A and B), 7 weeks old with 6 kg average weight were used [28]. These animals were acquired from Gestión Cinegética Integral SL farm (Segovia, Spain).

Group A, wild boars 1 to 3, were postnatally CSFV PI animals; they were intranasally infected in the first 24 h after birth with 2.5 ml of 10^4TCID$_{50}$/ml of the CSFV Cat01 strain [24]. These wild boars remained apparently healthy at 7 weeks old, but were viraemic and lacked CSFV-specific cellular and humoral responses [24], similar to CSFV PI piglets that were infected postnatally [25].

The second group (Group B, animals 4 to 6), housed in an independent isolation unit at the BSL-3 facility of CReSA, (animals 4 to 6), was used as control; these animals tested pestivirus-free throughout the experiment.

All the wild boars were fed with a conventional piglet starter diet and pellets until the end of the trial (Startrite 100, Kwikstart and Prestarter; SCA Iberica S.A., Zaragoza, Spain) and were handled according to previous studies conducted in CReSA [24, 34]. After a 5-day acclimation period, all the animals were experimentally infected by intramuscular (i.m.) injection in the neck with a dose of 10^4 TCID$_{50}$ ASFV E75 strain. In previous studies, this viral dose caused acute ASF and often induced death within a week post-infection [17]. Sera and nasal and rectal swabs were collected at 0, 3, 5, 7 and 10 days post infection (dpi). Blood samples for the isolation of PBMCs were collected in EDTA tubes at 0 dpi and at the time of euthanasia (10 dpi).

A trained veterinarian recorded the clinical signs daily in a blinded manner [35]. The clinical signs compatible with CSFV and after ASFV infection were previously described ([17, 31, 36–38]). Moreover, the clinical statuses registered in both experimental groups were scored from 0 to 6 as follows: 0: no signs; 1: mild pyrexia; 2: pyrexia plus mild clinical signs; 3: mild-to-moderate clinical signs; 4: moderate clinical signs; 5: moderate-to-severe clinical signs and 6: death. For ethical reasons, the animals were euthanized when the clinical score reached 5 or developed any of the following symptoms: fall of the hindquarters, inability to drink or feed, prostration or moderate nervous disorders. After euthanasia, an exhaustive necropsy was conducted, in which the presence of pathological findings in different organs was evaluated and tissues (spleen, lung and tonsil) were obtained. Euthanasia was performed according to European Directive 2010/63/EU, using a pentobarbital overdose of 60–100 mg/kg administered via the anterior vena cava. Animal care and procedures were in accordance with the guidelines of the Good Experimental Practices (GEP), under the supervision of the Ethical and Animal Welfare Committee of the Autonomous University of Barcelona (UAB), and they were approved under number 8804, according to existing national and European regulations. Additionally, the biosafety level of the viruses used in this study was stated as biosecurity level 3, as approved by the Biosafety Committee of the UAB, with registration assignment AR-296-15.

Detection of CSFV RNA

CSFV RNA was extracted from sera, nasal and recta swabs, and tonsil, spleen and lung tissues using th NucleoSpin RNA isolation kit (Macherey-Nagel), ac cording to the manufacturer's instructions. The presenc of CSFV RNA was analysed by a CSFV qRT-PCR [39] Positive results were considered for threshold cycl values (Ct) equal to or less than 42, when fluorescence i no longer detected. Samples in which fluorescence wa undetectable were considered negative.

Detection of ASFV DNA

ASFV DNA was extracted from sera, nasal and recta swabs and tissue samples (tonsil, spleen and lung) usin the NucleoSpin blood kit (Macherey-Nagel, Düren Germany) according to the manufacturer's recommenda tions. The presence of viral DNA was analysed by ASFV qRT-PCR technique using a Universal Probe Librar [40]. Positive results were considered for threshold cycl values (Ct) equal to or less than 40, when fluorescence i no longer detected. Samples in which fluorescence wa undetectable were considered negative.

Specific CSFV and ASFV antibodies detection

For CSFV-specific antibody detection, sera from 0 dpi, 7 dpi and 10 dpi were tested with neutralisation peroxidase-linked assay (NPLA) [41], and the titres were expressed as the reciprocal dilution of serum that neu tralised 100 TCID$_{50}$ of the Cat01 strain in 50% of the culture replicates. The detection of CSFV E2-specific antibodies was performed using a commercial ELISA kit (HerdChek CSFV Ab, IDEXX) following the manufac turer's recommendations. The samples were considered positive when the blocking percentage was ≥40%. Fo ASFV-specific antibody detection, a blocking ELISA assay technique was conducted using a commercia ELISA kit (INGEZIM PPA Compac, Ingenasa) following the manufacturer's recommendations. This ELISA test i validated by the European Union Reference Laborator for ASF (EURL-ASF, CISA-INIA, Spain).

ELISA detection of serum soluble factors

Sera collected at days 0, 7 and 10 dpi were analysed for the detection of several serum soluble factors. A house-ELISA was used to evaluate the serum IFN-α levels. Anti-IFN-α monoclonal antibodies (K9 and K17) and IFN-α recombin ant protein (PBL Biomedical Laboratories, Piscataway, New Jersey, USA) were employed in the ELISA assay using a previously described protocol [14, 25, 42]. On the othe hand, commercial ELISA tests were used for the detection of tumour necrosis factor-α (TNF-α) (TNF alpha ELISA

Kit, Porcine, Life Technology), interleukin-10 (IL-10) (IL-10 ELISA Kit, Porcine, Life Technology), IFN-γ (IFN-γ ELISA Kit, Porcine, Life Technology) and interleuking-6 (IL-6) (IL-6 ELISA Kit, Porcine, Life Technology). The results were expressed as units per millilitre (U/ml) for IFN-α. For IFN-γ, IL-6, TNF- α and IL-10, the results were expressed in pg/ml. Finally, soluble CD-163 (sCD163) was quantified by a formerly described ELISA using lysates from CD-163-transfected Chinese hamster ovary (CHO) cells as standard [43].

PBMC collection and phenotype analysis

To address the effect of ASFV infection on the PBMC populations in both experimental groups, a comparative study of the expression of different porcine surface markers was carried out by flow cytometry, using cells collected before and after ASFV infection (end-point lifetime after ASFV infection). PBMCs were separated from whole blood by density-gradient centrifugation with Histopaque 1077 (Sigma). The number and viability of the PBMCs were determined by staining with Trypan Blue [36]. To phenotype these cells, flow cytometry was performed using the corresponding monoclonal antibody (mAbs). The mAbs for porcine CD4 (74–12-4, IgG2b) Alexa Fluor 647 conjugate (BD Pharmingen) and CD8-α (76–2-11, IgG2a) FITC-labelled (BD Pharmingen) were used. Further, anti-CD172a mAb (BA1C11, IgG1) produced in our laboratory was used in indirect labelling, with goat anti-mouse IgG Alexa Fluor 647 conjugated (Jackson ImmunoResearch) as a secondary antibody. The staining protocols were performed as previously described [17, 25, 42]. Finally, the cells were analysed by flow cytometry, using a FACSCalibur (Becton Dickinson FACSAria I) (Becton Dickinson, San Jose, California, USA), and the positive percentages were analysed by FACSDiva software, version 6.1.2 [25, 42].

Statistical analysis

All statistical analyses were performed using SPSS software, version 15.0 (SPSS Inc., Chicago, Illinois, USA). The significance level (α) was set at $P < 0.05$. Throughout the trial, a non-parametric test (Mann-Whitney) was chosen to compare values obtained from the clinical and virological parameters, PBMC phenotype and soluble factors parameters between Groups A and B. This non-parametric analysis was chosen due to the non-normality pattern observed for the studied parameters and the small number of animals used in each experimental group. Finally, a survival analysis was carried out to test differences in survival throughout the trial between Groups A and B.

Results

Clinical signs developed after E75 ASFV infection

After the E75-ASFV infection, one of the CSFV PI wild boars (CSFV-ASFV infected) from Group A showed mild clinical signs from 1 dpi to 3 dpi, consisting of mild pyrexia (40 °C - 40.5 °C) and mild apathy. No clinical signs were recorded in the pestivirus-free-ASFV infected wild boars (Group B) within this period; therefore, from 1 dpi to 3 dpi no statistical significant differences were found between both experimental groups (Fig. 1a–c). At 4 dpi, the three CSFV-ASFV infected animals from Group A presented mild apathy. Animal number 2 showed evidence of cyanosis and petechial haemorrhages in the ears and abdomen at five dpi; it suddenly died at 6 dpi. The rest of the infected wild boars from Group A showed signs of severe apathy, semi-prostration, cyanosis and haemorrhages in the skin, dyspnoea and tremors, for which reason they were euthanized at 7 dpi, reaching clinical score values from 1.5 to 5.5 (Fig. 1a–c). On the other hand, only pyrexia and mild apathy were registered from day 4 to 7 dpi in pestivirus-free-ASFV infected wild boars (Group B); nevertheless, two animals suddenly died at 8 dpi. On the contrary, only animal number 4 presented pyrexia (40 °C - 40.7 °C) and slight nasal secretions between 5 dpi and 8 dpi, remaining clinically asymptomatic from then on until the end of the experiment (Fig. 1a–c). Thus, statistical significant differences ($p < 0.05$) in terms of clinical signs between both experimental groups were found from 4 dpi to 7 dpi (Fig. 1c).

Despite the clinical differences observed between both groups, no statistical differences were found in the survival analysis. In this respect, the survival of CSFV-ASFV infected animals (Group A) was equal to the pestivirus-free-wild boars from Group B. Only animal 4 in Group B survived the ASFV infection until the end of the trial (10 dpi).

Although animals 5 and 6 of Group B suddenly died, several macroscopic lesions were observed after necropsy, which consisted of splenomegaly, splenic haemorrhagic, generalized lymphadenitis, moderate haemorrhagic enteritis, petechiae in the kidney and ascites. The surviving animal at the end of the study (animal 4 of Group B) had only a few petechiae in the kidney.

CSFV RNA detection after ASFV infection

Wild boars from Group A maintained similar CSFV RNA load during the whole trial even after ASFV infection. A high and constant CSFV RNA load in serum and swabs was found when examined by CSFV q-RT-PCR [39] (Fig. 2). A similar CSFV RNA load was detected in the tonsil and lung from these infected animals, with Ct values about 22–25 (data not shown). The samples analysed from Group B were CSFV RNA negative (data not shown).

ASFV DNA detection

ASFV DNA was detected in all samples analysed from both experimental groups. At 7 dpi, the animals from Group A (CSFV-ASFV infected) were found viraemic with a Ct value of around 17, corresponding with a high

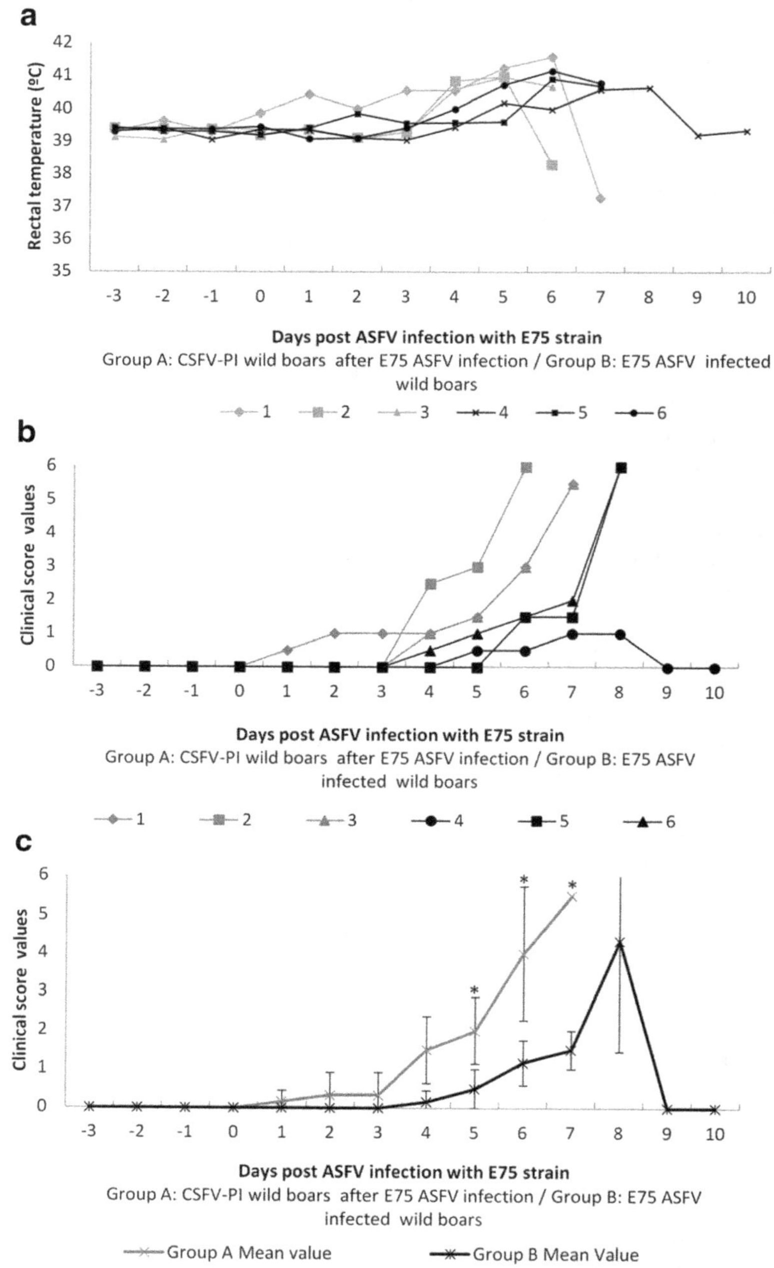

Fig. 1 Rectal temperature and clinical score values after ASFV infection. a The individual rectal temperature values that were detected after the ASFV strain infection. Temperatures greater than 40 °C were considered fevers. b The individual clinical score values that were detected after the E75 strain infection. c The mean and standard deviation of the clinical score values recorded after ASFV infection. An asterisk indicates statistical significance between the two groups from day 5 until day 7 ($p < 0.05$)

viral load in sera (Fig. 3a). In the case of ASFV-infected animals from Group B, similar Ct values were detected in two serum samples (animals 5 and 6). On the contrary, a lower DNA viral load (Ct value 24) was detected in the serum of animal 4. The ASFV DNA viral load detected in nasal and rectal swabs was comparable between both groups except for animal 4 (Group B), with a lower Ct value. At 10 dpi, the ASFV DNA viral load detected in the survivor (animal 4) considerably diminished with respect to day 7, with a Ct value of 26.25, 32.65 and 34.54 in sera, nasal and rectal swabs, respectively. Finally, similar results to those previously found in serum and swabs were obtained in tonsil, lung and spleen tissues in both experimental groups (Fig. 3b).

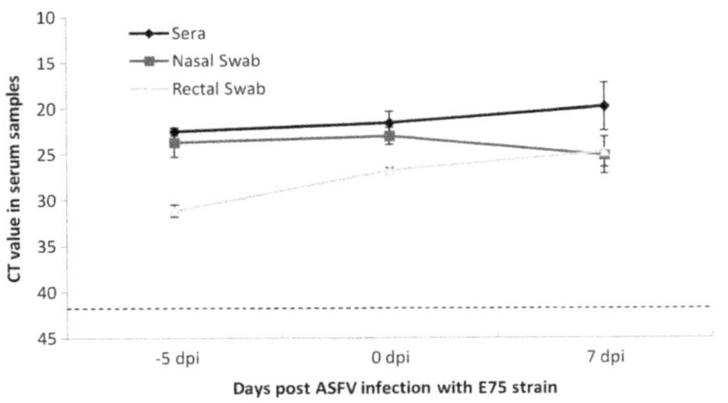

Fig. 2 Mean values and standard deviation values of the CSFV Catalonia strain RNA detection in serum, nasal and rectal swabs at different times before and after ASFV infection. CSFV Catalonia strain RNA detection in serum, nasal and rectal swabs samples in CSFV PI animals from Group A (numbers 1 to 3) at 5 days before ASFV infection, and at 0 and 7 days post ASFV infection. A dotted bar indicates the detection limit of the technique above 42 Ct

pecific CSFV and ASFV antibodies detection

era from all the animals in Groups A and B were negaive for the CSFV E2-specific antibodies and CSFV neuralising antibodies during the trial. For ASFV-specific ntibody response, only the surviving animal of Group B animal 4) was positive at 10 dpi, with a blocking perentage of 72%. The rest of the animals from Group B animals 5 and 6) and from Group A remained negative t all sampling times.

LISA detection of serum soluble factors

NF-α and IL-6 were not detected in any sample at 0 nd at 7 days post-ASFV infection. In contrast, high FN-α levels were found only in the samples from Group 3 after 7 days post-ASFV infection (Table 1), and signifiant differences ($p < 0.05$) were observed between Group A and B piglets at day 7 dpi. Within the B group, he IFN-α values observed for pigs 5 and 6 were approximately 30% higher than that detected in pig 4 Table 1). For IFN-γ, a variable response was detected in oth experimental groups after ASFV infection (7 dpi), s two out of three animals were positive in Group A nd one out of three was positive in Group B (Table 1). Additionally, IL-10 was detected only in Group B at 7 lpi. Finally, high levels of sCD163 were detected at 7 dpi n both Groups A and B (Fig. 4). For animal 4 (Group B) he level of sCD163 decreased to basal levels at 10 ASFV lpi (under 80,000).

BMC phenotype analysis after CSFV and ASFV infection

Before ASFV infection (0 dpi), the percentage of the T CD4$^+$ cell population was higher ($p = 0.08$) in the CSFV PI animals (Group A, animals 2 and 3) than in the nonnfected animals (pestivirus-free wild boars 4 to 6 from Group B). Further, the percentage of CD172a$^+$ was higher in the infected than in the non-infected animals (Group B). Unfortunately, animals 5 and 6 (Group B) died suddenly, and therefore, it was impossible to collect PBMCs after ASFV infection. Thus, the comparative study of the porcine surface markers expression included samples only from animals numbered 2 to 4 at 7 dpi. The results showed a marked effect on the CD4$^+$ and CD172a$^+$ populations in animals from Group A (1 and 2) after ASFV infection (Table 2). On the one hand, the percentage of T CD4$^+$ cell populations drastically decreased from 15 to 17% to 3% ($p = 0.10$). On the other hand, at the time of necropsy, the CSFV PI animals (Group A) showed a 20% increase in the CD172a$^+$ cell population after ASFV infection compared to their preinfection status. Moreover, the percentage of CD172a$^+$ cells in these animals 2 and 3 at 7 dpi was higher and statistically different ($p = 0.08$) than in the non-infected naive animals (wild boars from group B before ASFV infection). In contrast, the surviving ASFV-infected animal from Group B at 10 dpi (animal 4) presented around a 10% decrease in the CD172a$^+$ compared to the samples at day 0 (Table 2). In parallel, the forward versus scattered dot-plot side representation (FSC/SSC) indicated a high-complexity region that may correspond to immature granulocytes in the samples from Group A (data not shown).

Discussion

The ASF and CSF situation in Eastern Europe is of concern due to the current epidemiological complexity [7, 24, 25]. In this sense, the role of wild boar populations may be one of the main components in disease maintenance in these geographic areas [7, 24].

In the present work, we studied some virological and immunological parameters related to the innate and adaptive immune response in CSFV PI animals after ASFV infection, a virus that causes one of the most devastating diseases in swine. Likewise, we assessed the survival and disease progression in animals with CSF PI compared to those with ASFV infection. For this purpose, CSFV-PI wild boars were inoculated with a virulent ASFV strain. Finally, virological and immunological parameters after ASFV infection in naive wild boars were also assessed.

Even though the high infection rate of the Cat01 strain of CSFV PI wild boars was in accordance with previous studies, good health status was maintained before ASFV infection [24, 28]. Interestingly, the animals infected with a CSF persistent form (Group A) showed a progressive acute haemorrhagic disease after ASFV infection. In Group B, two pestivirus-free wild boars suddenly died shortly after ASFV infection (5 and 6 dpi), accordingly with previously published reports [44]. However, none of the pestivirus-free-ASFV infected wild boars (Group B)

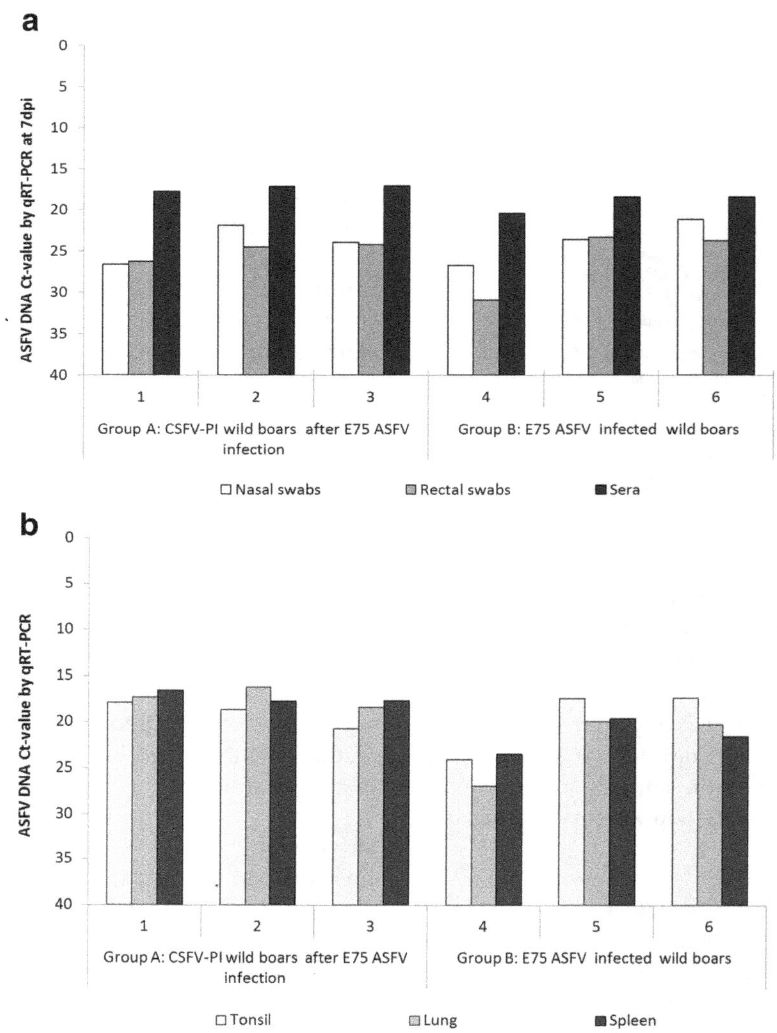

Fig. 3 ASFV E75 strain DNA detection in serum, nasal and rectal swabs and in tissues samples at different times after ASFV infection. **a** ASFV DNA detection in serum, nasal and rectal swabs samples in CSFV PI animals from Group A (numbers 1 to 3) and in pestivirus-free animals from Group B (numbers 4 to 6) at 7 days post ASFV infection. **b** ASFV DNA detection in tonsil, lung and spleen samples in both experimental Groups A and B. The detection limit of the technique was above 40 Ct

Table 1 Serum soluble factors detection at 7 days post ASFV infection

Experimental groups	Animal identifications	ELISA detection of serum soluble factors		
		IFN-α	IFN-γ	IL-10
CSFV-PI infected with ASFV E75	1	24	0	0
	2[a]	0	66	0
	3	40	915	0
Pestivirus Free- Infected with ASFV E75	4	122	0	39
	5	193	0	17
	6	184	213	149

[a]pig number 2 was sampled at 6 ASFV dpi (before necropsy)

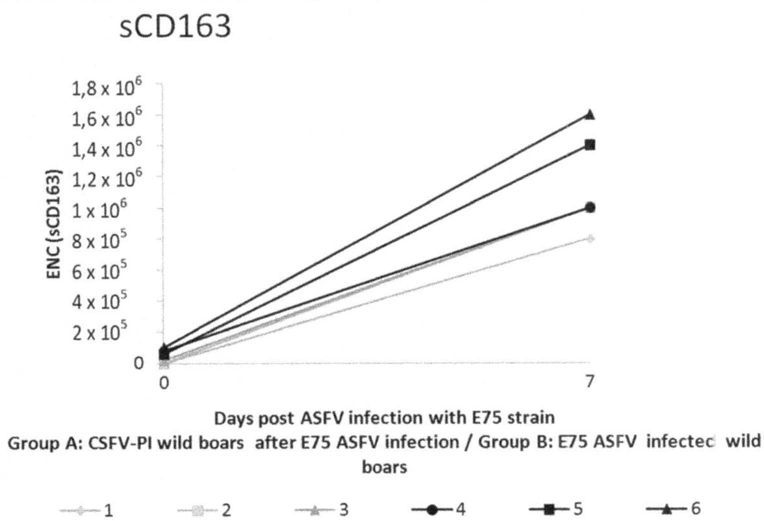

Fig. 4 sCD163 levels found before and after 7 days post ASFV infection in both experimental Groups A and B. The results are expressed as the equivalent number of CD-163-transfected cells

leveloped the haemorrhagic clinical form of the disease. Despite the different clinical pictures recorded between oth experimental groups, the survival rate after ASFV nfection was similar, suggesting that CSFV PI animals, egardless of their immunosuppression state, are equally usceptible towards ASFV infection as pestivirus-free anmals would be [24, 25].

Notably, the ASFV DNA load detected after infection n sera, swabs and tissue samples was high and similar or both groups, correlating with the ASF acute form 17, 44]. In addition, the CSFV RNA load in CSFV-ASFV-infected animals (Group A) remained unaltered fter ASFV infection during the trial [24, 42].

A recent report showed that vaccination against CSFV ould yield CSF progression in CSFV PI animals, although signs of cyanosis or haemorrhage were not previusly observed [42]. Considering this precedent, the ASFV infection could be a trigger factor for the haemorhagic disease progression in the CSFV PI wild boars. It s worth highlighting the high variability in the infection enerated by ASFV in swine [37]. Although only three animals per group were used in this study, our results suggest that the CSFV subclinical infection may also predispose animals to ASF disease and aggravate its progression, considering that the three animals from Group A showed cyanosis and severe haemorrhage in the skin. In agreement with the high variability generated by ASFV in swine, two of the pestivirus-free-ASFV infected wild boars from Group B suddenly died and one of them remained clinically asymptomatic until the end of the experiment. Although clinical signs were almost unapparent, this animal remained ASFV positive in the serum and excreted virus during the study. In addition, it was the only animal able to seroconvert against ASFV at 10 dpi. It is known that pigs that survive natural infection usually develop antibodies against ASFV from 7 to 10 days post-infection which persist for a long period of time [45]. Therefore, the detection of specific antibodies against ASFV is very useful for the diagnosis of inapparent forms of ASF [46]. Thus, despite the short duration of the experiment, this animal would represent an ASF subclinical case.

able 2 PBMC phenotype analysis after CSFV and ASFV infection

xperimental groups	Animal identification	Timing post-ASFV-infection					
		0 days post-ASFV-infection[a]			End-point lifetime after ASFV infection[a]		
		CD4$^+$	CD8$^+$	CD172a$^+$	CD4$^+$	CD8$^+$	CD172a$^+$
SFV-PI infected with ASFV E75	2	17	17	43	3	11	76
	3	15	14	63	3	21	73
estivirus Free- Infected with ASFV E75	4	7	16	30	11	26	19
	5	8	17	27			
	6	7	20	32			

Values expressed in %

It is known that ASFV activates monocytes/macrophages that secrete a wide range of mediators including pro-inflammatory cytokines such as IL-6 and TNF-α [47–49], which can trigger acute phase reactions, inflammation, activation of endothelial cells and apoptosis. Paradoxically, the absence of IL-6 and TNF- α was detected in the sera from both experimentally infected groups. On the other hand, it is also known that IL-10 inhibits a broad spectrum of immune responses, including the suppression of T cell proliferation, cytokine production and B cell responses [50–53]. Interestingly, all the ASFV-infected wild boars from group B showed detectable IL-10 levels in sera, a finding previously described in the ASF disease [48, 54]. In contrast, despite the ASFV replication in CSF-persistent animals, IL-10 levels in sera were not found, as previously reported in CSF-persistent disease [25].

Notably, the sCD163 is an activation macrophage marker that has been associated with acute ASF disease at 7 dpi [17]. Accordingly, high levels were found associated with ASFV infection in both experimental groups, with the highest values detected in the Group B animals that suddenly died. Interestingly, low levels of sCD163 were found in the survivor animal from Group B at 10 dpi, at which time a lower DNA ASFV load was detected.

In parallel, we analysed the capacity of ASFV to generate IFN-γ response in both infected groups. Notably, soluble IFN-γ was detected in some animals from both experimental groups. This finding is supported by data previously published in ASF-acute-infected domestic pigs [55] and suggests the swine immune system capability in CSFV PI animals to produce Type II IFN-γ against the unrelated viral infection. Otherwise, in the case of innate immune response against ASFV, as measured by type I IFN-α in the serum, it is worth mentioning that IFN-α was detected in all ASFV-infected animals from Group B, mainly in the animals that suddenly died. In this context, the IFN-α increase has been related to the cytokine storm after ASF disease [16, 17, 56]. Remarkably, lower IFN-α levels were found in the surviving ASFV-infected wild boar, correlating with its capability to control the infection. Strikingly, once again, the IFN-α response seemed to be impaired in CSFV PI animals, even after infection with the ASFV virus, which induces a potent effect on the innate immune system. The CSFV PI animals remained IFN-α negative, a cornerstone in the innate immune mechanisms; this fact might promote the maintenance of a high and constant CSFV load, as already described [28, 42]. Additionally, it may explain the CSFV ability to generate the SIE phenomenon previously described in swine [28].

The flow cytometry analysis showed that the percentage of CD8+ T cell populations were similar between both experimental groups before ASFV infection. Whereas, CD4$^+$ T cell populations were increased in CSFV PI animals, despite previously being in a state of immunosuppression [24, 25]. However, the CD4$^+$ T cell subset drastically decreased after ASFV infection, suggesting the incapacity to induce an effective immune response to ASFV [44, 57]. These results are underpinned by the capacity to overcome the disease in the ASFV survivor animal from Group B, in which the T cell populations remained almost within normal parameters. Finally, it is known that myeloid cells, granulocytes and monocyte/macrophages play a relevant role in ASFV and CSFV pathogenesis in swine. Considering this fact and in accordance with a previous report, the percentage of CD172a$^+$ cells found in the PBMCs from CSFV PI animals increased by 20% over the value found in naive wild boars [25]. It is also known that the progression of CSFV infection induced a clear imbalance in the proportion of blood cells towards enrichment in the CD172a$^+$ cells subset [36, 58]. This population, which has been identified as immature granulocytes [36], specifically 6D10$^+$ cells, were the predominant cell population in CSFV PI pigs [25]. Thus, in agreement with previous data, the 6D10$^+$ cell profile can explain the increase in the CD172a$^+$ cells after ASFV infection, due to the constant imbalance in the homeostasis in CSFV-ASFV infected wild boars, thereby hampering the immune response against ASFV. On the contrary, the lowering of CD172a$^+$ cells in ASFV-infected animal 4 correlates with the decrease in macrophages described after ASFV infections [57, 59].

Conclusion

Overall, our findings showed the development of a cellular homeostasis imbalance, and a type I Interferon blockade after ASFV infection of CSFV PI animals, which may explain how CSFV persists in the infected host. On the other hand, it should be noted that in terms of viral replication, ASFV infection does not produce any interference with CSFV replication, or vice versa. Despite the high DNA load generated after the ASFV infection, in CSFV PI animals, the CSFV RNA load remained high and unaltered during the trial. Additionally, ASFV infection could be a trigger factor for disease progression in the CSFV PI wild boars. Likewise, our results also suggest that the subclinical CSFV infection may be aggravating the ASF disease, considering that only the three CSFV persistently infected animals developed clinical haemorrhagic signs after ASFV infection. The survival rate against ASFV in CSFV PI animals was equal to those animals in the pestivirus-free ASFV-infected group; this fact may mean that there are relevant implications for CSF control in endemic countries, because they suggest the high resistance of these types of animals, even against a virus like ASFV. Finally, considering the co-existence of the increasing spread of ASF and the presence of CSF subclinical forms in endemic countries for both diseases, the possibility of ASFV and CSFV co-infection in swine cannot be ruled out and needs to be studied in greater depth.

bbreviations

SFV: African swine fever virus; BSL3: Biosecurity level 3; CD: Cluster of fferentiation; CHO cells: Chinese hamster ovary cells; CSFV: Classical swine fever rus; DMEM: Dulbecco's Modified Eagle Medium; DNA: Deoxyribonucleic acid; 3S: Foetal bovine serum; FITC: Fluorescein isothiocyanate; IFN: Interferon; : Immunoglobulin; IL: Interleukin; mAb: Monoclonal antibody; PI: Persistently fected; PLA: Peroxidase-linked assay; qRT-PCR: Quantitative reverse transcription olymerase chain reaction; RNA: Ribonucleic acid

cknowledgments

/e thank Claudia Pereira, Juan Carlos Prieto, Valentí Rosell, Iván Cordón and avid Solanes for their help in the animal facilities. The authors acknowledge aría Jesus Navas and Paula López-Monteagudo for their support.

unding

his research was supported by grants AGL2013-48998 and AGL2015-66907 from e Spanish government. S.M and A.C had a predoctoral fellowship FI-DGR 2014 om AGAUR, Generalitat de Catalunya.

uthors' contributions

G conceived and designed this study. SM, OC, AC, MP, RR, PM and LG erformed the experiments. SM, OC, FR, LF, JD and LG analysed data. LG, OC, , FR, RR and JD contributed reagents/material/analysis tools. SM, OC and G wrote the paper. SM, FR, JD and LG critically read the manuscript. All uthors read and approved the final manuscript.

onsent for publication

ot applicable

ompeting interests

he authors declare that the research was conducted in the absence of any ommercial or financial relationships that could be construed as a potential onflict of interest. The authors and their institutions never received payment services from a third party for any aspect of the submitted work.

uthor details

RTA, Centre de Recerca en Sanitat Animal (CReSA, IRTA-UAB), Campus de la niversitat Autònoma de Barcelona, 08193 Bellaterra, Spain. [2]Servei 'Ecopatologia de Fauna Salvatge, Departament de Medicina i Cirurgia nimals, Universitat Autònoma de Barcelona, 08193 Bellaterra, Spain. [3]OIE eference Laboratory for Classical Swine Fever, IRTA-CReSA, Campus de la niversitat Autònoma de Barcelona, 08193 Barcelona, Spain. [4]Departament Agricultura, Ramaderia, Pesca i Alimentació (DARP), Centre de Recerca en anitat Animal (CReSA, IRTA-UAB), Campus de la Universitat Autònoma de arcelona, 08193 Bellaterra, Spain. [5]Departament de Producció Animal, TSEA, Universidad de Lleida, 25198 Lleida, Spain. [6]Departamento de iotecnología, Instituto Nacional de Investigación y Tecnología Agraria y limentaria (INIA), 28040 Madrid, Spain.

eferences

Dixon LK, Abrams CC, Bowick G, Goatley LC, Kay-Jackson PC, Chapman D, et al. African swine fever virus proteins involved in evading host defence systems. Vet Immunol Immunopathol. 2004;100:117–34. doi:10.1016/j.vetimm.2004.04.002.

Moennig V, Floegel-Niesmann G, Greiser-Wilke I. Clinical signs and epidemiology of classical swine fever: a review of new knowledge. Vet J. 2003;165:11–20. Available at: http://www.ncbi.nlm.nih.gov/pubmed/12618065 [Accessed 16 Dec 2014]

3. Dixon LK, Escribano JM, Martins C, Fock DL, Salas ML, Wilkinson PJ. Asfarviridae in virus taxonomy. In: Fauquet CM, Mayo MA, Maniloff J, Desselberger U, Ball LA, editors. VIIIth report of the ICTV. London: Elsevier/Academic Press; 2005. p. 135–43.
4. Tulman ER, Delhon GA, Ku BK, Rock DL. African swine fever virus. Curr Top Microbiol Immunol. 2009;328:43–87 Available at: http://www.ncbi.nlm.nih.gov/pubmed/19216435 [Accessed 18 May 2016]
5. Gogin A, Gerasimov V, Malogolovkin A, Kolbasov D. African swine fever in the North Caucasus region and the Russian Federation in years 2007-2012. Virus Res. 2013;173:198–203. doi:10.1016/j.virusres.2012.12.007.
6. Costard S, Mur L, Lubroth J, Sanchez-Vizcaino JM, Pfeiffer DU. Epidemiology of African swine fever virus. Virus Res. 2013;173:191–7. doi:10.1016/j.virusres.2012.10.030.
7. De la Torre A, Bosch J, Iglesias I, Muñoz MJ, Mur L, Martínez-López B, et al. Assessing the risk of African swine fever introduction into the European Union by wild boar. Transbound Emerg Dis. 2015;62:272–9 doi:10.1111/tbed.12129.
8. Oganesyan AS, Petrova ON, Korennoy FI, Bardina NS, Gogin AE, Dudnikov SA. African swine fever in the Russian Federation: spatio-temporal analysis and epidemiological overview. Virus Res. 2013;173:204–11. doi:10.1016/j.virusres.2012.12.009.
9. Thiel H. Family Flaviviridae. In: Fauquet C, Mayo M. Maniloff J, Desselberger U, Ball L, editors. Virus taxonomy. Eighth report of the International Committee on Taxonomy of Viruses. San Diego: Elsevier Academic Press; 2005. p. 979–96.
10. Rümenapf T, Thiel H-J. Molecular biology of pestiviruses. In: Animal viruses: molecular biology; 2008. p. 39–96.
11. Summerfield A, Knötig SM, McCullough KC. Lymphocyte apoptosis during classical swine fever: implication of activation-induced cell death. J Virol. 1998;72:1853–61. Available at: http://www.pubmedcentral.nih.gov/articlerender.fcgi?artid=109475&tool=pmcentrez&rendertype=abstract [Accessed 14 Dec 2014]
12. Summerfield A, McNeilly F, Walker I Allan G, Knoetig SM, McCullough KC. Depletion of CD4(+) and CD8(high−) T-cells before the onset of viraemia during classical swine fever. Vet Immunol Immunopathol. 2001;78:3–19. Available at: http://www.ncbi.nlm.nih.gov/pubmed/11182144 [Accessed 4 Jan 2015]
13. Summerfield A, Alves M, Ruggli N, de Bruin MGM, McCullough KC. High IFN-alpha responses associated with depletion of lymphocytes and natural IFN-producing cells during classical swine fever. J Interf Cytokine Res. 2006;26:248–55. doi:10.1089/jir.2006.26.248.
14. Tarradas J, Argilaguet JM, Rosell R, Nofrarías M, Crisci E, Córdoba L, et al. Interferon-gamma induction correlates with protection by DNA vaccine expressing E2 glycoprotein against classical swine fever virus infection in domestic pigs. Vet Microbiol. 2010;142:51–8. doi:10.1016/j.vetmic.2009.09.043.
15. Afonso CL, Piccone ME, Zaffuto KM Neilan J, Kutish GF, Lu Z, et al. African swine fever virus multigene family 360 and 530 genes affect host interferon response. J Virol. 2004;78:1858–64. Available at: http://www.pubmedcentral.nih.gov/articlerender.fcgi?artid=369441&tool=pmcentrez&rendertype=abstract [Accessed 19 May 2016]
16. Fishbourne E, Abrams CC, Takamatsu H-H, Dixon LK. Modulation of chemokine and chemokine receptor expression following infection of porcine macrophages with African swine fever virus. Vet Microbiol. 2013;162:937–43. doi:10.1016/j.vetmic.2012.11.027.
17. Lacasta A, Monteagudo PL, Jiménez-Marín Á, Accensi F, Ballester M, Argilaguet J, et al. Live attenuated African swine fever viruses as ideal tools to dissect the mechanisms involved in viral pathogenesis and immune protection. Vet Res. 2015;46:135. doi:10.1186/s13567-015-0275-z.
18. Salguero FJ, Gil S, Revilla Y, Gallardo C, Arias M, Martins C. Cytokine mRNA expression and pathological findings in pigs inoculated with African swine fever virus (E-70) deleted on A238L Vet Immunol Immunopathol. 2008;124:107–19. doi:10.1016/j.vetimm.2008.02.012. Epub 2008 Feb 23
19. Ganges L, Núñez JI, Sobrino F, Borrego B, Fernández-Borges N, Frías-Lepoureau MT, et al. Recent advances in the development of recombinant vaccines against Classical swine fever virus: cellular responses also play a role in protection. Vet J. 2008;177:169–77. doi:10.1016/j.tvjl.2007.01.030.
20. van Oirschot JT, De Jong D, Huffels ND. Effect of infections with swine fever virus on immune functions. II. Lymphocyte response to mitogens and

enumeration of lymphocyte subpopulations. Vet Microbiol. 1983;8:81–95. Available at: http://www.ncbi.nlm.nih.gov/pubmed/6845636 [Accessed 14 Dec 2014]

21. Moennig V. The control of classical swine fever in wild boar. Front Microbiol. 2015;6:1211. Available at: http://www.ncbi.nlm.nih.gov/pubmed/26594202 [Accessed 18 May 2016]
22. Pérez LJ, Díaz de Arce H, Perera CL, Rosell R, Frías MT, Percedo MI, et al. Positive selection pressure on the B/C domains of the E2-gene of Classical swine fever virus in endemic areas under C-strain vaccination. Infect Genet Evol. 2012;12:1405–12. doi:10.1016/j.meegid.2012.04.030.
23. Weesendorp E, Backer J, Stegeman A, Loeffen W. Transmission of Classical swine fever virus depends on the clinical course of infection which is associated with high and low levels of virus excretion. Vet Microbiol. 2011; 147:262–73. doi:10.1016/j.vetmic.2010.06.032.
24. Cabezón O, Colom-Cadena A, Muñoz-González S, Pérez-Simó M, Bohórquez JA, Rosell R, et al. Post-natal persistent infection with classical swine fever virus in wild boar: a strategy for viral maintenance? Transbound Emerg Dis. 2015; doi:10.1111/tbed.12395.
25. Muñoz-González S, Perez-Simó M, Muñoz M, Bohorquez JA, Rosell R, Summerfield A, et al. Efficacy of a live attenuated vaccine in classical swine fever virus postnatally persistently infected pigs. Vet Res. 2015a;46:78. doi:10.1186/s13567-015-0209-9.
26. Bergua M, Zwart MP, El-Mohtar C, Shilts T, Elena SF, Folimonova SY. A viral protein mediates superinfection exclusion at the whole-organism level but is not required for exclusion at the cellular level. J Virol. 2014;88:11327–38. doi:10.1128/JVI.01612-14.
27. Folimonova SY. Superinfection exclusion is an active virus-controlled function that requires a specific viral protein. J Virol. 2012;86:5554–61. doi:10.1128/JVI.00310-12.
28. Muñoz-González S, Pérez-Simó M, Colom-Cadena A, Cabezón O, Bohórquez JA, Rosell R, et al. Classical swine fever virus vs. classical swine fever virus: the superinfection exclusion phenomenon in experimentally infected wild boar. PLoS One. 2016;11:e0149469. doi:10.1371/journal.pone.0149469.
29. Wensvoort G, Terpstra C, Boonstra J, Bloemraad M, Van Zaane D. Production of monoclonal antibodies against swine fever virus and their use in laboratory diagnosis. Vet Microbiol. 1986;12:101–8. Available at: http://www.ncbi.nlm.nih.gov/pubmed/2428160 [Accessed 14 Dec 2014]
30. Reed LJ, Muench H. A simple method of estimating fifty per cent endpoints. Am J Epidemiol. 1938;27:493–7. Available at: http://aje.oxfordjournals.org/content/27/3/493.extract [Accessed 14 Dec 2014]
31. Tarradas J, de la Torre ME, Rosell R, Perez LJ, Pujols J, Muñoz M, et al. The impact of CSFV on the immune response to control infection. Virus Res. 2014;185:82–91. doi:10.1016/j.virusres.2014.03.004.
32. Allepuz A, Casal J, Pujols J, Jové R, Selga I, Porcar J, et al. Descriptive epidemiology of the outbreak of classical swine fever in Catalonia (Spain), 2001/02. Vet Rec. 2007;160:398–403. Available at: http://www.ncbi.nlm.nih.gov/pubmed/17384291 [Accessed 14 Dec 2014]
33. Rodríguez F, Martín de las Mulas J, Herráez P, Sánchez Vizcaíno JM, Fernández A. Immunohistopathological study of African swine fever (strain E-75)-infected bone marrow. J Comp Pathol. 1996;114:399–406. Available at: http://www.ncbi.nlm.nih.gov/pubmed/8814534 [Accessed 19 May 2016]
34. Aragon V, Cerdà-Cuéllar M, Fraile L, Mombarg M, Nofrarías M, Olvera A, et al. Correlation between clinico-pathological outcome and typing of Haemophilus parasuis field strains. Vet Microbiol. 2010;142:387–93. doi:10.1016/j.vetmic.2009.10.025.
35. Tarradas J, Monsó M, Muñoz M, Rosell R, Fraile L, Frías MT, et al. Partial protection against Classical swine fever virus elicited by dendrimeric vaccine-candidate peptides in domestic pigs. Vaccine. 2011;29:4422–9. doi:10.1016/j.vaccine.2011.03.095.
36. Ganges L, Barrera M, Núñez JI, Blanco I, Frias MT, Rodríguez F, et al. A DNA vaccine expressing the E2 protein of Classical swine fever virus elicits T cell responses that can prime for rapid antibody production and confer total protection upon viral challenge. Vaccine. 2005;23:3741–52. doi:10.1016/j.vaccine.2005.01.153.
37. Gallardo C, Soler A, Nieto R, Cano C, Pelayo V, Sánchez MA, Pridotkas G, Fernandez-Pinero J, Briones V, Arias M. Experimental Infection of Domestic Pigs with African Swine Fever Virus Lithuania 2014 Genotype II Field Isolate. Transbound Emerg Dis. 2017;64:300–4. doi:10.1111/tbed.12346.
38. Galindo-Cardiel I, Ballester M, Solanes D, Nofrarías M, López-Soria S, Argilaguet JM, et al. Standardization of pathological investigations in the framework of experimental ASFV infections. Virus Res. 2013;173:180–90. doi 10.1016/j.virusres.2012.12.018.
39. Hoffmann B, Beer M, Schelp C, Schirrmeier H, Depner K. Validation of a real time RT-PCR assay for sensitive and specific detection of classical swine fever. J Virol Methods. 2005;130:36–44. doi:10.1016/j.jviromet.2005.05.030.
40. Fernández-Pinero J, Gallardo C, Elizalde M, Robles A, Gómez C, Bishop R, et al. Molecular diagnosis of African swine fever by a new real-time PCR using universal probe library. Transbound Emerg Dis. 2013;60:48–58. doi:10.1111/j 1865-1682.2012.01317.x.
41. Terpstra C, Bloemraad M, Gielkens AL. The neutralizing peroxidase-linked assay for detection of antibody against swine fever virus. Vet Microbiol. 1984;9:113–20. Available at: http://www.ncbi.nlm.nih.gov/pubmed/6375112 [Accessed 14 Dec 2014]
42. Muñoz-González S, Ruggli N, Rosell R, Pérez LJ, Frías-Leuporeau MT, Fraile L et al. Postnatal persistent infection with classical swine fever virus and its immunological implications. PLoS One. 2015b;10:e0125692. doi:10.1371/journal.pone.0125692.
43. Pérez C, Ezquerra A, Ortuño E, Gómez N, García-Briones M, Martínez de la Riva P, et al. Cloning and expression of porcine CD163: its use for characterization of monoclonal antibodies to porcine CD163 and development of an ELISA to measure soluble CD163 in biological fluids. Spanish J Agric Res. 2008;6:59. doi:10.5424/sjar/200806S1-374.
44. Blome S, Gabriel C, Beer M. Pathogenesis of African swine fever in domesti pigs and European wild boar. Virus Res. 2013;173:122–30. doi:10.1016/j.virusres.2012.10.026.
45. Cubillos C, Gómez-Sebastian S, Moreno N, Nuñez MC, Mulumba-Mfumu LK, Quembo CJ, Heath L, Etter EM, Jori F, Escribano JM, Blanco E. African swine fever virus serodiagnosis: a general review with a focus on the analyses of African serum samples. Virus Res. 2013;173:159–67. doi:10.1016/j.virusres.2012.10.021.
46. Nieto-Pelegrín E, Rivera-Arroyo B, Sánchez-Vizcaíno JM. First detection of antibodies against African swine fever virus in Faeces samples. Transbound Emerg Dis. 2015;62:594–602. doi:10.1111/tbed.12429.
47. Gómez del Moral M, Ortuño E, Fernández-Zapatero P, Alonso F, Alonso C, Ezquerra A, et al. African swine fever virus infection induces tumor necrosis factor alpha production: implications in pathogenesis. J Virol. 1999;73:2173–80 Available at: http://www.pubmedcentral.nih.gov/articlerender.fcgi?artid=104462&tool=pmcentrez&rendertype=abstract [Accessed 19 May 2016]
48. Gomez-Villamandos JC, Salguero FJ, Ruiz-Villamor E, Sánchez-Cordón PJ, Bautista MJ, Sierra MA. Classical swine fever: pathology of bone marrow. Ve Pathol. 2003;40:157–63. Available at: http://www.ncbi.nlm.nih.gov/pubmed/12637755 [Accessed 19 May 2016]
49. Murtaugh MP, Baarsch MJ, Zhou Y, Scamurra RW, Lin G. Inflammatory cytokines in animal health and disease. Vet Immunol Immunopathol. 1996; 54:45–55. Available at: http://www.ncbi.nlm.nih.gov/pubmed/8988847 [Accessed 19 May 2016]
50. Brady MT, MacDonald AJ, Rowan AG, Mills KHG. Hepatitis C virus non-structural protein 4 suppresses Th1 responses by stimulating IL-10 production from monocytes. Eur J Immunol. 2003;33:3448–57. doi:10.1002/eji.200324251.
51. Klinker MW, Lundy SK. Multiple mechanisms of immune suppression by B lymphocytes. Mol Med. 2012;18:123–37. doi:10.2119/molmed.2011.00333.
52. Selvarajah S, Keating S, Heitman J, Lu K, Simmons G, Norris PJ, et al. Detection of host immune responses in acute phase sera of spontaneous resolution versus persistent hepatitis C virus infection. J Gen Virol. 2012;93:1673–9. doi:10.1099/vir.0.041277-0.
53. Taoufik Y, Lantz O, Wallon C, Charles A, Dussaix E, Delfraissy JF. Human immunodeficiency virus gp120 inhibits interleukin-12 secretion by human monocytes: an indirect interleukin-10-mediated effect. Blood. 1997;89:2842–8. Available at: http://www.ncbi.nlm.nih.gov/pubmed/9108403 [Accessed 14 Dec 2014]
54. Gómez-Villamandos JC, Hervás J, Méndez A, Carrasco L, Martín de las Mulas J, Villeda CJ, et al. Experimental African swine fever: apoptosis of lymphocytes and virus replication in other cells. J Gen Virol. 1995;76:2399–405. doi:10.1099/0022-1317-76-9-2399.
55. Karalyan Z, Zakaryan H, Sargsyan K, Voskanyan H, Arzumanyan H, Avagyan H, et al. Interferon status and white blood cells during infection with Africa swine fever virus in vivo. Vet Immunol Immunopathol. 2012;145:551–5. doi:10.1016/j.vetimm.2011.12.013.
56. Alfonso P, Rivera J, Hernáez B, Alonso C, Escribano JM. Identification of cellular proteins modified in response to African swine fever virus infection

by proteomics. Proteomics. 2004;4:2037–46. Available at: http://www.ncbi.nlm.nih.gov/pubmed/15221765 [Accessed 18 May 2016]

7. Ramiro-Ibáñez F, Ortega A, Ruiz-Gonzalvo F, Escribano JM, Alonso C. Modulation of immune cell populations and activation markers in the pathogenesis of African swine fever virus infection. Virus Res. 1997;47:31–40. Available at: http://www.ncbi.nlm.nih.gov/pubmed/9037734 [Accessed 19 May 2016]

8. Summerfield A, Hofmann MA, McCullough KC. Low density blood granulocytic cells induced during classical swine fever are targets for virus infection. Vet Immunol Immunopathol. 1998;63:289–301. Available at: http://www.ncbi.nlm.nih.gov/pubmed/9656461 [Accessed 14 Dec 2014]

9. Sánchez-Torres C, Gómez-Puertas P, Gómez-del-Moral M, Alonso F, Escribano JM, Ezquerra A, Domínguez J. Expression of porcine CD163 on monocytes/macrophages correlates with permissiveness to African swine fever infection. Arch Virol. 2003;148:2307–23. Epub 2003 Sep 16

3

Understanding the early dynamics of the 2014 porcine epidemic diarrhea virus (PEDV) outbreak in Ontario using the incidence decay and exponential adjustment (IDEA) model

Amy L. Greer*, Kelsey Spence and Emma Gardner

Abstract

Background: The United States swine industry was first confronted with porcine epidemic diarrhea virus (PEDV) in 2013. In young pigs, the virus is highly pathogenic and the associated morbidity and mortality has a significant negative impact on the swine industry. We have applied the IDEA model to better understand the 2014 PEDV outbreak in Ontario, Canada. Using our simple, 2-parameter IDEA model, we have evaluated the early epidemic dynamics of PEDV on Ontario swine farms.

Results: We estimated the best-fit R_0 and control parameter (d) for the between farm transmission component of the outbreak by fitting the model to publically available cumulative incidence data. We used maximum likelihood to compare model fit estimates for different combinations of the R_0 and d parameters. Using our initial findings from the iterative fitting procedure, we projected the time course of the epidemic using only a subset of the early epidemic data. The IDEA model projections showed excellent agreement with the observed data based on a 7-day generation time estimate. The best-fit estimate for R_0 was 1.87 (95% CI: 1.52 – 2.34) and for the control parameter (d) was 0.059 (95% CI: 0.022 – 0.117). Using data from the first three generations of the outbreak, our iterative fitting procedure suggests that R_0 and d had stabilized sufficiently to project the time course of the outbreak with reasonable accuracy.

Conclusions: The emergence and spread of PEDV represents an important agricultural emergency. The virus presents a significant ongoing threat to the Canadian swine industry. Developing an understanding of the important epidemiological characteristics and disease transmission dynamics of a novel pathogen such as PEDV is critical for helping to guide the implementation of effective, efficient, and economically feasible disease control and prevention strategies that are able to help decrease the impact of an outbreak.

Keywords: Porcine epidemic diarrhea virus, PEDV, Swine, Pigs, Modeling, Epidemic, Disease dynamics, Forecasting

* Correspondence: agreer@uoguelph.ca
Department of Population Medicine, Ontario Veterinary College, University of Guelph, Guelph, ON N1G 2W1, Canada

Background

Porcine epidemic diarrhea virus (PEDV) is an alphacoronavirus and has circulated in Asian and European swine since 1971 with documented emergence of the virus into the Iowa swine industry in May 2013 where it rapidly spread to many North American locations [1–6]. The PEDV circulating in North American swineherds is highly pathogenic especially in non-immune, suckling piglets in which it causes watery, hemorrhagic diarrhea and sometimes vomiting with up to 100% morbidity creating a significant economic impact for the swine industry [6–9]. In older, weaned pigs, the disease causes similar symptoms along with anorexia, and lethargy and morbidity remains high (up to 90%), however mortality is significantly reduced with between zero and four percent of animals dying as a result of the infection [6, 9, 10]. It is also thought that the reproductive performance of PEDV infected animals is reduced resulting in smaller litter sizes [11].

Transmission of the virus is primarily via the oral-fecal route specifically due to shedding of infectious virus particles in the feces of infected animals [9]. In addition, transmission can occur via feces contaminated fomites such as boots, equipment, or transportation [12]. Environmental conditions (specifically cold and wet conditions) are believed to play an important role in the ability of the virus to persist within the environment and on fomites suitable for transmission [13]. In addition, data from some regions supports the hypothesis that infectious PEDV contaminated spray-dried plasma; a component of some swine feed products has been another route by which transmission of the virus has occurred [14, 15].

In the province of Ontario, Canada, PEDV emerged in January 2014 however, planning for the possible emergence of the virus in Canada had already begun due to the clinical severity of the disease, rapidity with which it spread widely in the United States in 2013, and the expected devastating economic and emotional toll that the emergence of the disease in Canada would take on the swine industry and Canadian farm families. The dynamics of the 2014 Ontario outbreak were distinct from those observed in the United States, because direct farm-to-farm transmission of the pathogen was not believed to be the route of transmission early in the outbreak [15]. Instead, a common source exposure linked to PEDV contaminated swine feed was believed to be the primary driver of the early outbreak dynamics [15]. Following a voluntary recall of the potentially contaminated feed products, subsequent PEDV cases within the province were believed to be the result of direct transmission between farms/premises.

The prevention and control of PEDV presents significant challenges for the swine industry. Pathogenicity appears to be dependent on a number of important factors including the age of animals affected, type of production system, biosecurity measures in place, the time at which the disease is detected (especially season), the herd size, the health status of the herd (e.g. presence of other co-occurring pathogens such as opportunistic bacterial infections), and the overall immune status of the herd [16–18]. Newborn piglets can be temporarily protected by maternal antibodies and therefore, the intentional exposure of sows to the virus especially within farrow to wean operations is a strategy that is used to quickly achieve some level of protective immunity for the newborn piglets [19].

Mathematical models are important tools for understanding the dynamics of infectious diseases within populations. This understanding contributes to our ability to identify disease prevention and control measures that will have the greatest likelihood of success and also allows for a thorough examination of the uncertainty associated with many epidemic processes. Many disease transmission models are mechanistic in nature and have been built for parsimony in order to present the simplest explanation for the observed data. Models are a mathematical representation of the health states considered to be relevant for the research question and population of interest. Parameter values describe the proposed way in which individuals move between the various health states (e.g. susceptible, infected, recovered). In the case of a mechanistic model, a significant amount of information related to the natural history of the disease, incidence within the population of interest, immune status of the population of interest and contact patterns between individuals and premises is required in order to appropriately parameterize such a model. The Incidence Decay and Exponential Adjustment (IDEA) model was first described in 2013 [20]. The model is not mechanistic in nature but rather is a simple, 2-parameter model that has shown significant promise as a descriptive tool capable of projecting epidemic processes within human populations using limited data [21, 22]. Here we apply the IDEA model to a veterinary infectious disease epidemic, specifically the Ontario PEDV outbreak in 2014. Our objectives were to assess the models ability to: 1) capture the documented patterns of PEDV epidemic growth in Ontario during the 2014 outbreak, 2) provide insight into the impact of different PEDV control measures, and 3) "near-cast" the final epidemic size and duration using only data from early in the outbreak.

Methods

Data source

Farm data were obtained from publically available reports published by the Ontario Ministry of Agriculture, Food, and Rural Affairs (OMAFRA) documenting all laboratory confirmed porcine epidemic diarrhea virus (PEDV) in the province of Ontario between January 2014 and January 2015 [23]. Ontario disease surveillance guidelines for PEDV requested that veterinarians visiting swine farms where animals showed signs of diarrhea submit samples to the University of Guelph, Animal Health Laboratory (AHL) for testing. Veterinarians were asked to submit a minimum of three pooled fecal samples (with each pooled sample containing feces from 5 different pigs from different litters or locations). Laboratory confirmation was based on a positive test result from the triplex porcine coronavirus polymerase chain reaction (PCR) test. Testing of diagnostic samples was completed at no cost to clients as part of the OMAFRA/AHL disease surveillance plan. Farms with laboratory confirmed PEDV were encouraged to undertake enhanced biosecurity measures in order minimize the risk to other farms. In addition, herd closures combined with feedback measures to rapidly expose the entire herd and establish herd immunity as quickly as possible were an important component of the response plans. Truck wash protocols (involving sanitation, disinfection, drying and downtime), and manure pumping protocols were put into place in order to minimize the risk of PEDV spread between facilities.

Available data include the date of laboratory confirmation, the county in which the confirmed positive farm was located and the type of swine production (e.g. finisher, nursery, farrow-to-finish, or farrow-to-wean) at the positive site. Due to the severity of the disease, rapid transmission within swine herds, and the critical nature of enhanced biosecurity, a liberal case definition is used whereby, a farm is defined as a confirmed case if the facility has had at least one animal sample confirmed as laboratory positive. The publically available data from OMAFRA do not include any suspected or probable cases and therefore, we do not expect the cumulative incidence to decrease between different time points due to suspect cases being ruled out through laboratory testing or other means.

The IDEA model

We used a previously described, 2-parameter model to evaluate the early epidemic dynamics of PEDV on Ontario swine farms. The "incidence decay and exponential adjustment" (IDEA) model was first described in 2013 and has since been used to examine the epidemic dynamics of the ongoing Ebola outbreak in West Africa and Middle East Respiratory Syndrome Coronavirus (MERS-CoV) in Saudi Arabia [20–22]. The first model parameter is an exponential growth term. Exponential growth is a function of the basic reproductive number (R_0) of the pathogen, which is defined as the (average) number of successful transmissions per infected individual within an entirely susceptible population, and the average serial interval [24]. In the case of PEDV and the farm-level nature of the OMAFRA dataset, we modify the definition slightly to consider the farm as the unit of observation. In this case, we define R_0 as the (average) number of successful farm-to- farm transmissions per infected farm within an entirely susceptible population of swine farms in Ontario. The average serial interval is defined as the time between laboratory confirmation in an index case/farm and laboratory confirmation in a secondary case/farm. The model also includes simultaneous exponential decay in the form of a control parameter (d). This parameter describes the slowing of the disease transmission process that is expected to occur as a result of interventions such as behavior change, increased immunity within the population or enhanced biosecurity. The model is not mechanistic and therefore is unable to identify between different prevention and control measures but rather, as a descriptive tool, permits us to identify the time point at which the epidemic begins to slow.

Previous exploratory work using the IDEA model has demonstrated its utility in describing epidemic processes in circumstances where the reproductive number (R_0) is low or moderate in size [20]. An important benefit of the model is the ability to fit the model to incidence or cumulative incidence data which is often the most easily accessible public data available in the early stages of an epidemic. In addition, unlike a mechanistic model, the IDEA model does not require extensive assumptions to be made regarding items such as the proportion of the population susceptible to the pathogen yet, appears to generate both epidemic size and duration projections that are in line with observations from a number of high-profile, human infectious disease outbreaks. The model has been shown to be able to detect abrupt changes in the epidemic curve due to disease control activities resulting from interventions. This is done by evaluating the change in the model control parameter (d) between each successive generation of the model.

The structure of the simple, 2-parameter model is as follows:

$$I_t = \left((R_0/(1+d)^t\right)^t \qquad (1.0)$$

Where, I_t is the number of incident cases in each model generation, R_0 is the basic reproductive number, d is a control parameter that allows for the decay of disease incidence over time and t is scaled in terms of the generation time. In the absence of any disease control interventions, we would expect the disease to increase over time with cases growing to the power of t. However, when control measures or interventions are implemented in the system, we expect that those controls act on the disease transmission parameter (R_0) by reducing it over time by a power of t^2. Best-fit model parameter values are obtained using maximum likelihood estimation (MLE) by fitting the model to the cumulative incidence data.

Model analyses

In order to derive an estimate of the generation time for the outbreak (time interval between successive generations of PEDV positive farms), we utilized publically available estimates of the incubation period (approx. 2 days) and the average infectious period (approx. 10 days) [25–28]. This allowed us to derive a mean generation time of seven days for PEDV based on the heuristic that the generation time (T) is the incubation period plus one half of the infectious period. However, due to the highly variable estimates for the incubation period and infectious period combined with a lack of detail regarding the potential connectivity of Ontario swine farms that would create opportunities for farm-to-farm transmission, we conducted sensitivity analyses that examined a range of possible generation times between 7 and 13 days.

Data used for the fitting of the IDEA model included only a subset of all laboratory confirmed PEDV positive farms in Ontario. Specifically, we used cumulative incidence data from February 20, 2014 to April 30, 2014. Twenty cases of PEDV occurred prior to this time period (between January 22, 2014 and February 19, 2014), however these cases have been excluded from our analyses, as it is believed that these initial cases in Ontario were linked to a point source exposure related to PEDV contaminated swine feed [15]. The contaminated feed was identified on February 9, 2014 and subsequently recalled by the manufacturer. As a result, we have excluded all cases prior to February 20th, 2014 since direct farm-to-farm transmission is not thought to have been the primary mechanism of transmission for this early time period. In addition, we have excluded five cases that were identified after April 30, 2014 because the time between these cases exceeded the possible generation times suggesting that these were sporadic cases and therefore, cases occurring after April 30, 2014 were also excluded from the analyses.

Initially, we estimated the best-fit R_0 and d parameters for the farm-to-farm transmission component of the PEDV outbreak (February 20 – April 30, 2014) by fitting the previously described IDEA model to cumulative incidence curves using the R statistical computing environment [29]. The IDEA model is not parameterized in terms of calendar date but rather generation time (epidemic generations) and therefore the observed case data were aggregated based on an estimated generation time of seven days. We also fit the IDEA model to the time series data describing cumulative cases over time in an iterative fashion. We did this by fitting the model to a dataset that included progressively more outbreak generations and comparing model fits using maximum likelihood estimates (MLE) for different combinations of values for R_0 and d. Lastly, we used the results from the iterative fitting procedure to examine the ability of the IDEA model to predict the projected time course of the observed epidemic using only model based estimates generated from the analysis of a small number of generations.

Alternate assumptions and sensitivity analyses

We conducted sensitivity analyses to examine alternate assumptions about the possible impact of a generation time that was greater than the base case estimate of seven days (7–13 days). In this case, we refit our model using 8-, 9-, 10-, 11-, 12-, and 13-day generation times. For each model fit, we examined the impact of the updated generation time on the estimated R_0 and d parameters. In addition, we considered the possible impact of under-reporting in the OMAFRA dataset. In our base case analysis, we assumed no under-reporting of cases. Given the emerging nature of the disease in Ontario as well as the clinical and economic severity of the disease this seemed a reasonable assumption to make. However, an alternative assumption exists which is that the dataset represents only the initial/index case within individual production systems (with some production systems being comprised of many individual farms or premises). To address the possibility of under-reporting in the dataset, we have fit the model examining a range of possible assumptions related to under-reporting (from 0% to 50% under-reporting).

Results

Descriptive epidemiology

The OMAFRA dataset describes 58 Ontario swine farms that were confirmed to have tested positive for PEDV between January 1st, 2014 and April 30th, 2014 (Fig. 1). The first confirmed case occurred on January 22, 2014 in Middlesex County and the last confirmed case in the dataset occurred on April 30, 2014 in the same county. All of the confirmed cases were found in southwestern Ontario with the exception of one case on February 14, 2014 that was located in eastern Ontario. Thirty-eight cases occurred during the period of time when transmission is thought to have been the result of direct transmission between farms (after February 19, 2014) rather than through a point source exposure (e.g. swine feed). In the post-recall period, the types of farms represented in the dataset-exhibited differences compared to the pre-recall period. During the pre-recall period, none of the documented cases occurred in finisher herds whereas, in the post-recall period, 61% of the cases occurred in finisher herds.

Estimation of the Basic Reproductive Number (R_0) and control parameter (d)

Using case data from the post-feed recall time period (after February 19, 2014), the model showed excellent agreement with the reported outbreak data using all available generations from February 20 to April 30, 2014

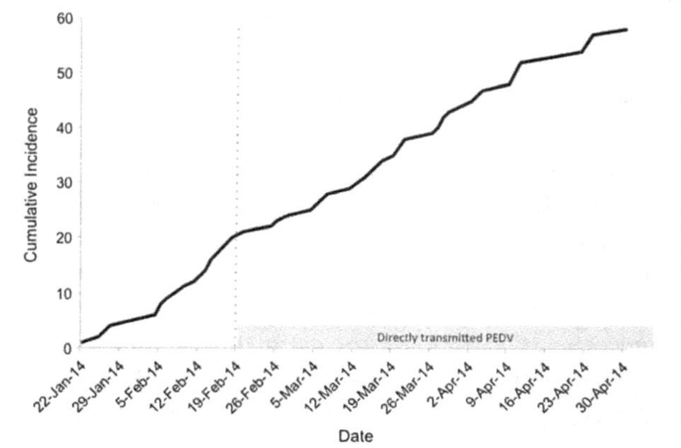

Fig. 1 Cumulative incidence data for the Ontario PEDV outbreak in 2014. Cases occurring prior to February 20, 2014 (*dashed line*) are assumed to be the result of a point source exposure through swine feed with cases occurring after February 20, 2014 being the result of direct farm-to-farm transmission

and using a generation time estimate of 7 days (Fig. 2). The best-fit estimate for R_0 was 1.87 (95% CI: 1.52 – 2.34). The best-fit model estimate for the control parameter (d) was 0.059 (95% CI: 0.022 – 0.117). Together these results suggest that the direct transmission period of the outbreak was not highly explosive ($R_0 < 2.5$) but was the focus of intensive and effective control measures ($d > 0.05$).

Using increasing numbers of successive outbreak generations, we found that there was a significant drop in the control parameter estimate (from 0.051 to 0.0150) in generation 4 (between March 6 and March 13, 2014) and then a return to intensive and effective control in subsequent generations (Fig. 3).

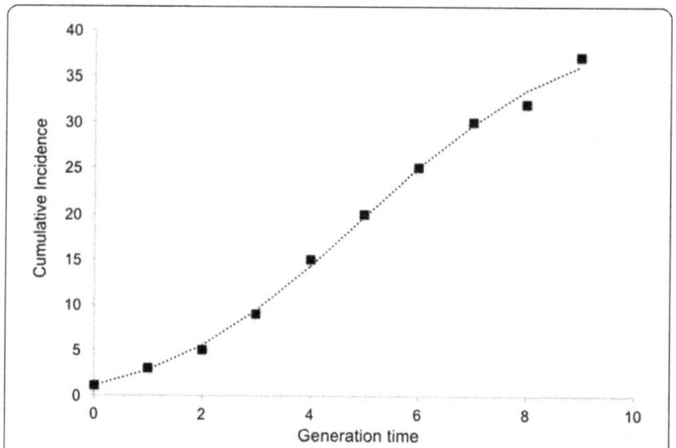

Fig. 2 Concordance between model fit (*curve*) and cumulative incidence data for the 2014 Ontario PED outbreak using a mean generation time estimate of 7 days using data from the post-recall time period (after February 19, 2014)

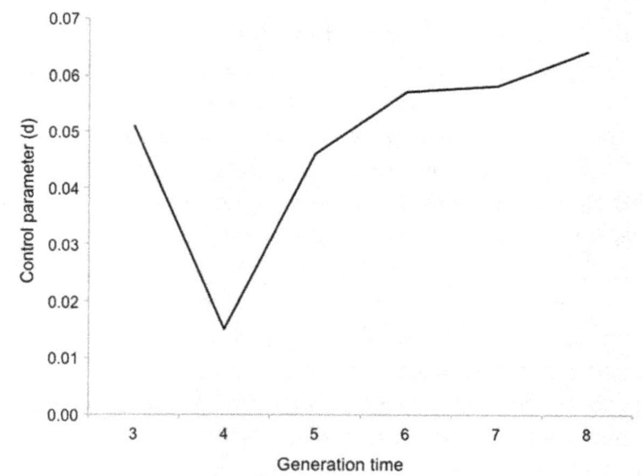

Fig. 3 Best fit values for the control parameter (d) at each epidemic generation assuming a 7-day generation time. Values greater than zero are indicative of epidemic slowing. Although the control parameter values were greater than zero from generation three onwards, the magnitude of the value changed over time. The control parameter dropped between generation 3 and 4 indicating epidemic acceleration followed by deceleration of the epidemic growth from generation 4 onwards

Short-term outbreak projection

Model-based estimates for R_0 and the control paramete (d) had stabilized sufficiently by generation three for th IDEA model to be able to project the future course o the outbreak with significant accuracy (Fig. 4). Usin only the data available after three generations (March 6 2014), the model projected that the peak of the outbrea would be reached by generation 12 (May 15, 2014), an that the expected number of cumulative cases would b

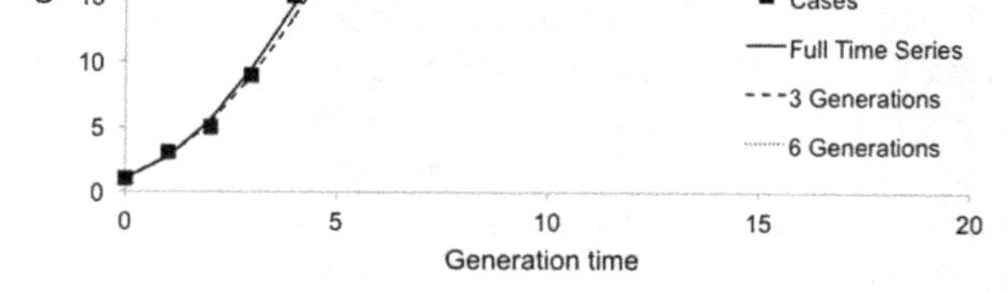

Fig. 4 Modeled cumulative incidence based on fitting the IDEA model to three or six epidemic generations assuming a seven day generation time. Squares represent the observed cumulative incidence by generation. The solid line represents the model fit to the entire time series. The dashed lines represent the model fit to only three or six outbreak generations (prior to the outbreak peak). Curves generated from data early in the outbreak are strongly representative of those resulting from fitting to the entire time series

1. This is an excellent approximation of the actual ob-erved number of cumulative cases on April 30, 2014 $N = 37$) predicting the overall final epidemic size within our cases and estimating the end of the outbreak within 5 days. Using six generations worth of data did not sig-ificantly improve the predictive ability of the model ompared to the estimates available at generation three Fig. 4).

ensitivity analyses and alternate assumptions

ensitivity analyses were conducted to examine the im-act of underestimating the potential generation time or the PEDV outbreak in Ontario. Compared to our ase case scenario with a generation time of seven days, ncreasing the possible generation time (to 10 and 3 days) aggregated the available data into fewer total pidemic generations for the period of time being inves-igated. As a result, best-fit model parameters for both R_0 and d were found to increase with increasing gener-tion time (Table 1) representing more explosive epi-emic growth but also most intensive intervention and ontrol. However, changing our assumption about the ossible generation time resulted in less accuracy when sing a small number of epidemic generations to predict nal outbreak size and timing (Fig. 5). Using a gener-tion time of 10 days, IDEA model projections of final utbreak size (48 cases) and timing (generation nine, May 21, 2014) when using only data from the first three pidemic generations, overestimated the epidemic by 11 ases and approximately 21 days (Fig. 5). In comparison, sing a generation time of 13 days, projections of final utbreak size (29 cases) and timing (generation five, April 26, 2014) when only using data from the first three pidemic generations, underestimated the epidemic tra-ectory by 8 cases and 4 days (Fig. 5). Suggesting that ur initial estimate of 7 days provides the most predict-ve fit available using minimal, publically available data nputs.

We also investigated the potential impact of PEDV nderreporting as the epidemic progressed (Table 1). In he case of potential under-reporting, our analyses demon-trate that 25% under-reporting results in an increased R_0

able 1 Sensitivity of IDEA model estimates to alternate ssumptions regarding the PEDV generation time and degree f under-reporting of cases

lternate assumption	R_0 (95% CI)	d (95% CI)
ase case	1.87 (1.52 - 2.34)	0.06 (0.02 - 0.12)
0-day generation time	3.34 (2.28 - 4.47)	0.19 (0.09 - 0.40)
3-day generation time	4.92 (3.07 – 6.01)	0.30 (0.13 – 0.66)
utbreak 25% under-reported	2.21 (1.78 – 2.81)	0.16 (0.11 - 0.27)
utbreak 50% under-reported	2.8 (2.21 – 3.65)	0.12 (0.06 – 0.19)

I confidence interval

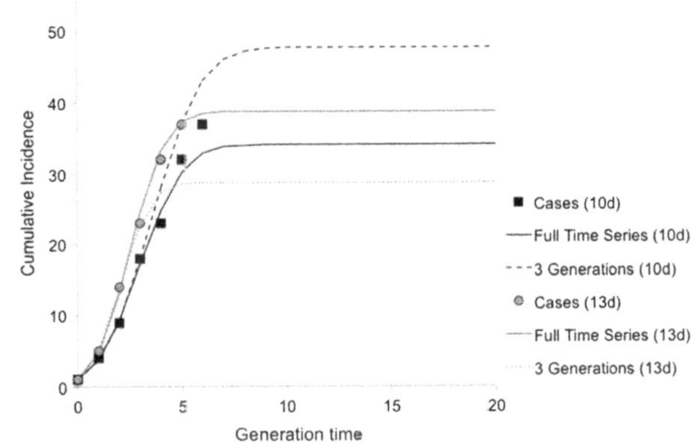

Fig. 5 Modeled cumulative incidence based on fitting the IDEA model to three epidemic generations assuming a longer generation time than the base case scenario (10 or 13 days). Squares represent the observed cumulative incidence by generation assuming a 10-day generation time and circles represent a 13-day generation time. Solid lines represent the model fit to the entire time series (black = 10 days, and gray = 13 days). The dashed lines represent the model fit based on only three outbreak generations (prior to the outbreak peak). In this case, curves generated from data early in the outbreak are less representative of those resulting from fitting to the entire time series

estimate of 2.21 (95% CI = 1.78 – 2.81) and d estimate of 0.16 (95% CI = 0.11 – 0.27). Increasing the level of under-reporting from 25% to 50% further increased the estimated R_0 to 2.8 (95% CI = 2.21 – 3.65) and reduced d to 0.12 (95% CI = 0.06 – 0.19).

Discussion

The emergence and subsequent spread of PEDV within the province of Ontario in 2014 represents an important agricultural emergency and the disease remains a threat to the swine industry, and the Canadian economy [15, 30]. Developing an understanding of the important epidemiological characteristics and disease transmission dynamics of a novel pathogen such as PEDV is critical for helping to guide the implementation of effective, efficient, and economically feasible disease control and prevention strategies that are able to help decrease the impact of an outbreak. The ability to obtain short-term projections of epidemic growth and contraction using simple, case-count time series data represents an important capacity that has not been readily available prior to the development of the Incidence Decay and Exponential Adjustment (IDEA) model [20].

Using publically available data from the Ontario Ministry of Agriculture and Rural Affairs (OMAFRA) on the occurrence of PEDV in Ontario in winter 2014 and our previously described IDEA model [20], we have estimated the direct, farm-to-farm, basic reproductive number (R_0) for the 2014 PEDV outbreak in Ontario. Our estimate of 1.87 (95% CI: 1.52 – 2.34), indicates that the introduction of PEDV into Ontario had the potential to cause an epidemic.

The second parameter of the IDEA model is the control parameter (d). We found that the best-fit control parameter value was 0.06 (95% CI: 0.02 – 0.12). Control parameter values greater than zero indicate that effective control measures were occurring within the province to help slow epidemic growth during the course of the outbreak. In a descriptive sense, an increasing control parameter indicates that the epidemic growth dynamic is slowing [20–22]. There are a variety of possible mechanistic explanations for slowing epidemic growth within the context of the PEDV outbreak including decreased rate of contact between farms (e.g. decreased truck movements), greater farm-level biosecurity, depletion of susceptible farms/premises within the province, environmental conditions which are less favorable for the persistence of the pathogen on vectors of transmission such as trucks and equipment, or any other factor which could act to reduce the force of infection. Despite this limitation, the model does permit the user to identify acceleration or deceleration of the epidemic dynamic based on the available data, including early in the course of an outbreak.

An interesting observation found during the course of this study was that a significant drop in the control parameter (d) was observed in generation four and then the control parameter appeared to rebound in subsequent generations. There is no obvious explanation for this observation however; this period of decreased "control" (and therefore a short period of epidemic acceleration between generation three and four) could be the result of environmental conditions. PEDV is a cold tolerant virus and it is believed that in Ontario, one way that the virus was spread between farms was on PEDV contaminated trucks [12, 13, 31]. Although Ontario implemented rigorous disinfection protocols for vehicles moving between farms, disinfection protocols are less effective in very cold temperatures as it is difficult to properly clean and dry trucks in freezing conditions allowing a cold tolerant virus to persist in the truck environment for longer periods of time and facilitating possible spread between premises [7, 12].

There is significant variability in the documented incubation period and infectious period for PEDV within the published literature [7, 23, 25]. It is thought that some proportion of animals can continue to shed the virus for up to 20–30 days after infection [25]. In this case, the expected generation time would be longer than the seven days that we have used in this study. However, we expect that the highest risk of direct farm-to-farm transmission likely occurs during the initial infection period for a farm/herd when infection rates are still low, clinical symptoms have not yet become widespread, a veterinarian has not yet submitted samples to the laboratory, and therefore enhanced biosecurity measures are not yet in place. This likely describes the first seven days of a farm level outbreak and therefore, this is how we justify our lower limit generation time of seven days. We would expect that as the outbreak becomes more obvious within a specific herd even though shedding may continue to occur for long periods of time, between farm transmission risk is decreased due to enhanced biosecurity.

The to approximate the epidemic final size, epidemic trajectory, and time at which the final size would be reached using only 3 generations worth of simple case count data assuming a generation time of seven days (Fig. 4). For veterinary epidemiologists and others tasked with providing situational awareness and updates to industry during an infectious disease outbreak, the ability to reasonably project forward in time an estimate of the total number of cases expected and the time at which the epidemic is expected to peak would be an incredibly useful application. In this instance, the ability to "near cast" with some certainty would better allow emergency operations personnel to budget the physical and human resources that would be required to see an outbreak through to completion. Given the uncertainty around the possible generation time estimates, we also examined two alternative scenarios whereby we assumed a longer generation time of 10 or 13 days. In both cases, we found that the model was less accurate at projecting the expected course of the PEDV outbreak using three generations of data assuming a generation time of 10 or 13 days than in the base case that assumed a generation time of seven days (Figs. 4 and 5). This suggests that even without accounting for the possibility of a prolonged duration of viral shedding within some swine, the lower generation time estimate is sufficient to capture the dynamics of the outbreak.

Lastly, it has been proposed that the publically reported data available through OMAFRA may in fact be under-reported by virtue of the fact that for some producers, the laboratory confirmed status documented in the dataset represents only the initial or index farm case within individual production systems (with some production systems being comprised of many individual farms or premises). For instance, a farrow-to-wean farm may test positive for PEDV and some of those infected pigs may move to other farms within the production system causing downstream infections at receiving facilities (e.g. finisher herds etc.). These subsequent downstream farms that become infected may not appear in the OMAFRA dataset as the movement of pigs and subsequent clinical disease in other farms within the same production system occur within a system that is already aware of the PEDV status of the index farm within the production system. The treatment of downstream pigs and enhanced biosecurity would likely be addressed without the submission of additional samples to the laboratory. To address the possibility of under-reporting in the dataset, we examined the potential impact of 25% and 50% under-reporting and found that even if the data represent only a subset of infected farms within Ontario, the model parameter estimates for R_0 and d remain relatively stable (Table 1) suggesting that the model is not overly sensitive to mild to moderate levels of under-reporting.

As is the case with all epidemiological and mathematical modeling studies, this work has certain limitations, which include the quality of the available data, the specific assumptions that have been made regarding generation time estimates and assumptions related to under-reporting. However, we feel that our findings have demonstrated consistency even when confronted with alternative assumptions and scenarios. It is possible that generation times may differ depending on the type of farm (e.g. farrow-to-weaning vs. farrow-to-finisher). However, for our analysis, the two dominant herd types were finisher herds (61%) and farrow-to-finish herds (21%) suggesting that there was consistency in the type of herds throughout the time period considered which likely minimizes the potential impact of this variability. While it may in fact be the case that the publically reported data available online through the OMAFRA website may underrepresent the true number of PEDV positive farms in Ontario during this time period, the use of publically available data has a clear advantage of allowing for rapid and transparent analysis which would likely not be possible during times of emergency if obtaining data directly from the swine industry was the only way to conduct such analyses.

Conclusions

Using a simple mathematical model that considers only two parameters, we have demonstrated that the epidemic growth of the 2014 swine PEDV outbreak in Ontario, Canada was to be expected with a reproductive number that exceeded one. However, our analyses also demonstrated that the outbreak began to quickly decelerate ($d > 0$) as a result of enhanced disease control efforts relatively quickly. Our successful application of the IDEA model to a case study of livestock infectious disease outbreak data is encouraging and suggests that despite some critical differences in the interpretation of the key model parameters and in the individual unit of study (farms/herds/premises vs. individuals), the model can provide useful information for decision-makers in the early stages of an infectious disease outbreak. We encourage the veterinary epidemiology community to continue to assess the usefulness of this simple model in the context of other emerging diseases of veterinary importance. In the case of real-time application and use of the model within an emergency management context, it is our hope that the model may be able to allow for the rapid identification of whether or not interventions are working to control the epidemic spread of the disease.

Abbreviations

IDEA: Incidence decay and exponential adjustment; OMAFRA: Ontario Ministry of Agriculture, Food, and Rural Affairs; PEDV: Porcine epidemic diarrhea virus

Acknowledgments

The authors wish to thank Drs. Ashleigh Tuite and David Fisman for discussion regarding the potential applicability of the IDEA model to a non-human, infectious disease case study and for suggestions on implementing the model code in R.

Funding

The Canada Research Chairs Program and the Natural Sciences and Engineering Research Council (NSERC) funded this research. Ms. Spence is supported by an Ontario Graduate Scholarship (OGS), and an Ontario Veterinary College Scholarship. Dr. Gardner is supported by an Ontario Veterinary College Fellowship. The funders had no role in the design of the study, collection, analysis, and interpretation of data or in the writing of the manuscript.

Authors' contributions

ALG, KS, and EG conceived the study and collected, analyzed and interpreted the data, and wrote the manuscript. All authors read and approved the final manuscript.

Competing interests

The authors declare that they have no competing interests.

Consent for publication

Not applicable.

References

1. Tian P-F, Jin Y-L, Xing G, Qv L-L, Huang Y-W, Zhou J-Y. Evidence of recombinant strains of porcine epidemic diarrhea virus, United States, 2013. Emerg Infect Dis. 2014;20:1735–8.
2. Huang YW, Dickerman AW, Piñeyro P, Li L, Fang L, Kiehne R, et al. Origin, evolution, and genotyping of emergent porcine epidemic diarrhea virus strains in the united states. MBio. 2013;4:1–8.
3. Chen Q, Li G, Stasko J, Thomas J, Stendland W, Pillatzki A, et al. Isolation and characterization of porcine epidemic diarrhea viruses associated with the 2013 disease outbreak among swine in the United States. J Clin Microbiol. 2014;52:234–43.
4. Oldham J. Letter to the Editor. Pig Farming. 1972;10:72–3.
5. Pensaert M, De Bouck P. A new Coronavirus-like particle associated with diarrhea in swine. Arch Virol. 1978;58:243–7.
6. Stevenson GW, Hoang H, Schwartz KJ, Burrough ER, Sun D, Madson D, et al. Emergence of Porcine epidemic diarrhea virus in the United States: clinical signs, lesions, and viral genomic sequences. J Vet Diagn Invest. 2013;25:649–54.
7. EFSA Panel on Animal Health and Welfare. Scientific Opinion on porcine epidemic diarrhoea and emerging porcine deltacoronavirus. EFSA J. 2014;12:1–68.
8. Song D, Park B. Porcine epidemic diarrhoea virus: a comprehensive review of molecular epidemiology, diagnosis, and vaccines. Virus Genes. 2012;44:167–75.
9. Martelli P, Lavazza A, Nigrelli AD, Merialdi G, Alborali LG, Pensaert MB. Epidemic of diarrhoea caused by porcine epidemic diarrhoea virus in Italy. Vet Rec. 2008;162:307–10.
10. Lin C-N, Chung W-B, Chang S-W, Wen C-C, Liu H, Chien C-H, et al. US-like strain of porcine epidemic diarrhea virus outbreaks in Taiwan, 2013–2014. J Vet Med Sci. 2014;76:1297–9.

11. Olanratmanee EO, Kunavongkrit A, Tummaruk P. Impact of porcine epidemic diarrhea virus infection at different periods of pregnancy on subsequent reproductive performance in gilts and sows. Anim Reprod Sci. 2010;122:42–51.
12. Lowe J, Gauger P, Harmon K, Zhang J, Connor J, Yeske P, et al. Role of transportation in spread of porcine epidemic diarrhea virus infection, United States. Emerg Infect Dis. 2014;20:872–4.
13. Jung K, Chae C. Effect of temperature on the detection of porcine epidemic diarrhea virus and transmissible gastroenteritis virus in fecal samples by reverse transcription-polymerase chain reaction. J Vet Diagn Invest. 2004;16:237–9.
14. Dee S, Clement T, Schelkopf A, Nerem J, Knudsen D, Christopher-Hennings J, et al. An evaluation of contaminated complete feed as a vehicle for porcine epidemic diarrhea virus infection of naïve pigs following consumption via natural feeding behavior: proof of concept. BMC Vet Res. 2014;10:176.
15. Pasick J, Berhane Y, Ojkic D, Maxie G, Embury-Hyatt C, Swekla K, et al. Investigation into the role of potentially contaminated feed as a source of the first-detected outbreaks of porcine epidemic diarrhea in Canada. Transbound Emerg Dis. 2014;61:397–410.
16. McOrist S. PED - Epidemiology and risk factors for transmision in east Asia. Chicago: Int. Conf. Swine Enteric Coronavirus Dis; 2014. Available from: https://www.aphis.usda.gov/animal_health/animal_dis_spec/swine/downloads/meeting/presentations/24%20-%202%20-%20McOrist.pdf.
17. Dufresne L, Robbins R. Field experience with porcine epidemic diarrhoea. Am Assoc Swine Veterinarians. 2014;613–16.
18. Williamson S, Strugnell B, Thomson J, Webster G, McOrist S, Clarke H. Emergence of severe porcine epidemic diarrhea in pigs in the USA. Vet Rec. 2013;173:146–8.
19. Bandrick M, Theis K, Molitor TW. Maternal immunity enhances Mycoplasma hyopneumoniae vaccination induced cell-mediated immune responses in piglets. BMC Vet Res. 2014;10:124.
20. Fisman DN, Hauck TS, Tuite AR, Greer AL. An IDEA for short term outbreak projection: nearcasting using the basic reproduction number. PLoS One. 2013;8:e83622.
21. Fisman D, Khoo E, Tuite A. Early epidemic dynamics of the West African 2014 ebola outbreak : estimates derived with a simple two-parameter model. PLOS Curr Outbreaks. 2014.
22. Majumder M, Rivers C, Lofgren E, Fisman D. Estimation of MERS-coronavirus reproductive number and case fatality rate for the spring 2014 Saudi Arabia outbreak: insights from publicly available data. PLOS Curr Outbreaks. 2014.
23. Ontario Ministry of Agriculture and Rural Affairs. Porcine Epidemic Diarrhea. OMAFRA Website. 2015. Available from: http://www.omafra.gov.on.ca/english/food/inspection/ahw/PED-advisory.html. Accessed 19 Dec 2014.
24. Vynnycky E, White RG, Fine PEM. An Introduction to Infectious Disease Modelling. New York: Oxford University Press; 2010.
25. World Organisation for Animal Health (OIE). Infection with porcine epidemic diarrhoea virus. 2014.
26. Geiger J, Connor J. Porcine Epidemic Diarrhea, Diagnosis, and Elimination. Univ. Minnesota, Coll. Vet. Med. webpage. 2013. p. 1–4. Available from: https://www.aasv.org/aasv%20website/Resources/Diseases/PED/13-05-29PEDWhitePaper.pdf.
27. Linden J. Porcine epidemic diarrhea. Pig Site. 2014.
28. Hank Harris D. Porcine Epidemic Diarrhea. Merck Vet. Man. 2013. Available from: http://www.merckvetmanual.com/mvm/digestive_system/intestinal_diseases_in_pigs/porcine_epidemic_diarrhea.html.
29. R Core Team. R: A language and environment for statistical computing. Vienna: R Foundation for Statistical Computing; 2013.
30. MacDougald D. Lessons Learned From PEDV. London: London Swine Conf. - Position. Success; 2014. p. 19–21.
31. Thomas PR, Karriker LA, Ramirez A, Zhang J, Ellingson JS, Crawford KK, et al. Evaluation of time and temperature sufficient to inactivate porcine epidemic diarrhea virus in swine feces on metal surfaces. J Swine Heal Prod. 2015;23:84–90.

4

A novel multiplex qPCR targeting 23S rDNA for diagnosis of swine dysentery and porcine intestinal spirochaetosis

Anna Borgström*, Simone Scherrer, Constanze Kirchgässner, Sarah Schmitt, Daniel Frei and Max M. Wittenbrink

Abstract

Background: A multiplex qPCR targeting a 128 bp region on the 23S rDNA gene was developed for detection of *Brachyspira (B.) hyodysenteriae* and *B. pilosicoli*, the agents of swine dysentery (SD) and porcine intestinal spirochaetosis (PIS), together with a triplet of apathogenic *Brachyspira* spp. (*B. innocens, B. intermedia, B. murdochii*) in porcine feces. The multiplex qPCR was evaluated against a duplex PCR (La et al., J Clin Microbiol 41:3372–5, 2003).

Results: Using DNA extracted from fecal culture, the multiplex qPCR showed excellent agreement with the duplex PCR (κ = 0.943 and 0.933). In addition, thanks to the three probes whereof one detecting the apathogenic *Brachyspria* spp., a more diversified overview of the brachyspiral flora in porcine fecal samples can be delivered as a part of the routine diagnostic. The multiplex qPCR with a limit of detection of 5–10 genomic equivalents (GE) per reaction (6×10^2 GE per gram) allows reliable detection of *Brachyspira* species directly from fecal swab DNA. In line with this, analysis of 202 fecal swabs in comparison with culture-based qPCR showed a high agreement for the causative agents of SD (*B.hyodysenteriae:* κ = 0.853, sensitivity 87% specificity 98%).

Conclusion: The novel multiplex qPCR is robust and has a high analytical sensitivity and is therefore suitable for high-throughput screening of porcine fecal swabs for the causative agents of SD. This assay can therefore be used for the direct proof of the pathogenic *B.* spp. in fecal swabs within the scope of a monitoring program.

Keywords: Swine dysentery, *Brachyspira hyodysenteriae*, 23S rDNA, Multiplex Real-time PCR, Swabs

Background

Brachyspira (*B.*) *hyodysenteriae* is the causative agent of swine dysentery (SD), a severe mucohaemorrhagic diarrheal disease of weanling to finishing pigs [1]. SD occurs worldwide and causes significant economic loss in affected pig production systems. Aside from *B. hyodysenteriae,* other *Brachyspira* species are found in the porcine intestine. *B. pilosicoli* causes the porcine intestinal spirochaetosis (PIS), an enteric disease in weaning pigs clinically resembling SD, but with milder symptoms [2]. To date, three additional species have been described in pigs, namely *B. innocens, B. intermedia* and *B. murdochii.* Although *B. intermedia* has been suspected to cause colitis and diarrhea in swine [3–5], experimental infections of pigs failed at all points [6, 7]. Therefore, *B. innocens, B. intermedia* and *B. murdochii* are still considered as only mildly pathogenic or as commensals in pigs [8, 9]. PIS has been observed in Switzerland for over a decade [10]. However, etiologically confirmed cases of SD were diagnosed for the first time as late as 2008 [11]. Since then the agent is spreading throughout Switzerland. Currently *B. hyodysenteriae* is diagnosed in nearly 2% of all pig herds served by the Swiss Pig Health [12]. To further monitor the spreading and clinical significance of *B. hyodysenteriae* in the Swiss pig population, large scale analyses on porcine fecal specimens for *Brachyspira* are necessary.

Standard procedure for the bacteriological diagnosis of SD/PIS consists of selective culture of anaerobic spirochetes from clinical specimens (feces, colonic tissue) [13] and subsequent classification of spirochetal isolates to the species level by PCR targeting the brachyspiral

Correspondence: anna.borgstroem@vetbakt.uzh.ch
Institute of Veterinary Bacteriology, Vetsuisse Faculty, University of Zurich, Winterthurerstrasse 270, CH 8057 Zurich, Switzerland

16S rDNA and NADH Oxidase (*nox*) gene [14], respectively. However, culture-coupled PCR to detect pathogenic *Brachyspira* often requires six days or longer to be completed [15], and its workflow can be tedious compared to modern real-time PCR assays, a major drawback of this approach when a large series of specimens should be analyzed. In two previous studies comparing direct fecal-PCR with culture coupled PCR it was found that direct fecal PCR assays are nearly a 100-fold less sensitive than culture coupled PCR, and are, therefore, not suitable for the reliable identification of infected pigs [15, 16]. Moreover, conventional PCR assays do not contain internal controls making false negative result a possible problem, especially when analyzing difficult fecal samples. Thus, it is of particular interest to improve the analytic sensitivity of PCR detection methods for large scale analyses of porcine fecal specimens for *Brachyspira.* In the present study, we describe the evaluation of a novel 23S rDNA multiplex qPCR on a diversified panel of fecal specimens from pig herds suspected of SD.

Methods

Brachyspira strains and growth conditions

Twelve reference strains representing six *Brachyspira* species were included in this study: *B. hyodysenteriae* B78 ATCC 27164, *B. hyodysenteriae* B204 ATCC 31212, *B. hyodysenteriae* WA-1 ATCC 49526, *B. pilosicoli* P43/6/78 ATCC 51139, *B. pilosicoli* 102/06[1] *B. innocens* B256 ATCC 29796, *B. innocens* 8244/05[2], *B. murdochii* 56-150 ATCC 51284, *B. murdochii* 403-2x/06[2], *B. intermedia* PWS/A ATCC 51140, *B. intermedia* 863/06[2] and *B. alvi-nipulli* 91-1207/C1 ATCC 51933. The strains were cultured on selective Tryptose Soy Agar (TSA) as described elsewhere [17, 18].

Fecal samples

Rectal swabs were collected from feeder pigs on 17 farms from 18 different Swiss Cantons (Fig. 1). All samples were routine submissions during a SD monitoring program and were collected between August 2009 and September 2015. Swabs with fecal matter were inserted into Amies transport medium in airtight screw cap plastic vials (VWR, Dietikon, Switzerland) and transported to the laboratory under cooled conditions within 18 h. Swabs were cultured for *Brachyspira* spp. as cited above. Afterwards, the swabs were stored at −20° until DNA extraction. Areas of weak or strong beta-hemolysis on the TSA plates were examined for spirochetal growth by dark-field microscopy of surface scrapings resuspended in a small volume of 0.15 M NaCl. Spirochetal isolates were subcultured anaerobically on Colombia sheep blood agar (Oxoid, Pratteln, Switzerland). For PCR analyses, spirochetal surface growth was directly transferred from Colombia sheep blood agar into 1 ml sterile distilled water.

Sample groups

Overall, a panel of 453 swabs with a positive culture of *Brachyspira* spp. was arbitrarily selected from diagnostic samples. Samples were divided into two groups fo

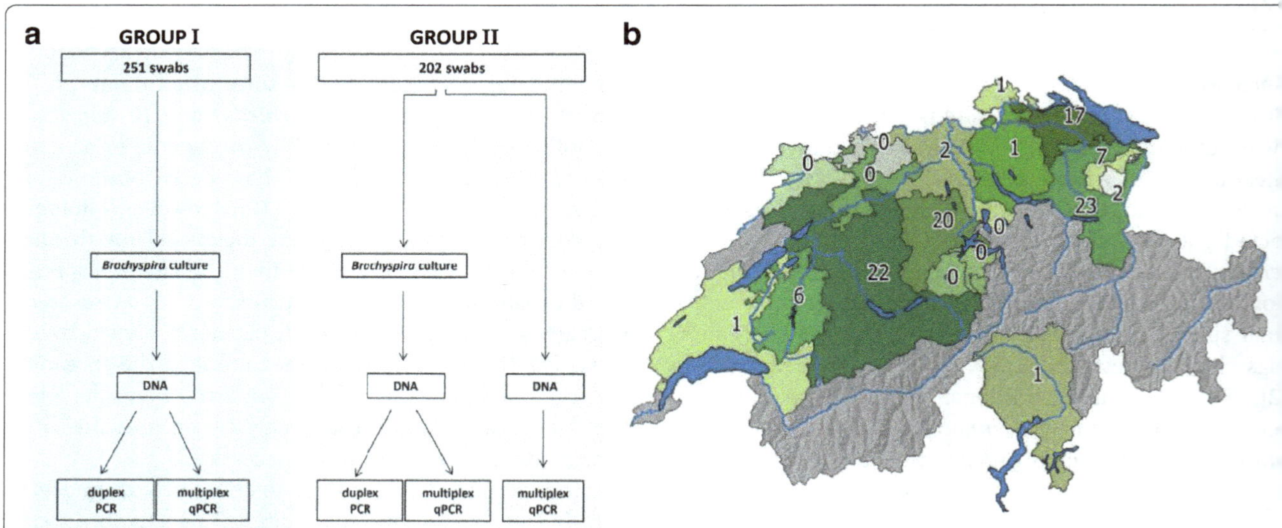

Fig. 1 Sample groups and origin of collected samples. The 453 samples in this study were divided into two different samples groups (1–2). Group 1 consisted of cultured samples compared with the duplex PCR, Group 2 contained DNA samples directly extracted from the swabs without the culture step, and the same samples after culture of the swabs. All samples results were compared between the multiplex qPCR and the conventional duplex PCR (**a**). Map of the Swiss cantons from which the samples were collected. Colored cantons were included in the study and the total of *B.hyodysenteriae* positive samples detected with the multiplex qPCR are marked in each region (**b**). For 11 of the *B. hyodysenteriae* positive samples data about origin was not provided

omparison of culture and PCR methods as outlined in 'ig. 1. Group 1 consisted of 251 fecal swabs that were nalyzed by culture coupled duplex PCR and multiplex PCR. Group 2 contained 202 swabs for the comparison f culture coupled PCR assay and direct fecal multiplex PCR.

NA extraction

'or DNA extraction the total bacteria lawn from the gar plate was harvested in 1 ml sterile distilled water nd with the use of a drigalski spatula. DNA was ex-racted from *Brachyspira* reference strains as well as ecal isolates by using the InstaGene Matrix (Bio Rad, 'ressier, Switzerland) according to the manufacturer's nstructions. For DNA extraction of fecal swabs, first an vernight incubation step at 56 °C in ATL buffer supple-nented with proteinase K (60 mAU/ml, Qiagen, Basel, witzerland) was carried out, followed by DNA extrac-ion with the QIAcube system and the Cador Pathogen NA extraction protocol (Qiagen) with additional Car-ier RNA (1 μg per 100 μl, Qiagen) added to the VXL uffer. The DNA was measured at 260 nm using a NanoDrop 2000c Spectrophotometer (Thermo Scien-ific, Reinach, Switzerland) for the determination of con-entration, diluted to 20 ng/μl and stored at −20 °C until se.

uplex PCR

'he duplex PCR for the detection of *B. hyodysenteriae* nd *B. pilosicoli* was performed as described by La et al. 14], (Table 1) on a Veriti® 96 -well thermal cycler (Ap-lied Biosystems, Life Technologies, Zug, Switzerland). Primers were synthesized by Microsynth (Balgach, Switzerland). PCR products were analyzed by QIAxcel capillary electrophoresis with the screening cartridges (Qiagen).

Development of the multiplex real-time PCR

Primers, probes and PCR settings

Primers and probes were selected using CLC Main Workbench software (Vers. 7.5.1, Qiagen) from align-ments of the available sequences of the 23S rDNA gene (NCBI databank). The selected primers amplify the same 128-bp fragment on the 23S rDNA gene of all five differ-ent *Brachyspira* spp. (*B. hyodysenteriae*, *B. pilosicoli*, *B. intermedia*, *B. innocens*, *B. murdochii*). On the 128-bp amplicon, target sequences for three DNA probes spe-cific for (i) *B. hyodysenteriae*, (ii) *B. pilosicoli* and (iii) a triplet of three apathogenic species (*B. intermedia*, *B. innocens*, *B. murdochii*) were identified (Table 1, Add-itional file 1: Figure S1). BLAST searches of both primer and probe sequences were conducted to confirm gene and species specificity. Oligonucleotide primers were synthesized by Microsynth (Balgach, Switzerland). DNA probes were provided by Eurogentec S.A. (Seraing, Belgium). All probes are quenched by black-hole non-fluorescent quenchers either at the 3′-end (probe_pilo) or coupled internally (probe_hyo, probe_apathogen, Table 1). Rox dye, as a component of the Fast Universal PCR Master mix (Applied Biosystems) was used as pas-sive reference for normalization purposes.

An internal amplification control (IAC) was added to each reaction well for signalling presence of PCR inhibi-tory substances. Five femtogram (fg) of a 712 base pair

able 1 Oligonucleotide primer and probe sequences with their respective reporter dye and quencher used in this study

rimer or probe ame	Target	Concentration	Sequence 5′→3′	Amplicon
Aultiplex qPCR				
Primer for	23S rDNA	0.4 μM	TTCGATGGAATGACACAGATTGT	128 bp
Primer rev	23S rDNA	0.4 μM	CCGAAAGCCCAGTCACTATC	
Probe_hyo	*B.hyodysenteriae*	100 nM	6-FAM-CCTTAACCTTAAAGAAGCAAGCAT(BHQ-1)TTGACTCACCTCAAG-SpacerC3	
Probe _pilo	*B.pilosicoli*	100 nM	Yakima Yellow-AGGTGATGGTTATCCTCGTCGAAT-BHQ-1	
Probe_ pathogen	*B. intermedia/ B. innocens/ B. murdochii*	25 nM	Dragonfly Orange-CCTCAACCTTAAAGCAACAAGCAT(BHQ-2)TTTACTCATCACAAG-SpacerC3	
eGFP for	enhanced GFP	0.2 μM	GACCACTACCAGCAGAACAC	177 bp
eGFP rev	enhanced GFP	0.2 μM	GAACTCCAGCAGGACCATG	
Probe_eGFP	enhanced GFP	25 nM	ATTO 647N-AGCACCCAGTCCGCCCTGAGCA-BHQ-3	
uplex PCR [12]				
B.hyo_for	*nox*	0.5 μM	ACTAAAGATCCTGATGTATTTG	345 bp
B.hyo_rev	*nox*	0.5 μM	CTAATAAACGTCTGCTGC	
B.pilo_for	16S rDNA	0.17 μM	AGAGGAAAGTTTTTTCGCTTC	823 bp
B.pilo_rev	16S rDNA	0.17 μM	GCACCTATGTTAAACGTCCTTG	

fragment of the enhanced green fluorescent protein (eGFP) gene was used, and a 177 base pair long amplicon [19] was generated by amplification with specific eGFP forward and eGFP reverse primers and detected by the eGFP-probe with ATTO 647 N reporter dye (Table 1). DNA samples from three ATCC reference strains (*B. hyodysenteriae* 4000 fg, *B. pilosicoli* 40 fg, *B. intermedia* 4000 fg) were used as positive controls in each PCR run. The PCR was performed on an ABI7500 Instrument (Applied Biosystems) using the TaqMan® Fast Universal PCR Master Mix (2x), no AmpErase® UNG (Applied Biosystems). Each reaction contained 5 μl master mix, 1 μl primer mix with eGFP primer (2 μM) and 23S rDNA primer (4 μM), 1 μl of probe mix consisting of 100 nM Yakima Yellow labeled probe, 100 nM 6-FAM labeled probe, 25nM Dragonfly Orange labeled probe, 25 nM ATTO 647 N labeled probe, 1 μL internal control eGFP DNA (5 fg), 2 μl template DNA (20 ng/μl). The cycling conditions were 20 s at 95 °C, followed by a two-step cycling stage of 45 cycles of 15 s at 95 °C and 60 s at 62 °C. The ramp in the cycling stage was set at 80% in order to ensure an efficient hybridization of primers and probes to the template DNA. Samples were considered positive when presenting a typical amplification curve with a C_t value of ≤38. The concentration of the IAC was adjusted to have a C_t value around 27 to allow reliable amplification of the target gene. Analyses of samples with IAC C_t values >32 were repeated after reduction of PCR-inhibitory substances by 1:2 and 1:10 dilution.

Analytical sensitivity and specificity

Analytical sensitivities of the multiplex qPCR were determined by plotting standard curves (C_t values against quantified genomic equivalents, GE) in ten-fold dilution from 4×10^7 to 4×10^3 GE. With an estimated genome size of 3 Mb for *B. hyodysenteriae,* 2.6 Mb for *B. pilosicoli,* and 3.2 Mb for the apathogenic species [20], the following DNA quantities for 1 GE were calculated: *B. hyodysenteriae* 3.3 fg, *B. pilosicoli* 2.8 fg, and *B. intermedia/B. murdochii/B. innocens* 3.5 fg. The slope of the linear relationship of this curve was used to calculate the amplification efficiency [21]. The minimum detectable bacterial concentrations were determined as the quantification limits of the multiplex qPCR. For each reference strain twelve replicates of samples containing 50, 25, 15, 10, 5, 2, 1 GE per 10 μl PCR reaction were analyzed. Primers and probes were confirmed specific for each *Brachyspira* species in the monoplex real-time set up. The multiplex format was optimized in terms of probe and primer concentrations and annealing temperature by comparing the efficiencies of PCR runs. To determine the specificity of the optimized multiplex qPCR, a variety of DNA mixtures from different *Brachyspira* spp. as well as a variety of 26 spirochetal and non-spirochetal bacteria were used (Additional file 2: Figure S2).

Data analysis/statistics

The agreement between the conventional duplex PCR and the multiplex qPCR of swabs or cultured isolate was evaluated by Cohen's kappa index using the IBM SPSS Statistics 22 Software. The strength of agreemen was ranked accordingly: Poor (<0.00), Slight (0.00–0.20), Fair (0.20–0.40), Moderate (0,41–0.60), Substantia (0.61–0.80), Almost perfect (0.81–1.00) [22].

Results

Sensitivity and specificity of the multiplex qPCR

The efficiency of the multiplex qPCR was determined by the use of serial dilution standard curves. The linear correlation coefficient r^2 for the three different target within 23S rDNA was between 0.98 and 0.99, showing a significant linearity of the multiplex qPCR assay (Additional file 3: Figure S3). The amplification efficiencie were 97% for *B. pilosicoli*, 92% for *B. hyodysenteriae* and 103% for *B. intermedia.* Furthermore, the limit of detection (LOD) of each target was evaluated for the multiplex qPCR. The LOD was defined as the lowest numbe of GE which gave rise to a detectable signal in all of the 12 replicate samples. The LODs were set at 10 GE for *B. hyodysenteriae* and *B. pilosicoli* (equal to 33 and 28 fg DNA), while the detection limit for the triplet of apathogenic *Brachyspira* spp. was set at 5 GE (17.5 fg DNA). The sensitivity and specificity of the assay was calculated for the two pathogens in both sample groups (Table 2).

The performance of the optimized multiplex qPCR with different strains of the targeted *Brachyspira* taxon demonstrated no unspecific reactions with other bacteria spp. or cross amplification between the different target species. The multiplex qPCR was shown to simultaneously detect all three *Brachyspira* targets in one reaction and the C_t values did not show any significant shift as a result of the multiplex setup compared with those of the monoplex reactions (data not shown). No template controls as well as the panel of 26 heterologou bacteria consistently scored negative.

Evaluation of the multiplex qPCR

Comparison of the duplex and multiplex PCR using DNA from culture samples

DNA from a total of 251 cultured harvests was analyzed with the multiplex qPCR in parallel with the conventional duplex PCR (Fig. 1, Group I). The multiplex qPCR identified a total of 76 out of 251 samples (30.3%) *B.hyodysenteriae*-positive. One sample was found negative for *B.hyodysenteriae* with the multiplex qPCR while classified as positive with the duplex PCR. In contrast, the multiplex qPCR found five new *B.hyodysenteriae*

able 2 Sensitivity and specificity calculated for the multiplex qPCR assay, compared to the gold standard duplex PCR

ethod		Total samples (n)	Target spp.	Sensitivity (%) (95% CI)	Specificity (%) (95% CI)
roup 1	multiplex qPCR	251	*B.hyodysenteriae*	93 (86–97)	97 (94–99)
			B.pilosicoli	93 (93–100)	96 (96–100)
roup 2	multiplex qPCR	202	*B.hyodysenteriae*	100 (90–100)	98 (94–100)
			B.pilosicoli	94 (87–98)	98 (94–100)
	swabs[a]	202	*B.hyodysenteriae*	87 (72–96)	98 (94–99)
			B.pilosicoli	65 (54–76)	96 (91–99)

[a]wab-coupled multiplex qPCR analysis compared with culture-coupled multiplex qPCR

ositive samples which were not detected by the duplex CR. The multiplex qPCR detected 93 of 251 samples 37.1%) as *B.pilosicoli* positive, while seven samples were lassified as negative in the multiplex qPCR although being positive in the duplex PCR. Regarding the detection f *B.hyodysenteriae* and *B.pilosicoli* both PCR methods howed a significant agreement with κ-values of 0.943 nd 0.933 respectively (Table 3).

In 91 samples (36.3%) the multiplex qPCR was able to emonstrate the presence of *Brachyspira* i.e. the triplet of apathogenic *Brachyspira spp.* Another panel of 86 samples from the multiplex qPCR analysis exhibited different combinations of mixed infections with *B.hyodysenteriae*, *B.pilosicoli* and apathogenic *Brachyspira*.spp. With the multiplex assay ten mixed infections of *B.hyodysenteriae* and *B.pilosicoli* (4.0%) were detected. The duplex PCR was able to confirm four cases (1.6%) of these *B.hyodysenteriae* and *B.pilosicoli* mix infections (Table 3).

able 3 Result from the multiplex qPCR analysis of culture erived DNA in Group 1 (A). Agreement between the multiplex PCR and the duplex PCR calculated with the kappa test (B). The trength of agreement was ranked accordingly: Poor (<0.00), light (0.00–0.20), Fair (0.21–0.40), Moderate (0,41–0.60), Substantial).61–0.80), Almost Perfect (0.81–1.00). B.hyo = *B.hyodysenteriae*; .pilo = *B.pilosicoli*

roup 1				
pecies distribution				
		Culture DNA % (n)		
hyodysenteriae		19.5% (49)		
pilosicoli		10% (25)		
pathogen		36.6% (92)		
ixes		33.9% (85)		
B.hyo + apathogen		6.8% (17)		
B.pilo + apathogen		23.1% (58)		
B.hyo + *B.pilo*		2.4% (6)		
B.hyo + *B.pilo* + apathogen		1.6% (4)		
otal samples		total =251		
ultiplex vs. Duplex on fecal culture (*n* = 251)				
		Duplex PCR		Kappa index
		+	-	
ultiplex qPCR				
B.hyodysenteriae	+	71	5	0.943
	-	1	174	
B.pilosicoli	+	92	1	0.933
	-	7	151	

Comparative PCR analysis using DNA from cultured samples and from swabs

A total of 202 fecal swabs were examined for *Brachyspira* spp. by comparative PCR analysis of DNA from culture harvests and DNA directly extracted from the swabs (Fig. 1, Group 2). Using DNA from culture harvests, both PCR methods were again in excellent agreement in detecting *B. hyodysenteriae* and *B. pilosicoli* (κ-values of 0.932 and 0.928, Table 4). A direct comparison of both PCR methods on direct swab DNA was not feasible since the vast majority of samples analyzed by duplex PCR were negative due to the substantially lower LOD in comparison to the multiplex qPCR. Comparative analysis of both swab and culture harvest DNA in the multiplex qPCR revealed that the detection rate of *B. hyodysenteriae* was 18% (37–38 positive) in either type of specimen. *B. pilosicoli* was detected in 81 DNA samples from culture harvests (40.1%), whereas swab DNA was found positive in 58 cases (28.7%). The results obtained by comparative multiplex qPCR analysis of swab and culture harvest DNA were in large agreement regarding the detection rate of *B. hyodysenteriae* and the triplet of apathogenic *Brachyspira* spp. alone or in different combinations (Fig. 2). Overall, the detection rates for *B. hyodysenteriae* and *B. pilosicoli* were ranked as "almost perfect" and in "substantial" agreement, respectively (κ-values of 0.853 and 0.643, Table 4). In addition, DNA from 75 fecal swabs, which were evaluated *Brachyspira* negative by microscopy evaluation of culture growth, were analyzed with the multiplex qPCR. Fifty-one of these samples were negative in the multiplex qPCR analysis, however, 23 samples (30.7%) were positive for apathogen *Brachyspira* spp. and one sample was

Table 4 Species distribution of samples in Group 2 (A). Agreement between the multiplex qPCR and the duplex PCR using the kappa index (Group 2) (B). The second panel displays the detection of *B.hyodysenteriae* and *B.pilosicoli* and the agreement between culture derived DNA vs swab derived DNA using the multiplex qPCR assay (C)

Group 2				
A				
Species distribution				
		Culture DNA % (n)		
B.hyodysenteriae		10.4% (21)		
B.pilosicoli		8.9% (18)		
apathogen		47% (95)		
negative for *Brachyspira*		7.4% (15)		
mixes		26.3% (53)		
B.hyo + apathogen		6.5% (13)		
B.pilo + apathogen		18% (37)		
B.hyo + *B.pilo*		0.5% (1)		
B.hyo + *B.pilo* + apathogen		1% (2)		
Total samples		total =202		
B				
Multiplex vs. Duplex on fecal culture ($n = 202$)				
		Duplex PCR		Kappa index
		+	-	
Multiplex qPCR culture				
B.hyodysenteriae	+	34	4	0.932
	-	0	164	
B. pilosicoli	+	79	2	0.928
	-	5	116	
C				
Multiplex qPCR culture vs. swabs ($n = 202$)				
		Culture		Kappa index
		+	-	
Swabs				
B.hyodysenteriae	+	33	4	0.853
	-	5	160	
B.pilosicoli	+	53	5	0.643
	-	28	116	

positive for *B. pilosicoli* and apathogen spp. with a C_t-value close to the threshold (C_t: 37.8 for *B. pilosicoli)*. Two additional samples from the same herd as the *B. pilosicoli* positive sample were submitted to our laboratory for analysis. Both samples were evaluated *B.pilosicoli* positive by duplex PCR and multiplex qPCR.

Discussion

In this study, a total of 453 fecal samples from pigs originated from a cross-section of the Swiss cantons in which

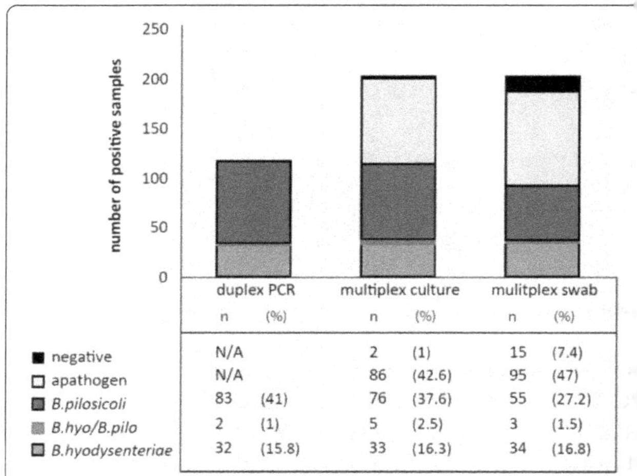

Fig. 2 Comparison of result between the duplex PCR and the qPCR with culture derived DNA and swab DNA (Group 2). N/A: not applicable

pig breeding and pig farming is carried out (Fig. 1), wer analyzed for *Brachyspira* spp. to evaluate a novel multiplex qPCR, designed to simultaneously detect *B. hyodysenteriae, B. pilosicoli* and a triplet of apathogeni *Brachyspira* spp. *(B. intermedia, B. murdochii, B. innocens*). Using spirochetal DNA from fecal anaerobic cultures as a target, the multiplex qPCR displayed a almost perfect agreement with the reference duplex PC with kappa index values of 0.943 and 0.933 for *B.hyodysenteriae* and *B.pilosicoli,* respectively. Regarding the advantage of identifying the two significant pathogeni *Brachyspira* spp. from cultures of porcine fecal specimens in one PCR run, the novel multiplex qPCR can definitively replace the more labor-intensive duplex PCR The latter one is relying on the amplification of two different genes (*nox* and 16S rDNA gene) for the detectio of *B.hyodysenteriae* and *B.pilosicoli* [14]. Our novel assa on the contrary is based on one single target sequenc (namely the 23S rDNA gene), a fact which increases th efficiency of the PCR and additionally avoids competition for the PCR reagents between different targets Traditionally 16S rDNA sequencing has been used fo the differentiation between different bacteria species, bu members of the genus *Brachyspira* have been reporte difficult to differentiate solely based on this gene sequence [23]. The 23S rDNA on other hand, comprise of longer regions of hypervariability [24] and has previously been used for specific detection of *B. hyodysenteriae* and two other groups of weakly beta-hemolyti procine *Brachyspira* [25]. Another benefit of the multiplex qPCR is the internal control which informs abou PCR inhibitor factors, and thereby helps avoiding false negative samples.

In other studies on the detection of porcine *Brachyspira* using a variety of PCR protocols minimal detectio mits between 10^2 and 10^4 cells or DNA copies per ram specimen (depending on study) has been demonstrated [25–27]. Even with a moderate analytic sensitivity PCR should reliably identify pigs with clinical SD. Iowever, the detection of the epidemiologically important asymptomatic carriers, which according to experince shed only low numbers of *Brachyspira,* is severely mited [13]. The analytic sensitivity of our multiplex PCR was determined to 5–10 GE which corresponds to detectable minimum bacterial load of minimum 6×0^2 and on average 1×10^3 GE per g specimen. The lack hole quencher used in this assay is providing a low ignal-to-noise ratio and thereby also providing a higher ensitivity compared to traditional probes with a secondry fluorescent dye as quencher. Thus, in comparison rith suitable data from the literature, our multiplex PCR hows a promising analytic sensitivity which should be dequate to identify *Brachyspira* spp. in DNA directly xtracted from fecal swabs. Interestingly, *Brachyspira* pp. patterns obtained by PCR analysis of culture-erived DNA only slightly differed from the patterns obained from the corresponding swab DNA with exception of *B. pilosicoli* (Fig. 2). DNA samples derived lirectly from fecal swabs are expected to display the natural distribution of *Brachyspira* spp. By comparison,)NA from culture harvests may not reflect the original rachyspiral spectrum in a fecal specimen since the culure conditions may either stimulate or even delay the rowth rate of a single *Brachyspira* sp. in a brachyspiral nixture. Accordingly, *B.pilosicoli* appeared to be more usceptible to a cultural enrichment. In our study *B.pilosicoli* either alone or in mixed infection was detected at significant higher frequency in DNA samples from culure harvests than in swab DNA (81 vs. 58, $p < 0.05$, Chi quare test). It is however important to consider that the wabs used in this study had already been used streaking ut on TSA, consequently less material is available for he direct swab DNA extraction. Extracting DNA from he swabs directly after delivery might improve the result nd lead to an increased concordance with the cultured)NA analyzed with the reference duplex PCR or our ovel multiplex qPCR. As a step in the evaluation of the nultiplex qPCR we tested 75 swabs evaluated by culture o be *Brachyspira* negative. Thirty percent of the samles were positive for *Brachyspira* spp. when analyzed vith our assay. This high number of *Brachyspira* spp. indings in culture negative swabs confirms the high senitivity of the novel multiplex qPCR even in comparison vith culture.

With PCR analysis of DNA from swabs, without culuring the samples, the result can be delivered already fter 1 day. This is a substantial improvement compared o the conventional microbiological culture methods vhere 3 to 6 days of culture is needed until DNA can be extracted and the analysis for pathogenic *Brachyspira* spp. can be achieved. Both the culture and swab samples methods show high specificity, however, the culture coupled qPCR has the highest sensitivity, especially in the case of *B.pilosicoli* detection due to its fast growth rate in culture. Therefore, we recommend these two analysis approaches in different setups: high-throughput screening of fecal swabs and the culture-coupled approach to identify *B.hyodysenteriae* infected individuals within qPCR positive herds with the purpose to establish pathogen *Brachyspira* strains e.g. for antimicrobial susceptibility testing. We are currently evaluating the effect of a short incubated enrichment broth on further increasing the sensitivity of the swab-based multiplex qPCR for *B.hyodysenteriae* and *B.pilosicoli* to close the small, but still evident, sensitivity gap between culture-harvest and swab DNA analysis.

Conclusion

In comparison to a widely used reference PCR a novel multiplex qPCR targeting a 128 bp region on the 23S rDNA gene allows the sensitive simultaneous detection of *B. hyodysenteriae* and *B. pilosicoli* and three apathogenic *Brachyspira* spp in fecal swabs. The multiplex qPCR provides more detailed insights into the composition of the porcine brachyspiral fecal due to the concurrent detection of pathogenic and apathogenic *Brachyspira* spp. We propose this assay as a robust diagnostic tool with the ability to decrease the work load and improve the diagnostic results readout.

Endnotes

[1]Footnote: Strains were kindly provided by Dr. Judith Rhode, Institute for Microbiology, University of Veterinary Medicine Hanover, Hanover, Germany.

Additional files

Additional file 1: Figure S1. Consensus sequence alignment of the target DNA region within 23S ribosomal DNA. Primers (Brachy primer for. and Brachy primer rev.) on the target DNA are marked in grey. The probe for *B. hyodysenteriae* (Probe_hyo) is highlighted in yellow, the probe for *B. pilosicoli* (Probe_pilo) in purple, and the probe for the *B. intermedia/B. innocens/B. murdochii* (probe inter) in green. Differences in single residues are marked in red.

Additional file 2: Figure S2. A panel of 26 spirochetal and non-spirochetal bacteria used for specificity testing of the multiplex qPCR. ATCC, American Type Culture Collection; DSM, German Collection of Microorganisms [Deutsche Sammlung von Mikrooganismen]. (PDF 258 kb)

Additional file 3: Figure S3. Plotting of standard curves for the three probes.

Abbreviations

PIS: Porcine intestinal spirochaetosis; SD: Swine dysentery

Acknowledgments

We thank Ella Hübschke, Natasha Carroli and Andreas Lehmann for their excellent technical assistance in the diagnostic laboratory.

Funding

No funds were received for this research.

Author's contributions

AB, SiS, MMW conceived and designed the experiments. AB, SiS, DF performed the experiments. AB, SiS analyzed the data. AB, MMW drafted the manuscript. Bacteria culture and microscopy: SaS, CK. All the authors have read and approved the final manuscript.

Competing interests

The authors declare that they have no competing interests.

Consent for publication

Not applicable.

References

1. Taylor DJ, Alexander TJ. The production of dysentery in swine by feeding cultures containing a spirochaete. Br Vet J. 1971;127:58–61.
2. Taylor DJ, Simmons JR, Laird HM. Production of diarrhoea and dysentery in pigs by feeding pure cultures of a spirochaete differing from Treponema hyodysenteriae. Vet Rec. 1980;106:326–32.
3. Binek M, Szynkiewicz ZM. Physiological properties and classification of strains of Treponema sp. isolated from pigs in Poland. Comp Immunol Microbiol Infect Dis. 1984;7:141–8.
4. Fellström C, Gunnarsson A. Phenotypical characterisation of intestinal spirochaetes isolated from pigs. Res Vet Sci. 1995;59:1–4.
5. Komarek V, Maderner A, Spergser J, Weissenböck H. Infections with weakly haemolytic Brachyspira species in pigs with miscellaneous chronic diseases. Vet Microbiol. 2009;134:311–7.
6. Hudson MJ, Alexander TJ, Lysons RJ. Diagnosis of swine dysentery: spirochaetes which may be confused with Treponema hyodysenteriae. Vet Rec. 1976;99:498–500.
7. Jensen TK, Møller K, Boye M, Leser TD, Jorsal SE. Scanning electron microscopy and fluorescent in situ hybridization of experimental Brachyspira (Serpulina) pilosicoli infection in growing pigs. Vet Pathol. 2000; 37:22–32.
8. Stanton TB. Proposal to change the genus designation Serpula to Serpulina gen. nov. containing the species Serpulina hyodysenteriae comb. nov. and Serpulina innocens comb. nov. Int J Syst Bacteriol. 1992;42:189–90.
9. Stanton TB, et al. Recognition of two new species of intestinal spirochetes: Serpulina intermedia sp. nov. and Serpulina murdochii sp. nov. Int J Syst Bacteriol. 1997;47:1007–12.
10. Litzenberger B, Corboz L, Hoelzle LH, Wittenbrink MM. Detection of Brachyspira pilosicoli in the intestine of pigs in Switzerland. 2004.
11. Speiser SA, et al. [Swine dysentery eradication in a grower-finisher farm in Switzerland]. Schweiz Arch Tierheilkd. 2011;153:14–8.
12. Figi, Goldinger, Fuschini, Hartnack, Sidler. [Eradication of swine dysentery as modified partial depopulation in a nucleus sow breeding farm]. Schweiz Arch Tierheilkd. 2014;156:373–80.
13. Fellström C, Zimmerman U, Aspan A, Gunnarsson A. The use of culture, pooled samples and PCR for identification of herds infected with Brachyspira hyodysenteriae. Anim Health Res Rev. 2001;2:37–43.
14. La T, Phillips ND, Hampson DJ. Development of a duplex PCR assay for detection of Brachyspira hyodysenteriae and Brachyspira pilosicoli in pig feces. J Clin Microbiol. 2003;41:3372–5.
15. Wilberts BL, Warneke HL, Bower LP, Kinyon JM, Burrough ER. Comparison of culture, polymerase chain reaction, and fluorescent in situ hybridization for detection of Brachyspira hyodysenteriae and 'Brachyspira hampsonii' in pig feces. J Vet Diagn Invest. 2015;27:41–6.
16. Råsbäck T, Fellström C, Gunnarsson A, Aspán A. Comparison of culture and biochemical tests with PCR for detection of Brachyspira hyodysenteriae and Brachyspira pilosicoli. J Microbiol Methods. 2006;66:347–53.
17. Dünser, M., Sweighardt, H., Pangerl, R., Awad-Masalmeh, M. and Schluh, M. Swine dysentery and spirochetal darrhea - a comparative study of enteritis cases caused by Serpulina. [GE]. Wien. Tierarztl. Monatsschr. 1997;84:151-16
18. Prohaska S, et al. MALDI-TOF MS for identification of porcine Brachyspira species. Lett Appl Microbiol. 2014;58:292–8.
19. Hoffmann B, Depner K, Schirrmeier H, Beer M. A universal heterologous internal control system for duplex real-time RT-PCR assays used in a detection system for pestiviruses. J Virol Methods. 2006;136:200–9.
20. Wanchanthuek P, et al. The complete genome sequence of the pathogenic intestinal spirochete Brachyspira pilosicoli and comparison with other Brachyspira genomes. PLoS One. 2010;5:e11455.
21. Klein D, et al. Proviral load determination of different feline immunodeficiency virus isolates using real-time polymerase chain reaction: Influence of mismatches on quantification. Electrophoresis. 1999;20:291–9.
22. Landis JR, Koch GG. The measurement of observer agreement for categorical data. Biometrics. 1977;33:159–74.
23. Stanton, T. In *Prokaryotes Volume 7* (eds. Dworkin, M., Falkow, S., Rosenberg E. & Schleifer, K.-H.) 330–356. New York: (Springer, 2006).
24. Ludwig W, Schleifer KH. Bacterial phylogeny based on 16S and 23S rRNA sequence analysis. FEMS Microbiol Rev. 1994;15:155–73.
25. Leser TD, Møller K, Jensen TK, Jorsal SE. Specific detection of Serpulina hyodysenteriae and potentially pathogenic weakly beta-haemolytic porcine intestinal spirochetes by polymerase chain reaction targeting 23S rDNA. Mc Cell Probes. 1997;11:363–72.
26. La T, Collins AM, Phillips ND, Oksa A, Hampson DJ. Development of a multiplex-PCR for rapid detection of the enteric pathogens Lawsonia intracellularis, Brachyspira hyodysenteriae, and Brachyspira pilosicoli in porcine faeces. Lett Appl Microbiol. 2006;42:284–8.
27. Song Y, Hampson DJ. Development of a multiplex qPCR for detection and quantitation of pathogenic intestinal spirochaetes in the faeces of pigs and chickens. Vet Microbiol. 2009;137:129–36.

5

Development of a stochastic agent-based model to evaluate surveillance strategies for detection of emergent porcine reproductive and respiratory syndrome strains

A. G. Arruda[1*], Z. Poljak[1], D. Knowles[2] and A. McLean[2]

Abstract

Background: The objective of the current study was to develop a stochastic agent-based model using empirical data from Ontario (Canada) swine sites in order to evaluate different surveillance strategies for detection of emerging porcine reproductive and respiratory syndrome virus (PRRSV) strains at the regional level. Four strategies were evaluated, including (i) random sampling of fixed numbers of swine sites monthly; (ii) risk-based sampling of fixed numbers, specifically of breeding sites (high-consequence sites); (iii) risk-based sampling of fixed numbers of low biosecurity sites (high-risk); and (iv) risk-based sampling of breeding sites that are characterized as low biosecurity sites (high-risk/high-consequence). The model simulated transmission of a hypothetical emerging PRRSV strain between swine sites through three important industry networks (production system, truck and feed networks) while considering sites' underlying immunity due to past or recent exposure to heterologous PRRSV strains, as well as demographic, geographic and biosecurity-related PRRS risk factors. Outcomes of interest included surveillance system sensitivity and time to detection of the three first cases over a period of approximately three years.

Results: Surveillance system sensitivities were low and time to detection of three first cases was long across all examined scenarios.

Conclusion: Traditional modes of implementing high-risk and high-consequence risk-based surveillance based on site's static characteristics do not appear to substantially improve surveillance system sensitivity. Novel strategies need to be developed and considered for rapid detection of this and other emerging swine infectious diseases. None of the four strategies compared herein appeared optimal for early detection of an emerging PPRSV strain at the regional level considering model assumptions, the underlying population of interest, and absence of other forms of surveillance.

Keywords: Stochastic agent-based model, Porcine reproductive and respiratory syndrome control, Porcine reproductive and respiratory syndrome surveillance, Risk-based surveillance, Surveillance system sensitivity

* Correspondence: goncalvesarruda.1@osu.edu
[1]Department of Population Medicine, Ontario Veterinary College, University of Guelph, 50 Stone Rd East, Guelph, ON N1G 2W1, Canada
Full list of author information is available at the end of the article

Background

Porcine reproductive and respiratory syndrome (PRRS) is an endemic infectious swine disease caused by an RNA virus and is responsible for considerable economic losses in North America and many European countries [1, 2]. The syndrome is characterized by decreased growth in pigs across all ages (mainly due to respiratory disease and secondary infections) and reproductive failure in adult female pigs. Even though strategies for PRRS control and elimination have been previously investigated and described [3], it remains a challenge for the swine industry. Factors related to the current characteristics of the North American swine industry contribute to the maintenance of PRRS within a country or region. Among these are the high degree of connectivity between swine sites, the constant exchange of subpopulations of animals that are at higher risk for disease transmission between sites (e.g. weaned piglets and culled sows), the high turnover rates of animals within farms, and the segregated nature of the different phases of production [4].

Currently, in Canada, the most commonly used approach for PRRSV surveillance is the submission of specimens from suspected clinical cases to diagnostic laboratories. This is commonly complemented by other activities that include: (i) detection of PRRSV cases through on-going monitoring when expected prevalence is low (e.g., nursery sites from specific production systems), (ii) certification of absence of infection using minimum pre-specified level, or (iii) specific regional studies or programs conducted to assess trends in disease prevalence or incidence over time. With the advent of regional disease control programs for PRRS, a frequently posed question relates to the design of effective surveillance strategies when one of the objectives is detection of new cases due to circulation of a novel PRRSV strain. In this context, risk-based surveillance strategies have been widely used and justified as effective and efficient strategies. The main idea behind this approach is that it targets subpopulations of animals that are at increased risk for the occurrence of infection due to the presence of known risk factors [5]. Although implementation of risk-based approaches to sampling in food animal veterinary medicine is relatively frequent under field conditions, its quantitative assessment has been relatively limited to cases of supporting declaration of freedom from infection in a jurisdiction [6], or for comparisons between alternative surveillance strategies before a recommendation is made [7]. Typically, assessment of surveillance systems has been accomplished using stochastic scenario tree modelling (STM). This methodology models the process of disease detection while including factors that affect probability of infection or detection of a surveillance system [8].

Risk-based approaches could be considered when detection of emerging strains of an endemic pathogen is important. However, the framework for the quantitative assessment of alternative surveillance approaches for such situation is not well described in the relevant literature. Velasova et al. [9] used a stochastic STM approach to evaluate the expected performance of a passive monitoring system for detection of novel strains of PRRSV in the United Kingdom. Even though STM appears a logical extension when the main objective is detection of cases due to circulation of a novel PRRSV strain for endemic situations, its uniform application in all situations is limited due to two main reasons. Firstly, the goals and approaches to surveillance within endemic scenarios could vary greatly (e.g. monitor disease trends over time, detecting new cases and possibly novel pathogen strains, etc.), and secondly the modern swine production systems are hierarchically structured and networks have been identified as important contributors to disease spread [10, 11], representing yet another layer of risk factors that would be difficult if not impossible to incorporate using STM. These risk factors would be difficult to incorporate in a typical STM, and an alternative is to develop agent-based models (ABM) with swine sites as agents. Such an approach is particularly appealing in the context of disease control projects because observed data on risk factors can be easily incorporated at the site level, together with contact structure among swine sites. In addition, performance of high-risk surveillance strategies could be compared to high-consequence surveillance strategies in a natural manner, since the directed flow of infected animals could be incorporated in such models explicitly [12].

The goal of the current study was to develop a stochastic ABM that would allow for the evaluation of different surveillance strategies for detection of emerging PRRSV strains at the regional level. Four surveillance strategies were evaluated, including (i) random sampling of fixed numbers of swine sites monthly; (ii) risk-based sampling of fixed numbers of specifically breeding swine sites (high-consequence sites); (iii) risk-based sampling of fixed numbers of low biosecurity sites (high-risk sites); and (iv) risk-based sampling of breeding sites that are also characterized as low biosecurity sites (high-risk/high-consequence sites). The main outcome of interest was the sensitivity of the surveillance systems evaluated, i.e. the probability of the systems in detecting infected sites. Furthermore, the time to detection of the three first cases was also described, and sensitivity analysis was conducted to evaluate the impact of the target design prevalence (level of disease that the system aims to detect) used for sample size calculation (1%, 2% or 5%) in the main outcomes of interest.

Methods

A stochastic agent-based model was created and implemented using the software Anylogic® version 7.1.2 (XJ Technologies, St Petersburg, Russia). The model description outlined in the next paragraphs follows general reporting guidelines from the standardized overview, design concepts, and details (ODD) protocol as described by Grimm et al. [13].

Purpose

The main purpose of the model was to simulate the dynamics of a representative sample of Ontario swine sites and the spread of PRRSV between these sites using empirical data from the PRRS Area Regional Control and Elimination (ARC&E) projects in Ontario, Canada. The model would allow for the evaluation of regional PRRS surveillance strategies to detect emerging PRRS virus cases within this population of interest.

State variables and scales

The model features a collection of swine sites that can transfer PRRSV infections through their trucking, production system, and feed networks. A swine site was defined as one or more barns built close together that housed pigs in a specific physical location. A total of 816 swine sites were enrolled in a provincial PRRS control project when this study was conducted and this corresponded to our population of interest.

Swine sites were given characteristics described by parameters, which were extracted from the Ontario Swine Health Advisory Board regional control program database from a standardized questionnaire answered by swine producers as they enrolled in the project. This database was privately owned and maintained by the Ontario Swine Health Advisory Board, and the authors were given permission to access it by this entity. These parameters were modelled as being static, and therefore were not allowed to change over time. Characteristics included were animal flow (continuous animal flow or all-in all-out animal flow), number of neighbors (categorized into zero neighbors, one to five neighbors, and more than five neighbors), presence of a shower in facility (yes or no), number of animals (categorized into up to 500 animals, from 500 to 2000 animals, and more than 2000 animals), and production type (breeding site, nursery site, and growing pig site, the last included wean-to-finish and finishing operations). For a relatively small percentage of sites, the information regarding one or more parameters was missing, and for those the model was set to randomly assign a category for the parameters. This occurred for 85 sites (10%) for the parameter 'presence of shower facility', 23 sites (3%) for number of animals, and 217 sites (27%) for animal flow. These characteristics were selected because they have been previously reported as risk factors for PRRS [14, 15] and because the information was readily available from the control program.

The increase or decrease in the risk of PRRSV infection according to those risk factors was specified at model start according to values found in Table 1. At receipt of an 'exposure', a non-infected swine site would become infected with a 10% probability. This was then multiplied by the relative risk of infection factors relevant to the model, animal flow, number of neighboring facilities, presence of showers, number of animals at the facility, and immunity status (Table 1).

Swine sites were eligible to be part of up to three different static undirected networks: production system, truck, and feed networks. Sites were considered connected through each of these networks if the swine producer (site owner) had named a common ownership structure (for production system), a common transportation company (for the truck network), and a common feed company (for the feed network) as other swine producer(s). This information was collected during administration of the same questionnaire previously mentioned and corresponded to 'static' relationships (no frequency of contact information collected). A simplified visualization of the model with site characteristics and network connections is shown in Fig. 1.

The model proceeded in daily time steps, with the new PRRSV strain introduced on day 3 after model start and a follow-up time of approximately 2 years and 8 months (1000 days). It was assumed that this population of 816 swine sites was stable for the time evaluated, with no swine sites being added or removed from the population.

Process overview and scheduling

Swine sites included in this model were characterized by mutually exclusive PRRS immunological status that included 'completely susceptible', 'partially susceptible', and 'completely immune'. The nomenclature given to this so-called 'immunity status' refers to the likelihood of infection with the new virus strain that was purposely introduced as a 'challenge' in order to evaluate the surveillance strategies. Detailed rules for such classification are presented in Table 2. In summary, swine sites within the 'completely susceptible' compartment corresponded to sites containing a naïve animal population, characterized by being both seronegative and virus negative, therefore reflective of no previous or current PRRSV exposure. Sites within the 'partially susceptible' compartment corresponded to swine sites that were serologically positive or positive by virus detection, which meant that the population of animals within these sites was at a lower risk for infection with a new PRRSV strain

Table 1 Definition of parameters and values used for model simulations

Parameter	Value (unit)
Time to PRRSV[a] elimination for breeding sites	385 (days)[b]
Time to PRRSV elimination for AIAO[c]nurseries	56 (days)
Time to PRRSV elimination for AIAO finishers/ wean-to-finish sites	112 (days)
Baseline probability of infection with PRRSV (new strain)	10% per ye
Percent of the swine sites considered "completely susceptible"	63%[d]
Relative Risks for getting infected with PRRSV	
Relative risk of getting infected with PRRSV for nurseries compared to breeding sites	1.2
Relative risk of getting infected with PRRSV for finishers/ wean-to-finish sites compared to breeding sites	1.5
Relative risk of getting infected with PRRSV for sites with no shower in facility compared to sites with shower	1.3
Relative risk of getting infected with PRRSV for sites with continuous flow compared to sites with AIAO	1.5
Relative risk of getting infected with PRRSV for sites with medium number of neighbours compared to sites with no neighbours	1.5
Relative risk of getting infected with PRRSV for sites with high number of neighbours compared to sites with no neighbours	2.0
Relative risk of getting infected with PRRSV for sites with medium number of animals compared to sites with reduced number of animals	1.5
Relative risk of getting infected with PRRSV for sites with high number of animals compared to sites with reduced number of animals	2.0
Relative risk of getting infected with PRRSV for naïve sites compared to sites with complete immunity	2.0
Relative risk of getting infected with PRRSV for sites infected with other PRRSV strains (partial immunity) compared to sites with complete immunity	1.5

Formula for probability of infection
0.10* (relative risk [RR]) animal flow* (RR) number of neighbors* (RR) presence of shower* (RR) number of animals* (RR) production type* (RR) immunity status

[a]Porcine reproductive and respiratory syndrome virus
[b]Linhares et al., 2014 [21]
[c]All-in, all-out animal flow
[d]Arruda et al., 2015 [22]

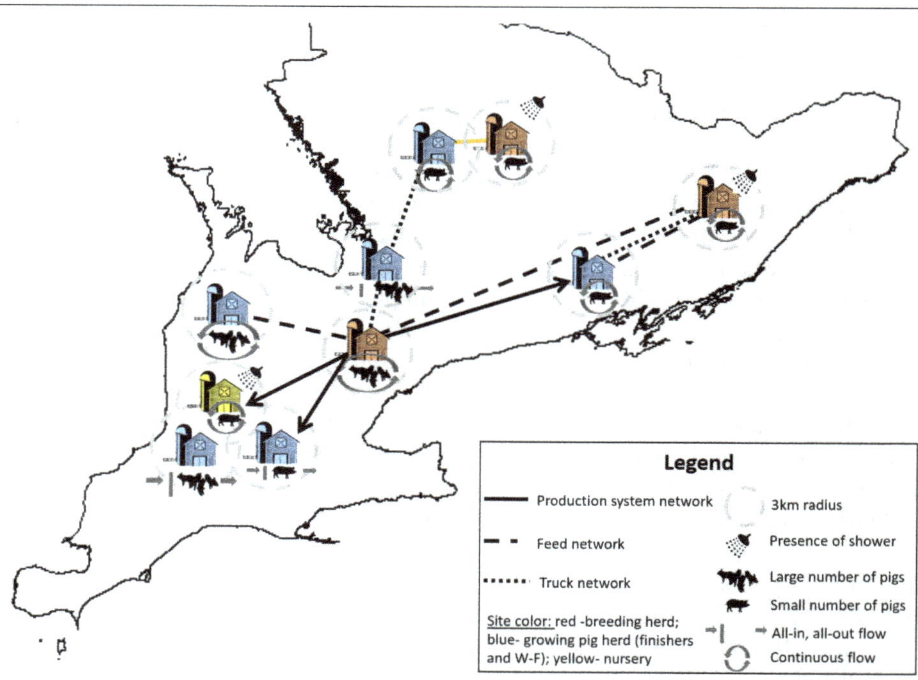

Fig. 1 Model scheme using ten hypothetical swine sites characteristics and locations in Southern Ontario. Underlying immunity of swine sites are not shown due to their dynamic nature. A link between swine sites represented a common service provider within the specific network

able 2 Definition of site immune status according to the PRRS control program and model assumptions for underlying immunity

				Breeding sites	Growing pig sites
nmunity level[a]	OSHAB classification	Serology[b]	Virus detection[c]	Comments	Comments
ompletely susceptible	Confirmed negative	Negative	Negative	Series testing	Series testing
artially susceptible	Confirmed positive	At least one positive		Parallel testing	Parallel testing
ompletely susceptible	Presumed negative	-	-	Sample size not met, sample of downstream growing pig sites	Sample size not met, sample of upstream sow sites
artially Susceptible	Presumed positive	-	-	Downstream sites confirmed positive by diagnostic test, veterinarian assessment of site	Upstream sites confirmed positive by diagnostic test, veterinarian assessment of site

ᴬs defined by the current model (underlying swine site immunity)
ᴱvidence of previous exposure to porcine reproductive and respiratory syndrome virus (PRRSV), measured through ELISA testing for antibody detection in serum · oral fluids
ᴱvidence of current virus infection, measured via PCR testing in serum, oral fluids or tissue samples

ompared to the naïve population due to partial immun-y conferred by antibodies produced against a heterol-gous PRRSV strain. As a proportion of swine sites may hoose to eliminate PRRS viruses from their herds (i.e. nove from the compartment 'partially susceptible' to ompletely susceptible'), and as a proportion of negative ites get infected yearly according to a baseline PRRS in-idence rate (i.e. move from the compartment 'com-letely susceptible' to 'partially susceptible'), immunity tatuses were allowed to change over time (Fig. 2a).

At model start, none of the sites were classified as ompletely immune' because it was assumed that the irus introduced into the population was completely ew to the population of animals within sites. Swine ites would transition into that immunological compart-nent if animals within those sites were infected with the new virus strain as model progressed. In this case, it was assumed that a sufficient percentage of animals were exposed to the new virus and sufficiently protected so that the site was considered 'completely immune' for a limited period of time, and therefore could not get re-infected while in this compartment. Sites could also opt for and successfully eliminate the virus and return to the 'completely susceptible' compartment at rates that varied according to production type (Figure 2a; Table 1).

Design concepts

Interactions between agents (indirect contacts among swine sites) were modeled using the three above-mentioned networks. At model start, networks were loaded in Anylogic® as symmetric matrices extracted

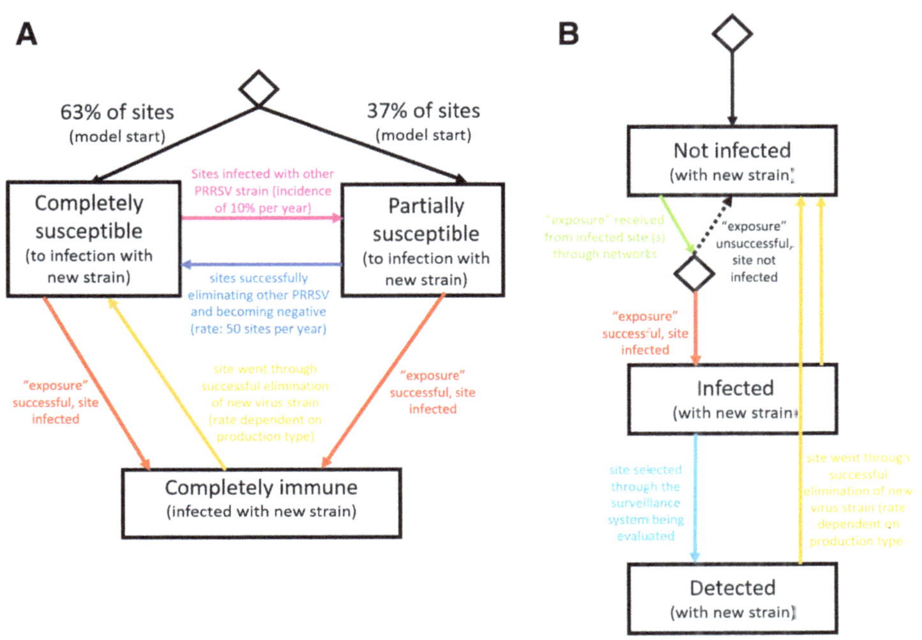

Fig. 2 Compartmental states for swine sites. **a**. Underlying immunity state chart considering infection with other porcine reproductive and respiratory syndrome virus (PRRSV) strains; and **b**. New infections and new detections state chart

from network analysis using UCINET 6 [16]. Each of the three matrices contained site identifiers and "1" in case the two sites had an indirect contact through the specific network, and "0" otherwise. Networks were represented separately, and the frequency of contact between swine sites through these networks was considered more intense for the production system network (a contact was assumed to occur one time per week), followed by the truck network (one contact every two weeks) and the feed network (one contact per month). The role of the production system network was to reflect the movement of people, personnel, equipment, and animals between sites, and two sites that were linked through this network could be connected directly or indirectly, depending on the nature of the movement (considering site type). For the truck and feed networks, however, connections between sites were always indirect. Due to the type of service involved (movement of genetic stock, deadstock, slaughterhouse transportation, besides others for the truck network; and delivery of feed for the feed network), it was assumed that the truck network would be heavier in the "disease transmission scale" compared to the feed network.

Transmission of disease between sites was modelled through communications via the use of Anylogic© 'messages' reflecting exposure to the virus (opportunity for infection) that could result in infection or not. The virus was introduced into the population of sites through random selection of one site in the population to be infected. Following this, the infected site would expose other sites within its networks at the frequencies established above. At receipt of an 'exposure', non-infected swine site's characteristics were considered and a stochastic process was carried out using the formula on Table 1 to determine whether a site would be infected or not. This described process was modelled using compartments within a state chart as shown in Fig. 2b. It is important to note that, uniquely for the production system network, the direction of 'exposure' was taken into account. The production type for the site being the source of the 'message' (the infected site exposing others, or the sender of the 'message') was assessed, as well as the production type of site that was receiving the exposure (site at risk for infection, or receiver of the 'message'). In cases where the exposure was between two sites of the same production type, the risk of infection was considered relatively small, since it would be most commonly reflective of indirect transmission through sharing of site personnel, equipment, etc. On the other hand, when the direction of exposure was from a breeding herd to a nursery or growing pig operation, as well as if it was from a nursery to a growing pig operation, the likelihood of infection was assumed to be higher because there could be movement of animal in such direction, which would be indicative of direc PRRSV transmission. The comparison between thos numbers can be obtained in Table 1. Finally, it wa assumed that swine sites had one outbreak ever 20 years due to modes of transmission non-specifie in this model (including but not limited to airborn transmission).

Initialization

At model start, surveillance system screenings were set t occur through Anylogic© 'events', triggered at regular in tervals (monthly, or every 30 days) starting on day zerc The number of swine sites to be checked (inspected) fo infection with the emerging PRRSV depended on th pre-determined design prevalence (Table 3).

The evaluation of each regional surveillance strateg began after the challenge-virus introduction on day 3 fo each simulation. The model ran for three days befor virus introduction to assure loading of network an parameters datasets.

Inputs

Model inputs were obtained from the peer-reviewe literature whenever possible, and when not availabl

Table 3 Description of porcine reproductive and respiratory syndrome site-level surveillance scenarios investigated

Scenario[a]	Type of sampling	Design prevalenc (number of sites sampled)
Random_1	Random	1% (23)
Random_2	Random	2% (13)
Random_5	Random	5% (5)
HR_1	Risk based - High-risk[b]	1% (23)
HR_2	Risk-based - High-risk[b]	2% (13)
HR_5	Risk-based - High-risk[b]	5% (5)
HC_1	Risk-based - High-consequence[c]	1% (23)
HC_2	Risk-based - High-consequence[c]	2% (13)
HC_5	Risk-based - High-consequence[c]	5% (5)
HR/HC_1	Risk-based - High-risk and high-consequence[d]	1% (23)
HR/HC_2	Risk-based - High-risk and high-consequence[d]	2% (13)
HR/HC_5	Risk-based - High-risk and high-consequence[d]	5% (5)

[a]Each scenario consisted of 1000 simulations
[b]High-risk based sampling consisted of sampling of swine sites that were considered at the highest risk of being infected: sites that had low biosecurity (no shower-in facility and continuous animal flow)
[c]High-consequence based sampling consisted of sampling of swine sites that were considered at the highest risk of infecting other sites: breeding sites
[d]High-risk and high-consequence based sampling consisted of sampling of swine sites that had a combination of the highest risk of getting infected as well as the highest risk of infecting others: breeding herds that had low biosecurity (no shower-in facility and continuous animal flow) herds

hey were obtained from discussions with experts in the rea of swine production. A list of inputs used in the nodel is shown in Table 1.

Iodel calibration and statistical analysis of outcomes

'he model was calibrated to reproduce plausible values n terms of the underlying immunological status of the opulation for an endemic disease such as PRRS in Iorth America. The aim was to produce a mean PRRS revalence between 30 and 40% within the two-year eriod evaluated. There is no available information to ne knowledge of the authors concerning the quantifica- ion of system sensitivity for any surveillance strategy; herefore, it was unfeasible to compare current model esults with expected outcomes. The outcomes mea- ured herein included daily total number of sites that vere infected with the new PRRS virus strain, total num- er of infected sites that were detected and total number f non-infected sites. Data processing was conducted sing Excel® (2012, Microsoft Corporation) and Stata 13 Stata-IC version 13; StataCorp, 2007, College Station, 'exas, USA); descriptive analyses, surveillance sensitiv- ies, Kaplan-Meier survival functions and median urvival times were conducted and calculated using tata 13. For the construction of survival curves, only imulations that had at least three cases were eligible o have the outcome of interest (time to detection of irst three cases). The median survival time was com- ared across scenarios, which refers to the time by vhich 50% of the eligible simulations (simulations vith at least three cases) achieved detection of a ninimum number of three cases.

imulation experiments

 total of 1000 simulations were run for each of the valuated scenarios using a random seed. Twelve scenar- os were investigated, as described on Table 3. Site sur- eillance was programmed through cyclic events. Four nain scenarios were investigated that are detailed in the ollowing paragraphs, and the fixed number of swine ites to be sampled varied according to the desired de- ign prevalence: 1% (n = 23 sites per month), 2% (n = 13 ites per month), or 5% (n = five sites per month). Sam- le sizes were calculated with the objective of demon- trating freedom of infection at the population level, and vere calculated using the online tool "FreeCalc" (AusVet nimal Health Services©) [17] considering 100% herd evel specificity, 95% herd level sensitivity, type I error of .05, a population size of 816 and the modified hyper- eometric exact calculation method. Sample sizes were alculated using annual specified design prevalence, and hen the total number to be sampled was divided by 12 o give the monthly number of sites to be sampled. For ll scenarios, it was assumed that, even when a swine site was detected with the new PRRSV strain, trans- mission to other sites was still possible which is re- flective of field conditions for PRRSV and other endemic viral pathogens. It was further assumed that sampling size requirements for detection of PRRSV within herds was met in all cases (no false positives among sites selected for sampling and sufficient num- ber of animals sampled to detect pre-specified within herd design prevalence).

Baseline scenario

The baseline scenario consisted of random sampling a fixed number of swine sites each month (varying accord- ing to desired design prevalence), based on sampling with replacement (swine sites were eligible for selection in the next sampling event, unless they were detected).

High-risk scenario

The high-risk scenario targeted as sampling units swine sites that had low biosecurity measures: a combination of both continuous animal flow and the absence of a shower facility in the site. The sampling consisted of a random sampling of fixed numbers of swine sites (vary- ing according to desired design prevalence) that met both criteria described above (n = 342, number is approximate due to the fact that sites with missing infor- mation were randomly assigned to an equal distribution of the possible responses).

High-consequence scenario

The high-consequence scenario targeted as sampling units swine sites that were considered to have high con- sequence if infected, i.e. they could potentially spread disease to multiple sites. This population of sites corre- sponded to breeding herds (n = 259).

High-risk/ high-consequence scenario

The final scenario corresponded to the targeted sampling of sites that met both high-risk/high-consequence criteria, therefore the eligible pool were sites that were breeding herds with low biosecurity (both absence of a shower facil- ity and continuous animal flow), number of eligible sites varied from 62 to 157, depending on how sites with miss- ing information were assigned to characteristics during model runs). For all evaluated scenarios, once sites were detected as infected by the surveillance system, they were excluded from the pool of sites eligible for selection.

Results

Results from the model were that, under the conditions specified, all evaluated surveillance strategies showed relatively low overall mean sensitivity in detecting an emergent PRRSV strain over an approximate three-year period (Table 4). It is, however, important to note that

Table 4 Mean (%), standard deviation (%), minimum (%) and maximum (%) surveillance system sensitivities; and median total of infected sites according to surveillance scenarios evaluated

Scenario[a]	Surveillance system sensitivity[b]				Median of total infected sites (IQR
	Mean	SD	Minimum	Maximum	
Random_1	17.6	21.7	0	100.0	26.0 (100.0)
Random_2	7.5	11.3	0	50.0	18.0 (69.0)
Random_5	10.7	25.9	0	100.0	21.0 (101.0)
HR_1	14.1	23.4	0	100.0	24.0 (101.5)
HR_2	18.2	30.8	0	100.0	22.0 (100.0)
HR_5	6.9	19.5	0	100.0	24.0 (100.0)
HC_1	20.4	29.4	0	100.0	26.0 (101.0)
HC_2	7.9	18.3	0	100.0	24.0 (101.0)
HC_5	3.6	5.3	0	23.0	23.0 (139.0)
HR/HR_1	7.2	18.2	0	100.0	20.0 (101.0)
HR/HC_2	7.9	18.4	0	100.0	18.0 (94.0)
HR/HC_5	9.9	24.9	0	100.0	24.0 (100.0)

[a]Each scenario consisted of 1000 simulations; please refer to Table 3 for detailed scenario definitions
[b]Calculated as the fraction of number of cases detected divided by the total of infected cases, for each simulation, considering in a period of approximately three years
[c]Interquartile range

the surveillance sensitivity distribution across simulations within the different surveillance strategies was highly right-skewed, with a small number of simulations yielding high sensitivity for almost all strategies (Fig. 3); these cases were in majority cases in which a small number of sites were infected. The number of simulations at which the mean surveillance system sensitivity and the variance stabilized varied according to scenario, but approximately after 100 simulations this happened across all scenarios (data not shown).

As expected, for all scenarios, as design prevalenc decreased (and number of sites sampled per month in creased), system sensitivity also tended to increase which is reasonable given the increase in the likelihoo of sampling infected sites. Interestingly, this observatio was not evident for the high-risk or high-risk/ high consequence scenarios (Table 4 and Fig. 3).

Kaplan-Meier survival functions showed that, regard less of design prevalence, the random sampling surveil lance strategy was the one for which detection of th three first cases was faster over an approximate tim

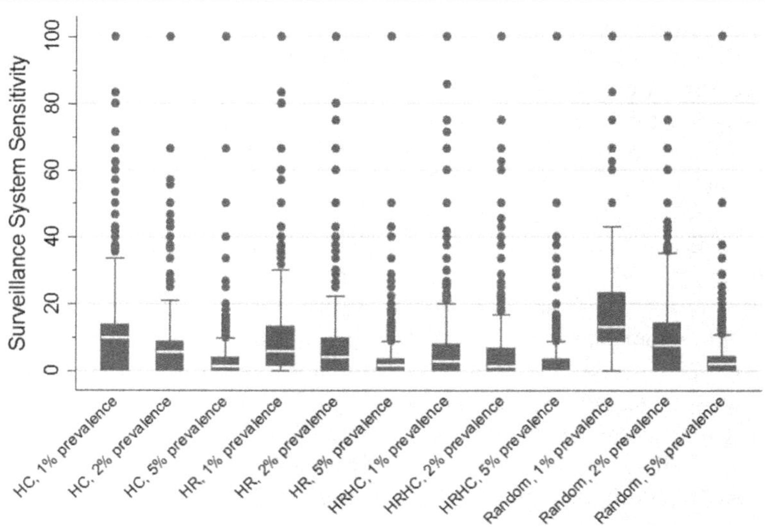

Fig. 3 Surveillance sensitivity boxplots for the total of simulations, by surveillance strategy. HC: high consequence, HR: high risk, HRHC: high risk- high consequence

eriod of three years when compared to the other strat-gies (Fig. 4).

Under the 1% design prevalence scenario, median urvival time was 271 days (SE: 18.79) for the random ampling strategy and 481 days for both the high-onsequence (SE: 30.87) and high-risk (SE: 27.85) cenarios. For the 2% prevalence scenario, the median urvival time was 511 days (SE: 42.19) for the random sampling strategy, 631 days (SE: 53.74) for the high-consequence scenario, and 961 days (SE: 11.00) for the high-risk scenario. The median survival time was not reached for the 5% prevalence scenario, regardless of surveillance strategy examined. The high-risk/ high-consequence strategy only reached a median survival time under the 1% prevalence scenario, and this point was reached in 871 days (SE: 68.92).

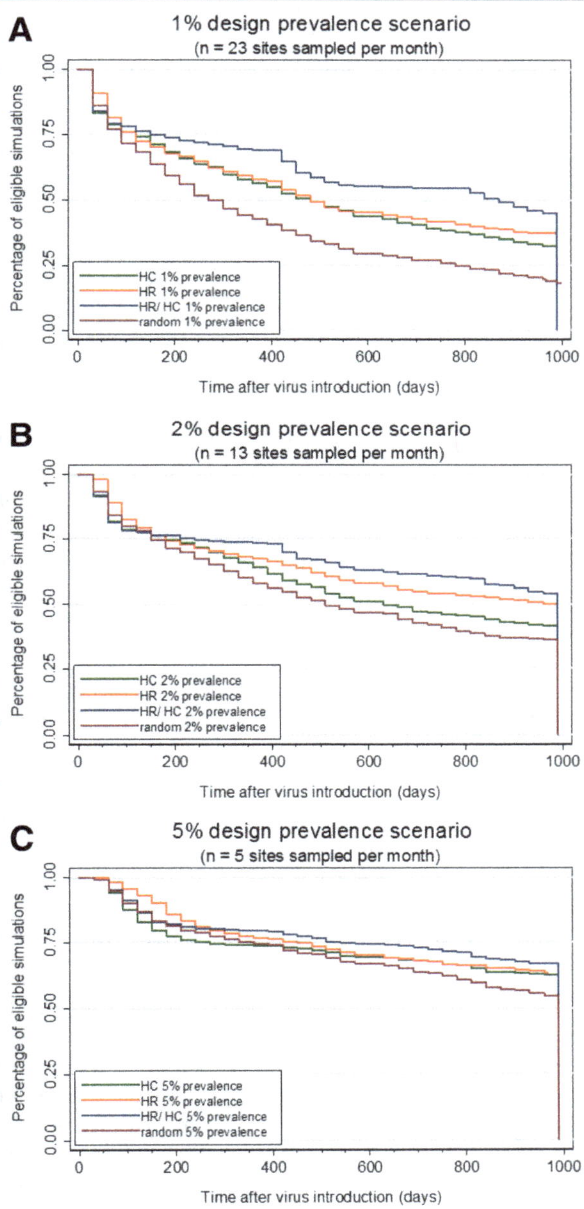

Fig. 4 Kaplan-Meier survival functions showing time to detection of first three cases; according to different sample sizes calculated for 1% (**a**), 2% (**b**) and 5% (**c**) design prevalence, and stratified by surveillance strategies. HC: high consequence, HR: high risk, HR/HC: high risk- high consequence. Only simulations with at least three infected sites were eligible for this outcome

Discussion

The model developed herein simulates transmission of a hypothetical emerging PRRSV strain between swine sites through three important industry networks; production system, truck and feed networks. Importantly, this model considers sites' underlying immunity due to past or recent exposure to heterologous PRRSV strains, as well as the different likelihood of infection due to previously described demographic, geographic and biosecurity-related PRRS risk factors [14, 15]. The present study fulfilled its main objective of development of a tool for the evaluation of surveillance systems for situations where emergent cases (e.g. emerging genotype) of a certain disease are to be detected within a specific area in which the disease is already endemic; in such the emphasis of the system should be on timely detection of new cases [18]. Many times such evaluation is both financially and logistically unfeasible to complete under field conditions.

While there are numerous arguments in favor of risk-based sampling for disease detection [19], the low surveillance system sensitivities found for all the risk-based sampling scenarios (as implemented in this study), was not unexpected considering what has been previously reported on the occurrence of PRRS within the Ontario swine industry. Previous work has shown that given the unique nature of such an industry, focusing on demographics or biosecurity characteristics of individual sites for risk-based surveillance would not yield the most impactful strategies because the most important determinant of PRRS status has been reported to be the production system and not site characteristics on their own [11].

The authors suggest that the target of risk-based sampling needs to be reconsidered and strategies need to be developed considering how production systems are connected, the importance of sites in the different networks, and the number of sites within network components. Additionally, it would be worthwhile to evaluate the manner by which downstream site status should be handled in cases where breeding sites are detected as infected. The current approach for PRRS ARC&E projects in Ontario is to automatically declare downstream sites from positive breeding herds as positive by animal flow, a measure that can result in false positive classifications.

An alternative would be to prioritize sampling of downstream growing pig sites, action which could result in rapid depletion of resources in cases breeding sites from large production systems are infected. These additional scenarios were not evaluated herein, but are examples of a future research area that is very applicable under field conditions. To the best knowledge of the authors, there is no available information on quantification of active surveillance system sensitivity for PRRS in endemic disease contexts that would allow for comparison to current study results.

In general, all survival times (time to detection of the first three cases) for examined scenarios were long. We therefore conclude that none of the compared strategies were optimal for early detection of this disease given model assumptions, the underlying population, and absence of other forms of surveillance. The median survival time was never reached for the 5% design prevalence scenario, which supports the fact that, regardless of the strategy examined, if sample size is limited, prompt detection of potential outbreak cases will very likely not occur (considering such sampling is the only strategy in place to detect new infection cases).

There are important limitations to the current study that need to be acknowledged. Firstly, data were obtained from a limited portion of the Ontario swine industry (estimated at approximately 30% of all sites), and therefore the service providers network is not complete. Even though there is no reason to believe that the sample of sites are selectively biased in any form, the possibility exists that connections from absent sites could potentially change the structure in meaningful ways, and that could impact disease spread in unpredictable ways. Given this limitation, it is important to restate that the focus of this study was primarily the development of the methodology and the comparison among surveillance strategies themselves. Another important issue is the lack of data for PRRS parameter estimations such as the baseline probability of infection given exposure and relative risks presented on Table 1, as well as the fact that authors relied on expert opinion for the selection of risk factors for disease introduction (e.g. animal flow and number of neighbors). It is important to consider these assumptions when interpreting results of the model.

Furthermore, passive surveillance systems were not taken into consideration in the current study, and in the case where the challenge PRRSV was a highly virulent strain, the role of passive surveillance might have been particularly important and increased disease recognition and control efforts. However, sensitivity of passive surveillance is difficult to estimate. In England, the probability of infected farms being detected through passive surveillance for PRRS was reported as low, with a mode of 7.4% assuming 35% active PRRS infection prevalence [9]. This varied when regional pig density and use of vaccination were considered, with farms in a low pig density area and not using a vaccine having the lowest detection probability. Sensitivity analysis conducted in that study showed that an important parameter, as expected, was the probability that an infected pig would show clinical signs [9]. In a different context, during detection of the PRRS outbreak in Sweden in 2007 [20], active surveillance had a major role, and that particular outbreak was detected from the annual surveillance program and not due to clinical suspicion, even though animals from the whole country were naïve to the virus. The authors of the current study were interested not in quantifying the passive surveillance system per se, but in evaluating which of other active surveillance strategies would optimize disease detection.

An important assumption of the model was that transmission was possible even after swine sites were detected as infected by the surveillance systems. The authors acknowledge that this is to a certain extent contradictory to the core intention of surveillance for early detection, but argue that it is a plausible assumption given the current structure of this dynamic industry. Most of the time it is simply logistically impossible to stop animal movement or coordinate and schedule service providers according to PRRS status in a timely matter. However, it is important to note that if detection were to in fact prevent transmission and mitigate risk, the system sensitivities calculated herein would had been underestimated.

Lastly, our calculated sample size was not adjusted for sampling with replacement. In large populations such adjustment is not needed, but considering the study example population of 816, for the 1% design prevalence strategy, a considerable proportion of the population would had been sampled (approximately 33%), which could have impacted the number of farms detected. Even though this was a limitation of the study, it should not influence comparison between surveillance strategies.

Future directions for prospective projects include the expansion of this tool for evaluation of different surveillance scenarios. For example, one could propose an active surveillance strategy based on monthly risk-based slaughterhouse sampling and evaluate how that compares to current methodologies, as well as assess the cost-benefit of such and other approaches. Finally, the mathematical modelling approach supports collaboration between multiple branches such as the private sector, swine veterinarians, academic researchers and governmental agencies, since input and feedback is needed from all involved parts to test new hypotheses and strategies that are relevant at the same time as logistically and economically viable to all mentioned parties. Eventually, the development of the methodology could e applied for other emerging pathogens, and within dif- erent regions of the country or country-wide.

onclusions

n conclusion, the model developed herein integrates the nowledge of the complex swine industry and character- stics of PRRSV transmission between herds to develop a omprehensive framework that could be used to test ther hypotheses in the future regarding surveillance pproaches for this and other emerging swine infectious iseases.

bbreviations

BM: Agent-based model; ARC&E: Area Regional Control and Elimination; DD: Overview, design concepts, and details; PRRS: Porcine reproductive and spiratory syndrome; PRRSV: Porcine reproductive and respiratory syndrome rus; STM: Scenario tree modelling

cknowledgements

ne authors would like to extend their appreciation to the participating vine producers, veterinarians and area leaders who assisted with sampling nd data entry.

unding

raduate student funding provided by the Natural Sciences Engineering esearch Council (NSERC) and the Ontario Graduate Scholarship (OGS). ne Ontario Ministry of Agriculture, Food and Rural Affairs (OMAFRA), the ntario Swine Health Advisory Board (OSHAB), the Canadian Swine Health oard (CSHB), Ontario Pork, the Agricultural Adaptation Council (AAC), and ne Animal Health Laboratory (AHL) of the University of Guelph provided nancial support for the PRRS ARC&E projects.

uthors' contributions

GA: This paper was written in partial fulfilment of the requirements of a nD in Epidemiology degree. AGA conceptualized the project, conducted mpirical data management, planned model construction, carried model mulations, analyzed the output data, wrote the first draft of this paper nd had the main role during the publication process. ZP: ZP is the primary dvisor for AGA's PhD, and contributed with project conceptualization, nodel extension and improvement, interpretation of results, critical review nd revision of the manuscript. DK: DK was one of the instructors for an gent-based modelling course in which the primary author was enrolled. K contributed with initial model framework development, model coding, xtension and improvement, critical review, and revision of the manuscript. M: AM was a teaching assistant from the same modelling course above- nentioned. AM contributed with model building including conceptualization nd coding, model extension and improvements, critical review, revision of ne manuscript and final approvals. All authors read and approved the final nanuscript.

ompeting Interests

ne authors declare that they have no competing interests.

onsent for publication

ot applicable

Author details

[1]Department of Population Medicine, Ontario Veterinary College, University of Guelph, 50 Stone Rd East, Guelph, ON N1G 2W1, Canada. [2]Department of Computer Science, Computational Epidemiology and Public Health Informatics Lab, University of Saskatchewan, 176 Thorvaldson Bldg, 110 Science Place, Saskatoon, SK S7N 5C9, Canada.

References

1. Holtkamp DJ, Kliebenstein JB, Neumann EJ, Zimmerman JJ, Rotto HF, Yoder TK, et al. Assessment of the economic impact of porcine reproductive and respiratory syndrome virus on United States pork producers. J Swine Health Prod. 2013;21:72–84.
2. Nieuwenhuis N, Duinhof TF, van Nes A. Economic analysis of outbreaks of porcine reproductive and respiratory syndrome virus in nine sow herds. Vet Rec. 2012;170:225.
3. Corzo CA, Mondaca E, Wayne S, Torremorell M, Dee S, Davies P, et al. Control and elimination of porcine reproductive and respiratory syndrome virus. Virus Res. 2010;154:185–92.
4. Perez AM, Davies PR, Goodell CK, Holtkamp D., Mondaca-Fernandez E, Poljak Z, et al. Lessons learned and knowledge gaps about the epidemiology and control of porcine reproductive and respiratory syndrome virus in North America. J Am Vet Med Assoc. 2015;246: 1304–17.
5. Stark K, Regula G, Hernandez J, Knopf L, Fuchs K, Morris R, et al. Concepts for risk-based surveillance in the field of veterinary medicine and veterinary public health: Review of current approaches. BMC Health Serv Res. 2006;6: 20–7.
6. Hadorn DC, Rufenacht J, Hauser R, Stark KDC. Risk-based design of repeated surveys for the documentation of freedom from non-highly contagious diseases. Prev. Vet. Med. 2002;56:179–92.
7. Bessell PR, Orton R, O'Hare A, Mellor DJ, Logue D, Kao RR. Developing a frameqork for risk-based surveillance of tuberculosis in cattle: a case study of its application in Scotland. Epidemiol Infect. 2013;141:314–23.
8. Martin PAJ, Cameron AR, Greiner M. Demonstrating freedom from disease using multiple complex data sources 1: A new methodology based on scenario trees. Prev. Vet. Med. 2007;79:71–97.
9. Velasova M, Alarcon P, Williamson S, Wieland B. Risk factors for porcine reproductive and respiratory syndrome virus infection and resulting challenges for effective disease surveillance. BMC Vet Res. 2012;8:184.
10. Kwong GP, Poljak Z, Deardon R, Dewey CE. Bayesian analysis of risk factors for infection with a genotype of porcine reproductive and respiratory syndrome virus in Ontario swine herds using monitoring data. Prev. Vet. Med. 2013;110:405–17.
11. Arruda AG, Friendship R, Carpenter J, Hand K, Poljak Z. Characterization of multiple swine site networks, cluster and risk factor analyses for porcine reproductive and respiratory syndrome. Prev. Vet. Med. 2016;128:41–50.
12. Cameron AR. The consequences of risk-based surveillance: Developing output-based standards for surveillance to demonstrate freedom for disease. Prev. Vet. Med. 2012;105:280–6.
13. Grimm V, Berger U, Bastiansen F, Eliassen S, Ginot V, Giske J, et al. A standard protocol for describing individual-based and agent-based models. Ecol Model. 2006;198:115–26.
14. Lambert ME, Arsenault J, Poljak Z, D'Allaire S. Epidemiological investigations in regard to porcine reproductive and respiratory syndrome (PRRS) in Quebec, Canada. part 2: Prevalence and risk factors in breeding sites. Prev. Vet. Med. 2012;104:84–93.
15. Pitkin A, Otake S, Dee S. In: Biosecurity protocols for the prevention of spread of porcine reproductive and respiratory syndrome virus. Swine Disease Eradication Center. University of Minnesota College of Veterinary Medicine. 2009. https://www.aasv.org/aasv/PRRSV_BiosecurityManual.pdf . Acessed 8 June 2017.
16. Borgatti SP, Everett MG, Freeman LC. Ucinet for Windows: Software for Social Network Analysis. 1st ed. Analytic Technologies: Harvard; 2002.
17. FreeCalc: estimate sample size for freedom testing with imperfect tests, AusVet Animal Health Services©. http://epitools.ausvet.com.au/content.php?page=FreeCalc2 . Accessed 8 June 2017.
18. Cano JP, Polson D, Mondaca E, Batista L, Philips R, Diaz E. PRRS surveillance program: a regional approach. Proc 2012 Allen D. Leman Swine Conference. 2012;39:198.

19. Reist M, Jemmi T, Stark KDC. Policy-driven development of cost-effective, risk-based surveillance strategies. Prev. Vet. Med. 2012;105:176–84.
20. Frossling J, Agren EC, Eliasson-Selling L, Lewerin SS. Probability of freedom from disease after the first detection and eradication of PRRS in Sweden: Scenario-tree modelling of the surveillance system. Prev. Vet. Med. 2009;91: 137–45.
21. Linhares DC, Cano JP, Torremorell M, Morrison RB. Comparison of time to PRRSV-stability and production losses between two exposure programs to control PRRSV in sow herds. Prev Vet Med. 2014;116:111–9.
22. Arruda AG, Poljak Z, Friendship R, Carpenter J, Hand K. Descriptive analysis and spatial epidemiology of porcine reproductive and respiratory syndrome (PRRS) for swine sites participating in area regional control and elimination programs from three regions of Ontario. Canada Can J Vet Res. 2015;79: 268–78.

6

Hunters' acceptability of the surveillance system and alternative surveillance strategies for classical swine fever in wild boar

Katja Schulz[1*], Clémentine Calba[2], Marisa Peyre[2], Christoph Staubach[1] and Franz J. Conraths[1]

Abstract

Background: Surveillance measures can only be effective if key players in the system accept them. Acceptability, which describes the willingness of persons to contribute, is often analyzed using participatory methods. Participatory epidemiology enables the active involvement of key players in the assessment of epidemiological issues. In the present study, we used a participatory method recently developed by CIRAD (Centre de Coopération Internationale en Recherche Agronomique pour le Développement) to evaluate the functionality and acceptability of Classical Swine Fever (CSF) surveillance in wild boar in Germany, which is highly dependent on the participation of hunters. The acceptability of alternative surveillance strategies was also analyzed. By conducting focus group discussions, potential vulnerabilities in the system were detected and feasible alternative surveillance strategies identified.

Results: Trust in the current surveillance system is high, whereas the acceptability of the operation of the system is medium. Analysis of the acceptability of alternative surveillance strategies showed how risk-based surveillance approaches can be combined to develop strategies that have sufficient support and functionality. Furthermore, some surveillance strategies were clearly rejected by the hunters. Thus, the implementation of such strategies may be difficult.

Conclusions: Participatory methods can be used to evaluate the functionality and acceptability of existing surveillance plans for CSF among hunters and to optimize plans regarding their chances of successful implementation.

Keywords: Classical swine fever, Surveillance, Participatory epidemiology, Acceptability, Wild boar

Abbreviations: CSF, Classical Swine Fever; FLI, Friedrich-Loeffler-Institute; LUA, Central Laboratory of Rhineland-Palatinate; MV, Mecklenburg-Western Pomerania; RP, Rhineland-Palatinate

Background

The emergence of Classical Swine Fever (CSF) within a wild boar population is a highly undesirable event. This is mainly due to the potential transmissibility of the infectious agent from wild boar into domestic pig populations [1–3]. Also, strict movement regulations affecting domestic pig holdings are implemented for the holdings in the restriction zone around a CSF outbreak according to EU and national legislation.

Correspondence: katja.schulz@fli.de
[1]Friedrich-Loeffler-Institut, Federal Research Institute for Animal Health, Institute of Epidemiology, Südufer 10, 17493 Greifswald, Insel Riems, Germany
Full list of author information is available at the end of the article

CSF is caused by an enveloped single-stranded RNA pestivirus, which belongs to the family of *Flaviviridae* [4]. The course of disease is determined by several factors such as viral virulence, the age of the infected animal and its immune status [5]. Both the acute and chronic forms of disease cause non-specific clinical signs including fever, inappetence and weakness resulting in increased mortality in the affected population [5–7]. Consequently, introduction of the virus into commercial pig holdings usually entails huge economic consequences [8, 9].

Since the first occurrence of the CSF-virus in 1833 in the United States, the disease has spread through the American and European continents [10]. In the 1970s,

Germany had several years without any detected CSF-cases within the wild boar population. However, from the beginning of the 1980s until the most recent cases in 2009, the disease has occurred in a number of German federal states [1, 11–13]. Since 2012, Germany has been recognized as officially free from CSF [13]. To demonstrate freedom from CSF on a regular basis, which is prerequisite for participating in international trade, Germany has to implement regular surveillance for the disease in the wild boar population which fulfils the requirements of the current legislation in the European Union (Commission Decision 2002/106/EG).

Private hunters typically conduct sampling of harvested wild boar in Germany. However, in times of freedom from disease this happens on a voluntary basis, since hunters are often private persons and there is no legal requirement based on which hunters can be forced to support surveillance activities in times of disease freedom. In a few federal states, they are compensated for their financial expenses and their time [14]. However, neither in Rhineland-Palatinate nor in Mecklenburg-Western Pomerania, from where hunters were recruited in the present study, compensations are paid. Many surveillance activities for CSF thus rely on the involvement of hunters, in particular in relation to sampling shot wild boar. It is therefore essential that hunters accept the necessity of these surveillance activities and contribute to their implementation. Their front-line role in the system makes it equally important to consider their concerns during the development of new or the modification of existing surveillance strategies.

Meynard et al. [15] defined acceptance as the willingness of a person or an institution to participate in the implementation of a surveillance system. By evaluating acceptability, one can identify clues for improving the operation of the system [16]. Acceptance is often measured using participatory methods [17, 18].

Participatory epidemiology originates from the fields of social sciences and public health [19]. It comprises of a new range of methods and tools, which can also be used in the field of veterinary epidemiology. So far, participatory epidemiology has been mainly used in developing countries but it has been recently applied in the European Union (EU) to develop a method to assess the acceptability of surveillance systems (AccEPT) [20–23]. Its principle is based on the active participation of concerned parties in problem-solving, process-optimization and the development of new concepts. Visualization tools are used to facilitate discussions between involved persons or stakeholders [23]. Tools such as proportional piling, where categories can be formed and scored, make it possible to evaluate outcomes not only qualitatively but also quantitatively. By including participatory epidemiology in the design of new or the evaluation of existing surveillance strategies, there is a chance to integrate surveillance actors' knowledge or experience, which coul otherwise remain inaccessible (23). Moreover, participatory epidemiology can help to prevent surveillance fron failing due to lack of acceptability by key players. Since number of studies have shown that the application of participatory methods could improve the outcome of anima health surveillance in developing countries, it is hypothesized that the use of these methods could be beneficial t industrialized countries [23–26].

The aim of the study was to evaluate the acceptabilit of the currently implemented surveillance strategy fo CSF in wild boar using the AccEPT method (23). Additionally, alternatives to the conventional strategy wer constructed on the basis of risk-factors for a highe probability of CSF virus infection and detection in wil boar in Germany. The acceptability of these strategies b hunters was also evaluated.

Methods

Recruitment of hunters

From April 2015 to June 2015, hunters were recruited fron districts of the federal states of Mecklenburg-Wester Pomerania (MV) and Rhineland-Palatinate (RP) by contacting the responsible hunting authorities at the distric level (Landkreis) via email and contacts with the so calle "Kreisjagdmeister" were established. The Kreisjagdmeiste is elected by the hunters of a district and represent the hunters in the communication with the distric hunting authority. With the help of the Kreisjagdmeister, hunters were contacted and meetings arrange with those who were willing to participate. It wa planned to recruit 3–5 hunters, who formed a focu group, per participating district.

Five groups of hunters were interviewed in RP an three in MV. The group discussions took place betwee the 16 June and the 7 July 2015. On average, the meetings lasted approximately two hours. The biggest grou consisted of seven hunters whereas only two hunter took part in the smallest discussion group. In total, 2 male hunters and one female hunter participated. Fo the majority of participants, hunting was a hobby. A hunters stated that they hunted several times a week The estimated average age was above 50 years; mos hunters had thus been actively involved, when CSF outbreaks occurred in the respective federal states.

Surveillance system of CSF in wild boar

To illustrate the processes and the responsibilitie within the surveillance system for CSF in wild boa an information flow diagram was developed. This wa done by interviewing experts and by using information from the German contingency plan for CS (Tierseuchenbekämpfungshandbuch) [27].

By creating a diagram of the information flow within the surveillance system for CSF in wild boar, it became obvious that hunters play a key role in this system (Fig. 1). In times of freedom from disease, hunters take samples from wild boar and deliver the samples to the veterinary authority. The central state laboratory (Landesuntersuchungsamt, LUA) plays another key role. It collects and analyses samples from the 36 local district veterinary authorities. Negative results are reported back to the local veterinary authorities, whereas samples that tested inconclusive or positive are sent to the Friedrich-Loeffler-Institute (FLI) for further investigation. The FLI reports results back to the LUA and simultaneously to the local veterinary authorities. Subsequently, the local veterinary authorities report the results to the intermediate authority, which is an interposed authority between the authorities of the district and the supreme authority, and back to the hunters. The intermediate authority reports the results to a group of experts, the supreme veterinary and the supreme hunting authority of the federal state. Finally, the group of experts evaluates the surveillance results and reports these evaluations back to the supreme veterinary and hunting authority of the federal state (Fig. 1).

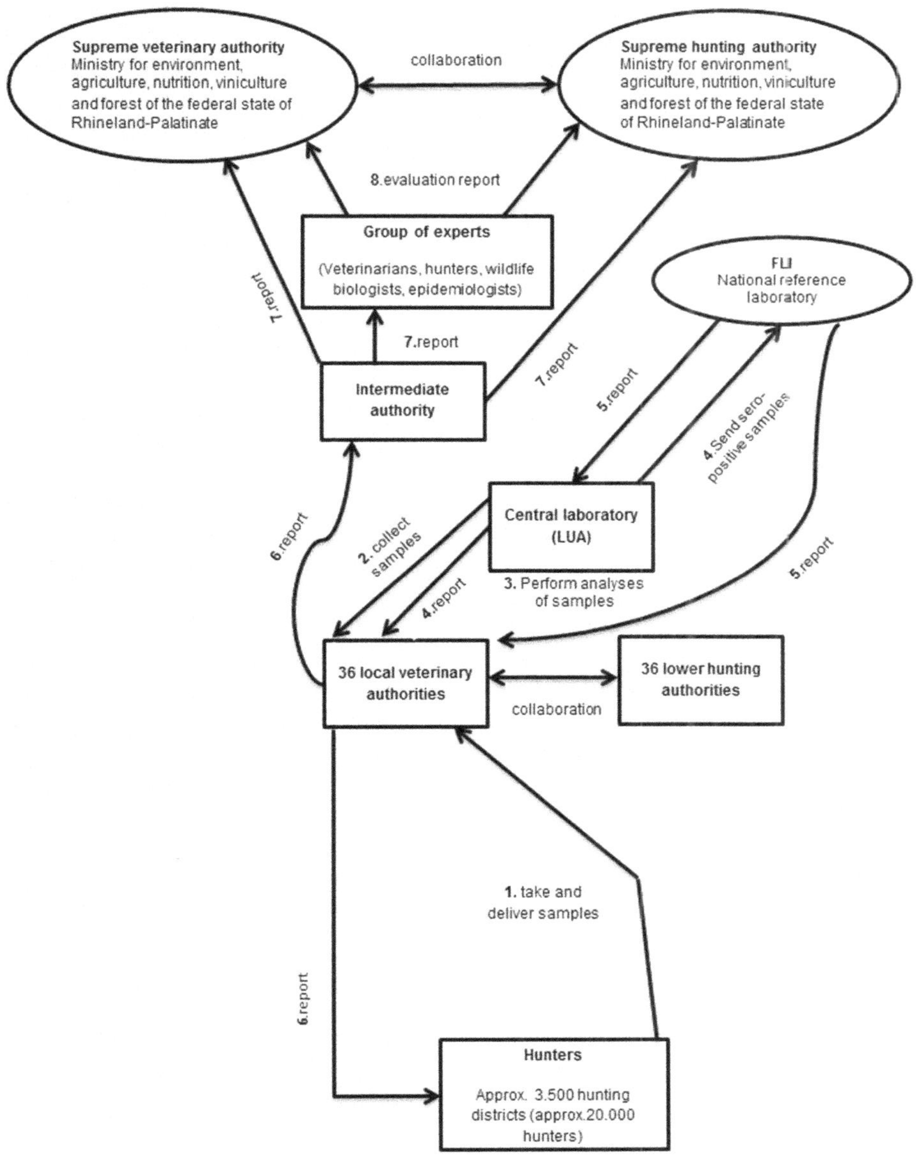

Fig. 1 Information flow (*bottom up*) within the surveillance system of the currently implemented, active surveillance for Classical Swine Fever in wild boar in times of disease freedom on the basis of the federal state of Rhineland-Palatinate

To avoid any biased responses, the generated information flow diagram was not presented to the hunters.

Implementation of participatory methods

Focus group discussions were conducted. The meetings were performed always by the same scientist and recorded with an Olympus dictation machine with the participants' consent.

Acceptability of the current surveillance system

The method used was adapted from the AccEPT method recently developed [23]. Where not stated differently, analyses of the discussions were done by qualitative as well as semi-quantitative analyses by using the scoring system of [23].

For further analysis, the results of the group discussions of hunters of each federal state were first summarized. For the final evaluation, all group discussions were analyzed together.

The investigation of the acceptability of the surveillance system was divided into three parts:

After the implementations of each part, the hunters were asked to explain their choices and motivations. These discussions were part of the descriptive analyses.

1. Evaluation of the acceptability of the operation of the system.
   These investigations were subdivided into:
   a) Satisfaction of the hunters with their own role in the surveillance system.
   An information flow diagram was created by the hunters. The hunters were asked to state, which institution they would contact in case of a suspicious wild boar and what they thought would happen with this information. The analysis of the satisfaction of the hunters with their own role was done through a semi-quantitative analysis of the discussions during the creation of the flow diagram as well as through a merely qualitative analysis of the discussions. The scoring system of the semi-quantitative analysis is described in detail in the study of [23].
   b) Satisfaction of the hunters with their social relationships within the hunting network.
   A relational diagram was used to identify the persons or institutions the hunters were in contact with regarding their hunting activities. The hunters were asked to name persons or institutions within their hunting network. In addition to [23], we used smileys to visualize the satisfaction with the named persons/institutions. After reaching an agreement, the groups were asked to put one smiley to each of the listed persons/institutions. By assigning scores to each smiley used, satisfaction could be analyzed in a semi-quantitative way (Table 1).
   c) Consequences for the hunters in the case of a suspicion of CSF in wild boar.
   By creating an impact diagram as described in the study of [23], the hunters were asked to list consequences they were expecting for themselves in the case of a CSF outbreak in wild boar. They were motivated to distinguish between negative and positive consequences. Afterwards, they were asked to explain their choice. To score the named consequences, proportional piling was implemented. The method and also the analyses are described in detail in [23].
   The scores of parts a–c were summed up and arithmetic means calculated to determine the acceptability of the operation of the system by the hunters (Table 2).
2. Evaluation of acceptability of the objective of the surveillance system.
   The hunters were asked to describe to the best of their knowledge the information flow to be observed if they find a dead wild boar or an animal-suspected being CSF-infected. The acceptability of the objective of the surveillance system, which is demonstrating freedom from disease, was investigated by asking the hunters directly after the creation of the information flow diagram. It was asked, what, in their opinion, is the objective of the currently in Germany implemented surveillance system for CSF in wild boar. The results of the discussions were analyzed in a semi-quantitative way using the scoring system described by [23].
3. Evaluation of the trust in the surveillance system

Table 1 Assessment of the satisfaction of hunters with the relationships within the hunting network

	Score
very unhappy	-2
unhappy	-1
neutral	0
happy	1
very happy	2

Mean	Level	Score
[-2; -0.7]	Low	-1
]-0.7; 0.7]	Medium	0
]0.7; 2]	High	1

able 2 Assessment of the level of acceptability of the peration of the surveillance system

evel	Score
ow	[−1; −0.33]
ledium	]−0.33; 0.33]
igh	] 0.33; 1]

The trust of the hunters in the functionality of the surveillance system of CSF in wild boar was assessed by using proportional piling [23] after creation the flow diagram. One hundred small tokens were presented to the hunters and they were asked to pile these in relation to their trust either in a field for "Trust" or in another field for "Distrust". It was asked, whether the hunters believed that different key players in the system and their work are expedient and reliable and if the system works effectively. After they had allocated the tokens to the two fields, the hunters were asked to pile the stones of the field "Trust" proportional to their trust into the different persons within the flow diagram.

cceptability of alternative surveillance systems

)ue to time restrictions and in the interest of maintain-ng a good working relationship with the hunters, only a nanageable number of alternative surveillance strategies ould be presented.

Alternative strategy 1 (Table 3) was presented assum-ng that there is an increased probability of detecting SF in animals identified through passive surveillance. nfected animals are more likely to be involved in road raffic accidents and an increased mortality of infected nimals has been demonstrated, particularly in the be-inning of an outbreak [6, 28, 29]. The acceptability of lternative strategy 2 was examined as it can be expected hat sampling in only 4 months of the year would result n less cost and work load. Alternative strategy 3 was presented to the hunters because the probability of detecting CSF-specific antibodies in older animals is higher due to the cumulatively increased seroprevalence in the boar population [30–32]. In the alternative strategy 4, active and passive sampling elements were combined. As it is recommended in Commission Decision 2002/106/EG to examine also all animals found through passive surveillance, it was important to establish if a surveillance strategy consisting of active and passive elements would be accepted by the hunters.

The method used to evaluate the hunters' acceptability of the conventional surveillance strategy and of the alternative surveillance strategies for CSF in wild boar (A_s, $s \in$ {strategy 1, alternative strategy 1, alternative strategy 2, alternative strategy 3 and alternative strategy 4}) (Table 3), was newly developed and is described in detail in the following section.

Five strategies were presented to the hunters (Table 3). Each hunter got five smileys, i.e. one smiley for each level of satisfaction (m =5) (Table 1). The hunters were asked to distribute these smileys on the presented strategies depending on their level of acceptance. For each strategy, the arithmetic mean was calculated according to

$$A_s = \frac{\sum_{i=1}^{m} x_i \cdot sc_i}{n}$$

where $i = 1$ represents the level of satisfaction, x_i the number of hunters giving score i (sc_i) and n the total number of hunters. The scoring values sc_i for each smiley are shown in Table 1. All hunters were asked to state reasons for their choice. The discussions were analyzed descriptively.

able 3 Chosen strategies for CSF surveillance in wild boar for vhich the acceptability of hunters were evaluated

. Currently implemented (strategy 1) 59 samples of the whole hunting bag per district within one year
. Passive (alternative strategy 1) Sampling of wild boar found dead, shot sick or involved in a road traffic accident
. Quarterly (alternative strategy 2) 59 samples of the whole hunting bag per district within one year; sampling only quarterly e.g. January, April, July, October
Sub-adults (alternative strategy 3) 59 samples, only from sub-adults, of the whole hunting bag per district within one year
Strategy 1 combined with 50 % passive (alternative strategy 4) Sampling 50 % of all wild boar which were found dead, shot sick or were involved in a road traffic accident plus 59 samples of the whole hunting bag per district within one year

Results

Acceptability of the current surveillance system

1. Acceptability of the operation
   a) By creating a flow diagram, all groups could identify the local veterinary authorities as the institution that should be directly contacted in the case of suspicion of CSF in a wild boar. Knowledge about the processes above the veterinary authority differed between the groups (Fig. 2). Good cooperation with the closest institution was stated as a positive reflection of the status quo, whereas a lack of transparency regarding the processes within the supreme authorities was named as a negative aspect. During the preparation of the flow diagram, mainly positive discussions points were noted in half of the groups. For the others, positive and negative points were balanced. The scoring of the

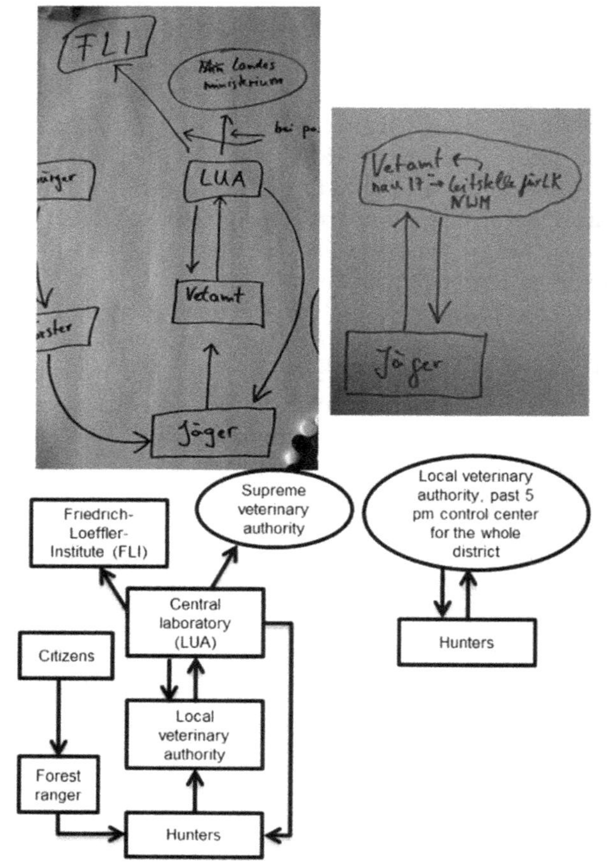

Fig. 2 Two original examples of flow diagrams to evaluate the satisfaction of the hunters with their own role within the surveillance system for CSF in wild boar (English translation subjacent). Left: The group could illustrate the information flow very detailed. Right: The group could only identify the local veterinary authority as the closest institution

discussion points is described in [23]. The satisfaction of the hunters with their own role within the system resulted in a medium score of 0.45 (Table 4).

b) By generating a relational diagram, a total of 29 persons or institutions were named by the different groups as those, with which they had contact within the network of hunting. The lower hunting authority was named by all eigh groups. Forestry authorities, farming and veterinary authorities were mentioned by seven groups. Eleven persons or institutions including the media and meat consumers were listed by a single group. During the discussions, all groups emphasized that they found it difficult to make generally applicable statements concerning the quality of contacts as it was believed to be highly dependent on the individual correspondents. The relationship to authorities that were closed to the hunters, such as the lower hunting or the local veterinary authority was described as very good. By contrast, the relationship to farmers, forest officers or the public was regarded as difficult. Problems were mainly seen as a consequence of conflicts of interest.
c) During the development of the impact diagram, all hunters had difficulties naming a positive consequence for them after the discovery of a wild boar suspected of being infected with CSF. Two groups failed to list positive consequences. Named positive consequences included a learning effect and the reduction of the wild boar population due to CSF and its control. Among the negative consequences, it was mentioned by all eight groups, that a CSF-suspected boar resulted in higher workload, increased expenses and hunting restrictions.

By summarizing these three parts for both study areas, a medium level of acceptability of the operation of the surveillance system was calculated with a score of −0.1 (Table 4, Fig. 3).

2. Acceptability of the objective of the system
No group could exactly define the objective "demonstrating freedom from disease". Consequential, the calculated level for the acceptability of the objective of the surveillance system for CSF in wild boar (demonstrating freedom from disease) by all hunters was a score of −0.4 (Table 4, Fig. 3).

Table 4 Results of the calculations of the acceptability of the surveillance system of CSF by hunters

	Acceptability of the operation of the system			Trust in the system	Acceptability of the objective of the syster
	satisfaction with their own role (RP 0.6) (MV 0.3) (Mean 0.45)	satisfaction with the relationships (RP 0) (MV 0.7) (Mean 0.35)	consequences in a suspicious case (RP−1) (MV−1) (Mean−1)		
RP		−0.1		0.8	−0.6
MV		0		0.7	0
All hunters		−0.1		0.8	−0.4

Abbreviations: *RP* indicates Rhineland-Palatinate, *MV* indicates Mecklenburg-Western Pomerania

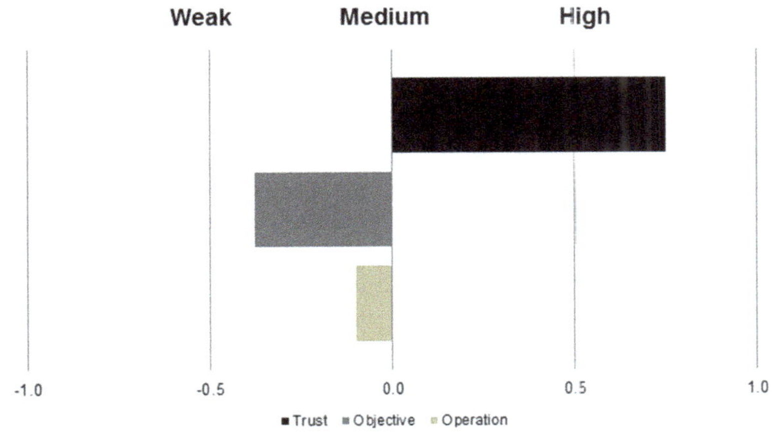

Fig. 3 Level of acceptability of the objective and the operation of the CSF surveillance system as well as the level of trust in the surveillance system by hunters from Mecklenburg-Western Pomerania and Rhineland-Palatinate

3. Evaluation of the trust in the surveillance system
   The trust in the surveillance system was high in all groups and resulted in a score of 0.8 (Table 4, Fig. 3). This was mainly justified by the argument that "past outbreaks showed that the system works" (focus group with hunters, 16.06.2015). The greatest trust was assigned to the authorities working close to the hunters like the lower hunting authority and the local veterinary authority. However, the trust in the hunters themselves was low, which was explained by the heterogeneity of the group of all hunters. It was mentioned that some hunters might ignore a dead wild boar for convenience or due to lack of time. Also, due to lack of transparency, the trust in the supreme authorities of the respective federal states was regarded as relatively low.

Acceptability of alternative surveillance systems

Summarizing the results and the discussions in the eight groups of hunters, the currently implemented strategy (strategy 1) was well accepted and resulted in a score of 0.9. Alternative strategy 1 (Table 3) showed the lowest level of acceptability with a score of −1.3 (Fig. 4). The hunters stated that dead animals are very often not found. Additionally they avoid sampling dead animals due to disgust and the effort, which is unprofitable to them. Alternative strategy 3 resulted in the best score of 1 (Fig. 4), also because sub-adults represent the group from which animals are shot most often anyway. Alternative strategies 2 and 4 were moderately accepted. The former scored −0.4 (Fig. 4); quarterly sampling was criticized as "too complicated" (focus groups with hunters, 16.06. and 17.06.2015) and the hunters emphasized that shooting wild boar is not predictable, especially in the

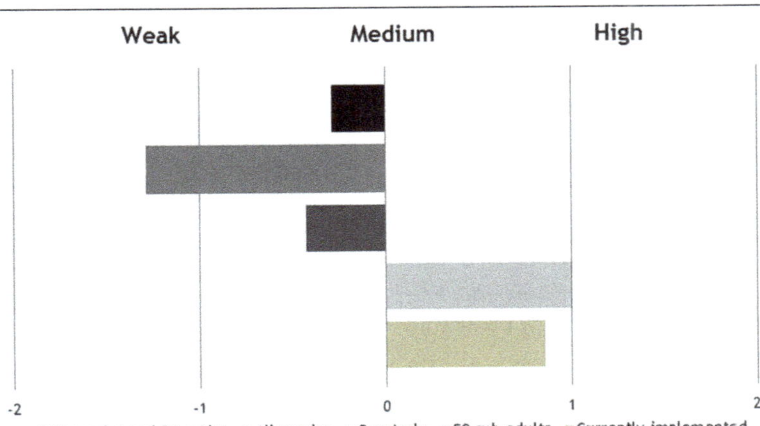

Fig. 4 Level of acceptability of different CSF surveillance strategies by all hunters of Rhineland-Palatinate and Mecklenburg-Western Pomerania

summer months. Similarly, the latter alternative received a score of −0.3, which was mainly due to the passive element of the strategy.

Discussion

Participatory methods are still rarely used in the field of veterinary epidemiology, particularly in industrialized countries [23, 33]. This is, among other reasons, due to difficulties in interpreting results since the analyses have often to be done in a qualitative way. The interpretation of discussions brings the danger of subjectivity, which is why it is recommended for more than one scientist to conduct the studies. In the present study, only one scientist could hold the meetings due to time and cost restrictions. However, for transparency, all discussions were recorded.

Only hunters from two federal states (MV and RP) were recruited. Both federal states have been affected by CSF in the past and most of the recruited hunters were estimated to be older than 50 years and practiced hunting in times of CSF outbreaks [13]. Thus, it cannot be assumed that the experience and knowledge of this group regarding CSF is representative of the national average for all hunters. Presumably, experience and knowledge regarding CSF in wild boar were above average. To avoid these inherent bias factors, it would be necessary to disperse the selection of hunters more widely. However, the number of interviews in this study was limited due to restricted resources.

A cause of bias in all participatory studies is the method of participant selection [23]. By contacting the lower hunting authority, it is likely that we reached hunters who were in contact with the authorities anyway. These hunters are more likely to be interested and to cooperate with the authorities.

This study included only a small sample size. Only 28 of approximately 400,000 registered German hunters participated (https://www.jagdverband.de/content/jagdscheininhaber-deutschland). Qualitative studies aim to reach "theoretical saturation" meaning that no new information can be obtained from interviewees [34]. Although this theory was not implemented consciously, no new information was added after the third group discussion, which may indicate that theoretical saturation had already been reached.

In spite of the listed limitations, our study clearly demonstrates that the acceptability of the current CSF surveillance system in German wild boars is only rated as medium by hunters, a major stakeholder group within the surveillance program.

Major determinants of this score were that the knowledge of the procedure in the event of discovering a wild boar suspected of CSF was excellent and that trust in these immediate contacts was high. However, the hunters could not define the overarching objective of the program and lacked trust in the transparency of operations at the supreme level of each federal state. Furthermore, some hunters could not identify even a single positive outcome for reporting a CSF-suspicious carcass; this is clearly problematic for a scheme run on a voluntary basis. These findings correlate with the hypothesis of [26] that communication between stakeholders and executing key players needs to be improved. Better communication and more information from the supreme authorities could help to increase the acceptability of the system and thereby the functionality.

The analysis of the acceptability of the different surveillance strategies showed that there is a need to improve the willingness to sample animals resulting from passive surveillance since it is known that the probability of detecting CSF in these animals is higher [28, 29]. To sample quarterly (alternative strategy 2) was not well accepted by the hunters. It is assumed that this strategy would be cost-effective as transportation and sample handling are more concentrated in time. However, according to the hunters, it is impractical due to the seasonal variation of the numbers of hunted boar. These findings strongly emphasize the advantages of participatory methods. Even if a surveillance strategy shows a theoretical advantage such as high detection probability or low costs, it will be hard to apply when hunters are not willing or capable of supporting it because they have strong arguments against a certain strategy. The high acceptability for sampling only in the age-class of sub-adult animals demonstrates the additional potential for combining risk-based surveillance strategies with participatory methods.

Conclusions

The acceptability among German hunters regarding a surveillance system for CSF in wild boar was evaluated by participatory methods recently adapted to evaluation of surveillance systems. The methods were well accepted by all interviewed groups of hunters. It was shown that acceptability is an attribute that can be used to gain important knowledge and to take experience of key players into account, which is often overlooked in the planning of surveillance strategies. Therefore, participatory epidemiology can be considered as an additional tool to inform decision-making on the improvement of surveillance strategies to inform disease freedom status.

Acknowledgements

The authors wish to thank all participating hunters and staff from the lower hunting authorities of the federal states of Rhineland-Palatinate and Mecklenburg-Western Pomerania for the successful co-operation. We are thankful to Conor O'Halloran for reviewing the English.

unding

nis study was performed under the framework of the RISKSUR project and ceived funding from the European Community's Seventh Framework P7/2007–2013) under grant agreement no. 310806. The funding body had o influence on the design of the study and collection, analysis, and terpretation of data and in writing the manuscript.

uthors' contributions

S carried out the data collection and data analyses and drafted the anuscript. CC participated in the study design and reviewed the anuscript. MP and CS coordinated the project. CS, MP and FJC gave itical review of the different drafts. All authors read and approved the nal manuscript.

ompeting interests

ne authors declare that they have no competing interests.

onsent for publication

ot applicable.

thics approval and consent to participate

ll hunters participated voluntarily in the group discussions and were formed about the objectives of the study. Formal consent or ethics pproval was not required for this study as it did neither include clinical ials in humans, where ethical approval would have been required ccording to paragraph 40 of the German "Arzneimittelgesetz" or aragraph 20 of the German "Medizinproduktegesetz" nor animal xperiments, where ethical approval would have been required ccording to paragraph 15 of the German "Tierschutzgesetz" Animal Health Act).

uthor details

riedrich-Loeffler-Institut, Federal Research Institute for Animal Health, stitute of Epidemiology, Südufer 10, 17493 Greifswald, Insel Riems, ermany. [2]Centre de Coopération Internationale en Recherche Agronomique our le Développement (CIRAD), Département ES, UPR AGIRs, TA C22/E, ampus International de Baillarguet, 34398 Montpellier Cedex 5, France.

eferences

Fritzemeier J, Teuffert J, Greiser-Wilke I, Staubach C, Schlüter H, Moennig V. Epidemiology of classical swine fever in Germany in the 1990s. Vet Microbiol. 2000;77:29–41.

Laddomada A. Incidence and control of CSF in wild boar in Europe. Vet Microbiol. 2000;73:121–30.

Kaden V, Steyer H, Schnabel J, Bruer W. Classical swine fever (CSF) in wild boar: the role of the transplacental infection in the perpetuation of CSF. J Vet Med B Infect Dis Vet Public Health. 2005;52:161–4.

Lindenbach BD, Murray CL, Thiel HJ, Rice CM. Flaviviridae. In: Knipe DM, Howley PM, editors. Fields virology. Vol. I. Philadelphia: Lippincott-Raven; 2013; 712–746.

Moennig V, Floegel-Niesmann G. Greiser-Wilke I Clinical signs and epidemiology of classical swine fever: A review of new knowledge. Vet J. 2003;165:11–20.

Artois M, Depner KR, Guberti V, Hars J, Rossi S, Rutili D. Classical swine fever (hog cholera) in wild boar in Europe. Rev Sci Tech. 2002;21:287–303.

World Organisation for Animal Health. Classical swine fever (hog cholera). In: Manual of Diagnostic Tests and Vaccines for Terrestrial Animals. Paris: OIE; 2009.

Saatkamp HW, Dijkhuizen AA, Geers R, Huirne RBM, Noordhuizen J, Goedseels V. Economic evaluation of national identification and recording systems for pigs in Belgium. Prev Vet Med. 1997;30:121–35.

9. Meuwissen MPM, Horst SH, Huirne RBM, Dijkhuizen AA. A model to estimate the financial consequences of classical swine fever outbreaks: principles and outcomes. Prev Vet Med. 1999;42:249–70.
10. Edwards S. Survival and inactivation of classical swine fever virus. Vet Microbiol. 2000;73:175–81.
11. Wolf P. Zur Strategie und Taktik der Verhütung und Bekämpfung der klassischen Schweinepest beim Schwarzwild in den Bezirken Rostock, Neubrandenburg und Schwerin. Humboldt Universität Berlin.1986.
12. Kaden V. Classical swine fever in wild boars—situation in the European Community and selected aspects of transmission of the disease. Berl Munch Tierarztl Wochenschr. 1998;111:201–7.
13. Staubach C, Höreth-Böntgen D, Blome S, Fröhlich A, Blicke J, Jahn B, Teuffert J, Kramer M. Descriptive summary of the classical swine fever control in wild boar in Germany since 2005. Berl Munch Tierarzt Wochenschr. 2013;126:491–9.
14. Sächsisches Staatsministerium für Umwelt und Landwirtschaft. Hinweise für Jäger zum Überwachungsprogramm von Wildschweinen auf Klassische und Afrikanische Schweinepest des Sächsischen Ministeriums für Soziales und Verbraucherschutz. 2014. http://www.lua.sachsen.de/download/lua/LUA_VM_Informationsblatt_Jaeger.pdf.
15. Meynard JB, Chaudet H, Green AD, Jefferson HL, Texier G, Webber D, Dupuy B, Boutin JP. Proposal of a framework for evaluating military surveillance systems for early detection of outbreaks on duty areas. BMC Public Health. 2008;8:146.
16. Calba C, Goutard FL, Hoinville L, Hendrikx P, Lindberg A, Saegerman C, Peyre M. Surveillance systems evaluation: a systematic review of the existing approaches. BMC Public Health. 2015;15:448.
17. Bronner A, Henaux V, Fortane N, Hendrikx P, Calavas D. Why do farmers and veterinarians not report all bovine abortions, as requested by the clinical brucellosis surveillance system in France? BMC Vet Res. 2014;10:93.
18. Mckerr C, Lo YC, Edeghere O, Bracebridge S. Evaluation of the National Notifiable Diseases Surveillance System for Dengue Fever in Taiwan, 2010–2012. PLoS Negl Trop Dis. 2015;9:e0003639.
19. Chambers R. The origins and practice of Participatory Rural Appraisal. World Dev. 1994;22:953–69.
20. Malak AK, Mpoke L, Banak J, Muriuki S, Skilton RA, Odongo D, Sunter J, Kiara H. Prevalence of livestock diseases and their impact on livelihoods in Central Equatoria State, southern Sudan. Prev Vet Med. 2012;104:216–23.
21. Roeder P, Mariner J, Kock R. Rinderpest: the veterinary perspective on eradication. Philos Trans R Soc Lond B Biol Sci. 2013;368:20120139.
22. Reix CE, Dikshit AK, Hockenhull J, Parker RMA, Banerjee A, Burn CC, Pritchard JC, Whay HR. A 2-Year Participatory Intervention Project with Owners to Reduce Lameness and Limb Abnormalities in Working Horses in Jaipur, India. PLoSs One. 2005;10:e0124342.
23. Calba C, Antoine-Moussiaux N, Charrier F, Hendrikx P, Saegerman C, Peyre M, Goutard F. Applying participatory approaches in the evaluation of surveillance systems: a pilot study on African swine fever surveillance in Corsica. Prev Vet Med. 2015;122:389–98.
24. Bradley JE, Mayfield MV, Mehta MP Rukonge A. Participatory evaluation of reproductive health care quality in developing countries. Soc Sci Med. 2002; 55:269–82.
25. Catley A, Alders RG, Wood JLN. Participatory epidemiology: Approaches, methods, experiences. Vet J. 2012;191:151–60.
26. Pfeiffer DU. Epidemiology Caught in the Causal Web of Bovine Tuberculosis. Transbound Emerg Dis. 2013;60:104–10.
27. Anonymous, 2015. Tierseuchenbekämpfungshandbuch. https://tsbh.fli.bund.de/Default.aspx?tabid=61. Accessed 17 Nov 2015.
28. von Rueden S, Staubach C, Kaden V, Hess RG, Blicke J, Kuhne S, Sonnenburg J, Frohlich A, Teuffert J, Moennig V. Retrospective analysis of the oral immunisation of wild boar populations against classical swine fever virus (CSFV) in region Eifel of Rhineland-Palatinate. Vet Microbiol. 2008;132:29–38.
29. Blome S, Gabriel C, Beer M. Viral diseases in pigs: Classical swine fever. Prakt Tierarzt. 2012;93:18–20.
30. Kern B, Depner KR, Letz W, Rott M, Thalheim S, Nitschke B, Plagemann R, Liess B. Incidence of classical swine fever (CSF) in wild boar in a densely populated area indicating CSF virus persistence as a mechanism for virus perpetuation. J Vet Med B Infect Dis Vet Public Health. 1999;46:63–7.
31. Kaden V, Heyne H, Kiupel H, Letz W, Kern B, Lemmer U, Gossger K, Rothe A, Bohme H, Tyrpe P. Oral immunisation of wild boar against classical swine fever: concluding analysis of the recent field trials in Germany. Berl Munch Tierarztl Wochenschr. 2002;115:179–85.

32. Rossi S, Pol F, Forot B, Masse-Provin N, Rigaux S, Bronner A, Le Potier MF. Preventive vaccination contributes to control classical swine fever in wild boar (Sus scrofa sp.). Vet Microbiol. 2010;142:99–107.
33. Calba C, Ponsich A, Nam S, Collineau L, Min S, Thonnat J, Goutard FL. Development of a participatory tool for the evaluation of Village Animal Health Workers in Cambodia. Acta Trop. 2014;134:17–28.
34. Glaser B, Strauss A. The Discovery of Grounded Theory: Strategies for Qualitative Research. New York: Aldine; 1967.

7

Molecular characterization of US-like and Asian non-S INDEL strains of porcine epidemic diarrhea virus (PEDV) that circulated in Japan during 2013–2016 and PEDVs collected from recurrent outbreaks

Nguyen Van Diep, Masuo Sueyoshi, Junzo Norimine, Takuya Hirai, Ohnmar Myint, Angeline Ping Ping Teh, Nida Zahli Izzati, Naoyuki Fuke and Ryoji Yamaguchi*

Abstract

Background: Since late 2013, porcine epidemic diarrhea virus (PEDV) has reemerged in Japan and caused severe economic losses to the swine industry. Although PEDV vaccines have been used widely, the disease has swept rapidly across the county, and is commonly observed in PED-vaccinated farms, and has recurred in domestic herds. To better understand PEDVs responsible for the reemerging outbreaks in Japan, full-length spike (S), membrane (M), and nucleocapsid (N) genes of 45 PEDVs collected in Japan during 2013–2016, were sequenced and analyzed.

Results: Phylogenetic analysis based on S gene sequences revealed that all the recent field PEDVs were genetically distinct from the classical Japanese strains, and were classified into three genotypes: North American (NA), S INDEL, and Asian non-S INDEL. Our data suggested a possibility that multiple parental PEDV strains were introduced into Japan from abroad at the same time or similar times. The newly identified Japanese strains showed the closest relationship to the US strains. Two sublineages of Japanese strains circulating in Japan were similar to two sublineages identified in the US, suggesting common ancestors for these strains. In comparison with two vaccine strains used in Japan, the field strains had various changes in epitope regions, glycosylation sites, and phosphorylation sites. These substitutions, particularly observed in epitope regions of the S (521, 553, 568, and 570), M (5), and N (123, 252, and 255) proteins, may have affected antigenicity and vaccine efficacy, resulting in an unsuccessful PEDV control. Sequence comparisons between PEDVs collected from primary and secondary outbreaks in three herds revealed that the disease has developed to an endemic stage in which PEDV could persist for nearly two years in the herds or local regions, causing subsequent epidemics.

Conclusions: These results elucidate the genetic characteristics, origin, and molecular epidemiology of PEDVs circulating in Japan, as well as the PEDV strains causing recurrent outbreaks. This study provides a better insight into the PEDVs responsible for recent outbreaks in Japan, and could potentially help to develop measures for controlling and preventing the disease.

Keywords: Porcine epidemic diarrhea virus, PEDV, Spike gene, M gene, N gene, Genetic heterogeneity

Correspondence: a0d402u@cc.miyazaki-u.ac.jp
Department of Veterinary Medicine, Faculty of Agriculture, University of Miyazaki, Gakuen-kibanadai-nishi-1-1, Miyazaki 889-2192, Japan

Background

Porcine epidemic diarrhea virus (PEDV) is the etiologic agent of porcine epidemic diarrhea (PED), an acute enteritis disease that is characterized by vomiting and watery diarrhea and usually leads to high morbidity and mortality, especially in piglets [1]. The disease was first recognized in England in 1971 [2], and the prototype virus, which was designated as PEDV CV777, was identified in Belgium [3]. Subsequently, PEDV has been reported in several other European countries, causing only sporadic outbreaks. Since the 1980s, it has been widespread in Asia and has become an economic concern for the swine industry in many Asian countries such as Japan, China, South Korea, Thailand, and Taiwan [1, 4]. In late 2010, new Chinese strains of PEDV were detected. These new strains were clinically more severe than the classical strains, resulting in 80%–100% illness among infected swine herds and a 50%–100% mortality rate among infected suckling piglets [5]. In April 2013, a PEDV outbreak was confirmed in the US for the first time. It swept across more than 30 states in the country, causing deaths of more than 8 million newborn piglets during the one-year-epidemic period, and subsequently spread throughout North America, including Canada and Mexico [6]. Afterward, US-like PED epidemics have been reported in South Korea, Taiwan, Japan, Germany, France, and Belgium [4, 7].

Belonging to the *Coronaviridae* family in the *Nidovirale* order, PEDV has a single-stranded positive-sense RNA genome of approximately 28 kb in size that encodes four structural proteins (S, E, M, and N) and non-structural proteins (1a, 1ab, and ORF3) [1]. Among the viral proteins, the S glycoprotein is the most diverse [8], and plays a critical role in the process of inducing neutralizing antibodies and binding specific receptors [9]. At least two B cell epitopes (SS2 and SS6) and two regions containing neutralizing epitopes (COE and 2C10) have been identified on this protein [10–12]. The S gene is also associated with growth adaptation in vitro and attenuation of virulence in vivo [13], and was used as an important component in studies for understanding genetic relatedness among PEDV isolates, the epidemiological status, and vaccine development [14, 15]. The M protein is the most abundant component of viral protein in the envelope, and is responsible for morphogenesis, assembly, and budding [16]. The N protein of coronavirus interacts with viral genomic RNA, serving as the critical basis for the helical nucleocapsid during the viral assembly [17]. Two antigenic epitopes (NEP-D4 and NEP-D6) have been identified in the N protein of PEDV [18].

In Japan, the PED-like disease was observed from late 1982 to early 1983, but was not reported again until the outbreaks that occurred between September 1993 and June 1994 [19]. In an epidemic of diarrhea caused by a PEDV infection in 1996, more than 39,000 suckling pigs died [20]. Afterward, there were no PED cases reported from 2006 until the first half of 2013 [21, 22]. PED outbreaks first reemerged in October 2013 from a southern location (Okinawa Island) and spread rapidly throughout the country. Until May 2016, PEDV infections were reported from more than 1000 farms in 39 of 47 prefectures; the infections affected over 1.5 million pigs and led to the death of half a million pigs, according to the Ministry of Agriculture, Forestry, and Fisheries of Japan (http://www.maff.go.jp). Currently, PEDV infections and piglet mortality has decreased significantly. However, PED still occurred and frequently recurred in pig farms in Japan. Therefore, better insight into the causes for the reemergence of PED outbreaks is required for more efficient control and prevention of the disease. Toward this goal, we sequenced and analyzed the full-length S, M, and N genes of the Japanese field PEDVs in comparison with those of vaccine strains used in Japan, classical Japanese PEDV strains, and isolates from other countries.

Methods

Sample collection, RNA extraction, and PEDV detection

Small intestine or stool specimens were obtained from suckling piglets, post-weaning piglets, and sows presenting acute watery diarrhea at pig farms in Japan, between December 2013 and February 2016. Intestinal samples were collected from dead piglets, and fecal samples were non-invasively collected immediately after excretion. Thus, no aggressive actions toward the pigs were carried out for sampling purpose. Samples of two major vaccine strains that have been employed in Japan, P5-V (Nisseiken Co., Ltd) and 96-P4C6 (Kaketsuken Co., Ltd., Japan), were collected from commercial vaccine bottles used in the swine farms. Sample preparation, RNA extraction, and PEDV detection were performed as previously described [23]. Japanese field samples may contain both PEDV variants with large deletions in the 5′ terminus of the S gene and PEDV strains with an intact S gene [24]. Due to the complexity in discriminating, isolating, and individually sequencing PEDV strains, only specimens containing PEDVs with an intact S gene were used in our study. Finally, 45 PEDV-positive field samples were collected from 37 farms, located in five different prefectures in Japan. These samples, along with the two vaccine samples described above, were sequenced to determine the full-length sequence of the S, M, and N genes (Table 1). All these field PEDVs were confirmed to possess an intact 5′-terminus of the S gene, showing only the expected prominent single DNA band from PCR products on a 1.2% agarose gel [24].

Table 1 Forty-five Japanese field PEDVs and two vaccine strains were used in this study

No	Strain	Age group	Collection time	Geographic origin	Accession No of genes		
					S gene	M gene	N gene
	14JM-01	Suckling	2014/Mar	Miyazaki	KY619734	KY619830	KY619781
	14JM-07	Post-weaning	2014/Apr	Miyazaki	KY619735		KY619782
	14JM-40	Suckling	2014/Apr	Hokkaido	KY619736		KY619783
	14JM-118	Suckling	2014/Mar	Miyazaki	KY619737		KY619784
	14JM-119	Suckling	2014/Apr	Miyazaki	KY619738		KY619785
	14JM-123	Suckling	2014/Mar	Miyazaki	KY619739		KY619786
	14JM-126	Suckling	2014/Mar	Miyazaki	KY619740		KY619787
	13JM-127	Suckling	2013/Dec	Miyazaki	KY619741	KY619831	KY619788
	13JM-128	Suckling	2013/Dec	Miyazaki	KY619742	KY619832	KY619789
0	14JM-138	Suckling	2014/Mar	Miyazaki	KY619743		KY619790
1	14JM-139	Suckling	2014/Mar	Miyazaki	KY619744		KY619791
2	14JM-140	Suckling	2014/Mar	Miyazaki	KY619745		KY619792
3	14JM-142	Suckling	2014/Mar	Miyazaki	KY619746		KY619793
4	14JM-143	Suckling	2014/Feb	Miyazaki	KY619747		KY619794
5	14JM-144	Suckling	2014/Mar	Miyazaki	KY619748	KY619833	KY619795
6	14JM-146	Suckling	2014/Apr	Miyazaki	KY619749		KY619796
7	14JM-147	Suckling	2014/May	Miyazaki	KY619750		KY619797
8	14JM-150	Suckling	2014/Mar	Miyazaki	KY619751		KY619798
9	14JM-152	Suckling	2014/Mar	Miyazaki	KY619752		KY619799
0	14JM-157	Suckling	2014/May	Aichi	KY619753		KY619800
1	14JM-168 [farm 1]	Suckling	2014/May	Aomori	KY619754		KY619801
2	14JM-179 [farm 2]	Suckling	2014/May	Miyazaki	KY619755		KY619802
3	14JM-181 [farm 2]	Suckling	2014/May	Miyazaki	KY619756		KY619803
4	14JM-199 [farm 3]	Suckling	2014/May	Miyazaki	KY619757		KY619804
5	14JM-200 [farm 3]	Suckling	2014/May	Miyazaki	KY619758		KY619805
6	14JM-205	Suckling	2014/Jun	Hokkaido	KY619759		KY619806
7	14JM-208	Suckling	2014/Jun	Aichi	KY619760	KY619834	KY619807
8	14JM-210	Sow	2014/Jul	Aichi	KY619761		KY619808
9	14JM-216	Sow	2014/Jul	Aichi	KY619762	KY619835	KY619809
0	14JM-226	Suckling	2014/Jul	Kagoshima	KY619763		KY619810
1	14JM-236	Suckling	2014/Jul	Miyazaki	KY619764	KY619837	KY619811
2	14JM-242	Suckling	2014/May	Miyazaki	KY619765		KY619812
3	14JM-248	Suckling	2014/Jane	Miyazaki	KY619766		KY619813
4	14JM-268	Suckling	2014/May	Miyazaki	KY619767		KY619814
5	13JM-291	Suckling	2013/Dec	Kagoshima	KY619768		KY619815
6	13JM-293	Suckling	2013/Dec	Kagoshima	KY619769		KY619816
7	14JM-297	Suckling	2014/Apr	Aichi	KY619770		KY619817
8	14JM-311	Suckling	2014/Apr	Aichi	KY619771		KY619818
9	15JM-315	Suckling	2015/Jun	Aichi	KY619772		KY619819
0	16JM-319 [farm 3]	Suckling	2016/Feb	Miyazaki	KY619773	KY619836	KY619820
1	16JM-323 [farm 3]	Suckling	2016/Feb	Miyazaki	KY619774		KY619821
2	16JM-325 [farm 2]	Suckling	2016/Feb	Miyazaki	KY619775		KY619822
3	16JM-326 [farm 2]	Suckling	2016/Feb	Miyazaki	KY619776		KY619823

Table 1 Forty-five Japanese field PEDVs and two vaccine strains were used in this study *(Continued)*

No	Strain	Age group	Collection time	Geographic origin	Accession No of genes		
					S gene	M gene	N gene
44	16JM-334 [farm 1]	Suckling	2016/Feb	Aomori	KY619777	KY619838	KY61982
45	16JM-339 [farm 1]	Suckling	2016/Feb	Aomori	KY619778	KY619839	KY61982
46	96P4C6	Nisseiken Co	2013/Dec		KY619779	KY619828	KY61982
47	P5-V	Kakatsuken Co	2014/Apr		KY619780	KY619829	KY61982

- The following Japanese field strains have the same S gene sequences: 14JM-127 and 14JM-311; 14JM-01, 14JM-119, and 14JM123; 14JM-138, 14JM-142, and 14JM-150; 14JM-208 and14JM-216; 14JM-146, 14JM-147, and 14JM-199; 16JM-334 and 16JM-339; 16JM-319, 16JM-323, and 16JM-325
-The following Japanese field strains have the same M gene sequences: 14JM-01, 14JM-07, 14JM-40, 14JM-118, 14JM-119, 14JM-123, 14JM-126, 14JM-138, 14JM-139, 14JM-140, 14JM-142, 14JM-143, 14JM-146, 14JM-147, 14JM-150, 14JM-152, 14JM-157, 14JM-168, 14JM-179, 14JM-181, 14JM-199, 14JM-200, 14JM-205, 14JM-210, 14JM-226, 14JM-242, 14JM-248, 14JM-268, 13JM-291, 13JM-293, 14JM-297, 14JM-311, and 15JM-315; 16JM-319, 16JM-323, 16JM-325, and 16JM-326; 13JM-12 and 13JM-128; 14JM-208 and 14JM-216; 16JM-334 and 16JM-339
- The following Japanese field strains have the same N gene sequences: 13JM-127, 13JM-128, 14JM-142, 14JM-143, 14JM-157, 14JM-208, 14JM-216, 14JM-248, an 13JM-291; 14JM-01 and 14JM-119; 14JM-07, 14JM-126, and 14JM-123; 14JM-138, 14JM-150, and 14JM-226; 14JM-139, 14JM-152, and 14JM-242; 14JM-146, 14JM-147,14JM-179, 14JM181, 14JM-199, 14JM-200, 14JM-236, and 14JM-311; 14JM-268 and 13JM-293; 16JM-319 and 16JM-323; 16JM-334 and 16JM-339; 16JM-325 and 16JM-326

Sequencing of S, M, and N genes

After producing cDNA, as previously described [23], the full-length S gene of PEDV was amplified using the primer pair FS-F/FS-R (Table 2) and KOD FX Kit (Toyobo Co., Japan). The PCR products were used as templates for nested PCR reactions that amplified five DNA fragments spanning the entire S gene using 5 primer sets (CS1-CS5), as previously reported [24]. The M and N genes of the PEDV were also amplified from the cDNA using two newly designed primer sets, fMF/fMR and fNF/fNR (Table 2). EmeraldAmp MAX PCR Master Mix kit (Takara Bio, Japan) was used for PCR amplifications of the CS1-CS5 fragments, as well as the M and N genes. The amplified PCR products were purified using a FastGene Gel/PCR Extraction Kit (NIPPON Genetics Co., Ltd., Japan) according to the manufacturer's protocol. All sequencing reactions were carried out in duplicate, and sequences were determined in both directions using BigDye® Terminator v3.1 Cycle Sequencing Kits (Applied Biosystems, CA, USA). Products were analyzed using ABI PRISM 3130xl Genetic Analyzers (Applied Biosystems).

Sequence analysis

Nucleotide (nt) and deduced amino acid (aa) sequences were edited, assembled, and aligned using Geneious v9.1.6 software (http://www.geneious.com), and per centage sequence divergences at the nt and aa level were further calculated by using the same software. Th obtained nt sequences were deposited in GenBan under the following accession numbers: KY619734- KY619839 as shown in Table 1. Unrooted phylogeneti trees were constructed using molecular evolutionar genetics analysis (MEGA) software, version 6.06 [25 with the maximum likelihood method and bootstra tests of 1000 replicates. The best-fit nt substitutio models for analysis were assessed. Phylogenetic tree based on the nt sequences of the full-length S and N genes were generated using the Tamura-Nei substitutio model with a discrete gamma distribution (TN93 + G). A phylogenetic tree based on the nt sequences of the M gene was created using the Kimura 2-parameter sub stitution method with a discrete gamma distributio (K2 + G). N-glycosylation sites were predicted using service available on http://www.cbs.dtu.dk/services NetNGlyc. Phosphorylation sites were predicted usin the NetPhos 3.1 server (http://www.cbs.dtu.dk/ser vices/NetPhos) and NetPhosBac 1.0 server (http:/ www.cbs.dtu.dk/services/NetPhosBac-1.0). Predictio of antigenic regions was performed using the EMBOS protein analysis tool [26] integrated into the Geneiou software.

Table 2 Primers used in this study

Primer	Nucleotide sequence (5'-3')	Target gene (fragment size, bp)	Position[a]
FS-F	TCCATTAGTGATGTTGTGTTAGG	Full-length S gene (4371)	20,530–24,90
FS-R	ACTACATTRAGCTCCAACTC		
fMF	CTTGTCACCGGTTGTGTAATAG	Full-length M gene (826)	25,567–26,39
fMR	CTGACAGAAGCCATAAAGTTTCTG		
fNF	ACTGGTTGGGCTTTCTATGTC	Full-length N gene (1507)	26,263–27,76
fNR	CTCAGTAATAACAGTGTAATGGCAC		

[a]Numbers correspond to positions within the Colorado/USA/2013 genome

esults

nalysis of the S gene

hylogenetic and sequence analyses of the S gene

dentical nt sequences of the S gene were distin-uished and excluded, resulting in the identification f 34 individual sequences from the 45 total collected eld strains. Phylogenetic analysis based on the S ene sequences from the Japanese strains and refer-nce strains identified from various countries revealed two major clusters: genogroup G1 divided into subgroups G1a and G1b, and genogroup G2 divided into subgroups G2a and G2b (Fig. 1).

All 45 Japanese field PEDVs in the present study fell into 3 subgroups G2a, G2b, and G1b. The most dominant strains belonged to G2b, which comprised 42 of 45 current Japanese strains, along with the highly virulent (North American type) PEDVs isolated in the US, Canada, Mexico, South Korea, and Taiwan. Two PEDV

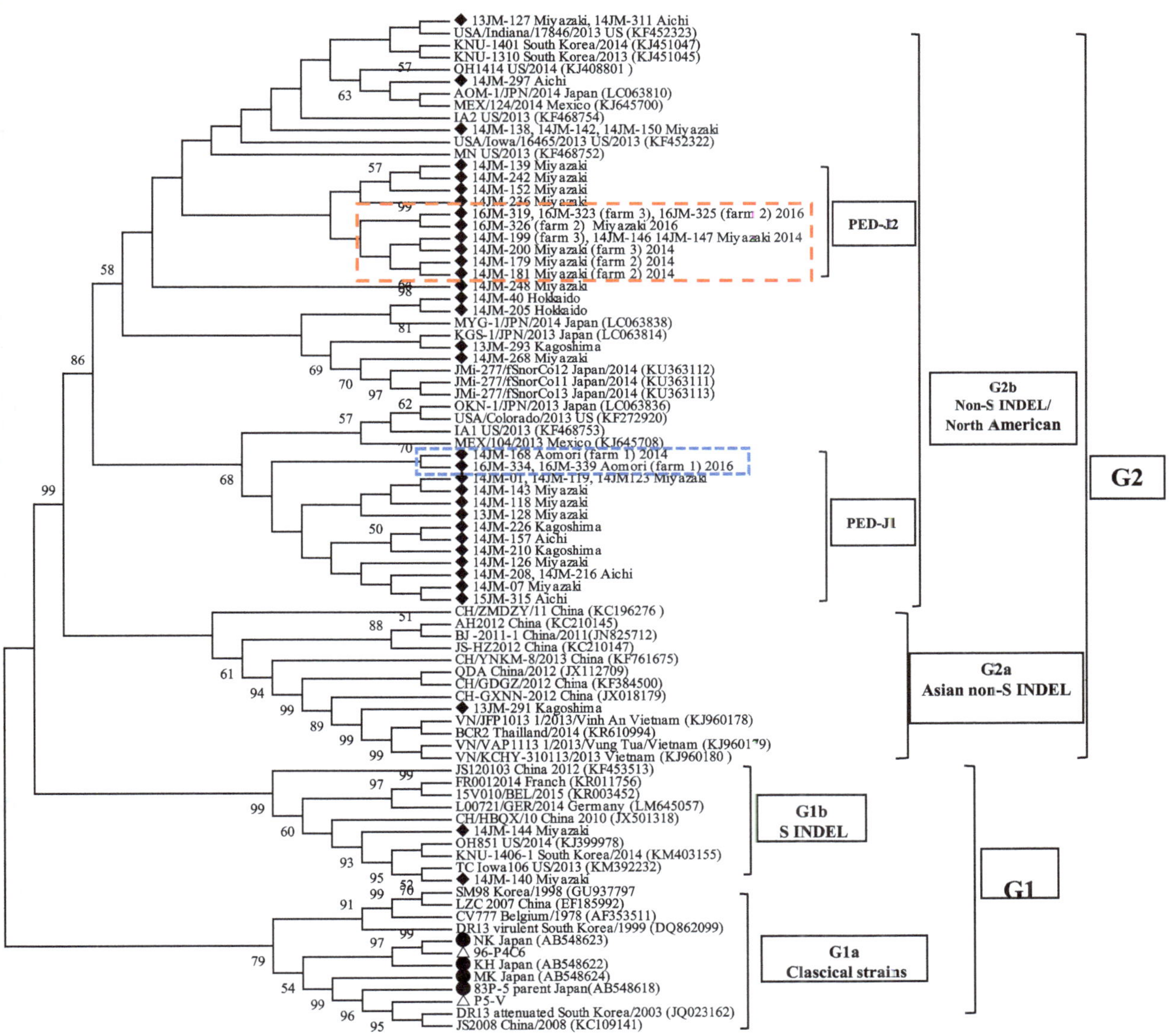

Fig. 1 Phylogenetic tree of PEDVs based on the nucleotide sequences of the entire S gene. The tree was constructed by the maximum likelihood method using the Tamura-Nei substitution model with a discrete gamma distribution in the MEGA v.6.05 program. Numbers at nodes represent the percentage of 1000 bootstrap replicates (values < 50 are not shown). Names of strains, countries and years of isolation, and GenBank accession numbers are shown. The Japanese field PEDV strains identified in this study are marked by solid diamond symbols and accompanied by the corresponding prefectures where they were collected. The classical Japanese strains identified prior to 2013 are marked by solid round symbols and the vaccine strains being used in Japan are marked by hollow triangle symbols. PEDV strains collected from farm 1 (14JM-168, 16JM334, and 16JM-339) were marked in a blue box; strains collected from farms 2 and 3 (14JM-179, 14JM-181, 14JM-199, 14JM-200, 16JM-319, 16JM-323, 16JM-325, 16JM-326 are marked in a red box

strains (14JM-140 and 14JM-144) were clustered into G1b, which included the new S INDEL strains that have been detected since 2013 in the US, Germany, France, Belgium, South Korea, Japan, and China. Isolate 13JM-291 fell into G2a, which included PEDV strains identified from PEDV outbreaks that occurred after 2010 in Vietnam, Thailand, and China. The two vaccine strains (P5-V and 96-P4C6) clustered into the G1a subgroup, which primarily consisted of classical strains, such as CV777, KH, NK, LZC, SM98, and DR13 parent.

Pairwise alignment of the 45 field PEDVs in this study revealed that their S genes were heterogeneous. The S gene nt (aa) sequences had 94.36%–100% (94.45%–100%) identity with each other, but only 93.24%–95.91% (92.01%–96.17%) identity with the two Japanese vaccines. Most of the Japanese PEDVs belonging to G2b had 99.16%–100% nt among themselves, and shared a high (98.27%–100%) nt identity with other highly virulent PEDVs. Interestingly, 13JM-127 from the first PED outbreak in Miyazaki prefecture (South Japan, December 2013) shared the same sequence with 14JM-311 (Aichi prefecture, north-central Japan, April 2014) and US strains, such as USA/Indiana/17846/2013 (from the first reported PED case in the US) [27], USA/Colorado/2013, OH1414, and IA1. No relatedness were found between the two farms from where 13JM-127 and 14JM-311 were collected. Additionally, 14JM-01 has 100% nt sequence identity with two other US strains (NPL-Pedy/2013 US and USA/Minnesota127/2014) and a Canadian strain (ON-007).

Of the 45 field PEDVs, 14JM-01 from Miyazaki and 16 other strains from Aomori, Aichi, Kagoshima, and Miyazaki were grouped into a monophyletic branch designated as PED-J1, and they shared high nt and aa sequence identities (99.69%–100% and 99.35%–100%, respectively) with each other. Another subclade, designated as PED-J2, including 14 Japanese strains collected in Miyazaki were also clustered into a segregated branch as shown in Fig. 1. The strains 14JM-140 and 14JM-144 showed 98.99%–99.92% nt sequence identity with other S INDEL strains within G1b. The S gene of 14JM-144 had the highest (99.93%) nt sequence identity with OH851 which was the first reported S INDEL strain in the US. The S gene from 13JM291 shared 97.64%–99.35% nt sequence identity to those of other G2a strains, with the highest nt identity (99.3%) to those of VN/VAP1113_1/2013/VungTua/Vietnam and VN/KCHY_310113/2013/KhoaiChau/HungYen from Vietnam, BCR2 from Thailand, and CH/GXNN/2012 from China.

The sequence data revealed that S genes from the Japanese field PEDVs are of 4152–4161 nt long, and encode proteins with 1381–1386 aa residues. This consequence was due to the presence of several deletions or insertions that accumulated primarily in the N-terminus of the S protein. Multiple alignments of the S gene demonstrated that 14JM-140 and 14JM-144 exhibited insertions and deletions (1-nt, 11-nt, and 3-nt deletions at positions 167, 176, and 416, respectively, and a 6-nt insertion between positions 474 and 475), which are typical for S INDEL strains [28, 29].

Compared to the two vaccine strains, all Japanese field PEDVs were highly conserved in epitopes 2C10 and SS2 except for strain 13JM-293 that had an aa substitution (L1375I) within 2C10 (Fig. 2). Additionally, compared to the vaccine strains, all the Japanese field PEDVs had two aa changes (L768S and D770S) in the epitope SS2, and three serine substitutions (A521S, T553S, and G598S) in the neutralizing domain COE (excluding 13JM291 and 14JM-268). Notably, the aa substitutions at positions 521 and 553 resulted in predictable phosphorylation sites in the S protein of the Japanese field strains. Furthermore, different amino acids were found at the 12 sites within the COE domain (Fig. 2).

Regarding the prediction of high-specificity N-glycosylation sites in the S protein, most Japanese strains belonging to G2b exhibited eight N-glycosylation sites over the entire S protein (Additional file 1: Table S1). 14JM-268 had one additional N-glycosylation site at residue 557, and 14JM-242 possessed an additionally unique N-glycosylation site at position 382 of the aa chain. Two Japanese S INDEL strains (14JM-140 and 14JM-144) had seven N-glycosylation sites, while 13JM-291 had eight N-glycosylation sites. Compared with the vaccine strain, 96-P4C6, most of the Japanese non-S INDEL strains in G2b lost three N-glycosylation sites (at 132, 557, and 1233) and gained another N-glycosylation site (at 60). Compared with P-5 V, these G2b Japanese strains lost three N-glycosylation sites (at 117, 132, and 515) and gained four other N-glycosylation sites (at 60, 119, 325, and 1262).

Analysis of the M gene

The M gene sequences from all the Japanese field PEDVs and the two vaccine strains consisted of 681 nucleotides encoding a protein of 226 aa. Identical nt sequences were distinguished and excluded, resulting in the identification of seven unique sequences from the 45 total collected PEDVs (Table 2). A phylogenetic tree based on the M gene of the Japanese strains and reference strains revealed that all the sequences were divided into two groups (G1 and G2); G2 was further divided into two subgroups G2a and G2b (Fig. 3a). All the current Japanese PEDVs fell into G2, and showed the closest relatedness to the NA strains and emerging strains identified in Europe, South Korea, and China. These field PEDVs were phylogenetically distant from the vaccine strains and a classical Japanese strain (JMe2) of G1. The M genes of field PEDVs had 99.56%–100% nt identity to

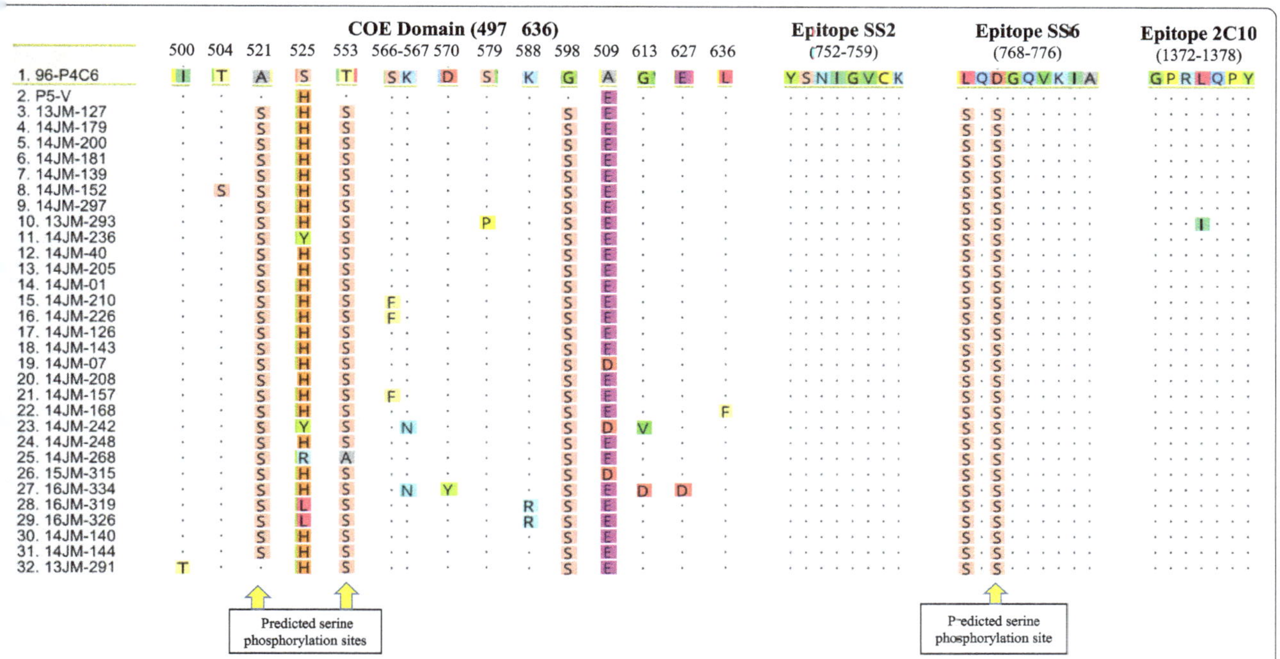

Fig. 2 Amino acid substitutions in the S protein epitope regions of the field and vaccine strains. The twelve substitutions between the Japanese field strains and vaccine strains were I500T, T504S, H/S525Y/R/L, S566F, K567 N, D570Y, S579P, K588R, A/E509D, V613D/V, E627D, and L636F. Predicted serine phosphorylation was occurred at positions 521, 553, and 770

ach other and 97.5%–98.24% nt identity with the vac-ine strains.

The B cell epitope, WAFYVR [30], located at position 95–200 of the M protein, was conserved in all field and accine strains. Compared with the vaccine strains, all apanese field strains had an aa substitution (A214S) be-onging to an antigenic region (aa 205–223), as predicted y the EMBOSS protein analysis tool (Additional file 2: igure S1A). Strain 14JM-236 had a different aa (S213 N) eading to the loss of a predicted serine phosphorylation ite. In another predicted epitope region (aa 5–15), the eld PEDVs had one different aa (V12I) compared to P-V, and two aa substitutions (F5S and Q13E) compared o 96-P4C6. These substitutions (F5S) resulted in gaining predicted high-specificity N-glycosylation site.

nalysis of the N gene

'he N gene of all the field PEDVs and vaccine strains vas 1326 nt in length encoding a protein of 441 aa. dentical nt sequences of the N gene were distinguished nd excluded, resulting in the identification of 19 unique equences. Phylogenetic analysis based on the N genes rom the Japanese strains and reference strains revealed he classification of PEDV strains into three groups: G1, G2, and G3 (Fig. 3b). All Japanese field strains were losely clustered together into subgroup G3 with other JS and US-like strains. The Japanese field PEDVs shared 8.72%–100% N gene nt sequence identity to each other and 95.70%–96.76% to the vaccine strains. Strain 13-JM127 from the first outbreak in Miyazaki had 100% nt identity to eight other field strains collected in Miyazaki, Aichi, and Kagoshima, and this is likely to be the most dominant sequence of N gene among the field strains. Compared to the vaccine strains, all the field strains in the present study had 9 aa substitutions (Additional file 2: Figure S1B); the substitution K123 N resulted in forming a predicted N-glycosylation site on the N protein from the field strains, while the aa substitutions A142T and N255S observed in field strains formed two predicted phosphorylation sites. Of note, the substitutions K123 N and N255S belong to the reported antigenic epitopes NEP-D4 (aa 18–133) and NEP-D6 (aa 252–262), respectively [18].

Comparison between strains collected from primary and secondary outbreaks

There were three swine farms where PED outbreaks first occurred in 2014, and then recurred in 2016, as shown in Table 3. Farm 1 is located in Aomori prefecture, while farms 2 and 3 are located in the same town in Miyazaki prefecture. Phylogenetic analysis based on the S gene sequences revealed that three PEDV strains (14JM-168, 16JM-334, and 16JM-339) collected from two different outbreaks on farm 1 were closest to each other and segregated into a distinct minor branch. PEDVs from the primary PED outbreaks on farm 2 (14JM-179, 14JM-

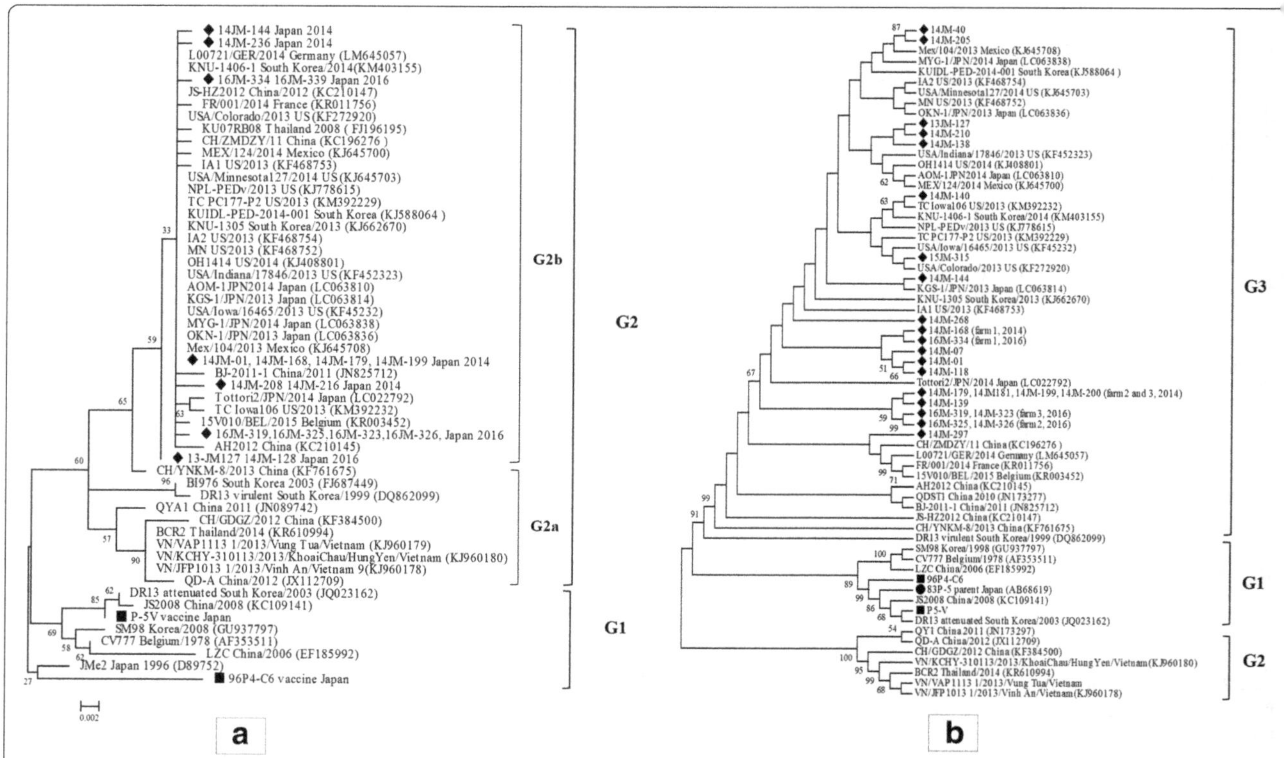

Fig. 3 Phylogenetic trees of PEDVs based on nucleotide sequences of entire M and N genes. Phylogenetic trees based on the M gene (**a**) and the N gene (**b**) were constructed using the maximum likelihood method in the MEGA program. Numbers at nodes represent the percentage of 1000 bootstrap replicates. The scale bars indicate the number of nucleotide substitutions per site. Names of strains, countries and years of isolation, and GenBank accession numbers are shown. The Japanese field PEDV strains identified in this study are marked by solid diamond symbols and the vaccine strains used in Japan are marked by solid square symbols

181) and farm 3 (14JM199 and 14JM-200) grouped closest together, along with two other strains (14JM-146 and 14JM-147) from different pig farms in Miyazaki prefecture in 2014. Likewise, strains from recurrent outbreaks on farm 2 (16JM-325 and 16JM-326) and farm 3 (16JM-319, 16JM-323) were also grouped into a monophyletic branch. All the PEDV strains collected from the primary and recurrent outbreaks on farms 2 and 3 were clustered into the minor group PED-J2, along with several strains collected from PED outbreaks that occurred on other pi farms in Miyazaki in 2014. Similar phylogenetic related ness among PEDVs obtained from primary and recurren outbreaks was observed, based on the phylogenetic tree o the N gene.

On farm 1, the S, M, and N genes of PEDVs identifie from the recurrent outbreak (16JM-334 and 16JM-339 shared the highest (99.66%, 100%, and 99.55% respectively nt sequence identities to a strain (14JM-168) collecte

Table 3 Information of primary and recurrent PED outbreaks occurred in the three pig farms in this study

	Farm 1		Farm 2		Farm 3	
	Primary outbreak	Recurrent outbreak	Primary outbreak	Recurrent outbreak	Primary outbreak	Recurrent outbreak
Outbreak time	May-2014	Feb-2016	May-2014	Feb-2016	May-2014	Feb-2016
Scale of farm	2000 sows	2000 sows	580 sows	600 sows	700 sows	700 sows
Vaccination	No	Yes	Yes	Yes	Yes	Yes
Morbidity (%)	100	60	100	70	100	70
Mortality (%)	100[a]	50[b]	70[a]	30[a]	70[a]	30[a]
Sample	14JM-168	16JM-334, 16JM-339	14JM-179, 14JM-181	16JM-325, 16JM-326	14JM-199, 14JM-200	16JM-319, 16JM-32

[a]Mortality rate of piglets less than two weeks-old; [b]Mortality rate of the piglets less than one-week-old
All the information for mortality and morbidity was kindly supplied by the veterinarians responsible for these farms

om the primary outbreak. The S genes of PEDVs from ne primary outbreak on farms 2 and 3 had high (99.92%–9.98%) nt identity to each other. These strains also had lentical sequences for the M and N genes. In the second-ry outbreaks, PEDVs from farms 2 and 3 also shared ighly homologous genes. The S and M genes of two trains (16JM-319 and 16JM-323) from farm 3 shared 00% nt sequence identities with those of a strain (16JM-25) from farm 2.

Compared with the strain collected from the primary utbreak on farm 1, two strains from the recurrent utbreak had 11 aa substitutions in their S proteins Additional file 3: Figure S2). Notably, the substitution 722 N lead to the loss of a predicted serine phosphoryl-tion site. These recurrent strains also had two aa sub-titutions (R166S and T413 N) in the N protein; the 166S substitution formed a predicted serine phosphor-lation site. Comparison to PEDVs from the primary utbreak on farms 2 and 3, PEDVs from the recurrent utbreaks had 13 aa substitutions in the S proteins, in ddition to a single aa change (A42V) in the M protein nd two aa changes (L18I and S31F) in the N protein. Iotably, the substitutions L18I and S31F occurred in the eported epitope NEP-D4 (18–133) of the N protein.

iscussion

ince late 2013, massive PED outbreaks have recurred in apan causing tremendous financial losses in the swine ndustry. Despite the nationwide use of available attenu-ted vaccines developed decades ago [21], PEDV has apidly swept across the county. Our sequencing data re-ealed that the prevailing Japanese PEDVs are genetically eterogeneous and can be classified into 3 genotypes: JA, S INDEL, and Asian non-S INDEL. Both the NA nd S INDEL types, which have been identified in recent tudies in Japan [21–23, 31] were also responsible for re-ent outbreaks in the US and South Korea. In our study, esides the two previously reported PEDV types, we lentified another type of Japanese PEDV (designated as sian non-S INDEL) that is closely related to the 'ietnamese, Thai, and Chinese strains. The Asian non-S NDEL type was collected from an early PED epidemic hat occurred in southern Japan where the recent PED andemic began spreading. Moreover, the Asian non-S NDEL type appeared at a similar time to the appearance f the NA and S INDEL types in Japan [21]. Together vith the absence of PED cases from 2007 to 2012 in apan [21, 22], we speculated a possibility that the three ypes of Japanese PEDV originated from one source and merged at the same or similar time in the southern re-ion of Japan before spreading across the country.

The result of this study revealed that all the field EDV strains (except 13JM-291) were closely related to merging strains identified in the US, South Korea, Taiwan, and in European countries. Of note, the Japanese PEDVs were genetically most closely related to the US strains; some even had identical S gene. Since the recent PED pandemics in Japan started to reemerge six months after those in the US, the close genetic relationship indicated that the current Japanese PEDV might have been introduced directly from the US, or both the US and Japanese PEDVs were derived from one source of origin.

Since April 2013, the NA type of PEDV has emerged in the US. The NA strains were identified subsequently in South Korea, Taiwan, and Japan from late 2013. Another PEDV type possessing typical insertions and deletions in the N-terminus of the S gene when compared to the prototype NA type was first discovered in Ohio in the US [29]. This PEDV type, therefore, was designated as S INDEL. The S INDEL PEDVs were also identified later in recent outbreaks in Japan, South Korea, Canada, Belgium, France, Germany, Portugal, Slovenia, and the Netherlands [4]. Both highly virulent and S INDEL PEDVs prevailing in the US are supposed to be derived from Chinese PEDVs as a result of recombinant events [4, 28, 32]. In accordance with these findings, our sequence analysis showed that the S INDEL strains, such as CH/HBQX/10 and JS120103, had already appeared in Chinese PED outbreaks during 2010–2012 [33, 34]. With the prevalence of both NA and S INDEL strains in the US, South Korea, and Japan since 2013, we suggested that there are two major possibilities of origin for the reemerging Japanese PEDV strains. First, US-like strains have been directly transmitted to Japan from the US or South Korea. Second, the same source of the US strains could have introduced the PEDV into Japan, from China, shortly after the US outbreaks. However, our study revealed the prevalence of the Asian none-S IDEL PEDV strain in Japan, which has not been reported in the US or South Korea. Thus, we incline toward the possibility that multiple parent PEDV strains have been introduced into Japan, from China or China's neighboring countries (such as the Southeast Asian region), causing the recent PED pandemic. Further investigation and surveillance are required to specifically identify the source of origin for the reemerging Japanese PEDVs.

Sixteen PEDV strains from four different prefectures including Miyazaki, Kagoshima, Aomori, and Aichi formed a well-supported subclade (PED-J1). Fourteen PEDV strains from various farms in Miyazaki prefecture were also grouped into a distinct subclade (PED-J2). These results suggested that strains of those Japanese sublineages (PED-J1 and PED-J2) may derive from two common ancestral PEDVs whose progeny have spread in the regions. Two genetic sublineages of US strains, namely IA1-Co/13 and MN-IA2 [32], were identified from the US outbreaks in 2013. Notably, the Japanese PEDV of the Japanese sublineage PED-J1 in this study showed a close relationship with the US sublineage IA1-Co/13, and PEDVs of the Japanese sublineage PED-J2 showed close relatedness with the US sublineage MN-IA2. This data revealed the common pattern of genetic diversity as well as the close relationship between the Japanese strains and the US strains, suggesting a common ancestor for these strains.

In our previous study [23], by sequencing a partial S gene containing a neutralizing epitope region (COE domain), we suggested that 14JM-140 may belong to the S INDEL type that has been circulating in Japan together with the highly virulent US-like strains. In this study, by sequencing the full-length S gene, we confirmed 14JM-140 to be an S INDEL strain. We also identified another strain that belonged to the S INDEL type, 14JM-144, although it was not predicted to be an S INDEL PEDV in the previous study. This discrepancy arose due to the region of the partial S gene utilized in the previous report that lack the typical insertions and deletions of the S INDEL type. Our data revealed the circulation of S INDEL strains in PED outbreaks occurring in Japan, but these strains compose only a minor population of the reemerging Japanese PEDVs. These results are consistent with two recent reports of Japanese PEDV [21, 22].

Phosphorylation of viral proteins is a reversible post-translational modification that can have major impacts on viral infection, replication, and cytotoxicity in a host cell [35]. For infectious bronchitis virus, belonging to the coronaviruses, the phosphorylation of the nucleocapsid protein has a dramatic influence on RNA binding capability and the recognition of viral RNA from non-viral RNA in the process of viral replication [36]. Along with phosphorylation, glycosylation is another post-translational modification that often strongly affects the protein functions of viruses. N-glycosylation sites in the spike gene of the severe acute respiratory syndrome coronavirus were demonstrated to be crucial for viral infection [37]. On the other hand, mutations observed in the neutralizing regions have been proposed as presenting a viral evolution, allowing escape from antibodies developed against vaccine or classical PEDV strains [38]. In this study, we characterized differences in epitope regions, high-specificity N-glycosylation and phosphorylation sites, between the vaccine and recent field strains. Various substitutions observed in the S (521, 553, 568, and 570), M (5), and N (123, 252, and 255) proteins may have affected the antigenicity, conferring the capacity for immune evasion in the PEDV field strains, and consequently, influencing the efficacy of the vaccines. In fact, despite vaccination, PEDV infections still spread rapidly and are commonly observed on PED-vaccinated farms in Japan [23]. Vaccination showed very low efficacy and could not mitigate the severe losses caused by PED [39]. Based on the antigenicity analysis of the vaccine and field strains, as well as the recent performance of th PED vaccines on the Japanese pig farms, we suggest tha the development of novel vaccines based on reemergin PEDVs is necessary to control current PED outbreaks.

The first PED epidemic on farm 1 was a severe occurrence in May 2014 (Table 3). Afterward, obvious clinica symptoms and death caused by PED were not observe in pigs of the herd until February 2016 when the subsequent outbreak recurred with less severity than the firs Although the pigs did not show any obvious symptom of PED, the presence of PEDV on this farm was detecte in piglets several times by RT-PCR during the perio from June 2014 to January 2016, according to the information supplied by veterinarians responsible for thi farm. Phylogenetic analysis based on the sequences c the S and N genes showed that PEDV strains from th primary and secondary outbreaks formed monophyleti branches. They also shared with each other the highes sequence identity of the S, M, and N genes compared t other strains used in this study. Additionally, PED outbreaks were not observed on other farms within a 5 kr radius of farm 1, and many strict measures for establishing a high level of security were implemented on thi farm. Taken together, we speculated that PEDV strain causing the primary outbreak induced partial protectiv immunity but persisted in the herd for nearly two year Subsequently, the persisted PEDVs caused the secondar epidemic. This is the first report of a two-year-long persistence of PEDV in a pig herd. It has been propose that the popular circulation of PEDV variants with larg deletions in the S gene is associated with the persistenc of the PEDV on the infected farms in Japan [24]. However, we did not detect the presence of the large S deletion variants in the fecal and intestinal samples collecte from this farm. Other factors, including the genetic variation of causative PEDV strains, may play a more important role in the disease recurrence.

On farms 2 and 3, PED first occurred in May 2014 despite all the sows receiving antepartum PEDV vaccinations in 2013. Afterward, the disease disappeared unti early 2016 when the subsequent outbreaks recurrec There was no detection of the PEDV during the interva between these two outbreaks. Phylogenetic analysi based on the S and N genes revealed that the strains collected from the first outbreaks on farms 2 and 3 forme a monophyletic branch. Moreover, these two farms wer located close to each other with a distance of 0.5 kn (separated by a small mountain), and the outbreaks occurred at the same time. This suggests that the PED strains introduced onto these farms that induced th first outbreaks were derived from a common source o PEDV. Likewise, in the secondary outbreaks, the strain collected from these two farms also have the highes genetic identity to each other and formed mino nonophyletic branches, as shown in the phylogenetic rees for the S and N genes. All the strains collected rom the primary and recurrent outbreaks on these arms were closely clustered into the subclade PED-J2, ogether with other strains collected from other farms ocated in Miyazaki prefecture (Fig. 1). This data suggested that the PEDV strains causing the subsequent utbreaks on farms 2 and 3 evolved from PEDVs that ad been circulating in the Miyazaki region since 2014. here are two possibilities for the origin of the strains hat caused the subsequent outbreaks on farms 2 and 3. irst, PEDVs may have persisted silently on these farms ince 2014, evolving, and then causing the subsequent utbreaks when suitable conditions arrived in early 016. Another possibility is that PEDVs may have persisted on other pig farms, circulating in the Miyazaki region since the 2014 PED occurrence, after which the EDVs were introduced again onto farms 2 and 3, causing the secondary epidemics. More data is needed to lucidate exactly the origin of these PEDVs strains. The ccurrence of PED in these herds has partially indicated he failure of using the current PEDV vaccines, which re based on old seed stock of classical Japanese strains. esides, the repeated outbreaks in these herds indicate hat the disease has developed to an endemic stage. hese results could be used to elucidate the prevalence f PEDVs and to contribute to the prevention of PED in he region.

onclusions

n conclusion, our study revealed that Japanese field EDVs causing PED outbreaks during 2013–2016 could e classified into three types, and these PEDVs might ave been introduced from overseas at the same time or uring similar periods. The disease has developed to an ndemic stage in which the PEDV can persist for a long me in these herds or these local regions causing subsequent epidemics. The distant genetic relationships and arious aa substitutions between the Japanese field EDVs and vaccine strains may be responsible for the nsuccessful PED control in Japan. Our findings will be seful in understanding the origin and molecular epidemiology of the PEDV, and helping to develop measures for the control of the disease.

dditional files

Additional file 1: Table S1. Highly-specific N-glycosylation sites in the spike protein of the vaccine and field strains.

Additional file 2: Figure S1. Amino acid substitutions in the M and N proteins between the field and vaccine strains. **A**: Amino acid substitutions in the M protein. The field strain 14JM-236 has an aa substitution, S213 N, resulting in the loss of a predicted phosphorylation site. The substitution at aa 5 in the M protein of the field strains may result in gaining a high-specificity N-glycosylation site (NGSI) compared with the vaccine strain 96-P4C6. **B**: Amino acid substitutions in the N protein. Two antigenic epitopes (NEP-D4 and NEP-D6) are marked by red bars. Compared with the vaccine strains, the Japanese field strains had 9 aa changes, including K123 N, A142T, T145A, M216 V, R241K, H242L, K 252 R, N255S, Q397L. A high-specificity N-glycosylation site (NFSQ) was predicted to occur at position 123 and a phosphorylation site was predicted to occur at positions 142, 166, and 255.

Additional file 3: Figure S2. Aligment of deduced S amino acid sequences of Japanese PEDVs from primary and recurent outbreaks. The deduced S protein of 14JM-168 had 11 amino acid substitutions (T211I, V312 M, A477S, K556 N, D569Y, G612D, E626D, F635 L, S722 N, T777 M, G888D) compared to those of 16JM-334 and 16JM-339. Deduced S proteins of 14JM-179, 14JM-181, 14JM-199, and 14JM-200 had 13 amino acid substitutions (Y6H, T24A, A311T, F345 V, T367 N. L416F, H524L, K587R, V674F, S925A, S968A, N1009S, and I1067M) compared to those of 16JM-319 and 16JM-326.

Abbreviations

aa: Amino acid; M: Membrane; N: Nucleocapsid; NA: North American; nt: Nucleotide; PED: Porcine epidemic diarrhea; PEDV: Porcine epidemic diarrhea virus; RT: Reverse transcription; S: Spike

Acknowledgements

Not applicable

Funding

The work was conducted with funding from the University of Miyazaki (grant number 2014–70) and Japan Society for the Promotion of Science (KAKENHI program, grant number 17H04639). The funders had no role in the design of the study and collection, analysis, and interpretation of data and in preparation of the manuscript.

Authors' contributions

RY and ND designed the study. RY, MS, ZN, and TH provided the viral samples and other materials. ND, NF, AT, UI, and OM conducted experiments. ND designed the primers interpreted the sequencing data and wrote the manuscript draft. RY, MS, ZN, TH, AT, UI, NF, and OM analysis the data and revise the manuscript. All authors prepared and approved the final manuscript.

Consent for publication

Not applicable

Competing interests

The authors declare that they have no competing interests.

References

1. Song D, Park B. Porcine epidemic diarrhoea virus: a comprehensive review of molecular epidemiology, diagnosis, and vaccines. Virus Genes. 2012;44(2): 167–75.
2. Oldham J. Letter to the editor. Pig Farming. 1972;10:72–3.
3. Pensaert MB, de Bouck P. A new coronavirus-like particle associated with diarrhea in swine. Arch Virol. 1978;58(3):243–7.
4. Lin CM, Saif LJ, Marthaler D, Wang Q. Evolution, antigenicity and pathogenicity of global porcine epidemic diarrhea virus strains. Virus Res. 2016;226:20–39.
5. Li W, Li H, Liu Y, Pan Y, Deng F, Song Y, Tang X, He Q. New variants of porcine epidemic diarrhea virus, China, 2011. Emerg Infect Dis. 2012;18(8): 1350–3.
6. Oka T, Saif LJ, Marthaler D, Esseili MA, Meulia T, Lin CM, Vlasova AN, Jung K, Zhang Y, Wang Q. Cell culture isolation and sequence analysis of genetically diverse US porcine epidemic diarrhea virus strains including a novel strain with a large deletion in the spike gene. Vet Microbiol. 2014;173(3–4):258–69.
7. Lee C. Porcine epidemic diarrhea virus: an emerging and re-emerging epizootic swine virus. Virol J. 2015;12(1):193.
8. Chen J, Liu X, Shi D, Shi H, Zhang X, Li C, Chi Y, Feng L. Detection and molecular diversity of spike gene of porcine epidemic diarrhea virus in China. Viruses. 2013;5(10):2601–13.
9. Bosch BJ, van der Zee R, de Haan CA, Rottier PJ. The coronavirus spike protein is a class I virus fusion protein: structural and functional characterization of the fusion core complex. J Virol. 2003;77(16):8801–11.

10. Chang SH, Bae JL, Kang TJ, Kim J, Chung GH, Lim CW, Laude H, Yang MS, Jang YS. Identification of the epitope region capable of inducing neutralizing antibodies against the porcine epidemic diarrhea virus. Mol Cells. 2002;14(2):295–9.
11. Cruz DJ, Kim CJ, Shin HJ. The GPRLQPY motif located at the carboxy-terminal of the spike protein induces antibodies that neutralize porcine epidemic diarrhea virus. Virus Res. 2008;132(1–2):192–6.
12. Sun D, Feng L, Shi H, Chen J, Cui X, Chen H, Liu S, Tong Y, Wang Y, Tong G. Identification of two novel B cell epitopes on porcine epidemic diarrhea virus spike protein. Vet Microbiol. 2008;131(1–2):73–81.
13. Sato T, Takeyama N, Katsumata A, Tuchiya K, Kodama T, Kusanagi K. Mutations in the spike gene of porcine epidemic diarrhea virus associated with growth adaptation in vitro and attenuation of virulence in vivo. Virus Genes. 2011;43(1):72–8.
14. Lee DK, Park CK, Kim SH, Lee C. Heterogeneity in spike protein genes of porcine epidemic diarrhea viruses isolated in Korea. Virus Res. 2010;149(2): 175–82.
15. Temeeyasen G, Srijangwad A, Tripipat T, Tipsombatboon P, Piriyapongsa J, Phoolcharoen W, Chuanasa T, Tantituvanont A, Nilubol D. Genetic diversity of ORF3 and spike genes of porcine epidemic diarrhea virus in Thailand. Infect Genet Evol. 2014;21:205–13.
16. Ujike M, Taguchi F. Incorporation of spike and membrane glycoproteins into coronavirus virions. Viruses. 2015;7(4):1700–25.
17. McBride R, van Zyl M, Fielding BC. The coronavirus nucleocapsid is a multifunctional protein. Viruses. 2014;6(8):2991–3018.
18. Wang K, Xie C, Zhang J, Zhang W, Yang D, Yu L, Jiang Y, Yang S, Gao F, Yang Z, et al. The identification and characterization of two novel epitopes on the Nucleocapsid protein of the porcine epidemic diarrhea virus. Sci Rep. 2016;6:39010.
19. Sueyoshi M, Tsuda T, Yamazaki K, Yoshida K, Nakazawa M, Sato K, Minami T, Iwashita K, Watanabe M, Suzuki Y, et al. An immunohistochemical investigation of porcine epidemic diarrhoea. J Comp Pathol. 1995;113(1):59–67.
20. Tsuda T. Porcine epidemic diarrhea: its diagnosis and control. Proc Jpn Pig Vet Soc. 1997;31:21–8.
21. Suzuki T, Murakami S, Takahashi O, Kodera A, Masuda T, Itoh S, Miyazaki A, Ohashi S, Tsutsui T. Molecular characterization of pig epidemic diarrhoea viruses isolated in Japan from 2013 to 2014. Infect Genet Evol. 2015;36:363–8.
22. Horie M, Kabemura M, Masatani T, Matsuu A, Ozawa M. Isolation and molecular characterization of porcine epidemic diarrhea viruses collected in Japan in 2014. Arch Virol. 2016;161(8):2189–95.
23. Van Diep N, Norimine J, Sueyoshi M, Lan NT, Hirai T, Yamaguchi R. US-like isolates of porcine epidemic diarrhea virus from Japanese outbreaks between 2013 and 2014. Spring. 2015;4:756.
24. Diep NV, Norimine J, Sueyoshi M, Lan NT, Yamaguchi R. Novel porcine epidemic diarrhea virus (PEDV) variants with large deletions in the spike (S) gene coexist with PEDV strains possessing an intact S gene in domestic pigs in Japan: a new disease situation. PLoS One. 2017;12(1):e0170126.
25. Tamura K, Stecher G, Peterson D, Filipski A, Kumar S. MEGA6: molecular evolutionary genetics analysis version 6.0. Mol Biol Evol. 2013;30(12):2725–9.
26. Rice P, Longden I, Bleasby A. EMBOSS: the European molecular biology open software suite. Trends Genet. 2000;16(6):276–7.
27. Stevenson GW, Hoang H, Schwartz KJ, Burrough ER, Sun D, Madson D, Cooper VL, Pillatzki A, Gauger P, Schmitt BJ, et al. Emergence of porcine epidemic diarrhea virus in the United States: clinical signs, lesions, and viral genomic sequences. J Vet Diagn Investig. 2013;25(5):649–54.
28. Vlasova AN, Marthaler D, Wang Q, Culhane MR, Rossow KD, Rovira A, Collins J, Saif LJ. Distinct characteristics and complex evolution of PEDV strains, North America, may 2013-February 2014. Emerg Infect Dis. 2014;20(10):1620–8.
29. Wang L, Byrum B, Zhang Y. New variant of porcine epidemic diarrhea virus, United States, 2014. Emerg Infect Dis. 2014;20(5):917–9.
30. Zhang Z, Chen J, Shi H, Chen X, Shi D, Feng L, Yang B. Identification of a conserved linear B-cell epitope in the M protein of porcine epidemic diarrhea virus. Virol J. 2012;9:225.
31. Yamamoto R, Soma J, Nakanishi M, Yamaguchi R, Niinuma S. Isolation and experimental inoculation of an S INDEL strain of porcine epidemic diarrhea virus in Japan. Res Vet Sci. 2015;103:103–6.
32. Huang YW, Dickerman AW, Pineyro P, Li L, Fang L, Kiehne R, Opriessnig T, Meng XJ. Origin, evolution, and genotyping of emergent porcine epidemic diarrhea virus strains in the United States. MBio. 2013;4(5):e00737-00713.
33. Zhao PD, Tan C, Dong Y, Li Y, Shi X, Bai J, Jiang P. Genetic variation analyse of porcine epidemic diarrhea virus isolated in mid-eastern China from 2011 to 2013. Can J Vet Res. 2015;79(1):8–15.
34. Zheng FM, Huo JY, Zhao J, Chang HT, Wang XM, Chen L, Wang CQ. Molecular characterization and phylogenetic analysis of porcine epidemic diarrhea virus field strains in Central China during 2010-2012 outbreaks. Bing Du Xue Bao. 2013;29(2):197–205.
35. Keating JA, Striker R. Phosphorylation events during viral infections provide potential therapeutic targets. Rev Med Virol. 2012;22(3):166–81.
36. Spencer KA, Dee M, Britton P, Hiscox JA. Role of phosphorylation clusters in the biology of the coronavirus infectious bronchitis virus nucleocapsid protein. Virology. 2008;370(2):373–81.
37. Han DP, Lohani M, Cho MW. Specific asparagine-linked glycosylation sites are critical for DC-SIGN- and L-SIGN-mediated severe acute respiratory syndrome coronavirus entry. J Virol. 2007;81(21):12029–39.
38. Hao J, Xue C, He L, Wang Y, Cao Y. Bioinformatics insight into the spike glycoprotein gene of field porcine epidemic diarrhea strains during 2011-2013 in Guangdong, China. Virus Genes. 2014;49(1):58–67.
39. Tsuji A, Yamamoto N, Toya R. Measure to mitigate loss caused by PED (porcine epidemic diarrhea) using maternal immunity. J Farm Anim Infect Dis. 2015;4(4):195–200.

Diagnosis of Swine Toxoplasmosis by PCR and Genotyping of *Toxoplasma gondii* from pigs in Henan, Central China

Haiyan Wang[1,2], Longxian Zhang[1*], Qinge Ren[1], Fuchang Yu[1] and Yurong Yang[1]

Abstract

Background: *Toxoplasma gondii*, a widely prevalent protozoan parasite, causes serious toxoplasmosis infections in humans and other animals. Among livestock, pigs are susceptible to *T. gondii* infection. Despite Henan being one of the biggest pig-raising provinces in China, little information exists on the epidemiology of toxoplasmosis in this location. Therefore, we molecularly characterized DNA samples from pigs in Henan. A total of 1647 samples, including 952 from dead piglets, 478 from seriously sick fattening pigs and 217 from abortion sows, were collected from different animal hospitals or pig farms from 10 different cities in Henan (2006–2008). Each pig corresponded to a separate pig farm. DNA was extracted from 3 to 5 g of the most severely affected pig tissue (liver, spleen, lung, hilar lymph nodes and amniotic fluid) after postmortem examination. The presence of the *T. gondii* B1 gene was detected using nested polymerase chain reactions (PCR). Genotyping was performed directly on DNA from the PCR-positive tissue samples using 11 PCR restriction fragment length polymorphism markers (SAG1, 5′- and 3′-SAG2, alternative SAG2, SAG3, BTUB, GRA6, L358, PK1, c22–8, c29–2, and Apico).

Results: Of all samples, thirty-four were positive for the *T. gondii* B1 gene (2.06%, 95% CI: 1.86%–2.26%) from four cities, including 31 from NanYang city, one (PgXY 1) from Xinyang City, one (PgZZ 1) from Zhengzhou City and one (PgZK1) from Zhoukou City. The prevalence was found to be highest in piglets than in fattening pigs and sows. And the difference was statistically significant (P<0.01). The following 32 samples were genotyped with complete data: 13 hilar lymph node tissue samples, seven liver tissue samples, seven lung tissue samples, four spleen tissue samples, and one amniotic fluid sample. Only one genotype, belonging to ToxoDB Genotype #9, was identified.

Conclusions: This is the first large-scale survey molecularly characterizing *T. gondii* from pigs in Henan. The results of the present study revealed that *T. gondii* infection is present in swine in Henan and is a potential source of foodborne toxoplasmosis in the investigated areas. Implementation of effective control measures for *T. gondii* to reduce the chance of zoonotic toxoplasmosis spreading from pig farms may be warranted. The results show that the ToxoDB #9 genotype may be the dominant *T. gondii* lineage in mainland China. These findings strengthen the limited Chinese *T. gondii* epidemiology database.

Keywords: Swine, Toxoplasmosis, PCR assay, Diagnosis, Molecular characterization, Henan

* Correspondence:
zhanglx8999@gmail.com; zhanglongxian8999@foxmail.com
[1]College of Animal Science and Veterinary Medicine, Henan Agricultural University, Zhengzhou 450002, Henan, People's Republic of China
Full list of author information is available at the end of the article

Background

Toxoplasma gondii, a common worldwide zoonotic protozoan parasite, infects a large number of warm blooded vertebrates. Humans become infected postnatally mainly by ingesting infectious oocysts from the environment or by consumption of undercooked or raw meat that contains tissue cysts. Although *T. gondii* generally causes a mild and self-limited infection in immunocompetent individuals, it can cause abortion, fetal abnormalities and prenatal death in pregnant women, and can be fatal to some immunocompromised patients such as those with AIDS or organ transplant recipients [1]. *T. gondii* infections in humans have recently been shown to be associated with an increased risk of schizophrenia [2]. It has been estimated that 33% of the world's population and 7.9% of the population in China have been exposed to this parasite [3, 4].

Among livestock, pigs are susceptible to infection with *T. gondii* and infected pigs are considered to be one of the most important sources of *T. gondii* infection in humans [5]. Therefore, the potential risk of transmission of the disease to humans by consumption of undercooked or raw pork is an important food safety issue.

Efforts have been made to genetically compare *T. gondii* strains from different animals with those from humans to reveal the transmission dynamics of the parasite and to gain better control of its spread. Based on multilocus restriction length polymorphism analysis (RFLP) or multilocus enzyme electrophoresis, three clonal lineages (type I, II and III) are predominant in Europe and North America [6]. However, recently, a few genetically diverse *T. gondii* isolates, designated as 'atypical' or 'exotic' have been found circulating in animals and humans in other geographical regions [7–9].

Despite the large literary data on toxoplasmosis worldwide, studies on the occurrence and genetic characterization of *T. gondii* isolates from pigs in China are rather scarce [10–16], although pork is one of the most popular meats, representing around 65% of meat consumption in this country [14]. Henan, central China, is one of the biggest producers of pork products in China. About 105 million pigs were reared in Henan in 2015, making Henan the country's second largest pork producer. However, information on toxoplasma in pigs is limited in Henan. Thus, the aim of this study was to diagnose swine toxoplasmosis in Henan by molecular methodology and to genetically characterize the causative agent of this serious parasitic zoonosis. The data obtained will augment the currently limited epidemiological database on *T. gondii* in China.

Methods

Collection area

Henan, which lies between latitude 31°23′–36°22′ degrees north and longitude 110°21′–116°39 degrees east, is also known as central China. The province is about 550 km from north to south, and about 580 kn from east to west (Fig. 1). It has a distinct temperat continental monsoon climate, with four clearly delineate seasons. The average annual temperature of the provinc is 12–16 °C, with the lowest temperature occurring i January (−5–3 °C) and the highest temperature occurrin in July (28–33 °C).

Sample collection

During the period from September 2006 to Decembe 2008, after permission was obtained from the anima hospitals and the pig farm owners, a total of 1647 sic or dead pigs, including 952 dead piglets, 478 seriousl sick fattening pigs and 217 abortion sows, were collecte from different animal hospitals or pig farms from 1 different cities in Henan (Table 1). Each pig correspond to a pig farm, including small peasant households an small- or large-scale intensive breeding farms. The ani mals were free-range or from semi-intensive rearing sys tems in rural areas. For each animal, 3–5 g of the mos seriously affected pathological tissues (liver, spleen, lung hilar lymph nodes and amniotic fluid), as determined b postmortem examination (subcutaneous hemorrhage enlargement and necrosis), were collected. Freshly col lected samples were placed into clean plastic bags an transported immediately to the laboratory where the were stored at −20 °C. The date of collection, age, an farm of origin for each animal was recorded in detail.

DNA extraction

The freshly collected samples were grinded up an digested in a trypsin solution for 2 h at 37 °C, and th

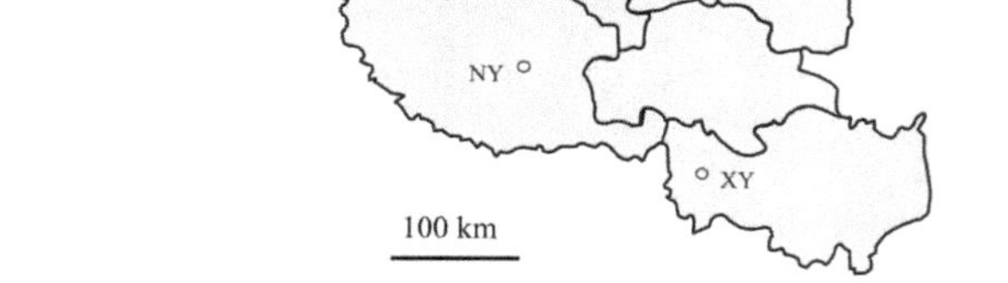

Fig. 1 Map showing Henan(HN), central China, where pigs from different animal hospitals or farms were sampled from Anyang City (AY), Xinxiang City (XX), Jiaozuo City (JZ), Luoyang City (LY), Zhengzhou City (ZZ), Pingdingshan City (PDS), Luohe City (LH), Zhoukou City (ZK), Nanyang City (NY) and Xinyang City (XY). The shadowed area of Henan is enlarged for clarity. The figure was generated using the softwares of MapInfo Professional 7.0, Microsoft PowerPoint 2007 and Adobe Photoshop 13.0

able 1 Prevalence of *T. gondii* by PCR in different cities in enan Province, China

ocation	No. positive/No. examined (%)			
	Piglets	Fattening pigs	Sows	Total
hengzhou	1/132(0.76)	0/86(0)	0/72(0)	1/290(0.34)
anyang	29/185(15.7)	0/102(0)	2/85(2.36)	31/372(8.33)
nxiang	0/98(0)	0/31(0)	0/7(0)	0/136(0)
ohe	0/64(0)	0/38(0)	0/16(0)	0/118(0)
aozuo	0/65(0)	0/20(0)	0/0(0)	0/85(0)
nyang	1/73(1.37)	0/95(0)	0/23(0)	1/191(0.52)
oyang	0/75(0)	0/35(0)	0/0(0)	0/110(0)
ngdingshan	0/80(0)	0/28(0)	0/2(0)	0/110(0)
nyang	0/98(0)	0/25(0)	0/0(0)	0/123(0)
houkou	1/82(0)	0/18(0)	0/12(0)	1/112(0.89)
otal	32/952(3.36)	0/478(0)	2/217(0.92)	34/1547(2.06)

ellets were stored at −20 °C until use. Genomic DNA vas extracted from the processed tissues using a tissue ien DNA kit (CWBIO, Beijing, China), according to the nanufacturer's recommendations. The DNA samples ere prepared after purification by silica gel column hromatography, eluted into 50 μL of elution buffer and tored at −20 °C until use.

CR analysis

nested PCR targeting the *T. gondii* B1 gene was erformed to detect possible infection with *T. gondii* 17]. A 194 bp fragment was PCR amplified using two rimer sets. The first fragment was amplified with the 1 (5′-TCTTTAAAGCGTTCGTGGTC-3′) and R1 (5′-GAACTGCATCCGTTCATGAG-3′) primer set, while he second fragment was amplified with the F2 (5′-GCGACCAATCTGCGAATACACC-3′) and R2 (5′-GCATAGGTTGCAGTCACTG-3′) primer set. The CRs were conducted in 25 μL volumes containing × PCR buffer (Takara Shuzo Co., Ltd., Otsu, Japan), .5 mM $MgCl_2$, 0.2 mM of each dNTP (Takara Shuzo o., Ltd), 0.4 μM of each primer, 1 unit of rTaq DNA olymerase (Takara Shuzo Co., Ltd.), and 2 μL of each ndividual DNA sample. The first amplification consisted f an initial denaturation step of 10 min at 94 °C, ollowed by 35 cycles of 10 s at 93 °C, 10 s at 62.5 °C nd 15 s at 72 °C, and a final extension step of 10 min at 2 °C. The second amplification consisted of an initial enaturation step of 10 min at 94 °C, followed by 35 cycles of 10 s at 93 °C, 10 s at 57 °C and 30 s at 72 °C, and final extension step of 10 min at 72 °C. Positive (RH train) and negative (distilled water) control samples vere included in each PCR run. The amplification products were electrophoretically separated on 1.5% agarose els containing ethidium bromide and then visualized on UV transilluminator.

Multilocus PCR-RFLP

Genetic characterization of all the *T. gondii*-positive samples was conducted using the multilocus PCR-RFLP method described by Su et al. [18]. In brief, the target DNA sequences were amplified by multiplex PCR using external primers for 11 genetic markers: SAG1, 5′ - and 3′ -SAG2, alternative SAG2, SAG3, BTUB, GRA6, L358, PK1, c22–8, c29–2, and Apico. The multiplex PCRs were each carried out in a 25 μL volume containing 1 × PCR buffer, 2 mM $MgCl_2$, 200 μM of each dNTP, 0.15 μM each of the external forward and reverse primers, 1 unit of FastStart DNA polymerase (Takara Shuzo Co., Ltd) and 1.5 μL of each DNA sample. The reaction mixture was heated to 95 °C for 4 min, followed by 30 cycles of 94 °C for 30 s, 55 °C for 1 min and 72 °C for 2 min. The multiplex PCR amplified products were diluted 1:1 by adding 25 μL of nuclease-free water. Then, 1 μL of each product served as the template DNA for nested PCR using the internal primers for each marker. The reaction mixture was heated at 95 °C for 4 min, followed by 35 cycles of 94 °C for 30 s, 60 °C for 1 min and 72 °C for 1.5 min (with an annealing temperature of 58 °C instead of 60 °C for the Apico marker). Each nested PCR product sample (5 μL) was digested with restriction endonucleases in a 20 μL volume and then resolved by 3% agarose gel electrophoresis to reveal the DNA banding pattern. The banding patterns of the samples were compared with the genotypes deposited in ToxoDB (http://toxodb.org/toxo/) to determine the *T. gondii* genotypes.

Results

In total, of the 1647 DNA samples we analyzed, 34 (2.06%, 95% CI: 1.86%–2.26%) from four cities were positive for the *T. gondii* B1 gene. These comprised 31 (PgNY 1–31) from Nanyang City, one (PgXY 1) from Xinyang City, one (PgZZ 1) from Zhengzhou City and one (PgZK1) from Zhoukou City. Nanyang City had the majority of *T. gondii*-positive farms. The prevalence was found to be highest in piglets than in fattening pigs and sows ($P<0.01$) (Table 1).

All the *T. gondii*-positive samples were identified by multilocus PCR-RFLP. The low DNA concentrations of the samples meant that only 32 of them generated complete genotyping results from the 11 PCR-RFLP markers. Two samples (PgNY 6 and 19) were genotyped at nine or fewer genetic loci. It is interesting that only one genotype (ToxoDB#9) from all the *T. gondii* samples from different cities in Henan was identified, while typical type I, II and III lineages, which are predominant in North America and Europe, were not found in our study. Table 2 shows the genotyping results for these samples and the ToxoD database reference information.

Table 2 Multilocus genotyping of *T. gondii* isolates from different porcine hosts and geographical locations worldwide by PCR-RFLP

Isolate ID	Host	Tissue	Location	Age	PCR RFLP genotype (genetic marker)											
					SAG1	5′ + 3′ SAG2	Alt. SAG2	SAG3	BTUB	GRA6	C22-8	C29-2	L358	PK1	Apico	Genotype
RH	Human		USA		I	I	I	I	I	I	I	I	I	I	I	Reference, ToxoDB #10 (type I)
PIH	Human		USA		II	II	II	II	II	II	II	II	II	II	II	Reference, ToxoDB #1 (type II)
CTG	Cat		USA		III	III	III	III	III	III	III	III	III	III	III	Reference, ToxoDB #2 (type III)
MAS	Human		France		u-1	I	II	III	III	III	u-1	I	I	III	I	Reference, ToxoDB #17
TgCgCa1	Cougar		Canada		I	I	II	III	III	II	II	u-1	I	u-2	I	Reference, ToxoDB #66
TgCatBr5	Cat		Brazil		I	III	III	III	II	III	I	I	I	u-1	I	Reference, ToxoDB #19
PgNY 1–5 (*n* = 5)	Pig	Liver	Ny, Henan	10–15 days	u-1	II	II	III	III	II	II	III	II	II	I	ToxoDB #9
PgNY 6	Pig	Liver	Ny, Henan	1–7 days	u-1	II	II	III	III	II	nd	III	II	nd	I	ToxoDB #9?
PgNY 20–31 (*n* = 12)	Pig	Hld	Ny, Henan	10–15 days	u-1	II	II	III	III	II	II	III	II	II	I	ToxoDB #9
PgNY 7–10,14 (*n* = 5)	Pig	Lung	Ny, Henan	1–7 days	u-1	II	II	III	III	II	II	III	II	II	I	ToxoDB #9
PgNY 11,16,17 (*n* = 3)	Pig	Spleen	Ny, Henan	20–30 days	u-1	II	II	III	III	II	II	III	II	II	I	ToxoDB #9
PgNY 12,15 (*n* = 2)	Pig	Lung	Ny, Henan	1–2 months	u-1	II	II	III	III	II	II	III	II	II	I	ToxoDB #9
PgNY 13,18 (*n* = 2)	Pig	Af	Ny, Henan	Sow	u-1	II	II	III	III	II	II	III	II	II	I	ToxoDB #9
PgNY 19	Pig	Spleen	Ny, Henan	20–30 days	u-1	nd	nd	III	III	II	II	III	II	nd	I	ToxoDB #9?
PgZK 1	Pig	Liver	Zk, Henan	20–30 days	u-1	II	II	III	III	II	II	III	II	II	I	ToxoDB #9
PgXX 1	Pig	Liver	Xy, Henan	1–2 months	u-1	II	II	III	III	II	II	III	II	II	I	ToxoDB #9
PgZZ 1	Pig	Hld	Zz, Henan	1–7 days	u-1	II	II	III	III	II	II	III	II	II	I	ToxoDB #9

nd, no data. u-1 and u-2 are unique RFLP genotypes
Hld and Af denote hilar lymph node and amniotic fluid, respectively
Ny, Zk, Xy and Zz denote the cities of Nanyang, Zhoukou, Xinyang and Zhengzhou, respectively

iscussion

nfection with *T. gondii* is relatively common in pigs. 'he prevalence of *T. gondii* differs greatly among ountries and regions within the same country. In the resent study, the prevalence of *T. gondii* was 2.06% in igs, a value lower than those reported in other studies ı China [11–13]. Because of the lack of existing epiemiological data on swine toxoplasmosis in the areas re investigated, we cannot speculate as to why a low oxoplasma prevalence rate was obtained. Prevalence ates can be affected by the detection methods used, the issue type sampled, sample sizes, animal age differences, nd animal housing conditions, along with many other nvironmental and farm management factors. The revalence rate was higher in Nanyang than in the other reas we tested, which could be related to Nanyang beıg the poorest city of those we investigated. Although it ossesses a substantial pig population, this population is ominated by small peasant households that breed pigs ı resource limited environments with poor animal mangement. The data from this region is similar to that in a atvia report where the prevalence of *T. gondii*-specific ntibodies was found to be greater in free-ranging doıestic pigs (6.2%, $P < 0.05$) than in intensively farmed igs (0.4%) [19]. Also, once *T. gondii* cysts have formed ı the brain and muscles, toxoplasmosis does not usually how any clinical signs or visible damage in immune ompetent animals, a situation that may lead to underesimates of the disease prevalence. Indeed, a study from nhui province, eastern China, found that a significant roportion (18.03%) of commercially available pork is ontaminated with *T. gondii* based on the real-time PCR esults [14].

In the present study, the prevalence of *T. gondii* was otably high in piglets. This might be explained by iglets being more susceptible to all kinds of opportunisc organisms, including *T. gondii*, and clinical manifesations may appear when their immunity declines under he poor animal management and the presence of some nmune system diseases (e.g. porcine circovirus or orcine reproductive and respiratory syndrome).

Our data show that swine toxoplasmosis exists in pig arms in Henan Province. Incorrect diagnosis or poor ıanagement of the disease may cause wider economic osses for swine herd production. Importantly, some symptomatic animals with *T. gondii* cysts in their brains nd muscle tissues may circulate in the fresh pork maret and become a source of foodborne toxoplasmosis, hus posing a food safety threat to public health. Thereore, integrated control strategies and measures should e implemented on farms to prevent *T. gondii* infection nd reduce the risk of spreading zoonotic toxoplasmosis.

The differential virulence of *T. gondii* strains has made he study of genetic diversity in *T. gondii* isolates an interesting and important research topic. Three predominant clonal types (i.e., I, II, and III) are commonly described in the scientific literature. Type I strains are highly virulent in mice, whereas type II and III strains are avirulent or non virulent [6]. Here, only one genotype (ToxoDB#9) was identified, while typical type I, II and III lineages, which have been predominantly described in pigs in North America and Europe [6], were not found in our study. This result is similar to the results reported by other authors in studies of *T. gondii* parasites isolated from pigs, yaks, cats, rats, mice, *Microtus fortis*, waterfowl and humans in eastern China (Anhui and Jiangsu) [14, 20, 21], southern China (Guangdong, Yunnan) [10, 22, 23], central China (Henan, Hubei and Jiangxi) [10, 11, 24–27], northern China (Beijing and Jilin) [28–30] and western China (Gansu, Yunnan and Guizhou) [12, 15, 31–35]. All current and past RFLP genotyping data for *T. gondii* isolates from China are summarized in Table 3. The compiled results provide solid evidence that genotype ToxoDB#9 has been, and remains, the predominant lineage in mainland China. Genotype ToxoDB#9 may also have a more worldwide distribution, circulating in South and North America, as well as in eastern Asia.

Conclusions

This is the first large-scale study to molecularly characterize *T. gondii* from pigs in central China. Our results have revealed that *T. gondii* infection is present in swine in Henan and may, therefore, pose a threat to public health via the consumption of raw or undercooked infected pork from this location. PCR-RFLP identified only one genotype (ToxoDB #9) in Henan. These findings augment the limited *T. gondii* epidemiology database in China. To better understand the molecular epidemiology and population structure of *T. gondii* in Henan, it will be necessary to sample a wider variety of animal hosts.

Abbreviations

RFLP: Restriction fragment length polymorphism; Hld: Hilar lymph node; Af: Amniotic fluid; nd: no data

Acknowledgements

The authors thank the laboratory staff in the animal hospitals of Henan Agricultural University and Henan University of Animal Husbandry and Economy for sample collection, and Professor Guosheng He from the Shanghai Veterinary Research Institute of the Chinese Academy of Agricultural Sciences for present the *T. gondii* RH strain.

Funding

This study was supported, in part, by the Key Program of the National Natural Science Foundation of China (31330079), the Innovation Scientists and Technicians Troop Construction Projects of Henan(134200510012), and the Key National Science and Technology Specific Projects (2012ZX10004220-001). The authors declare no conflict of interest associated with this study.

Table 3 Genetic PCR-RFLP *T. gondii* types in animals and humans in China

Host	No. of isolates	PCR RFLP genotype												References
		#10 (Type I)	#1 (Type II)	#2 (Type III)	#3 (Type II variant)	#3	#9	#18	#204	#205	#225	#213	#20	
Pig	65	15	0	0	1	4	43	0	0	0	0	2	0	[10, 11, 13–15, 25, 31, 36]
Cat	96	1	2	0	1	21	62	2	0	4	2	0	1	[30–33, 10, 15, 22–24, 28, 35]
yaks	2	0	0	0	0	0	2	0	0	0	0	0	0	[34]
Bird	6	0	0	0	4	0	2	0	0	0	0	0	0	[37]
Human	15	2	1	0	0	1	10	0	1	0	0	0	0	[10, 21, 32]
Sheep	1	0	1	0	0	0	0	0	0	0	0	0	0	[10]
Rat	4	0	0	0	0	0	4	0	0	0	0	0	0	[16]
Mouse	3	0	0	0	0	0	3	0	0	0	0	0	0	[16]
Goat	8	7	0	0	0	0	1	0	0	0	0	0	0	[36]
Vole	1	0	0	0	0	0	1	0	0	0	0	0	0	[31]
Chicken	1	0	0	0	0	0	0	0	0	0	1	0	0	[31]
Deer	6	0	0	0	0	0	6	0	0	0	0	0	0	[38]
Fox	5	2	0	0	0	0	3	0	0	0	0	0	0	[39]
Rabbit	1	0	0	1	0	0	0	0	0	0	0	0	0	[40]
Total	214	27 (12.6%)	4 (1.9%)	1 (0.5%)	6 (2.8%)	26 (12.1%)	137 (64.0%)	2 (0.9%)	1 (0.5%)	4 (1.9%)	3 (1.4%)	2 (0.9%)	1 (0.5%)	

uthors' contributions
onceived and designed the experiments: LXZ. Performed the experiments: YW and QER. Analyzed the data: FCY and YRY. Contributed to the writing the manuscript: HYW. All authors have read and approved the final anuscript.

ompeting interests
e authors declare no financial or commercial competing interest.

onsent for publication
ot applicable.

uthor details
College of Animal Science and Veterinary Medicine, Henan Agricultural niversity, Zhengzhou 450002, Henan, People's Republic of China.
Department of Animal Science, Henan Vocational College of Agriculture, hongmu, 451450 Henan, People's Republic of China.

eferences

Tenter AM, Heckeroth AR, Weiss LM. *Toxoplasma gondii*: from animals to humans. Int J Parasitol. 2000;30:1217–58.
Torrey EF, Bartko JJ, Lun ZR, Yolken RH. Antibodies to *Toxoplasma gondii* inpatients with schizophrenia: a meta-analysis. Schizophr Bull. 2007;33:729–36.
Weiss LM, Dubey JP. Toxoplasmosis: A history of clinical observations. Int J Parasitol. 2009;39:895–901.
Zhou P, Chen N, Zhang RL, Lin RQ, Zhu XQ. Food-borne parasitic zoonoses in China: perspective for control. Trends Parasitol. 2008;24:190–6.
Dubey JP. Toxoplasmosis in pigs–the last 20 years. Vet Parasitol. 2009;164:89–103.
Howe DK, Sibley LD. *Toxoplasma gondii* comprises three clonal lineages: correlation of parasite genotype with human disease. J Infect Dis. 1995;172:1561–6.
Khan A, Jordan C, Muccioli C, Vallochi AL, Rizzo LV, Belfort R Jr, et al. Genetic divergence of *Toxoplasma gondii* strains associated with ocular toxoplasmosis Brazil. Emerg Infect Dis. 2006;12:942–9.
Lehmann T, Marcet PL, Graham DH, Dahl ER, Dubey JP. Globalization and the population structure of *Toxoplasma gondii*. Proc Natl Acad Sci U S A. 2006;103:11423–8.
Dubey JP, Sundar N, Hill D, Velmurugan GV, Bandini LA, Kwok OC, et al. High prevalence and abundant atypical genotypes of *Toxoplasma gondii* isolated from lambs destined for human consumption in the USA. Int J Parasitol. 2008;38:999–1006.
). Zhou P, Zhang H, Lin RQ, Zhang DL, Song HQ, Su C, et al. Genetic characterization of *Toxoplasma gondii* isolates from China. Parasitol Int. 2009;58:193–5.
1. Zhou P, Nie H, Zhang LX, Wang HY, Yin CC, Su C, et al. Genetic characterization of *Toxoplasma gondii* isolates from pigs in China. J Parasitol. 2010;96:1027–9.
2. Zhou P, Sun XT, Yin CC, Yang JF, Yuan ZG, Yan HK, et al. Genetic characterization of *Toxoplasma gondii* isolates from pigs in southwestern China. J Parasitol. 2011;97:1193–5.
3. Jiang HH, Wang SC, Huang SY, Zhao L, Wang ZD, Zhu XQ, et al. Genetic Characterization of *Toxoplasma gondii* Isolates from Pigs in Jilin Province. Northeastern China Foodborne Pathog Dis. 2016;13:88–92.
4. Wang H, Wang T, Luo Q, Huo X, Wang L, Liu T, et al. Prevalence and genotypes of *Toxoplasma gondii* in pork from retail meat stores in Eastern China. Int J Food Microbiol. 2012;157:393–7.
5. Li YN, Nie X, Peng QY, Mu XQ, Zhang M, Tian MY, et al. Seroprevalence and genotype of *Toxoplasma gondii* in pigs, dogs and cats from Guizhou province. Southwest China Parasit Vectors. 2015;8:214.
6. Wang D, Liu Y, Jiang T, Zhang G, Yuan G, He J, et al. Seroprevalence and genotypes of *Toxoplasma gondii* isolated from pigs intended for human consumption in Liaoning province, northeastern China. Parasit Vectors. 2016;9:248.
7. Burg JL, Grover CM, Pouletty P, Boothroyd JC. Direct and sensitive detection of a pathogenic protozoan, *Toxoplasma gondii*, by polymerase chain reaction. J Clin Microbiol. 1989;27:1787–92.
18. Su C, Shwab EK, Zhou P, Zhu XQ, Dubey JP. Moving towards an integrated approach to molecular detection and identification of *Toxoplasma gondii*. Parasitology. 2010;137:1–11.
19. Deksne G, Kirjusina M. Seroprevalence of *Toxoplasma gondii* in domestic pigs (*Sus scrofa* domestica) and wild boars (*Sus scrofa*) in Latvia. J Parasitol. 2013;99:44–7.
20. Yan C, Liang LJ, Zhang BB, Lou ZL, Zhang HF, Shen X, et al. Prevalence and genotyping of *Toxoplasma gondii* in naturally-infected synanthropic rats (*Rattus norvegicus*) and mice (*Mus musculus*) in eastern China. Parasit Vectors. 2014;7:591.
21. Wang L, He LY, Meng DD, Chen ZW, Wen H, Fang GS, et al. Seroprevalence and genetic characterization of *Toxoplasma gondii* in cancer patients in Anhui Province. Eastern China Parasit Vectors. 2015;8:162.
22. Dubey JP, Zhu XQ, Sundar N, Zhang H, Kwok OC, Su C. Genetic and biologic characterization of *Toxoplasma gondii* isolates of cats from China. Vet Parasitol. 2007;145:352–6.
23. Tian YM, Huang SY, Miao Q, Jiang HH, Yang JF, Su C, et al. Genetic characterization of *Toxoplasma gondii* from cats in Yunnan Province. Southwestern China Parasit Vectors. 2014;7:178.
24. Chen ZW, Gao JM, Huo XX, Wang L, Yu L, Halm-Lai F, et al. Genotyping of *Toxoplasma gondii* isolates from cats in different geographic regions of China. Vet Parasitol. 2011;183:166–70.
25. Jiang HH, Huang SY, Zhou DH, Zhang XX, Su C, Deng SZ, et al. Genetic characterization of *Toxoplasma gondii* from pigs from different localities in China by PCR-RFLP. Parasit Vectors. 2013;6:227.
26. Qian WF, Yan WC, Wang TQ, Shao XD, Zhai K, Han LF, et al. Genetic characterization of *Toxoplasma gondii* from domestic animals in central China. Trop Biomed. 2015;32:540–4.
27. Yang Y, Ying Y, Verma SK, Cassinelli AB, Kwok OC, Liang H, et al. Isolation and genetic characterization of viable *Toxoplasma gondii* from tissues and feces of cats from the central region of China. Vet Parasitol. 2015;211:283–8.
28. Qian W, Wang H, Su C, Shan D, Cui X, Yang N, et al. Isolation and characterization of *Toxoplasma gondii* strains from stray cats revealed a single genotype in Beijing. China Vet Parasitol. 2012;187:408–13.
29. Zhang XX, Huang SY, Zhang YG, Zhang Y, Zhu XQ, Liu Q. First report of genotyping of *Toxoplasma gondii* in free-living *Microtus fortis* in northeastern China. J Parasitol. 2014;100:692–4.
30. Zhang FK, Wang HJ, Qin SY, Wang ZD, Lou ZL, Zhu XQ, et al. Molecular detection and genotypic characterization of *Toxoplasma gondii* in wild waterfowls in Jilin Province. Northeastern China Parasitol Int. 2015;64:576–8.
31. Wang L, Cheng HW, Huang KQ, Xu YH, Li YN, Du J, et al. *Toxoplasma gondii* prevalence in food animals and rodents in different regions of China: isolation, genotyping and mouse pathogenicity. Parasit Vectors. 2013;6:273.
32. Wang L, Chen H, Liu D, Huo X, Gao J, Song X, et al. Genotypes and mouse virulence of *Toxoplasma gondii* isolates from animals and humans in China. PLoS One. 2013;8 e53483.
33. Li M, Mo XW, Wang L, Chen H, Luo QL, Wen HQ, et al. Phylogeny and virulence divergency analyses of *Toxoplasma gondii* isolates from China. Parasit Vectors. 2014;7:133.
34. Qin SY, Zhou DH, Cong W, Zhang XX, Lou ZL, Yin MY, et al. Seroprevalence, risk factors and genetic characterization of *Toxoplasma gondii* in free-range white yaks (*Bos grunniens*) in China. Vet Parasitol. 2015;211:300–2.
35. Cong W, Meng QF, Blaga R, Villena I, Zhu XQ, Qian AD. Toxoplasma gondii, Dirofilaria immitis, feline immunodeficiency virus (FIV), and feline leukemia virus (FeLV) infections in stray and pet cats (*Felis catus*) in northwest China: co-infections and risk factors. Parasitol Res. 2016;115:217–23.
36. Miao Q, Huang SY, Qin SY, Yu X, Yang Y, Yang JF, et al. Genetic characterization of *Toxoplasma gondii* in Yunnan black goats (*Capra hircus*) in southwest China by PCR-RFLP. Parasit Vectors. 2015;8:57.
37. Cong W, Meng QF, Song HQ, Zhou DH, Huang SY, Qian AD, et al. Seroprevalence and genetic characterization of *Toxoplasma gondii* in three species of pet birds in China. Parasit Vectors. 2014;7:152.
38. Cong W, Qin SY, Meng QF, Zou FC, Qian AD, Zhu XQ. Molecular detection and genetic characterization of *Toxoplasma gondii* infection in sika deer (*Cervus nippon*) in China. Infect Genet Evol. 2016;39:9–11.
39. Zhang XX, Cong W, Ma JG, Lou ZL, Zhao Q, Meng QF, et al. First genetic characterization of *Toxoplasma gondii* infection in Arctic foxes (*Vulpes lagopus*) in China. Infect Genet Evol. 2016;44:127–9.

Experimental infection of pigs with H1 and H3 influenza A viruses of swine by using intranasal nebulization

Nobuhiro Takemae[1,2], Ryota Tsunekuni[1,2], Yuko Uchida[1,2], Toshihiro Ito[3] and Takehiko Saito[1,2,4*]

Abstract

Background: Experimental infection of pigs via direct intranasal or intratracheal inoculation has been mainly used to study the infectious process of influenza A viruses of swine (IAVs-S). Nebulization is known to be an alternative method for inoculating pigs with IAVs-S, because larger quantities of virus potentially can be delivered throughout the respiratory tract. However, there is very little data on the experimental infection of pigs by inhalation using nebulizer. In the current study, we used intranasal nebulization to inoculate pigs with 9 different IAVs-S—3 H1N1, 2 H1N2, and 4 H3N2 strains. We then assessed the process of infection by evaluating the clinical signs, nasal and oral viral shedding, and seroconversion rates of the pigs inoculated.

Results: Lethargy and sneezing were the predominant clinical signs among pigs inoculated with 7 of the 9 strains evaluated; the remaining 2 strains (1 H1N1 and 1 H1N2 isolate) failed to induce any clinical signs throughout the experiments. Significantly increased rectal temperatures were observed with an H1N1 or H3N2 strains between 1 and 3 days post-inoculation (dpi). In addition, patterns of nasal viral shedding differed among the strains: nasal viral shedding began on 1 dpi for 6 strains, with all 9 viruses being shed from 2 to 5 dpi. The detection of viral shedding was less sensitive from oral samples than nasal secretions. Viral shedding was not detected in either nasal or oral swabs after 10 dpi. According to hemagglutination–inhibition assays, all inoculated pigs had seroconverted to the inoculating virus by 14 dpi, with titers ranging from 10 to 320.

Conclusions: Our current findings show that intranasal nebulization successfully established IAV-S infections in pigs and demonstrate that clinical signs, viral shedding, and host immune responses varied among the strains inoculated.

Keywords: Influenza, Pig, Nebulization, Clinical sign, Viral shedding, Infection, Inoculation, Experimental

Background

Swine influenza, due to influenza A viruses of swine (IAVs-S), is a component of the porcine respiratory disease complex, which causes substantial economic losses in the pig industry. Swine influenza in pig farms typically is characterized by acute respiratory disease accompanied by fever, nasal discharge, cough, anorexia, and lethargy [1]. IAVs-S are spread among pigs through the nasopharyngeal route or by aerosols that are generated naturally through coughing and exhalation [2, 3]. Clinical signs quickly spread throughout piggeries or pig farms, and affected animals usually recover rapidly from illness [1]. In addition to the typical epizootic form showing clinical signs, IAVs-S have frequently been recovered from pigs without clinical signs, especially in the weaning and early-fattening stages [4–7]. Regardless of the severity, IAVs-S infection has adverse effects on the growth performance of pigs on farms [8].

Many experimental infection studies have been conducted to elucidate the infectious process of IAVs-S in pigs [9–15]. Pigs experimentally infected develop similar clinical signs as seen under natural infection [2], but different inoculation methods cause differences in pathogenicity, even among the same strain. Typically direct intranasal and intratracheal inoculation methods have been used to establish experimental infections in pigs

* Correspondence: taksaito@affrc.go.jp
[1]Division of Transboundary Animal Disease, National Institute of Animal Health, NARO, 3-1-5 Kannondai, Tsukuba, Ibaraki 305-0856, Japan
[2]Thailand–Japan Zoonotic Diseases Collaboration Center, Kasetklang, Chatuchak, Bangkok 10900, Thailand
Full list of author information is available at the end of the article

irect intranasal inoculation, in which the inoculum is elivered into the nasal cavity itself by using a syringe or ıucosal atomization device, is the easiest option, but it associated with variable efficacy in establishing infec-ons, because pigs may swallow most of the inoculum 2]. In contrast, intratracheal inoculation is believed to ıcrease the reliability and reproducibility of the course f infection in lung [16], but nasal shedding of virus ometimes is decreased in both titer and duration com-ared with direct intranasal inoculation of the same train [17]. Specifically, in the cited study, the duration f nasal virus shedding in the pigs inoculated intrana-ally with the avian-like IAV-S A/swine/Belgium/1/1998 H1N1) was 5 days, whereas that in pigs inoculated ıtratracheally with the same strain was 3 days [17]. In ddition, no respiratory disease symptoms occurred in igs inoculated intranasally with A/swine/Ghent/172/ 008 (H3N2), but swine inoculated intratracheally with he same strain developed prominent coughing, sneez-ıg, and nasal discharge [18]. Some researchers have dopted the mixed inoculation method [14, 19, 20]. For xample, Romagosa et al., infected the pigs intratrache-lly and intranasally with a total of 2 ml of the H1N1 AV-S at a titer of 1×10^6 $TCID_{50}$/ml [19].

Nebulization that may enable the delivery of large quan-ities of IAVs-S throughout the respiratory tract is ex-ected to be used for experimental infection with IAVs-S ı pigs [2]. However, the application of nebulization for xperimental inoculation of IAVs-S in pigs is limited [21–3], perhaps because this method is more labor-intensive han other methods. In the current study, we used intra-asal nebulization to infect pigs with several IAVs-S and hen assessed the infection process by measuring nasal nd oral viral shedding, determining seroconversion, and ıonitoring the clinical signs of infected pigs.

Methods

Influenza A viruses

To assess inoculation by the intranasal nebulization method, nine field strains of IAVs-S (Table 1) representing 7 genotypes were used and comprised two pandemic A(H1N1)2009 viruses (A(H1N1)pdm09v) [A/swine/Yamagata/11/2010(H1N1) (Yam10) and A/swine/Kagoshima/30/2015(H1N1) (Kag15)], a classical H1N2 IAVs-S [A/swine/Tochigi/1/2008(H1N2) (Toc08)], two H1 reassortants between classical H1 IAVs-S and A(H1N1)pdm09v [A/swine/Tochigi/1/2012(H1N2) (Toc12) and A/swine/Chiba/1-11/2015(H1N1) (Chi15)], a seasonal human-origin H3N2 IAVs-S [A/swine/Nagano/2000(H3N2) (Nag00)], an H3 reassortant between seasonal human-like H3N2 and A(H1N1)pdm09v (A/swine/Miyazaki/2/2013(H3N2) (Miy13)], and two North American Triple reassortant (TR) IAVs-S [A/swine/Yokohama/aq114/2011(H3N2) (Yok11) and A/swine/Minnesota/01146/2006(H3N2) (Min06)] (Table 1).

Four of these field strains (Yam10, Toc08, Toc12, and Miy13) were isolated from domestic pigs showing apparent clinical disease, such as sneezing, at pig farms. Strains Chi15 and Kag15 were isolated from domestic pigs without apparent clinical disease at pig farms. Nag00 that was isolated from a pig at a slaughterhouse was kindly supplied by the Nagano Environmental Conservation Research Institute, Japan. Yok11 that was isolated from a clinically healthy pig under quarantine at Animal Quarantine Office, Japan (Kanagawa, Yokohama, Japan) was submitted to the National Institute of Animal Health, Japan, for diagnosis. The other TR cluster IV strain, Min06 (kindly provided by Dr. Amy L. Vincent, US Department of Agriculture, Ames, IA, USA), was used for comparison with Japanese strains. All of the strains were isolated and grown by using MDCK cells before inoculation.

able 1 Gene constellation of influenza A viruses of swine used in this study

irus	Abbreviation	Subtype	H1 clade[c]	Genetic origin								Isolate ID or accession no.[d]
				HA	NA	PB2	PB1	PA	NP	M	NS	
/swine/Yamagata/11/2010[a]	Yam10	H1N1	1A.3.3.2	Pdm	Pdm	Pdm	Pdm	Pdm	Pdm	Pdm	Pdm	EPI_ISL_237800
/swine/Kagoshima/30/2015[a]	Kag15	H1N1	1A.3.3.2	Pdm	Pdm	Pdm	Pdm	Pdm	Pdm	Pdm	Pdm	EPI_ISL_237923
/swine/Chiba/1-11/2015[a]	Chi15	H1N1	1A.1	Cla	Pdm	Pdm	Pdm	Pdm	Cla	Pdm	Pdm	EPI_ISL_221941
/swine/Tochigi/1/2008[a]	Toc08	H1N2	1A.1-like	Cla	Hu	Cla	Cla	Cla	Cla	Cla	Cla	EPI_ISL_237796
/swine/Tochigi/1/2012[a]	Toc12	H1N2	1A.1-like	Cla	Hu	Pdm	Pdm	Pdm	Pdm	Pdm	Pdm	EPI_ISL_237798
/swine/Nagano/2000[a]	Nag00	H3N2	N/A	Hu	Hu	Hu	Hu	Hu	Hu	Hu	Hu	EPI_ISL_237795
/swine/Miyazaki/2/2013[a]	Miy13	H3N2	N/A	Hu	Hu	Pdm	Pdm	Pdm	Pdm	Pdm	Pdm	EPI_ISL_237794
/swine/Yokohama/aq114/2011	Yok11	H3N2	N/A	TR	TR	TR	TR	TR	TR	TR	TR	AB741020-AB741027
/swine/Minnesota/01146/2006[b]	Min06	H3N2	N/A	TR	TR	TR	TR	TR	TR	TR	TR	CY099035-CY099042

a classical swine lineage, *Hu* seasonal human-like lineage, *TR* North American triple-reassortant lineage
omplete genomic sequence was obtained during this study
Kindly provided by Dr. Amy L Vincent (US Department of Agriculture, Ames, IA, USA)
H1 clade was obtained by Swine H1 Clade Classification Tool [https://www.fludb.org/]. *N/A* not applicable
solate IDs from GISAID; accession numbers from GenBank

The complete genomic sequences of all isolates except for Yok11 and Min06 were obtained during the current study by using next-generation sequencing (Miseq, Illumina, San Diego, CA, USA) or Sanger sequencing (ABI model 3130, Applied Biosystems, Foster City, CA, USA) as previously described [24]. The complete genomic sequences of Yok11 were analyzed in our previous study [25] and those of Min06 had been already deposited in GenBank [https://www.ncbi.nlm.nih.gov/genbank/].

Animals and inoculation by nebulization

The study population comprised 40 specific pathogen-free (Large White × Landrace) crossbred pigs (obtained at 4 weeks of age; Zen-noh Premium Pig, Zen-Noh, Ibaraki, Japan) that were confirmed to be serologically negative for influenza A viruses (Influenza Ab Test Kit, IDEXX Laboratories, Westbrook, ME, USA) at 1 week prior to inoculation and were acclimated to Biosafety Level 3 housing (National Institute of Animal Health, Tsukuba, Ibaraki, Japan) for at least 5 days prior to inoculation. Four pigs were housed in each isolation unit (235 [w] × 365 [d] × 290 [h] cm; AIRTEC JAPAN, Tokyo, Japan), which were equipped with HEPA filters and passive airflow, throughout the experiment. Pigs in groups inoculated with Yam10, Toc08, or Toc12 were co-housed without partitions in each isolation unit, while all other pigs (including controls) were individually housed behind stainless-steel dividers in each isolation unit because the experimental rooms were renovated to assess the effect of IAV-S infection in individual pigs more accurately.

Just prior to inoculation, pigs (age, 5 weeks) were anesthetized with medetomidine (50 μg/kg IM; Domitor, Zenoaq, Fukushima, Japan) and midazolam (500 μg/kg IM; Dormicum, Astellas Pharma, Tokyo, Japan). Each strain was administered at a dose of 2×10^6 $TCID_{50}$/ml to 4 pigs by using a nebulizer unit (NE-U17, OMRON, Kyoto, Japan) with a fitted nose cone (Fig. 1). The device that is capable of generating aerosolized particle (diameter, 1 to 8 μm) by ultrasonic waves delivered th virus-containing particles at 0.5 ml/min for 4 min. Afte viral inoculation, anesthesia was reversed by using atipa mezole (5.0 mg/mL; Antisedan, Zenoaq). In additior four control pigs were inoculated with sterile PBS in th same manner.

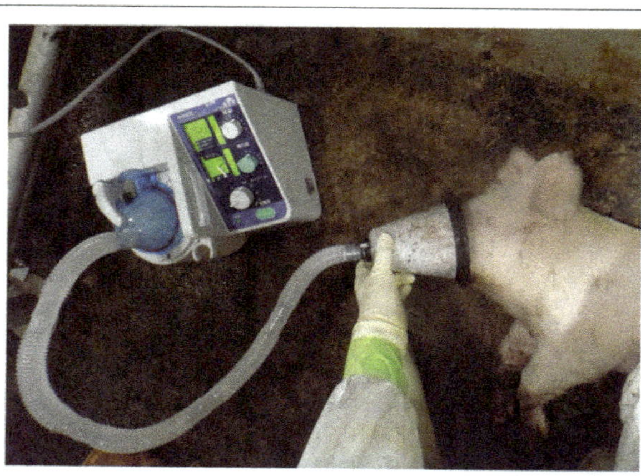

Fig. 1 Intranasal nebulization to inoculate pigs with IAVs-S by using the nebulizer unit

Clinical monitoring and sample collection

All of the pigs examined were observed every mornin for about 30 min for clinical signs of disease, such a sneezing, lethargy, and diarrhea until 14 dpi. The sneezing episode was defined either as a single sneeze or continuous sneezes. The lethargy was defined based on th response of each pig towards the investigators. The diarrhea was apparent when the rectal temperatures of the pigs were measured. The anorexia was defined b whether the pigs took the food or not. The pigs wer scored for the clinical signs as follows: sneezing [S] 0 – absent, 1 – present; lethargy [L] 0 – absent, 1 – present diarrhea [D] 0 – absent, 1 – present. All scores per pi group are accumulated for a total clinical score of eac individual pig. The score of anorexia was not accumulated because Yam10, Toc08, or Toc12 pig groups wer co-housed without partitions in each isolation unit which made unable to identify which pigs had anorexia.

Rectal temperatures of the pigs infected with Kag15 Chi15, Nag00, Miy13, Yok11, and Min06 and of the control pigs were measured in the morning at 0, 1, 2, 3 4, 5, 7, 10, and 14 dpi by using a thermometer (Thermoflex, Measure Technology, Taiwan). We were unable to obtain accurate rectal temperatures from the pigs inoculated with Yam10, Toc08, or Toc12 because these pig were able to move around freely before temperature assessment.

To evaluate viral shedding, nasal swab samples were collected individually from all pigs at 1, 2, 3, 4, 5, 7, 10 and 14 days post-infection (dpi) by using flocked swab with a plastic handle (Ex Swab 001, Denka Seiken Tokyo, Japan) and placed in 2 ml of medium (MEM containing penicillin [1000 unit/ml], streptomycin [1000 μg/ml], and Fungizone [25 μg/ml]; Thermo Fishe Scientific, Waltham, MA, USA], 0.01 M HEPES, and 0 5% bovine serum albumin); samples were centrifuged a 1400×*g* for 5 min, and supernatant was collected, aliquoted, and stored at – 80 °C until use.

In addition, oral swabs were collected at 1, 3, 5, 7, 10 and 14 dpi from the pigs infected with Kag15, Chi15 Yok11, Nag00, Miy13, and Min06, and rectal swabs were collected at 1, 2, 3, 4, 5, 7, 10, and 14 dpi from the pig infected with Yam10, Toc08, and Toc12. All of these samples were processed, aliquoted, and stored in the same manner as the nasal swab samples.

At 14 dpi, all pigs were anesthetized by using ketamine 30 mg/kg IM; Ketalar, Daiichi-Sankyo, Tokyo, Japan) nd euthanized by exsanguination. Then the lungs were emoved and evaluated macroscopically.

nalysis of viral shedding

'o remove any bacterial contaminants before use, super-atants from nasal, oral, and rectal swabs were thawed, ortexed, and filtered through polyvinylidene difluoride nembrane, which has low protein-binding ability (pore ize, 0.45 µm; catalog no. SLHVJ13SL, Millipore, Billerica, 1A, USA). Each sample was diluted ten-fold serially into erum-free MEM supplemented with 1 µg/ml TPCK-reated trypsin (Thermo Fisher Scientific) and antibiotics; 5 µl of each dilution was inoculated onto PBS-washed onfluent MDCK cells in 96-well plates. After 5 days of in-ubation at 37 °C under 5% CO_2, the $TCID_{50}$ of each sam-le was calculated according to hemagglutination activity y using 0.55% red blood cells from guinea pigs.

erologic assays

lood samples were collected at 3 days before inoculation nd at 14 dpi for use in ELISA and hemagglutination-nhibition (HAI or HI) assays. Sera were evaluated by LISA (Influenza Ab Test Kit, IDEXX Laboratories) ac-ording to the manufacturer's instructions. To remove onspecific hemagglutinin inhibitors from the samples be-ore their use in the HAI assay, sera were treated with a 0% suspension of kaolin (Sigma-Aldrich, St. Louis, MO, JSA) after heat inactivation at 56 °C for 30 min and then dsorbed to 0.55% guinea pig red blood cells for 20 min at oom temperature. HAI assays were conducted according o the WHO manual on Animal Influenza Diagnosis and urveillance [26].

tatistical analyses

Data were analyzed by using RStudio Version 1.0.136 [27]. n all analyses, the level of significance was $P < 0.05$.

esults

linical signs

noculation of IAVs-S by nebulization led to mild clinical igns in each group, except for those exposed to Yam10 r Toc08 (Table 2). The high clinical scores ranging rom 13 to 18 were observed in the Miy13, Yok11, Kag15, and Chi15 groups. All pigs from these groups emonstrated at least one clinical signs assessed. The Min06, Toc12, and Nag00 groups showed middle clinical cores ranging from 4 to 10. Two or three of the four igs showed at least one clinical sign in these groups. ethargy and sneezing were the most common signs mong the clinical signs observed and occurred between and 12 dpi in 18 and 15, respectively, of the 36 pigs in-culated with IAVs-S (Table 2). These clinical signs occurred most frequently in the Miy13 and Yok11 groups. Specifically, all pigs inoculated with Miy13 were lethargic and sneezing by 9 dpi, and 3 of the 4 pigs in the Yok11 group were similarly affected by 8 dpi (Table 2).

In addition, the clinical signs differed markedly between Yam10 and Kag15, although both are A(H1N1) pdm09 viruses (Table 1). Whereas all 4 pigs inoculated with Kag15 became lethargic between 3 and 7 dpi, those inoculated with Yam10 were clinically healthy throughout the experiments (Table 2). Overall, although clinical signs were most prevalent between 3 and 8 dpi, two pigs inoculated with Toc12 had diarrhea between 7 and 14 dpi (Table 2). In addition, one pig inoculated with Yok11 had anorexia from 10 to 12 dpi (Table 2).

We measured the body temperature of the pigs inoculated with Kag15, Chi15, Nag00, Miy13, Yok11, or Min06 and the control pigs. The normal body temperature (mean ± 1 SD on 0 dpi) of these 28 pigs was 38.9 ± 0.31 °C. Average rectal temperatures in 3 groups—those inoculated with Chi15, a reassortant H1 classical IAVs-S, and the 2 H3 TR IAVs-S, Yok11 and Min06—were higher than normal by 5 dpi ($P < 0.05$, Dunnet's test; Fig. 2). Specifically, 2 of the 4 pigs inoculated with Chi15 were febrile (that is, rectal temperature greater than 40 °C) at 2 and 3 dpi, as were 2 pigs in the Yok11 group. In addition, one of the pigs in the Yok11 group that had an increased temperature at 3 dpi later developed anorexia and a fever of 40.6 °C at 10 dpi (Table 2). In the Min06 group, the pigs' average rectal temperature was increased (39.4 °C ± 0.17) only at 1 dpi ($P < 0.05$, Dunnet's test). None of the groups inoculated with the A(H1N1)pdm09v Kag15 or the 2 human-like H3 IAVs-S, Nag00 and Miy13, developed a significantly increased rectal temperature throughout the experiment.

Viral shedding and macroscopic lesions

Inoculation of IAVs-S by inhalation using nebulizer unit evoked nasal viral shedding in all of the nine pig groups and the titer of each strain reached similar levels at titers of $10^{4.3}$ to $10^{5.4}$ $TCID_{50}$/ml at 4 dpi (Fig. 3). On the other hand, samples from the nasal swabs, except for those collected at 4 dpi, revealed different patterns of viral shedding among the evaluated strains (Fig. 3). Pigs typically began shedding virus at 1 dpi, but 2 pigs each in the Kag15 and Yok11 groups and 3 pigs in the Miy13 group did not shed any virus at 1 dpi. However all inoculated pigs shed virus at titers of $10^{1.2}$ to $10^{6.9}$ $TCID_{50}$/ml from 2 to 5 dpi. By 7 dpi, all the pigs except for 1 pig each in the Toc08 and Toc12 groups and 4 pigs in Min06 group had stopped shedding virus. No virus was shed from the inoculated pigs after 10 dpi.

According to nasal swab samples, the average virus titer did not differ between the groups inoculated with

Table 2 Clinical signs and clinical scores of each pig or pig group after inoculation with IAV-S by nebulization

Infected with	PigID	Day after infection												Total clinical scor
		3	4	5	6	7	8	9	10	11	12	13	14	
Yam10	1													0
	2													
	3													
	4													
Kag15	1	S, L		S		S, L					S			13
	2	L												
	3	S, L			L	L								
	4	L				L								
Chi15	1				L		L							13
	2	S		L	L		L							
	3			L	L		L							
	4			L	L	L	L							
Toc08	1													0
	2													
	3													
	4													
Toc12	1													7
	2	S												
	3												D	
	4					D	D	D		D			D	
Nag00	1			L	S	S		L						10
	2							L						
	3	S	S	S										
	4					S	S							
Miy13	1	S	S, L		L	S	S, L	S						18
	2		L				S, L							
	3				S		S, L							
	4			S			S, L	L						
Yok11	1			L	S				A	A	A			14
	2		S	L		L								
	3			L		L	L							
	4		S	L	S	L	S, L							
Min06	1													4
	2													
	3		S	S										
	4	S					S							

A anorexia, *L* Lethargy, *S* sneezing, *D* diarrhea

[a]Data for days 1 and 2 are not shown because none of the pigs in any group showed any clinical signs evaluated in this study

Yam10 and Kag15, the 2 A(H1N1)pdm09v strains, throughout the experiment. However, unlike those in the Kag15 group, all of the pigs in Yam10 group shed virus, at an average titer of $10^{2.7}$ $TCID_{50}$/ml, at 1 dpi (Fig. 3). The titers of the A(H1N1)pdm09 viruses were numerically lower than those of other classical H1 and H3N2 IAVs-S. The average titers of the Kag15 grou were lower than those of pigs inoculated with Toc08 Toc12, Chi15, or Nag00 at 1 dpi and lower than those o the Toc12, Miy13, and Min06 groups at 5 dpi ($P < 0.05$ Tukey HSD test) (Fig. 3). In addition, Yam10 titers wer lower than those of Chi15 and Min06 at 2 dpi and lowe

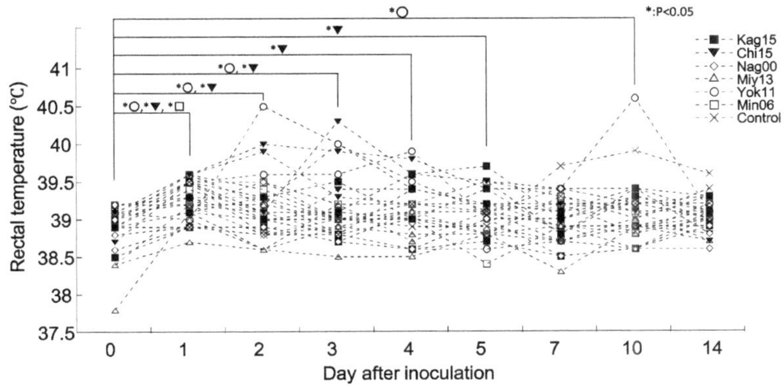

Fig. 2 Rectal temperatures of pigs from 0 to 14 days after inoculation. Pig groups in which the average body temperature was significantly ($P < 0.05$, Dunnet's test) higher than normal (38.9 ± 0.31 °C; calculated by using 0-dpi data from all pigs tested) are shown by asterisks

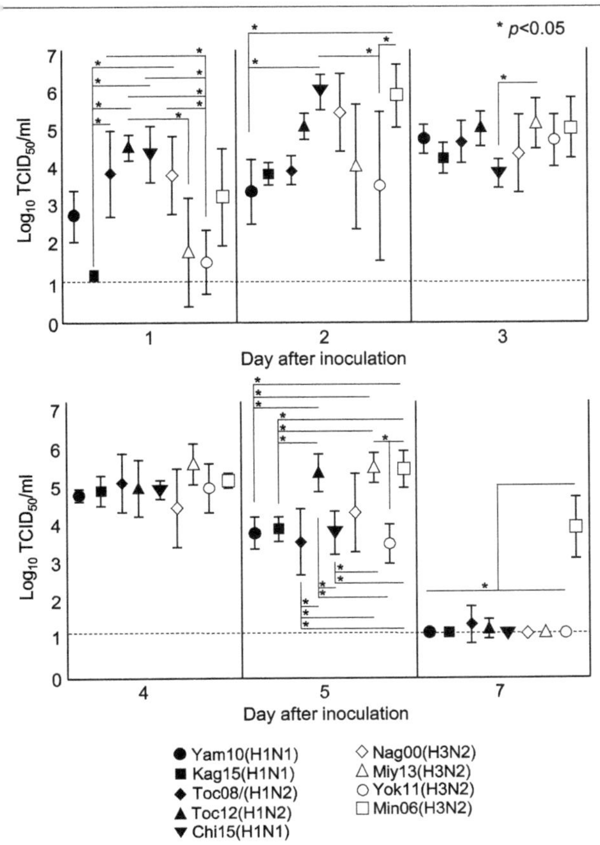

Fig. 3 Viral titers (mean ± 1 standard deviation) from nasal swabs of pigs inoculated with various IAVs-S by nebulization. No virus was shed from the control pigs throughout the experiment or from the inoculated pigs after 10 dpi. *, Significant difference ($P < 0.05$, Tukey HSD test) between groups on the same day; the dashed line indicates the limit of detection ($10^{1.1}$TCID$_{50}$/ml)

than those of Toc12, Miy13, and Min06 at 5 dpi ($P < 0.05$, Tukey HSD test) (Fig. 3). Among the groups inoculated with classical H1 virus, the titer of Toc12 peaked at $10^{5.2}$ TCID$_{50}$/ml at 5 dpi and was higher than the titers of Toc08 and Chi15 on the same day ($P < 0.05$, Tukey HSD test) (Fig. 3). No significant differences in virus titers occurred between the human-like H3 IAVs-S Nag00 and Miy13. Between the TR IAVs-S, the average titers of the Min06 group at 2, 5, and 7 dpi were higher than those of the Yok11 group ($P < 0.05$, Tukey HSD test) (Fig. 3). In addition, Min06 replicated the most efficiently among the IAVs-S tested; the average Min06 titer of $10^{3.8}$ TCID$_{50}$/ml at 7 dpi was higher than those of all other groups ($P < 0.05$, Tukey HSD test) (Fig. 3).

We also collected oral fluids from the pigs inoculated with Kag15, Chi15, Yok11, Nag00, Miy13, or Min06 to compare the viral shedding data between oral and nasal swab samples (Fig. 4). Viral titers determined from oral swabs were significantly lower than those from nasal

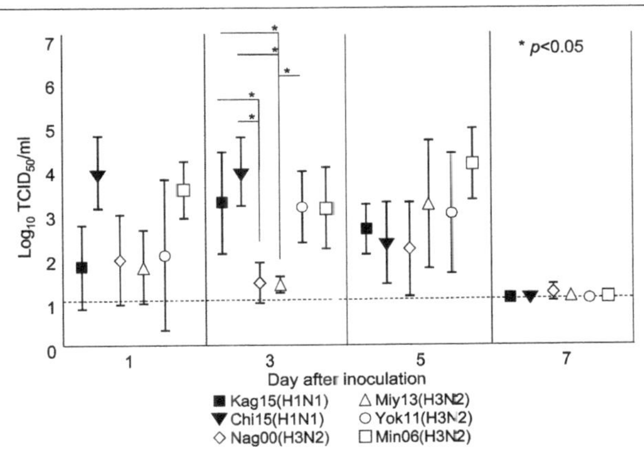

Fig. 4 Viral titers (mean ± 1 standard deviation) from oral swabs of pigs inoculated with Kag15, Chi15, Nag00, Miy13, Yok11, and Min06 by nebulization. No virus was shed from the inoculated pigs after 10 dpi. *, Significant difference ($P < 0.05$, Tukey HSD test) between groups on the same day; dashed line indicates the limit of detection ($10^{1.1}$TCID$_{50}$/ml)

swabs in all 6 groups at either 3 or 5 dpi. The average oral virus titers at 5 dpi were $10^{2.6}$ $TCID_{50}$/ml for Kag15, $10^{2.3}$ $TCID_{50}$/ml for Chi15, $10^{4.1}$ $TCID_{50}$/ml for Min 06, $10^{2.2}$ $TCID_{50}$/ml for Nag00, and $10^{3.2}$ $TCID_{50}$/ml for Miy13 and were lower than the nasal swab titers of $10^{3.8}$ $TCID_{50}$/ml, $10^{3.7}$ $TCID_{50}$/ml, $10^{5.3}$ $TCID_{50}$/ml, $10^{4.2}$ $TCID_{50}$/ml, and $10^{5.3}$ $TCID_{50}$/ml, respectively, at the same time point ($P < 0.05$; t-test). Yok11 yielded an oral virus titer of $10^{3.1}$ $TCID_{50}$/ml at 3 dpi, which was lower than the nasal virus titer with ($10^{4.6}$ $TCID_{50}$/ml) on the same day ($P < 0.05$, t-test). In addition, Nag00 yielded oral virus titers of $10^{1.9}$ $TCID_{50}$/ml at 1 dpi and $10^{1.4}$ $TCID_{50}$/ml at 3 dpi, which were significantly lower than the nasal virus titers with ($10^{3.8}$ $TCID_{50}$/ml and $10^{4.3}$ $TCID_{50}$/ml) on the same day ($P < 0.05$, t-test). Among the 6 groups, the average titers of the Nag00 and Miy13 groups were significantly lower than those of pigs inoculated with Kag15 or Chi15 at 3 dpi ($P < 0.05$, Tukey HSD test) (Fig. 4). The average titer of the Miy13 group was also significantly lower than that of pigs inoculated with Yok11 at 3 dpi ($P < 0.05$, Tukey HSD test) (Fig. 4). No virus was detected in the oral fluid of all the inoculated pigs after 10 dpi. Rectal swabs from pigs inoculated with Yam10, Toc08, or Toc12 failed to yield any virus throughout the study.

At 14 dpi, we removed the lungs from all pigs for macroscopic evaluation. Pneumonia-like lesions were present in one pig inoculated with Toc08. These lesions were purple to dark-red, consolidated areas in the apical parts of the cranial, middle, and caudal lobes (data not shown). In contrast, none of the other pigs (infected or control) had any macroscopic lung lesions at 14 dpi.

Serologic assays

By 14 dpi, all of the 36 inoculated pigs had seroconverted, according to results of HAI assays using each challenge strain as the antigen (Table 3). In contrast, the mean sample: negative ratios of the ELISAs at 14 dpi tended to be lower than the values before virus inoculation, such that 23 of the 36 virus-inoculated pigs were considered to be seronegative at 14 dpi (Table 3).

The kinetics of the immune responses differed among the IAVs-S we evaluated. For example, among the groups inoculated with classical H1 strains, the immune responses in pigs against Toc08 were relatively lower than those against the reassortant classical H1 IAVs-S (Toc12 and Chi15). Specifically, the geometric mean HAI titers at 14 dpi were 14, 95, and 113 in the Toc08, Toc12, and Chi15 groups, respectively. In addition, all of the pigs inoculated with Toc08 were considered seronegative according to ELISA, but at least 3 pigs each in the Toc12 and Chi15 groups were seropositive. In addition, whereas all of the H3N2-inoculated pigs had HAI titers greater than 80, only one pig in each of these groups

Table 3 Serologic analyses of sera obtained 3 days before (Pre) and 14 days post-infection (dpi)

Virus	Pig ID	HAI titer[a]		S:N of ELISA[b]		
		Pre	14 dpi	Pre		14 dpi
Yam10(H1N1)	1	< 10	80	0.95	–	0.72
	2	< 10	80	0.86	–	0.88
	3	< 10	80	0.97	–	0.68
	4	< 10	80	0.88	–	0.85
Kag15(H1N1)	1	< 10	20	0.96	–	0.73
	2	< 10	160	0.89	–	0.31
	3	< 10	160	0.91	–	0.61
	4	< 10	80	0.93	–	0.53
Toc08(H1N2)	1	< 10	20	1.04	–	0.76
	2	< 10	20	1.02	–	0.62
	3	< 10	10	0.91	–	0.66
	4	< 10	10	1.06	–	0.66
Toc12(H1N2)	1	< 10	80	0.85	–	0.71
	2	< 10	80	0.78	–	0.56
	3	< 10	160	0.96	–	0.39
	4	< 10	80	0.90	–	0.52
Chi15(H1N1)	1	< 10	160	1.08	–	0.59
	2	< 10	80	0.91	–	0.56
	3	< 10	160	0.87	–	0.55
	4	< 10	80	0.86	–	0.56
Nag00(H3N2)	1	< 10	160	0.94	–	0.79
	2	< 10	80	0.71	–	0.74
	3	< 10	80	0.70	–	0.72
	4	< 10	160	0.84	–	0.44
Miy13(H3N2)	1	< 10	320	0.72	–	0.78
	2	< 10	320	1.02	–	0.78
	3	< 10	160	0.70	–	0.59
	4	< 10	160	0.73	–	0.72
Yok11(H3N2)	1	< 10	320	0.93	–	0.74
	2	< 10	80	0.93	–	0.70
	3	< 10	160	0.95	–	0.62
	4	< 10	160	0.82	–	0.47
Min06(H3N2)	1	< 10	320	1.00	–	0.72
	2	< 10	320	0.68	–	0.96
	3	< 10	160	0.93	–	0.96
	4	< 10	80	0.75	–	0.49
Control	1	< 10	< 10	0.84	–	0.95
	2	< 10	< 10	0.82	–	0.93
	3	< 10	< 10	0.82	–	0.95
	4	< 10	< 10	0.86	–	0.95

[a]Homologous viruses were used as antigens in each group. Sera from control pigs were tested against classical H1 (Chi15), A(H1N1)pdm09v (Kag15), and triple-reassortant (Yok11) IAVs-S as antigens
[b]For swine sera, a sample:negative (S:N) ratio < 0.6 was considered positive (+; –, negative), according to the manufacturer's instructions

'as considered seropositive according to ELISA (Table 3) suggesting no clear correlation between HAI titers and LISA sample: negative values at 14 dpi.

iscussion

Ve demonstrated that nebulization successfully evoked iral shedding from nasal cavities and seroconversion in ll of the pigs inoculated with any of the IAVs-S evaluted in this study. As might have been expected [2], the ıtranasal nebulization method was highly effective for elivering the viruses to the upper respiratory tracts of igs. In fact, in humans and ferrets, aerosolized influenza iruses efficiently reach both the upper respiratory tract s well as deep into the lower regions [28, 29]. The ebulizer we used in the current study produces erosolized particles that are 1 to 8 μm in diameter. Vhereas aerosol particles larger than 6 μm are trapped referentially in the upper respiratory tract, those maller than 5 μm are efficiently deposited in the lower espiratory tract [28]. In one study, nebulization of swine (H1N1)pdm09v successfully infected pigs at a much ower dose than did direct intranasal administration 22]. Together these previous findings and our current esults support the idea that the nebulization method an deliver sufficient virus to establish IAV-S infection in igs.

The severity of clinical signs and duration of virus hedding in pigs appears to vary not only according to ne IAV-S inoculated but also according to protocols sed. In our present study, the severity of the clinical igns in pigs infected through nebulization differed mong the different strains of IAVs-S. For example, hi15 induced lethargy more often than did the other I1 IAVs-S, Toc08 and Toc12. In addition, among H3N2 AVs-S, Yok11 and Min06, but not Nag00 or Miy13, aused pigs to become febrile. Recent studies have reealed differences in virulence among IAVs-S strains isoıted after 2009. For example, 6 different TR H3N2 AVs-S that resulted from repeated spillover of A(H1N1) dm09v from humans to pigs demonstrated distinct paterns of viral shedding and different degrees of pathlogy in experimentally infected pigs [14]. In addition, isease characteristics, such as percentage of pneumonia nd viral titer in lungs, reportedly differed significantly mong H1 strains from the United States [12]. In the ited study, H1 IAVs-S isolated after 1999 tended to prouce more severe disease and greater viral shedding in igs than did classical strains, such as A/swine/Iowa/15/ 930 (H1N1).

In our current study, results from the HAI test and LISA assay were discordant in some cases. The Influnza Ab Test Kit (Idexx Laboratories) detects only the ntibodies produced against a highly conserved epitope f the influenza A nucleoprotein (NP) that binds virus RNA [30]. In contrast, HAI tests detect anti-HA antibodies, which predominate in the sera of animals infected with influenza A viruses. In general, HAI antibodies can be detected in the sera of pigs by 7 dpi and peak 2 to 3 weeks after primary infection [31, 32]. However, NP-specific IgG antibody responses after primary infection with IAVs-S arise later than HAI antibodies in pig serum. For example, the ELISA titers of pigs inoculated with 10^8 $TCID_{50}$/ml of avian-like H1N1 or H3N2 IAVs-S peaked 1 month after infection [33]. Together these data support our results in which ELISA titers were undetectable at 14 dpi in pigs that were shown to be infected in light of viral shedding.

Oral fluids collected from pigs by hanging a cotton rope in the pen have been proposed to be a useful tool for the detection of porcine circovirus 2 and porcine reproductive and respiratory syndrome virus in the context of increasing the cost-effectiveness and efficiency of sampling for surveillance of swine herds [34, 35]. However, for IAVs-S, our results indicate that virus titers from oral swabs are lower than those from nasal swabs, even when collected from the same pigs at the same time point by using flocked swabs. Similarly, other experiments have shown that the virus isolation rate from pigs experimentally inoculated with IAVs-S is lower from oral swabs than nasal swabs [36, 37]. However those studies relied on real-time RT-PCR analysis rather than virus isolation, suggesting that oral fluids might effectively be used for the detection of IAVs-S genes. In another study, viral RNA in pigs experimentally infected with A/swine/Gent/28/2010 (H1N1) was detectable in oral fluids at 21 dpi but in nasal swabs at 5 dpi [38]. Therefore, virus detection using pen-based oral fluid samples might decrease the cost and number of samples per farm compared with nasal swab collection from individual pigs. However, great care needs to be exercised during the genetic characterization of IAVs-S obtained from pen-based oral fluid samples, because whether the detected IAVs-S are reassortant viruses or multiple viruses derived from several pigs cannot be determined. That genetically different IAVs-S circulate concurrently within a single farm is unsurprising [6, 24, 39].

Conclusions

In conclusion, regardless of the strain, intranasal nebulization of IAVs-S successfully established infections in all of the inoculated pigs. The nebulization method is already well established for the experimental infection of horses with influenza A viruses [40, 41]. Our current study demonstrates that nebulization can be useful for the experimental infection of pigs as well. The application of this method to pigs has the potential to advance our understanding of the progression of IAVs-S infections within and between pigs and to facilitate vaccine efficacy tests in swine.

Abbreviations

A(H1N1)pdm09v: Pandemic A(H1N1)2009 virus; dpi: Days post-inoculation; IAV-S: Influenza A virus of swine; $TCID_{50}$: 50% of tissue infectious dose

Acknowledgments

We thank Drs. Amy Vincent (United States Department of Agriculture, Ames, IA, USA) and Mariko Kashiwabara (Zoetis Japan, Tokyo, Japan) for providing A/swine/Minnesota/01146/2006 (H3N2) and A/swine/Kagoshima/30/2015 (H1N1), respectively. We also thank Dr. Yuiko Hayakawa (Idias Swine Clinic, Chiba, Japan) for collecting the pig nasal swab samples from which the A/swine/Chiba/1-11/2015 (H1N1) was isolated.

Funding

This work is supported by the JRA Livestock Promotion Project.

Authors' contributions

TS and TI designed the study and coordinated the research. NT, RT, and YU performed the experiments and analyzed the data. NT and TS prepared the manuscript. All authors read and approved the final manuscript.

Consent for publication

Not applicable.

Competing interests

The authors declare that they have no competing interests.

Author details

[1]Division of Transboundary Animal Disease, National Institute of Animal Health, NARO, 3-1-5 Kannondai, Tsukuba, Ibaraki 305-0856, Japan. [2]Thailand–Japan Zoonotic Diseases Collaboration Center, Kasetklang, Chatuchak, Bangkok 10900, Thailand. [3]The Avian Zoonosis Research Center, Faculty of Agriculture, Tottori University, 4-101 Koyama-cho Minami, Tottori, Tottori 680-8550, Japan. [4]United Graduate School of Veterinary Sciences, Gifu University, 1-1, Yanagito, Gifu, Gifu 501-1112, Japan.

References

1. Olsen CW, Brown IH, Easterday BC, Van Reeth K. Swine influenza. In: Straw DJ, Zimmerman JJ, d'Alaaire S, Taylor DJ, editors. Diseases of swine. 9th ed. Oxford: Blackwell Publishing; 2006. p. 469–82.
2. Janke BH. Clinicopathological Features of Swine Influenza. In: Richt JA, Webby RJ, editors. Swine Influenza. Heidelberg: Springer Berlin Heidelberg; 2013. p. 69–83.
3. Alonso C, Raynor PC, Davies PR, Torremorell M. Concentration, Size Distribution, and Infectivity of Airborne Particles Carrying Swine Viruses. PLoS One. 2015;10:e0135675.
4. Takemae N, Shobugawa Y, Nguyen PT, Nguyen T, Nguyen TN, To TL, et al. Effect of herd size on subclinical infection of swine in Vietnam with influenza A viruses. BMC Vet Res. 2016;12:227.
5. Ozawa M, Matsuu A, Yonezawa K, Igarashi M, Okuya K, Kawabata T, et al. Efficient isolation of swine influenza viruses by age-targeted specimen collection. J Clin Microbiol. 2015;53:1331–8.
6. Corzo CA, Culhane M, Juleen K, Stigger-Rosser E, Ducatez MF, Webby RJ, et al. Active surveillance for influenza A virus among swine, Midwestern United States, 2009–2011. Emerg Infect Dis. 2013;19:954–60.
7. Takemae N, Parchariyanon S, Ruttanapumma R, Hiromoto Y, Hayashi T, Uchida Y, et al. Swine influenza virus infection in different age groups of pigs in farrow-to-finish farms in Thailand. Virol J. 2011;8:537.
8. Er C, Lium B, Tavornpanich S, Hofmo PO, Forberg H, Hauge AG, et al. Adverse effects of Influenza A(H1N1)pdm09 virus infection on growth performance of Norwegian pigs - a longitudinal study at a boar testing station. BMC Vet Res. 2014;10:284.
9. Landolt GA, Karasin AI, Phillips L, Olsen CW. Comparison of the Pathogenesis of Two Genetically Different H3N2 Influenza A Viruses in Pigs. J Clin Microbiol. 2003;41:1936–41.
10. Richt JA, Lager KM, Janke BH, Woods RD, Webster RG, Webby RJ. Pathogenic and antigenic properties of phylogenetically distinct reassortan H3N2 swine influenza viruses cocirculating in the United States. J Clin Microbiol. 2003;41:3198–205.
11. Choi Y, Goyal S, Joo H. Evaluation of transmission of swine influenza type A subtype H1N2 virus in seropositive pigs. Am J Vet Res. 2004;3:303–6.
12. Vincent AL, Lager KM, Ma W, Lekcharoensuk P, Gramer MR, Loiacono C, et al. Evaluation of hemagglutinin subtype 1 swine influenza viruses from the United States. Vet Microbiol. 2006;118:212–22.
13. Kitikoon P, Nilubol D, Erickson BJ, Janke BH, Hoover TC, Sornsen SA, et al. The immune response and maternal antibody interference to a heterologous H1N1 swine influenza virus infection following vaccination. Vet Immunol Immunopathol. 2006;112:117–28.
14. Rajão DS, Walia RR, Campbell B, Gauger PC, Janas-Martindale A, Killian ML, et al. Reassortment between Swine H3N2 and 2009 Pandemic H1N1 in the United States Resulted in Influenza A Viruses with Diverse Genetic Constellations with Variable Virulence in Pigs. J Virol. 2017;91:13 e01763–16
15. Ma W, Vincent AL, Lager KM, Janke BH, Henry SC, Rowland RRR, et al. Identification and characterization of a highly virulent triple reassortant H1N1 swine influenza virus in the United States. Virus Genes. 2009;40:28–36
16. Winkler GC, Cheville NF. Ultrastructural morphometric investigation of early lesions in the pulmonary alveolar region of pigs during experimental swine influenza infection. Am J Pathol. 1986;122:541–52.
17. De Vleeschauwer A, Atanasova K, Van Borm S, van den Berg T, Rasmussen TB, Uttenthal Å, et al. Comparative Pathogenesis of an Avian H5N2 and a Swine H1N1 Influenza Virus in Pigs. PLoS One. 2009;4:e6662.
18. Pomorska-Mol M, Kwit K, Markowska-Daniel I, Kowalski C, Pejsak Z. Local an systemic immune response in pigs during subclinical and clinical swine influenza infection. Res Vet Sci. 2014;97:412–21.
19. Romagosa A, Allerson M, Gramer M, Joo H, Deen J, Detmer S, et al. Vaccination of influenza a virus decreases transmission rates in pigs. Vet Re 2011;42:120.
20. Kitikoon P, Vincent A, Gauger P, Schlink S, Bayles D, Gramer M, et al. Pathogenicity and transmission in pigs of the novel A(H3N2)v influenza virus isolated from humans and characterization of swine H3N2 viruses isolated in 2010-2011. J Virol. 2012;86:6804–14.
21. Thacker EL, Thacker BJ, Janke BH. Interaction between Mycoplasma hyopneumoniae and Swine Influenza Virus. J Clin Microbiol. 2001;39:2525–30.
22. Hemmink JD, Morgan SB, Aramouni M, Everett H, Salguero FJ, Canini L, et al. Distinct immune responses and virus shedding in pigs following aerosol, intra-nasal and contact infection with pandemic swine influenza A virus, A(H1N1)09. Vet Res. 2016;47:103.
23. Swenson SL, Vincent LL, Lute BM, Janke BH, Lechtenberg KE, Landgraf JG, et a A Comparison of Diagnostic Assays for the Detection of Type a Swine Influenza Virus from Nasal Swabs and Lungs. J Vet Diagn Invest. 2001;13:36–42
24. Takemae N, Harada M, Nguyen PT, Nguyen T, Nguyen TN, Tol TL, et al. Influenza A Viruses of Swine (IAV-S) in Vietnam from 2010 to 2015: Multiple Introductions of A(H1N1)pdm09 Viruses into the Pig Population and Diversifying Genetic Constellations of Enzootic IAV-S. J Virol. 2017;91(1): e01490–16.
25. Matsuu A, Uchida Y, Takemae N, Mawataril T, Yoneyama S, Kasai T, et al. Genetic characterization of swine influenza viruses isolated in Japan between 2009 and 2012. Microbiol Immunol. 2012;56:792–803.
26. WHO.WHO Manual on Animal Influenza Diagnosis and Surveillance. In:WHO Global Influenza Programme. World Health Organization. 2002. http://www.who.int/csr/resources/publications/influenza/en/whocdscsrncs20025rev.pdf. Accessed 07 Apr 2017.
27. RStudio-Team.RStudio. In:Integrated Development for R. RStudio, Inc. 2015. http://www.rstudio.com/. Accessed 18 Apr 2017.
28. Raymond T. Review of Aerosol Transmission of Influenza A Virus. Emerg Infect Dis. 2006;12:1657.

9. Gustin KM, Belser JA, Wadford DA, Pearce MB, Katz JM, Tumpey TM, et al. Influenza virus aerosol exposure and analytical system for ferrets. Proc Natl Acad Sci U S A. 2011;108:8432–7.
0. IDEXX-Laboratories.Influenza A Ab Test Information Sheet. In:IDEXX Laboratories, Inc. 2010. https://www.idexx.com/en/livestock/livestock-tests/swine-tests/idexx-swine-influenza-virus-ab-test/. Accessed 22 Mar 2018.
1. Larsen DL, Karasin A, Zuckermann F, Olsen CW. Systemic and mucosal immune responses to H1N1 influenza virus infection in pigs. Vet Microbiol. 2000;74:117–31.
2. Van Reeth K, Labarque G, Pensaert M. Serological profiles after consecutive experimental infections of pigs with European H1N1, H3N2, and H1N2 swine influenza viruses. Viral Immunol. 2006;19:373–82.
3. Heinen P, De Boer-Luijtze E, Bianchi T. Respiratory and systemic humoral and cellular immune responses of pigs to a heterosubtypic influenza A virus infection. J Gen Virol. 2001;82:2697–707.
4. Ramirez A, Wang C, Prickett JR, Pogranichniy R, Yoon K-J, Main R, et al. Efficient surveillance of pig populations using oral fluids. Prev Vet Med. 2012;104:292–300.
5. De Regge N, Cay B. Comparison of PRRSV Nucleic Acid and Antibody Detection in Pen-Based Oral Fluid and Individual Serum Samples in Three Different Age Categories of Post-Weaning Pigs from Endemically Infected Farms. PLoS One. 2016;11:e0166300.
6. Detmer SE, Patnayak DP, Jiang Y, Gramer MR, Goyal SM. Detection of Influenza a Virus in Porcine Oral Fluid Samples. J Vet Diagn Invest. 2011;23: 241–7.
7. Goodell CK, Prickett J, Kittawornrat A, Zhou F, Rauh R, Nelson W, et al. Probability of detecting influenza A virus subtypes H1N1 and H3N2 in individual pig nasal swabs and pen-based oral fluid specimens over time. Vet Microbiol. 2013;166:450–60.
8. Decorte I, Steensels M, Lambrecht B, Cay AB, De Regge N. Detection and Isolation of Swine Influenza A Virus in Spiked Oral Fluid and Samples from Individually Housed, Experimentally Infected Pigs: Potential Role of Porcine Oral Fluid in Active Influenza A Virus Surveillance in Swine. PLoS One. 2015; 10:e0139586.
9. Abe H, Mine J, Parchariyanon S, Takemae N, Boonpornprasert P, Ubonyaem N, et al. Co-infection of influenza A viruses of swine contributes to effective shuffling of gene segments in a naturally reared pig. Virology. 2015;484: 203–12.
0. Mumford JA, Hannant D, Jessett DM. Experimental infection of ponies with equine influenza (H3N8) viruses by intranasal inoculation or exposure to aerosols. Equine Vet J. 1990;22:93–8.
1. Yamanaka T, Nemoto M, Bannai H, Tsujimura K, Kondo T, Matsumura T, et al. Assessment of antigenic difference of equine influenza virus strains by challenge study in horses. Influenza Other Respi Viruses. 2016;10:536–9.

10

Attenuated *Actinobacillus pleuropneumoniae* double-deletion mutant S-8Δ*clpP/apxIIC* confers protection against homologous or heterologous strain challenge

Fang Xie[†], Gang Li[†], Long Zhou, Yanhe Zhang, Ning Cui, Siguo Liu and Chunlai Wang[*]

Abstract

Background: *Actinobacillus pleuropneumoniae* is the etiological agent of porcine pleuropneumonia, which leads to large economic losses to the swine industry worldwide. In this study, S-8△*clpP*△*apxIIC*, a double-deletion mutant of *A. pleuropneumoniae* was constructed, and its safety and protective efficacy were evaluated in pigs.

Results: The S-8△*clpP*△*apxIIC* mutant exhibited attenuated virulence in a murine (BALB/c) model, and caused no detrimental effects on pigs even at a dose of up to 1.0×10^9 CFU. Furthermore, the S-8△*clpP*△*apxIIC* mutant was able to induce a strong immune response in pigs, which included high levels of IgG1 and IgG2, stimulated gamma interferon (IFN-γ), interleukin 12 (IL-12), and interleukin 4 (IL-4) production, and conferred effective protection against the lethal challenge with *A. pleuropneumoniae* serovars 7 or 5a. The pigs in the S-8△*clpP*△*apxIIC* immunized groups have no lesions and reduced bacterial loads in the lung tissue after challenge.

Conclusions: The data obtained in this study suggest that the S-8△*clpP*△*apxIIC* mutant can serve as a highly immunogenic and potential live attenuated vaccine candidate against *A. pleuropneumoniae* infection.

Keywords: *Actinobacillus pleuropneumoniae*, Live attenuated vaccine, Porcine pleuropneumonia

Background

Actinobacillus pleuropneumoniae is a highly adapted pathogen that causes porcine pleuropneumonia, which is an extremely contagious respiratory disease [1]. The disease is often fatal and characterized by fibrinous, hemorrhagic, and necrotic lung lesions, which remains an important global problem in the swine industry [2]. Transmission of the pathogen occurs through an aerosol route during close contact with diseased pigs or asymptomatic carriers, and it can infect pigs of different ages [3]. The clinical features can span from peracute disease with quick death to chronic infection leading to reduced growth rates, and the pigs frequently become asymptomatic carriers. To date, 16 serovars of *A. pleuropneumoniae* have been identified and all serovars can cause disease [4, 5]. Although the incidence of outbreaks has reduced in the developed countries, *A. pleuropneumoniae* remains one of the main causes of economic loss to the global swine production, especially in developing countries [6].

Antimicrobial therapy has been used to prevent and control porcine pleuropneumonia, but it results in the growing problems of multidrug-resistance and antibiotic residues in pigs [7–9]. Concern was raised that multidrug-resistance could be transmitted between different pathogens in pigs followed through the food chain to produce a risk to human health. Thus, vaccination becomes the most effective method of preventing *A. pleuropneumoniae* infection. It has been found that pigs surviving natural infection were protected against homologous and heterologous serovar infection [10]. It is speculated that live bacteria can induce in vivo expression of protective antigens and confer cross-protection. Thus, the application of an attenuated live vaccine is an

* Correspondence: chunlai.w@hvri.ac.cn
[†]Equal contributors
State Key Laboratory of Veterinary Biotechnology, Division of Bacterial Diseases, Harbin Veterinary Research Institute, Chinese Academy of Agricultural Sciences, Harbin, Heilongjiang, People's Republic of China

leal approach for vaccination against diversified sero-ars of *A. pleuropneumoniae* [11, 12].

ClpP protease is a family of ATP-dependent protease, hich plays a key role in the degradation of misfolded roteins and the stress tolerance in bacteria [13]. The ole of ClpP as an important virulence factor has been emonstrated in several pathogenic bacteria [14, 15]. A revious study of *Salmonella typhimurium* and *Salmon-lla enteritidis* also showed that the virulence of *clpP* de-tion mutants were remarkably decreased and that ese mutants can serve as live oral vaccine candidates 16]. In our previously study, the *clpP*-deleted mutant of . *pleuropneumoniae* serovar 7, a prevalent serovar in hina, was constructed and its physiological features ere analyzed. The ClpP protease mediates *A. pleurop-eumoniae* tolerance to multiple environmental tressors, affects the biofilm formation, and may play a ritical role in the virulence regulation [17]. The ApxII oxin is the most important virulence factor in *A. pleur-pneumoniae* serovar 7, and is encoded by the *apxIICA* ene cluster. The *apxIIA* gene encodes the ApxIIA toxin tructural protein, and the *apxIIC* gene encodes the ost-translational activating protein that is essential for ne ApxII toxin activation, thus disruption in the *apxIIC* ene of *A. pleuropneumoniae* results in secretion of the active ApxII toxin but with full antigenicity [18].

In the present study, we constructed the double-eletion mutant S-8△*clpP*△*apxIIC* of *A. pleuropneumo-iae* and evaluated the feasibility of its use as a live ttenuated negative marker vaccine based on the viru-nce, changes in clinical symptoms, immune responses, nd protective effects in pigs against challenge with the omologous and heterologous *A. pleuropneumoniae* trains.

lethods

xperimental animals

)ne hundred and ten 6-week-old female BALB/c mice Beijing Vital River Laboratory Animal Co., Ltd.) were sed in the study, with identical feeding conditions. A otal of 45 piglets were obtained for use in this study rom a farm that was free from *A. pleuropneumoniae* nd other respiratory pathogens including *Streptococcus uis*, *Haemophilus parasuis*, and porcine reproductive nd respiratory syndrome virus (PCR-negative for nasal nd tonsillar swabs and serological-negative in corre-ponding ELISA assays). The 45 piglets were randomly ivided into nine groups of same number and were eparately fed with same feeding conditions. The animal xperiment in this study was approved by the Animal thics Committee of Harbin Veterinary Research nstitute of the Chinese Academy of Agricultural ciences (CAAS) and carried out in strict accordance vith animal ethics guidelines and approved protocols.

Bacterial strains and growth conditions

A. pleuropneumoniae strains S-8 (serovar 7), Shope 4074 (serovar 1), K17 (serovar 5a), the S-8△*clpP* mutant and the S-8△*clpP*△*apxIIC* mutant were grown at 37 °C in tryptic soy broth (TSB) or tryptic soy agar (TSA) (Becton Dickinson, Franklin Lakes, NJ, USA) containing nicotina-mide dinucleotide (NAD, 10 μg/mL; Sigma-Aldrich).

Chromosomal inactivation of the apxIIC gene of S-8△clpP

Primers IICLF/IICLR, and IICRF/IICRR (Table 1) were used to amplify the two segments flanking with the *apxIIC* gene, IIC-L and IIC-R, as the recombination homologous arms. Using single-overlap extension PCR (SOE PCR), the fragment with a 270 bp internal deletion in the *apxIIC* gene (from nt 18 to 297) was generated, and cloned into the conjugative vector pEMOC2 [19] to construct plasmid pEM△*apxIIC*. Using *E. coli* β2155 and a single-step transconjugation system [20, 21], plasmid pEM△*apxIIC* was applied to introduce the *apxIIC* muta-tion into the S-8△*clpP* mutant. After two homologous recombination steps, the *A. pleuropneumoniae* S-8△*clpP*△*apxIIC* mutant strain was verified by PCR and sequencing using IICJDF/IICJDR primers.

Growth experiment and hemolytic assay

A. pleuropneumoniae wild-type strain S-8, the S-8△*clpP* mutant, and the S-8△*clpP*△*apxIIC* mutant were routinely grown in 3 ml of TSB for 16 h, then diluted to OD_{600} of 0.1. The fresh cultures were then inoculated in 30 ml of TSB and grown at 37 °C. The OD_{600} values were re-corded at an interval of 1 h using the Eppendorf BioPhotometer (Eppendorf, Germany).

A. pleuropneumoniae wild-type strain S-8, the S-8△*clpP* mutant, and the S-8△*clpP*△*apxIIC* mutant were respect-ively inoculated onto TSA plates supplemented with 5% defibrinated sheep erythrocytes, and incubated at 37 °C for 18 h. The hemolysis activity was assessed by visualizing clear zones around the colony.

Virulence studies in mice

To determine the residual virulence of the S-8△*clpP*△*ap-xIIC* mutant, various concentrations of *A. pleuropneumo-niae* strains S-8 and S-8△*clpP*△*apxIIC* mutant were injected intraperitoneally into mice. One hundred and ten 6-week-old female BALB/c mice (Beijing Vital River La-boratory Animal Co., Ltd.) were randomly divided into eleven experimental groups ($n = 10$). Five experimental groups were inoculated with 100 μL of PBS containing the S-8△*clpP*△*apxIIC* mutant (1.0×10^8 to 1.0×10^{10} CFU/mouse, Table 2). As a positive control, five experimental groups were inoculated with the wild-type strain S-8 (1.0×10^5 to 1.0×10^7 CFU/mouse, Table 2) using the identical method. Non-infected mice in the control group were inoculated with 100 μL of sterile PBS.

Table 1 Characteristics of bacterial strains, plasmids, and primers used in this study

Strains, plasmids, and primers	Characteristics or sequence	Source or reference
Strains		
E. coli β2155	*thrB1004 pro thi strA hsdS lacZ*ΔM15 (F′ *lacZ*ΔM15 *lacI^{q}traD36 proA$^+$ proB$^+$*)Δ*dap* :: *erm* (Erm^r))*recA* :: *RPA-2-tet*(Tc^r)::Mu-km (Km^r) λ*pir*	[21]
A.pleuropneumoniae S-8	*A. pleuropneumoniae* serotype 7 clinical isolate from the lung of a diseased pig in northern China	[17]
A.pleuropneumoniae S-8Δ*clpP*	Unmarked *clpP* gene knockout mutant of *A. pleuropneumoniae* S-8	[17]
*A.pleuropneumoniae S-8*Δ*clpP*Δ*apxIIC*	Unmarked *clpP/apxIIC* genes knockout mutant of *A. pleuropneumoniae* S-8	This work
Plasmids		
pEMOC2	Conjugative vector based on pBluescript SK with mob RP4, polycloning site, *Cm^r*, and transcriptional fusion of the *omlA* promoter with the *sacB* gene	Accession no. AJ86828 [19]
pEMΔ*apxIIC*	Conjugative vector pEMOC2 with a 270 bp deletion in the *apxIIC* gene which have a 1.4-kb upstream fragment and 1.4-kb downstream fragment	This work
Primers		
IICLF	5′ GCGTCGACATGACAACACCAATGATTGATTTAC 3′, upstream primer with internal SalI site (underlined)	This work
IICLR	5′ AATCCCCGAA**AGCATCATCC**CTCCCATTC 3′, downstream primer with reverse complement sequence(underlined) of sequence in bold from primer IICRF	This work
IICRF	5′ GGATGATGCT**TTCGGGGATT**CATCTCTATTG 3′, upstream primer with reverse complement sequence(underlined) of sequence in bold from primer IICLR	This work
IICRR	5′ TTGCGGCCGCGTTGTAATAAGTCCCGTAACACCAG 3′, downstream primer with internal NotI site (underlined)	This work
IICJDF	5′ GAAGAGCCATTACCCAACAAC 3′, upstream primer for identification of *apxIIC* gene deletion	This work
IICJDR	5′ ATACAATAGAGATGAATCCCCG 3′, downstream primer for identification of *apxIIC* gene deletion	This work

Table 2 Virulence of S-8Δ*clpP*Δ*apxIIC* and the wild-type strain S-8 of *A. pleuropneumoniae* in mice

Strains	Challenge dose[a] (CFU)	No. dead/ No.tested	Value of LD50[b] (CFU)	Fold attenuation[c]
S-8	1.0×10^7	10/10	5.62×10^5	1
	3.16×10^6	9/10		
	1.0×10^6	6/10		
	3.16×10^5	5/10		
	1.0×10^5	0/10		
S-8Δ*clpP*Δ*apxIIC*	1.0×10^{10}	10/10	1.12×10^9	1995
	3.16×10^9	8/10		
	1.0×10^9	5/10		
	3.16×10^8	1/10		
	1.0×10^8	0/10		
Control	PBS broth	0/10	-	-

[a] Groups of ten BALB/c mice were given intraperitoneal injections of 100 μL of bacterial suspension containing various quantities of *A. pleuropneumoniae* strains. Survival was recorded for 14 days after infection
[b] LD_{50} was calculated by the Karber's method [23]
[c] Fold attenuation was normalized to wild-type strain S-8

After infection, mice were monitored twice daily for a 14 day period and humanely euthanized if moribund [22]. The 50% lethal dose (LD_{50}) values of S-8 and S-8Δ*clpP*Δ*apxIIC* were calculated by Karber's method [23].

Virulence studies in pigs

Twenty-five 8-week-old pigs were randomly assigned into five experimental groups ($n = 5$). The pigs in group 1 were inoculated with 1×10^7 CFU of S-8Δ*clpP*Δ*apxIIC* via an intranasal (i.n.) route. The pigs in group 2 were injected with 1×10^7 CFU of S-8 via the i.n. route. The pigs in group 3 were injected with 1×10^9 CFU of S-8Δ*clpP*Δ*apxIIC* via the i.n. route. The pigs in group 4 were injected with 1×10^9 CFU of S-8 via the i.n. route. The pigs in group 5, the control group, were inoculated with an equivalent amount of PBS via the i.n. route. The rectal temperature, appetite, respiratory rate, and lethargywere recorded daily for 14 days after inoculation as described previously [24]. Pigs that showed severe respiratory distress during the observation period were euthanized. All of surviving pigs were euthanized at day 14 post-challenge, and the lung lesions were examined and scored as described previously [25]. Briefly, the lung lesion was determined by divided the complete lung into seven lobes, each lobe was scored 1-5 by assessing the pneumonic area.

rotection studies in pigs

'wenty 4-week-old pigs were randomly assigned into ɔur experimental groups ($n = 5$). The pigs in group 1 nd group 3 were immunized via an intramuscular (i.m.) ɔute with 1×10^7 CFU of S-8△*clpP*△*apxIIC* in 1 mL of 'BS. The pigs in group 2 and group 4 were inoculated vith 1 mL of PBS. The booster immunization was perɔrmed 21 days after the primary vaccination.

On day 14 following the booster immunization, the igs in groups 1 and group 2 were challenged with .0 × 10^9 CFU of *A. pleuropneumoniae* homologous erovar 7 (S-8) via the i.n. route. The pigs in groups and group 4 were challenged with 5.0×10^8 CFU of *A. leuropneumoniae* heterologous serovar 5a (K17) via the n. route. After challenge, the pigs from each group were bserved daily for clinical symptoms for 14-day period fter challenge as previously described [24]. Pigs that howed severe respiratory distress during the observation eriod were euthanized. At day 14 post-challenge, all surviving pigs were euthanized and lung lesions were examıed and scored as mentioned above [25].

ntibody measurements

erum samples were collected from pigs in different roups before the first immunization (day 0), before the ooster immunization (day 21) and before homologous r heterologous challenge (day 35). Antibodies against .pxII were examined using indirect ELISA as previously lescribed [26]. 96-well plates were coated with 5 μg/mL f ApxII in 50 mM sodium carbonate buffer (pH 9.6) at °C overnight. The wells were washed three times with 'BST buffer (PBS supplemented with 0.05% Tween-20) nd then blocked with PBS containing 5% bovine serum lbumin at 37 °C for 1 h. Serum samples diluted in PBS vere then added to the wells and incubated for 1 h at 7 °C. After the plates were washed, horseradish peroxdase (HRP)-conjugated goat anti-porcine IgG was diuted and added to the plates and incubated for 1 h at 7 °C. For determining the IgG isotypes, the sera were dded to the S-8△*clpP*△*apxIIC*-coated plates and incuated with mouse anti-pig IgG1 Monoclonal Antibody Clone K139 3C8, Thermo, United Kingdom) or mouse nti-pig IgG2 Monoclonal Antibody (Clone K68 Ig2, 'hermo, United Kingdom), followed by HRP-conjugated oat anti-mouse IgG (Abcam, United Kingdom). After hree washes, the substrate solution tetramethylbenzidine TMB) and H_2O_2 were added to the wells and incubated or 15 min, and the reaction was stopped by the addition of M sulfuric acid. The absorbance was measured at 450 nm ısing an ELISA reader. Each sample was tested in triplicate.

Determination of cytokines by ELISA

'erum samples at day 0, day 21, and day 35 were anayzed for swine gamma interferon (IFN-γ), interleukin 12 (IL-12) (R&D Systems, USA), and interleukin 4 (IL-4) (Invitrogen, USA) using ELISA kits performed according to the manufacturer's instructions. Concentrations of swine IFN-γ, IL-12, and IL-4 in tested sera samples were determined by extrapolation to the linear portion of the standard curve, which was generated with supplied reference standards.

Bacterial loads analysis

Pigs from each group were necropsied immediately after euthanasia and lung tissues were aseptically collected. Samples were weighed, suspended in 1 mL PBS, and homogenized using a tissue homogenizer. The tissue homogenates were serially diluted with sterile PBS. Viable counts in serial dilutions of homogenates were determined following culture on TSA plates for 18 h at 37 °C. Identification of *A. pleuropneumoniae* was conducted by colony PCR assay and expressed as $\log_{10}$ CFU/g.

Statistical analysis

All statistical analyses were conducted using GraphPad Prism version 5.01 (GraphPad Software Inc., USA). Student's *t*-test was used to evaluate the significance of the differences between multiple experimental groups. The data were expressed as the mean +/- standard deviation and values of $P < 0.05$ were considered to be significant.

Results

Construction of the S-8△clpP△apxIIC mutant strain

To construct the double-deletion mutant S-8△*clpP*△*apxIIC*, we deleted the *apxIIC* gene of *A. pleuropneumoniae* S-8△*clpP* mutant via the allelic exchange of the wild-type *apxIIC* gene with an unmarked, in-frame deletion lacking 270 bp of the *apxIIC* ORF (Fig. 1a and Fig. 1b). To test the stability of the in-frame deleted *apxIIC* gene in the genome of the *A. pleuropneumoniae* S-8△*clpP*△*apxIIC* mutant, a PCR assay was performed on the genomes of the mutant from 10 passages to detect a 294-bp DNA fragment characteristic of the in-frame deleted *apxIIC*. This fragment was observed in all 10 consecutive passages (Fig. 1c), suggesting a stable in-frame deletion in the *S-8△clpP△apxIIC* genome.

The growth curves of the S-8△*clpP* mutant, the S-8△*clpP*△*apxIIC* mutant, and the wild-type strain S-8 were similar at 37 °C (Fig. 2a). The hemolytic assay was examined in the wild-type strain S-8, the S-8△*clpP* mutant, and the S-8△*clpP*△*apxIIC* mutant. S-8 and the S-8△*clpP* mutant with the integrated *apxII* operon had hemolytic activity, as shown by clear zones around the colonies (Fig. 2b). However, the clear zones were absent in the S-8△*clpP*△*apxIIC* mutant, the result of deletion of the *apxIIC* gene rendered it unable to activate ApxII toxin, and thus lacking hemolytic activity.

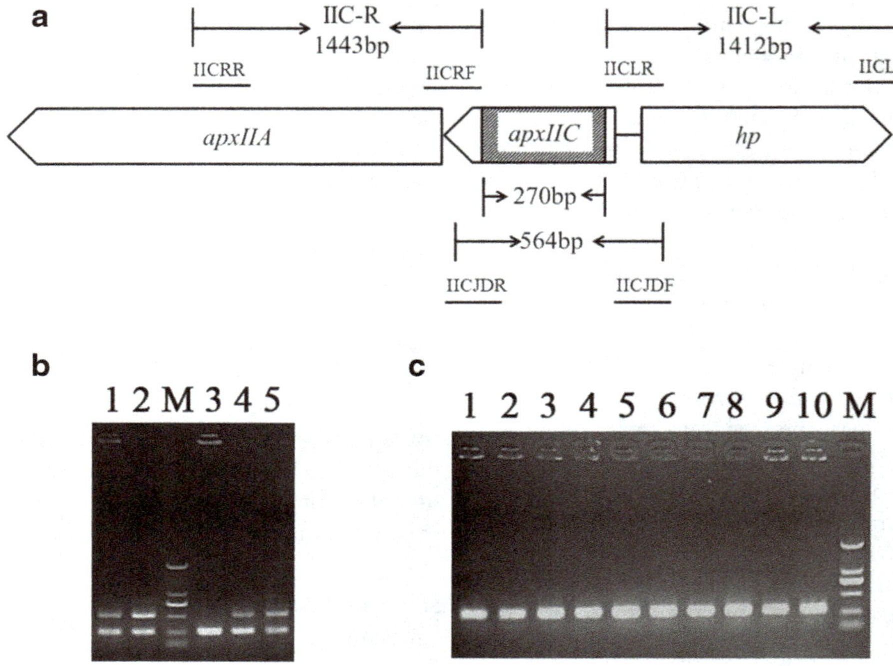

Fig. 1 Characterization of the *A. pleuropneumoniae* mutant S-8△*clp*△*apxIIC*. **a** Schematic representation of the *A. pleuropneumoniae apxIIC* locus. Binding locations for the primers IICLF/IICLR and IICRF/IICRR used to amplify the two flanking regions (1412 bp and 1443 bp, respectively) of the *apxIIC* gene were shown in the schematic, and primers IICJDF/IICJDR were used to identify the S-8△*clp*△*apxIIC* mutant (294 bp) and S-8△*clp* mutant (564 bp). The shadowed domain represents a 270 bp in-frame deletion in the *apxIIC* gene, hp indicates the encoding gene of the hypothetical protein. **b** PCR identification of the S-8△*clp*△*apxIIC* mutant using the primers IICJDF/IICJDR. For lane 3, the identified S-8△*clp*△*apxIIC* mutant (294 bp); for other lanes, the single crossover mutant (564 bp and 294 bp). **c** PCR identification of the 10 passages of the S-8△*clp*△*apxIIC* mutant. For lanes 1–10, 10 successive passages of the S-8△*clp*△*apxIIC* mutant; for lane M, DL2000 DNA molecular marker (from top to bottom: 2000, 1000, 750, 500, 250, and 100 bp)

Virulence of the S-8△clpP and S-8△clpP△apxIIC mutants in mice

The attenuation of virulence was investigated by determining the LD_{50} values of the S-8△*clpP*△*apxIIC* mutant, and the wild-type strain S-8 in BALB/c mice. The data showed LD_{50} values of 5.62×10^5 CFU per mouse for the wild-type strain S-8, and 1.12×10^9 CFU per mouse for the S-8△*clpP*△*apxIIC* mutant. Compared to the wild-type strain S-8, the S-8△*clpP*△*apxIIC* mutant was atten uated by approximately 1195-fold in mice. LD_{50} value showed that the S-8△*clpP*△*apxIIC* mutant was highl attenuated.

Virulence of the S-8△clpP△apxIIC mutant in pigs

The results of the safety study on the S-8△*clpP*△*apxIIC* mutant in pigs are listed in Table 3. Two of five pig

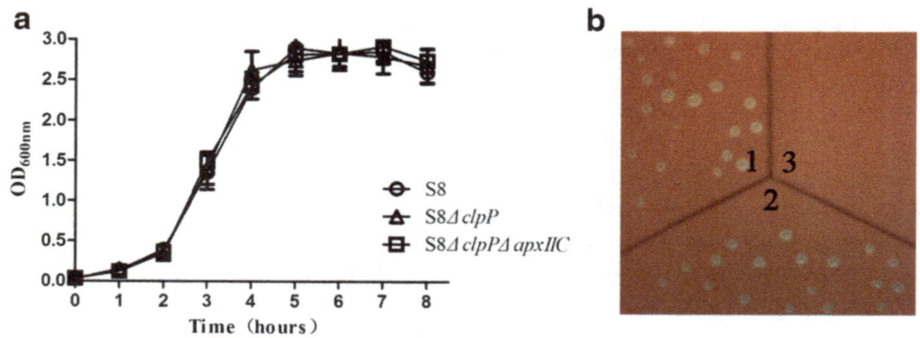

Fig. 2 Growth characteristics and hemolytic activities of the *A. pleuropneumoniae* mutants. **a** The growth curves of the S-8, S-8△*clp* and S-8△*clp*△*apxIIC* strains. Overnight cultures were inoculated into fresh TSB and then incubated at 37 °C. Growth was monitored by OD600 at an interval of 1 h. **b** Hemolytic activity test for the S-8, S-8△*clp* and S-8△*clp*△*apxIIC* strains. Section 1, S-8; section 2, S-8△*clp*; section 3, S-8△*clp*△*apxIIC*

able 3 Virulence of the *A. pleuropneumoniae* S-8△*clpP*△*apxIIC* mutant in pigs

roup	Strain for challenge	Challenge dose[a] (CFU)	Temperature (°C) [b]	Appetite[c]	Lethargy[c]	Dyspnea[c]	Lung lesion score [d]
	S-8△*clpP*△*apxIIC*	1.0×10^7	39.2 ± 0.3	0.2 ± 0.4*	0.1 ± 0.2**	0.2 ± 0.2**	1.8 ± 3.0**
	S-8	1.0×10^7	40.1 ± 0.4	1.8 ± 1.3	1.7 ± 0.7	1.9 ± 0.7	16.2 ± 8.5
	S-8△*clpP*△*apxIIC*	1.0×10^9	39.4 ± 0.5	0.4 ± 0.5*	0.3 ± 0.3**	0.4 ± 0.4**	3.0 ± 2.2**
	S-8	1.0×10^9	40.2 ± 0.6	2.4 ± 1.6	2.2 ± 0.6	2.5 ± 0.5	21.8 ± 5.8
	PBS	0	39.4 ± 0.3	0	0	0	0

Groups of five pigs were given intranasal inoculations with 1 mL of bacterial suspension containing various quantities of *A. pleuropneumoniae* strains. Survival as recorded for 14 days after infection

The average temperature value for each piglet during the observation period was calculated and the mean temperature value for each group was determined

Clinical signs were scored as described by Jolie et al [24]. Appetite was scored as follows: 0, did eat; and 1, did not eat. The total score equaled the number of 2-h periods of not eating over the 36-h observation period. Lethargy was scored as follows: 0, normal; 1, slight inactivity; 2, moderate; and 3, severe. Dyspnea as scored as follows: 0, normal; 1, slight; 2, moderate; and 3, severe. The final scores were obtained from the average of all of the data within the observation me and are expressed as arithmetic means ± SD; *, significance at a *P* value of <0.05; **, significance at a *P* value of <0.01

The lung lesion score was determined as described by Hannan et al [25]

noculated with 1.0×10^9 CFU of the S-8△*clpP*△*apxIIC* nutant via the i.n. route showed a slight increase in rectal temperatures (40.1 °C < body temperatures < 40.3 °C) fter 8–20 h post-infection and exhibited only mild linical symptoms of porcine pleuropneumonia, such as ecreased appetite. However, all of these pigs recovered uickly in 24 h and were in good health afterward. All f the five pigs inoculated with 1.0×10^7 CFU of the S-△*clpP*△*apxIIC* via the i.n. route exhibited no clinical igns of porcine pleuropneumonia. Compared to the roups inoculated with the S-8△*clpP*△*apxIIC* mutant, he groups inoculated with the S-8 strain exhibited nore severe clinical symptoms of porcine pleuropneumonia. Three of five pigs which were inoculated with .0 × 10^9 CFU of S-8 were euthanized because of severe linical symptoms. The lesions in their lungs were evere with massive hemorrhages and fibrinous nflammation was observed. Compared to serious lung esions of pigs in the S-8-inoculated groups, there are o or few lung lesions in the pigs of the S-8△*clpP*△*apxIIC*-inoculated groups (Fig. 3). The average lung lesion cores were 16.2 for 1.0×10^7 CFU and 21.8 for $1.0 \times$ 10^9 CFU of S-8 challenge. However, the groups inoculated with S-8△*clpP*△*apxIIC* showed significantly lower ung lesion scores, with 1.8 and 3.0 following challenge ith 1.0×10^7 CFU or 1.0×10^9 CFU, respectively Table 3).

nmune response of pigs to the S-8△clpP△apxIIC mutant

erum samples from pigs of each group were obtained rom blood via anterior vena cava venipuncture. igure 4a showed a significant increase in antibody titers n pigs immunized with S-8△*clpP*△*apxIIC* on days 21 nd 35, however, no antibody was detected in the PBS ontrol groups. The IgG isotype was determined to heck the specific antibody types against S-8△*clpP*△*apxIIC*. The levels of isotypes IgG1 and IgG2 in the immunized groups were significantly higher ($P < 0.01$) than that of PBS control groups (Fig. 4b, c).

Levels of IFN-γ in sera from S-8△*clpP*△*apxIIC* immunization groups were significantly higher than those of PBS control groups on days 21 and 35 ($P < 0.01$) (Fig. 5a). Levels of IL-12 in the S-8△*clpP*△*apxIIC* immunization groups were also significantly higher than those of control groups during the observation period ($P < 0.01$) (Fig. 5b). Both the IFN-γ and IL-12 concentrations in sera from S-8△*clpP*△*apxIIC* immunized animals increased substantially on day 21 and exhibited a smaller increase on day 35. While the IL-4 concentrations in sera from S-8△*clpP*△*apxIIC* immunized groups exhibited an approximately equal increase on day 21 and day 35, higher than in sera from the PBS control groups ($P < 0.01$) (Fig. 5c).

Protective efficacy in pigs

The protective efficacy of the S-8△*clpP*△*apxIIC* mutant against lethal challenge with *A. pleuropneumoniae* serovar 7 S-8 or serovar 5a K17 in pigs was evaluated in terms of body temperature, clinical signs, lung lesions, and survival rate. The results are summarized in Fig. 6 and Table 4. Pigs in the S-8△*clpP*△*apxIIC*-immunized groups showed slight or no lethargy, anorexia or dyspnea after challenge with *A. pleuropneumoniae* serovar 5a or serovar 7. Four immunized pigs had a transient increased body temperature (<40.3 °C) on day 0 upon challenge with *A. pleuropneumoniae* S-8 or K17 but recovered afterward. During the 14-day observation period, all immunized pigs survived with clinical symptoms ranging from none to only mild. All of the pigs in the PBS control groups developed anorexia, increased respiratory rate, and depression after challenge with *A. pleuropneumoniae* S-8 or K17. The average body temperature increased (41.2 °C) for at least 3 days. Four of ten pigs showed severe respiratory distress within

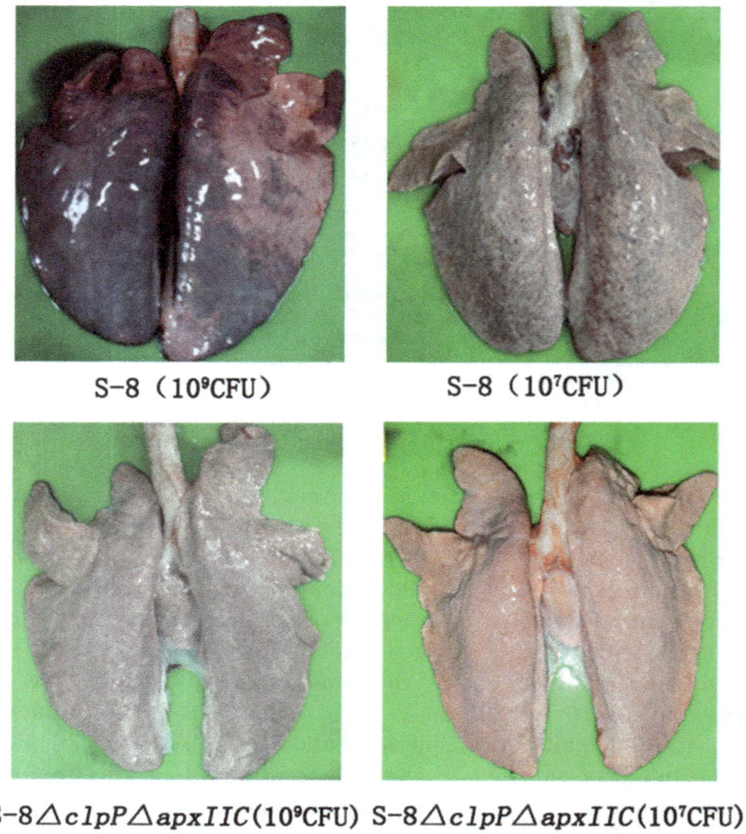

Fig. 3 Pathological changes of the lungs of pigs infected with *A. pleuropneumoniae*. Groups of pigs were inoculated with different doses of S-8 and S-8△*clp*△*apxIIC*. At 14 days post-infection, all pigs were euthanized and lungs were collected and subjected to pathological examination

48 h and were euthanized. Three pigs subsequently exhibited severe respiratory distress during the next four days and were euthanized. Only two pigs challenged with S-8 and one pig challenged with K17 in the control groups survived over the 14-day observation period.

At necropsy, the pigs in the PBS control groups showed severe lung lesions and pleuritis. Hemorrhage and fibrinous exudation on the lung and pleura were found in these pigs. The average lung lesion scores were 20.2 and 22.8 for challenge with *A. pleuropneumoniae* S-8 or K17, respectively. However, in comparison t the PBS control groups, the S-8△*clpP*△*apxIIC*-immunized groups showed significantly lower lung lesio scores of 1.4 and 1.8 for challenge with *A. pleurop neumoniae* S-8 or K17, respectively.

Bacteriological analysis of tissue homogenates

Bacterial loads in lung homogenates were counted afte challenge with *A. pleuropneumoniae* S-8 or K17 (Fig. 7) The numbers of CFUs recovered from the homogenize

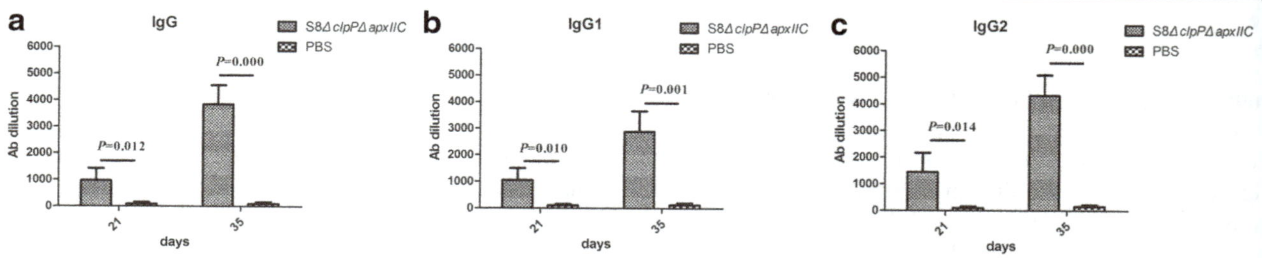

Fig. 4 Levels of IgG antibody (**a**), IgG1 (**b**), and IgG2 (**c**) in the sera of piglets. Blood samples were collected prior to and following immunization on days 0, 21, and 35 from the S-8△*clp*△*apxIIC* immunized groups and PBS control groups, and the antibody responses were determined by indirect ELISA. The results are expressed as the means ± SD

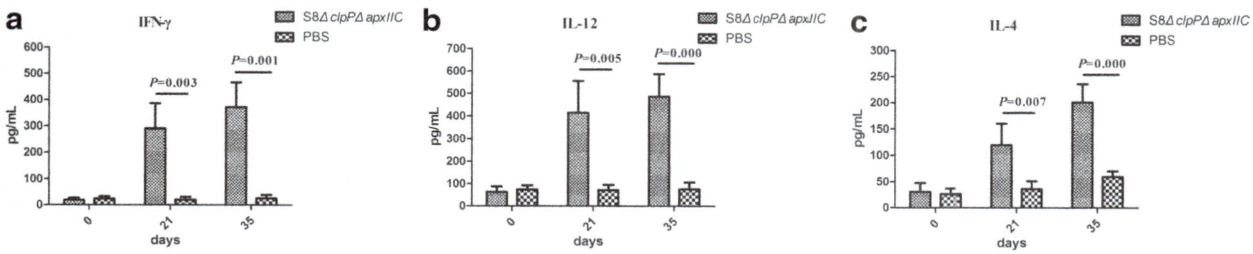

Fig. 5 Levels of IFN-γ, IL-12, and IL-4 in the sera of piglets. Blood samples were collected prior to and following immunization on days 0, 21, and 35 from the S-8△*clp*△*apxIIC* immunized groups and PBS control groups, and the levels of IFN-γ (**a**), IL-12 (**b**), and IL-4 (**c**) were determined by commercial kit. The results are expressed as the means ± SD

ıng tissues in S-8△*clpP*△*apxIIC* immunized groups were ignificantly lower ($P < 0.01$) than those of PBS control roups.

Discussion

With the growing emergence of drug resistance and the problem of antibiotic residues, vaccination becomes the nost effective method of preventing *A. pleuropneumoniae* infection [7, 11]. Previous studies found that pigs urviving natural infection of *A. pleuropneumoniae* ould be fully protected against homologous strain and partially against heterologous serovars, suggesting that ve bacteria likely induced in vivo expression of rotective antigens and conferred cross-protection [11]. Thus, an attenuated live vaccine is widely acknowledged s an ideal approach for vaccination against porcine leuropneumonia.

The ideal live vaccine of porcine pleuropneumonia hould be low virulent and cause minimum lung lesions 11]. Our previous study constructed S-8△*clpP*, an *A. pleuropneumoniae clpP* gene deletion mutant, and illusrated the important function of the ClpP protease in he stress response and biofilm formation of *A. pleuropneumoniae*, suggesting a putative role for ClpP protease n the virulence regulation [17]. Afterwards, the viruence of S-8△*clpP* was determined using the BALB/c nouse infection model. The finding that the S-8△*clpP* noderately attenuated by approximately 71-fold (data not shown) was unexpected as a previous study had found that *clpP* deletion strains of *S. typhimurium* and *S. enteritidis* were attenuated by approximately 10,000-fold [16]. Thus, in this study, we further deleted the *apxIIC* gene that encodes the ApxII activating protein, and rendered the double-deletion mutant S-8△*clpP*△*apxIIC* secreting unactivated ApxII toxins but with complete antigenicity [18]. Compared to the wild-type strain, S-8△*clpP*△*apxIIC* was greatly attenuated by approximately 1195-fold. We next evaluated the virulence of S-8△*clpP*△*apxIIC* in pigs via intranasal inoculation, with the results showing that pigs inoculated with 1.0×10^7 CFU of the S-8△*clpP* mutant displayed no clinical signs of porcine pleuropneumonia but exhibited only transient depression when inoculated with 1.0×10^9 CFU. Moreover, there are no or little lung lesions in the pigs of the S-8△*clpP*△*apxIIC*-inoculated group, which showed that the S-8△*clpP*△*apxIIC* mutant was adequately attenuated and has almost no detrimental effects on pigs that remained healthy throughout the experiment.

An essential characteristic for an effective attenuated live vaccine is that the strain should remain highly immunogenic [11]. Pigs vaccinated with the *A. pleuropneumoniae* S-8△*clpP*△*apxIIC* mutant exhibited a significantly increased ApxII-specific IgG Ab response compared to pigs injected with PBS. Interestingly, both *A. pleuropneumoniae*-specific IgG1 and IgG2 titers increased following the first immunization and booster immunization. The

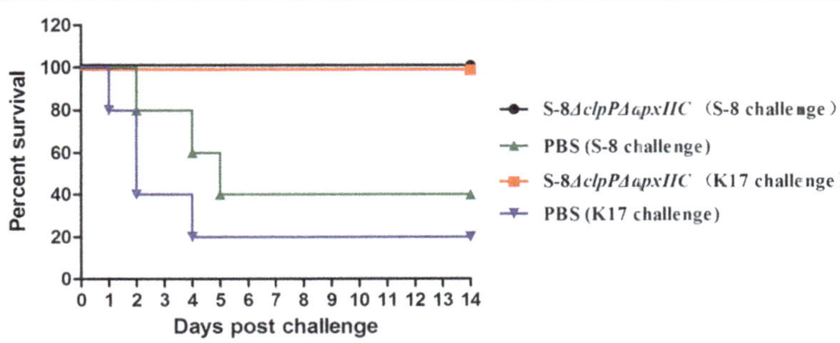

Fig. 6 Survival of pigs following intranasal challenge with *A. pleuropneumoniae* strains S-8 or K17

Table 4 Protective efficacy of the S-8△*clp*△*apxIIC* mutant against *A. pleuropneumoniae* S-8 and K17 challenge in pigs

Group	Immunogen	Strain for challenge	Temperature (°C) [a]	Appetite[b]	Lethargy[b]	Dyspnea[b]	Lung lesion score
1	S-8△*clpP*△*apxIIC*	S-8	39.4 ± 0.2	0.2 ± 0.3*	0.2 ± 0.3**	0.1 ± 0.2**	1.4 ± 2.2*
2	PBS	S-8	40.3 ± 0.5	2.4 ± 1.1	2.0 ± 0.6	2.3 ± 0.6	20.2 ± 11.9
3	S-8△*clpP*△*apxIIC*	K17	39.6 ± 0.3	0.3 ± 0.4*	0.3 ± 0.4**	0.4 ± 0.4**	1.7 ± 2.5**
4	PBS	K17	40.5 ± 0.4	2.6 ± 1.7	2.3 ± 0.5	2.6 ± 0.4	22.8 ± 9.3

[a] The average temperature value for each piglet during the observation period after challenge was calculated and the mean temperature value for each group was determined

[b] Clinical signs were scored as described by Jolie et al [24]. Appetite was scored as follows: 0, did eat; and 1, did not eat. The total score equaled the number of 12-h periods of not eating over the 36-h observation period. Lethargy was scored as follows: 0, normal; 1, slight inactivity; 2, moderate; and 3, severe. Dyspnea was scored as follows: 0, normal; 1, slight; 2, moderate; and 3, severe. The final scores were obtained from the average of all of the data within the observation time and are expressed as arithmetic means ± SD; *, significance at a P value of <0.05; **, significance at a P value of <0.01

[c] The lung lesion score was determined as described by Hannan et al [25]

production of IgG isotypes in pig is elicited by type 1 (IFN-γ, IL-12) and type 2 (IL-4) cytokines, which lead the responses to a cell-mediated or antibody-mediated immune response [27]. In pigs, IgG2 is linked to the production of IFN-γ and IL-12 and correlates with the Th1 response [27, 28]. Conversely, the production of the specific IgG1 antibody partially relies on the presence of the Th2 cytokine IL-4 [29]. In this study, we also found that on day 35, the levels of IFN-γ, IL-12, and IL-4 were significantly higher in sera from S-8△*clpP*△*apxIIC* immunized pigs than those in sera from PBS control groups, but IL-4 concentrations were lower than IFN-γ and IL-12 concentrations in sera from the immunization groups. These data suggested that immunization with *A. pleuropneumoniae* S-8△*clpP*△*apxIIC* generated a slight bias towards the Th1-type immune response. However, the IgG1 titers and IL-4 concentrations in the S-8△*clpP*△*apxIIC* immunized pigs were still much higher than those in the PBS control groups. These data showed that the Th2-type immune response also plays a partial role in immunization with live *A. pleuropneumoniae* S-8△*clpP*△*apxIIC*. Unlike the other *A. pleuropneumoniae* live attenuated mutant that is significantly biased toward a Th1-type immune response [30], S-8△*clpP*△*apxIIC* generated a more balanced and broader immune response.

Cross-protection is a crucial characteristic that is im portant to achieve widespread use of a vaccine. Ou findings demonstrated that immunization with the S 8△*clpP*△*apxIIC* mutant could induce acquired immunit and confer a marked resistance against the lethal chal lenge with *A. pleuropneumoniae* virulent homologou strain S-8 and heterologous serovar 5a. Although S 8△*clpP*△*apxIIC* exhibited good immune protection as live vaccine, a few pigs after challenge still had fev pathological lesions. As it is unlikely that the multiple gene deleted mutant can revert back to the wild-typ genotype, we will further delete other important viru lence genes of *A. pleuropneumoniae* in our future stud ies and construct a multiple-gene deleted mutant as safe, attenuated live vaccine to prevent and control *A* *pleuropneumoniae* infection.

Conclusion

In conclusion, data presented in this study indicated tha the immunizations with the candidate vaccine S 8△*clpP*△*apxIIC* were safe in pigs; and conferred efficien protection against the homologous or heterologous sero var infection. Overall, the S-8△*clpP*△*apxIIC* mutant of *A* *pleuropneumoniae* has the potential as a novel live atten uated vaccine against porcine pleuropneumonia, al though further trials are needed.

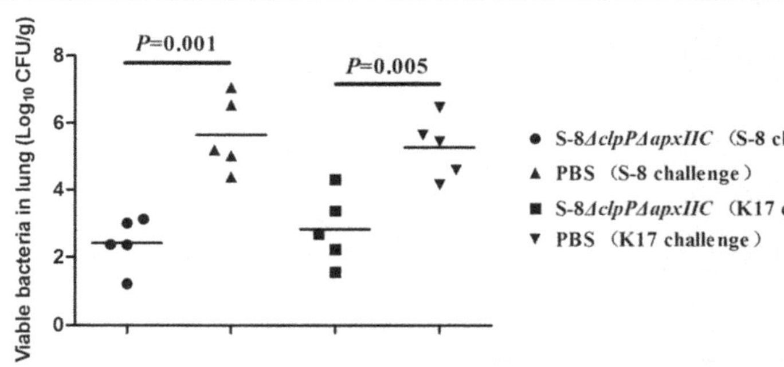

Fig. 7 Bacterial loads in lung homogenates after challenge with *A. pleuropneumoniae* strains S-8 or K17. The logarithm value (Log_{10}) of the CFU in each gram of tissue sample was recorded. The immunized groups were vaccinated with S-8△*clp*△*apxIIC* and the PBS control groups were injected with PBS. The results are expressed as the means ± SD

bbreviations

pleuropneumoniae: *Actinobacillus pleuropneumoniae*; ATP: Adenosine phosphate; CFU: Colony-forming unit; ELISA: Enzyme-linked immunosorbent say; IFN-γ: Gamma interferon; IgG: Immunoglobulin G; IL-12: Interleukin 12; -4: Interleukin 4; LB: Luria-Bertani; LD_{50}: Lethal dose 50% value; PCR: Polymerase nain reaction; *S. enteritidis*: *Salmonella enteritidis*; *S. typhimurium*: *Salmonella phimurium*; SOE PCR: Single-overlap extension polymerase chain reaction; ;A: Tryptic soy agar; TSB: Tryptic soy broth

cknowledgments

l the authors have seen and approved the content and have contributed gnificantly to the work.

unding

nis research was supported by grants from Special Fund for Agro-scientific esearch in the Public Interest (201303034), National Natural Science Founda- on of China (31100103), Natural Science Foundation of Heilongjiang Prov- ce of China (C2016067 and QC2016044), the project of Harbin Science and echnology innovative talents (2015RQQYJ073), and the State's Key Project Research and Development Plan (2016YFD0500700).

uthors' contributions

. and CW designed the experiments, FX and GL conducted experiments, Z, YZ and NC performed the experiments, FX and LZ analyzed the data and afted the manuscript, CW finalized the manuscript. All authors read and oproved the final manuscript.

ompeting interests

ne authors declare that they have no competing interests.

onsent for publication

ot applicable.

eferences

Fenwick B, Henry S. Porcine pleuropneumonia. J Am Vet Med Assoc. 1994; 204:1334–40.

Chiers K, De Waele T, Pasmans F, Ducatelle R, Haesebrouck F. Virulence factors of *Actinobacillus pleuropneumoniae* involved in colonization, persistence and induction of lesions in its porcine host. Vet Res. 2010;41:65.

Bosse JT, Janson H, Sheehan BJ, Beddek AJ, Rycroft AN, Kroll JS, et al. *Actinobacillus pleuropneumoniae*: pathobiology and pathogenesis of infection. Microbes Infect. 2002;4:225–35.

Blackall PJ, Klaasen HL, van den Bosch H, Kuhnert P, Frey J. Proposal of a new serovar of *Actinobacillus pleuropneumoniae*: serovar 15. Vet Microbiol. 2002;84:47–52.

Sarkozi R, Makrai L, Fodor L. Identification of a proposed new serovar of *Actinobacillus pleuropneumoniae*: serovar 16. Acta Vet Hung. 2015;63:444–50.

Subashchandrabose S, Leveque RM, Kirkwood RN, Kiupel M, Mulks MH. The RNA chaperone Hfq promotes fitness of *Actinobacillus pleuropneumoniae* during porcine pleuropneumonia. Infect Immun. 2013;81:2952–61.

Archambault M, Harel J, Goure J, Tremblay YD, Jacques M. Antimicrobial susceptibilities and resistance genes of Canadian isolates of *Actinobacillus pleuropneumoniae*. Microb Drug Resist. 2012;18:198–206.

Bosse JT, Li Y, Atherton TG, Walker S, Williamson SM, Rogers J, et al. Characterisation of a mobilisable plasmid conferring florfenicol and chloramphenicol resistance in *Actinobacillus pleuropneumoniae*. Vet Microbiol. 2015;178:279–82.

Bosse JT, Li Y, Walker S, Atherton T, Fernandez Crespo R, Williamson SM, et al. Identification of dfrA14 in two distinct plasmids conferring trimethoprim resistance in *Actinobacillus pleuropneumoniae*. J Antimicrob Chemother. 2015;70:2217–22.

). Nielsen R. *Haemophilus pleuropneumoniae* serotypes–cross protection experiments. Nord Vet Med. 1984;36(7-8):221–34.

. Ramjeet M, Deslandes V, Goure J, Jacques M. *Actinobacillus pleuropneumoniae* vaccines: from bacterins to new insights into vaccination strategies. Anim Health Res Rev. 2008;9:25–45.

2. Maas A, Meens J, Baltes N, Hennig-Pauka I, Gerlach GF. Development of a DIVA subunit vaccine against *Actinobacillus pleuropneumoniae* infection. Vaccine. 2006;24:7226 37.

13. Thomsen LE, Olsen JE, Foster JW, Ingmer H. ClpP is involved in the stress response and degradation of misfolded proteins in *salmonella enterica* serovar typhimurium. Microbiology. 2002;148:2727–33.

14. Raju RM, Unnikrishnan M, Rubin DH, Krishnamoorthy V, Kandror O, Akopian TN, et al. *Mycobacterium tuberculosis* ClpP1 and ClpP2 function together in protein degradation and are required for viability in vitro and during infection. PLoS Pathog. 2012;8:e1002511.

15. Frees D, Chastanet A, Qazi S, Sorensen K, Hill P, Msadek T, et al. Clp ATPases are required for stress tolerance, intracellular replication and biofilm formation in *Staphylococcus aureus*. Mol Microbiol. 2004;54:1445–62.

16. Tennant SM, Wang JY, Galen JE, Simon R, Pasetti MF, Gat O, et al. Engineering and preclinical evaluation of attenuated nontyphoidal salmonella strains serving as live oral vaccines and as reagent strains. Infect Immun. 2011;79:4175–85.

17. Xie F, Zhang Y, Li G, Zhou L, Liu S, Wang C. The ClpP protease is required for the stress tolerance and biofilm formation in *Actinobacillus pleuropneumoniae*. PLoS One. 2013;8:e53600.

18. Prideaux CT, Lenghaus C, Krywult J, Hodgson AL. Vaccination and protection of pigs against pleuropneumonia with a vaccine strain of *Actinobacillus pleuropneumoniae* produced by site-specific mutagenesis of the ApxII operon. Infect Immun. 1999;67:1962–66.

19. Baltes N, Tonpitak W, Hennig-Pauka I, Gruber AD, Gerlach GF. *Actinobacillus pleuropneumoniae* serotype 7 siderophore receptor FhuA is not required for virulence. FEMS Microbiol Lett. 2003;220:41–8.

20. Oswald W, Tonpitak W, Ohrt G, Gerlach G. A single-step transconjugation system for the introduction of unmarked deletions into *Actinobacillus pleuropneumoniae* serotype 7 using a sucrose sensitivity marker. FEMS Microbiol Lett. 1999;179:153–60.

21. Dehio C, Meyer M. Maintenance of broad-host-range incompatibility group P and group Q plasmids and transposition of Tn5 in *Bartonella henselae* following conjugal plasmid transfer from *Escherichia coli*. J Bacteriol. 1997;179:538–40.

22. Spindler KR, Fang L, Moore ML, Hirsch GN, Brown CC, Kajon A. SJL/J mice are highly susceptible to infection by mouse adenovirus type 1. J Virol. 2001;75:12039–46.

23. Finney DJ. Statistical methods in biological assays, 2nd ed. London: Charles Griffin & Company Limited; 1964.

24. Jolie RA, Mulks MH, Thacker BJ. Cross-protection experiments in pigs vaccinated with *Actinobacillus pleuropneumoniae* subtypes 1A and 1B. Vet Microbiol. 1995;45:383–91.

25. Hannan PC, Bhogal BS, Fish JP. Tylosin tartrate and tiamutilin effects on experimental piglet pneumonia induced with pneumonic pig lung homogenate containing mycoplasmas, bacteria and viruses. Res Vet Sci. 1982;33:76–88.

26. Nielsen R, van den Bosch JF, Plambeck T, Sorensen V, Nielsen JP. Evaluation of an indirect enzyme-linked immunosorbent assay (ELISA) for detection of antibodies to the Apx toxins of *Actinobacillus pleuropneumoniae*. Vet Microbiol. 2000;71:81–7.

27. Crawley A, Wilkie BN. Porcine Ig isotypes: function and molecular characteristics. Vaccine. 2003;21:2911–22.

28. Furesz SE, Wilkie BN, Mallard BA, Rosendal S, MacInnes JI. Anti-haemolysin IgG1 to IgG2 ratios correlate with haemolysin neutralization titres and lung lesion scores in *Actinobacillus pleuropneumoniae* infected pigs. Vaccine. 1998;16:1971–5.

29. Snapper CM, Paul WE. Interferon-gamma and B cell stimulatory factor-1 reciprocally regulate Ig isotype production. Science. 1987;236:944–7.

30. Fu S, Ou J, Zhang M, Xu J, Liu H, Liu J, et al. The live attenuated *Actinobacillus pleuropneumoniae* triple-deletion mutant DeltaapxIC DeltaapxIIC DeltaapxIV-ORF1 strain, SLW05, Immunizes pigs against lethal challenge with *Haemophilus parasuis*. Clin Vaccine Immunol. 2013;20:134–9.

11

Modeling the transboundary risk of feed ingredients contaminated with porcine epidemic diarrhea virus

Scott Dee[1*], Casey Neill[1], Aaron Singrey[2], Travis Clement[2], Roger Cochrane[3], Cassandra Jones[3], Gilbert Patterson[4], Gordon Spronk[1], Jane Christopher-Hennings[2] and Eric Nelson[2]

Abstract

Background: This study describes a model developed to evaluate the transboundary risk of PEDV-contaminated swine feed ingredients and the effect of two mitigation strategies during a simulated transport event from China to the US.

Results: Ingredients imported to the USA from China, including organic & conventional soybeans and meal, lysine hydrochloride, D-L methionine, tryptophan, Vitamins A, D & E, choline, carriers (rice hulls, corn cobs) and feed grade tetracycline, were inoculated with PEDV. Control ingredients, and treatments (ingredients plus a liquid antimicrobial (SalCURB, Kemin Industries (LA) or a 2 % custom medium chain fatty acid blend (MCFA)) were tested. The model ran for 37 days, simulating transport of cargo from Beijing, China to Des Moines, IA, US from December 23, 2012 to January 28, 2013. To mimic conditions on land and sea, historical temperature and percent relative humidity (% RH) data were programmed into an environmental chamber which stored all containers. To evaluate PEDV viability over time, ingredients were organized into 1 of 4 batches of samples, each batch representing a specific segment of transport. Batch 1 (segment 1) simulated transport of contaminated ingredients from manufacturing plants in Beijing (day 1 post-contamination (PC)). Batch 2 (segments 1 and 2) simulated manufacturing and delivery to Shanghai, including time in Anquing terminal awaiting shipment (days 1–8 PC). Batch 3 (segments 1, 2 and 3) represented time in China, the crossing of the Pacific and entry to the US at the San Francisco, CA terminal (day 1–27 PC). Batch 4 (segments 1–4) represented the previous events, including transport to Des Moines, IA (days 1–37 PC). Across control (non-treated) ingredients, viable PEDV was detected in soybean meal (organic and conventional), Vitamin D, lysine hydrochloride and choline chloride. In contrast, viable PEDV was not detected in any samples treated with LA or MCFA.

Conclusions: These results demonstrate the ability of PEDV to survive in a subset of feed ingredients using a model simulating shipment from China to the US. This is proof of concept suggesting that contaminated feed ingredients could serve as transboundary risk factors for PEDV, along with the identification of effective mitigation options.

Keywords: Transboundary, Porcine, Epidemic, Diarrhea, Virus, Antimicrobial, Ingredient, Lysine, Soybean meal, Choline

* Correspondence: sdee@pipevet.com
[1]Pipestone Applied Research, Pipestone Veterinary Services, 1300 Box188 Hwy 75 S, Pipestone, MN 56164, USA
Full list of author information is available at the end of the article

ackground

'orcine epidemic diarrhea virus (PEDV) is an enveloped ingle-stranded positive sense RNA virus belonging to ne Order *Nidovirales*, the family *Coronaviridae* and the enus *Alphacoronavirus* [1]. Following detection in the JS swine population during May, 2013 the virus spread apidly throughout the country [2]. During the initial utbreak, the American Association of Swine Veterinarans, the National Pork Producers Council and the JSDA Center for Epidemiology and Animal Health conucted an epidemiological investigation involving case nd control herds [3]. Of the 100 variables surveyed, 7 /ere significantly associated ($p < 0.05$) with having igher odds of acquiring PED, with all associated with ne process of feeding animals [3]. In 2014, the risk of ontaminated feed and feed ingredients was confirmed, /hen studies describing the ability of PEDV to survive or extended periods in feed (7 days in dry feed and 8 days in wet feed when stored at room temperature), nd proof of concept that contaminated complete feed nd feed ingredients could serve as vehicles for transnission to naïve pigs [4–6]. Shortly thereafter, the transnission of PEDV via ingestion of contaminated omplete feed was validated, along with calculation of ne minimum infectious dose of the virus in feed [7]. 'his information heightened the awareness of the need or strategies to mitigate the risk of contaminated feed, hrough thermal processing or chemical treatment. In egards to the latter approach, data are now available emonstrating the ability of a liquid antimicrobial prodct containing formaldehyde and propionic acid or a nedium chain fatty acid blend to successfully degrade 'EDV RNA in contaminated feed and prevent infection 8, 9].

Despite these advances at the domestic level, the risk f PEDV infection at the global level still exists, as the ource of the initial PEDV introduction to the US renains unidentified. During the widespread epidemic, the ole of feed in transboundary spread of the virus was ownplayed, based on lack of data supporting survival of 'EDV in feed ingredients over time and under conditions representative of trans-oceanic transport. Recently, xtended survival of PEDV in individual feed ingredients nder wintertime ambient conditions has been reported 10]. Most notably, survival of PEDV was demonstrated n soybean meal for 180 days, along with evidence of irus survival in lysine hydrochloride, choline chloride,)DGS and several porcine by-products for at least 0 days [10]. One feature that was consistent across sevral of these ingredients was that they are imported to he US from China. As the original PEDV detected in he US is closely related to a Chinese variant [11], it aises the question whether contaminated feed ingredints imported from China could have served as a source for viral entry to the US in 2013. Table 1 is a summary of data derived from the US International Trade Commission Harmonized Tariff Schedule website (www.hs.usitc.gov) which is a publicly available database that provides a transaction of specific trade commodities between the US and its international trading partners. These data provide insight into the types of and quantities of ingredients that entered the US from China during the height of the PED epidemic in 2013 and 2014 (G. Patterson, personal communication, May 2015). This collective information justifies renewed investigation into the transboundary risk of PEDV and the potential role that contaminated feed ingredients could play in the spread of disease during the process of trans-oceanic shipping. Therefore, the purpose of this study was to develop a model to evaluate the transboundary risk of PEDV-contaminated swine feed ingredients during a simulated shipment from China to the US, as well as test the effect of two mitigation strategies. The study was based on the hypothesis that while select non-treated ingredients could provide a protective effect on PEDV survival, mitigation would reduce risk.

Methods

Design of shipping model

Route and timetable

Based on the predominance of facilities processing agricultural feed ingredients for export in the eastern region of China, i.e., Shandong, Jilin, Henan, Hebei and Liaoning provinces (www.alibaba.com), and that the PEDV strain initially detected in the US most closely resembled a variant from the province of Anhui [11], the city of Beijing was designated as the starting point for the model. Here it was assumed that PEDV contamination of select ingredients would occur, either at the manufacturing plant or post-processing [4]. In an effort to determine if PEDV could be delivered in a viable state from Beijing to a major pork production region in the US,

Table 1 Summary of quantities (kg) of representative feed ingredients imported to the US from China in 2013 and 2014[a]

Ingredient	2013 (kg)	2014 (kg)
Soybeans (conventional and organic)	89,469,255	70,940,336
Lysine hydrochloride	21,469,477	5,382,454
Soybean meal (conventional and organic)	6,632,960	7,214,863
Feed-grade tetracycline	1,411,251	1,418,012
D-L methionine	377,495	1,790,280
Vitamin E	12,640	14,194
Choline chloride	11,284	23,572
Vitamin A	1156	1094
Vitamin D	1043	1052

[a]: Source = US Government Harmonized Tariff Schedule

Des Moines, IA was selected as the final destination. Based on these assumptions, a commercial website (SeaRates.com) was used to develop a representative route and timetable. Specifically, it was modeled that contaminated ingredients would travel for 1 day from Beijing to the Anquing terminal in Shanghai, where they would be held for 7 days in preparation for shipment to the US. Cargo would then travel across the Pacific Ocean over a 17 day period and enter the US at the port of San Francisco. Following a 7 day period to clear customs, it would then be transported for 2 days via Interstate 80 to Des Moines, where it would remain for 3 days, for a total transit period of 37 days (Table 2).

Compilation of environmental data

Once the 37-day timetable had been established, it was decided to model the shipping event over the period of December 23, 2012 to January 28, 2013. This decision was based on the timing of the initial detection of PEDV in the US (April 2013) and the availability of data summarizing temperature and % RH in shipping containers traveling from Asia to the US during the period of December 31, 2012 to January 16, 2013 [12]. Using this information, we designed a temperature and % RH curve for the oceanic segment of the study. In addition, we accessed historical meteorological data for the land segments of the model using Weather Underground (www.wunderground.com) encompassing the periods of December 23–30, 2012 and January 17–27, 2013, which were paired in conjunction with the oceanic transport period. To simulate the effect of daily fluctuation we collected historical temperature data at 4 designated times each day (6 AM, 12 PM, 6 PM, 12 AM) and at 3 designated times each day for % RH (8 AM, 12 PM, 4 PM). All data were then entered into the computer of an environmental chamber used to house samples during the model shipping period.

Processing of feed ingredients

A panel of 14 swine feed ingredients known to be imported to the US from China were selected for this study, including organic & conventional soybeans and soybean meal, lysine hydrochloride, D-L methionine, tryptophan, Vitamins A, D & E, choline chloride, two ingredient carriers (rice hulls or corn cobs) and feed grade tetracycline. In regards to the soy-based products the guaranteed analysis of conventional meal indicated a 48 % crude protein, 1 % fat and 3 % fiber while the organic product had lower protein (44 %) and higher fat and fiber (7.5 and 6.5 %, respectively). Furthermore, the process of manufacturing organic soybean meal was void of chemical (hexane) use and no chemical fertilizer had been used during the soybean growing period. Ingredients were screened by PCR to insure a PEDV-negative status prior to the onset of the study. The treatments selected for the study included a liquid antimicrobial (LA (SalCURB®, Kemin Industries, Des Moines, IA USA) or a medium chain fatty acid blend (MCFA). SalCURB® is a premix of aqueous formaldehyde solution 37 % (for maintenance of complete animal feeds or feed ingredients *Salmonella*-negative for up to 21 days) and propionic acid (as a chemical preservative for control of mold in feed or feed ingredients). While SalCURB® provide effective *Salmonella* control for up to 21 days, it is not approved for use by the U.S. Food & Drug Administration or the U.S. Department of Agriculture as a treatment for PEDV. The second treatment, MCFA, was a 2 % custom medium chain fatty acid blend of caproic caprylic and capric acids, blended at a 1:1 ratio [9]. Control ingredients were treated with sterile saline.

Sample management

Samples were organized into 1 of 4 identical batches each representing a specific segment of the 37-day shipping period. Batch 1 (segment 1) was designed to represent the transport of contaminated ingredients from manufacturing plants in Beijing to the Shanghai Anquing terminal (day 1 post-contamination (DPC)) Batch 2, a compilation of segments 1 and 2, simulated manufacturing and delivery to Shanghai, as well as time in the Anquing terminal awaiting shipment (1–8 DPC) Batch 3, a compilation of segments 1, 2 and 3 represented time in China, the crossing of the Pacific and arrival to the US at the San Francisco, CA terminal (1–2[illegible] DPC). Finally, batch 4 was a compilation of segments 1-4, thereby representing the entire process, including transport to and storage in, Des Moines, IA (1–37 DPC) On designated days post-contamination, a batch o

Table 2 Description of locations and events involved in the 37-day shipping model period

Day	Location	Events
1	Beijing	Ingredient manufacturing & contamination
2–8	Anquing terminal, Shanghai	Transport to Shanghai, awaiting shipment to U
9–25	Pacific ocean	Departure from China, crossing the ocean
26–32	San Francisco terminal, CA, US	Entry to the US, clearing customs
33–34	Interstate 80	Transport from California to Iowa
35–37	Des Moines, IA	Storage

amples was removed from the environmental chamber nd submitted for testing. Specifically, batch 1 was submitted on 1 DPC, batch 2 on 8 DPC, batch 3 on 27 DPC nd batch 4 on 37 DPC. In other words, the same samle was not repeatedly opened and tested, but rather a ew batch of samples was submitted on a designated ay. This method of sample management would insure hat all sample containers remained sealed from the time hey were inoculated until the time they were tested at he lab, minimizing the risk of cross-contamination, as vell as enhancing repeatability of results as several segnents were replicated across batches. Finally, to increase tatistical power, each of the 4 batches contained 2 replicates of each ingredient in the control group and 2 replicates of each ingredient within each treatment group, or a total of 90 samples per batch.

ample contamination procedures

. goal of the study was to limit the variability to the evel of the ingredient; therefore, the same quantity of ngredient, the same container type and the same environmental settings were used and samples were contaminated equally. To initiate this process, 30 g of each ngredient were added to food storage containers (Oxo 'ot Baby Blocks, Oxo International, El Paso, TX, USA) o simulate a shipping container [10]. Ingredients in the on-treated control group were treated with 0.1 mL of terile saline. Ingredients in the LA group were treated vith 0.1 mL of product, based on an inclusion rate of kg/ton of complete feed. Ingredients in the MCFA roup were treated with 0.6 g of product based on a 2 % nclusion rate. Individual treatments and saline placebo vere added to the designated samples using separate tuerculin syringes. To promote proper mixing, the feed as stirred manually for 10 clockwise rotations and 10 ounter-clockwise rotations using individual wooden aplicator sticks per ingredient. Following mixing, each inividual container was manually shaken vigorously (50 imes in a 10 s period). All samples were then inoculated vith 2 mL PEDV (passage 18, Ct = 17.15, total dose 91,520 FFU) and mixed as described. This quantity of EDV was selected in an effort to provide a final mean t value in feed ingredient of approximately 25 (range = 9–30) following mixing, based on data from actual field ases of PEDV-contaminated feed, a challenge level used n published studies [5, 8, 10].

ontrols

or the purpose of negative controls, 30 g samples of EDV-negative complete feed were inoculated with stere saline. Duplicate negative controls were included in ach of the 4 batches, across the control and treatment roups. For the purpose of positive controls, duplicate mL samples of stock PEDV in MEM (minimum essential media, Gibco, ThermoFisher Scientific, Waltham, MA, USA) were included in containers within each batch of ingredients in both control and treatment groups.

Sample storage

Once prepared, samples were stored in the environmental chamber. This instrument (Model 9005 L, Sheldon Manufacturing Inc., Cornelius, OR) had a programmable temperature range of 4–21^{C} C and a RH range of 40–95 %. In order for ingredients to be exposed to ambient air within the chamber, two holes, 0.318 cm in diameter were drilled into each plastic container (Fig. 1). Using the data from the historical temperature and % RH curve described above, the chamber computer was programmed to simulate fluctuation over time as previously described.

Diagnostic procedures

All diagnostic testing was conducted using protocols developed and validated by the South Dakota State University (SDSU) Animal Disease Research and Diagnostic Laboratory (ADRDL). Samples were submitted by code to the laboratory, so personnel were blinded as to batch, treatment versus non-treatment and ingredient type. It was originally planned to test all samples by PCR and virus isolation (VI), followed by the use of swine bioassay for samples determined to be PCR positive but VI negative.

Extraction of RNA

The MagMAX^{TM} 96 Viral Isolation Kit (Life Technologies, Waltham MA, USA) was used to obtain viral RNA from the samples, as described in the instructions provided (1836 M Revision F). A 175-µl volume of sample was used for the extraction. The magnetic bead extractions were completed on a Kingfisher96 instrument (Thermo Scientific, Waltham MA, USA).

Real-time PCR

A commercially available real-time, single tube RT-PCR multiplex assay for the detection of PEDV, porcine deltacoronavirus (PDCoV) and transmissible gastroenteritis virus (TGEV) was used in this study per kit instruction (Tetracore, Rockville, MD, USA). Briefly, 7 µl of the extracted RNA was added to 13 µl of the master mix. The one-step real-time RT-PCR amplification conditions started with 15 min at 48 °C, followed by 2 min at 95 °C. The final cycles consisted of 5 s at 95 °C and then 40 s at 60 °C (data collection step). The program was run for 38 cycles (Cycle time) with PEDV positive results indicated at ≤ 38 cycles. Positive and negative controls were included on each run. All amplification was completed on the ABI7500 instrumentation (Austin, TX, USA).

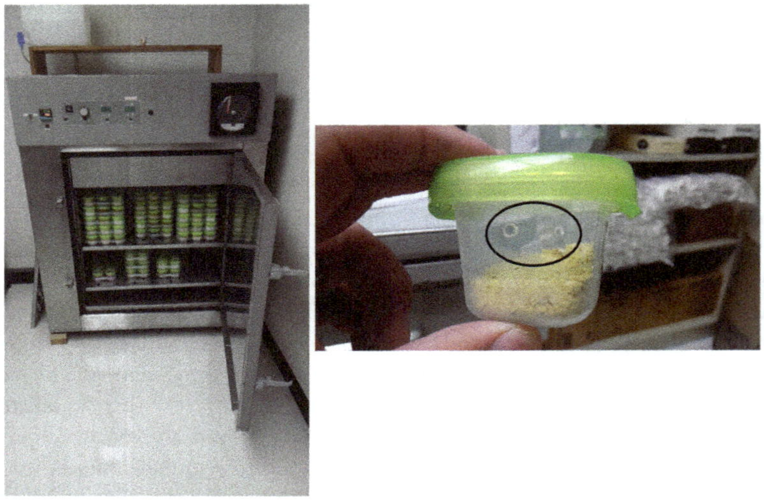

Fig. 1 Environmental chamber and sample containers. This figure depicts the environmental chamber loaded with sample containers as well as a close-up view of a container. Note the two 0.318 cm holes (*red circle*) drilled in the container to allow for contact of the ingredient with the chamber environment

PEDV stock virus propagation

For PEDV propagation, Vero 76 cells (ATCC CRL-1587) were maintained in MEM plus 10 % fetal bovine serum and antibiotics. Three-day old confluent monolayers of Vero 76 cells in 150 cm^2 flasks were washed 3 times with serum free minimum essential media (MEM) prior to inoculation. Monolayers were infected at ~0.1 moi of PEDV in MEM containing 2 *u*g/ml TPCK treated trypsin, incubated at 37 °C for approximately 48 h until obvious CPE was apparent. Flasks were frozen at −80 °C until needed.

Virus isolation

Once feed ingredient samples were tested for PEDV via PCR, the residual samples were tested for presence of viable virus. Samples were diluted in MEM containing 2 μg/ml TPCK-treated trypsin with a starting dilution of 1:2 and were two-fold serially diluted. Diluted samples were then added to washed confluent monolayers of Vero-76 cells in 96-well plates and incubated for 1 h at 37 °C. Plates were again washed and trypsin media replaced. After 24 h at 37 °C, plates were fixed with 80 % acetone and stained with FITC conjugated mAb SD6-29 to allow visualization of infected cells. Virus concentration was determined by calculating FFU/ml based on the number of fluorescent foci present in wells at selected dilutions using a previously published method adapted to PEDV [13]. Personnel reading the plates were blinded to the type of sample and the time of sampling.

Swine bioassay

Facilities and source of animals

The purpose of the swine bioassay was to determine whether viable PEDV was present in any feed ingredient sample that had tested positive on PCR but negative o VI. This study was conducted in a Biosafety Level 2 room at the Animal Resource Wing (ARW) at South Da kota State University. All procedures involving animal throughout the study were performed under the guid ance and approval of the SDSU Institutional Anima Care and Use Committee. Animals ($n = 24$, 5 day ol piglets) were sourced from a PEDV-naïve herd and wer tested on arrival to the ARW via blood sampling an collection of rectal swabs from each pig. Prior to anima arrival, all rooms (walls, ceilings, floors and drains) wer monitored for the presence of PEDV by PCR using sam pling procedures previously described [5, 8]. Piglets wer housed in one of 6 stainless steel gnotobiotic unit measuring 0.6 m W × 1.2 m L × 0.6 m H. Units were di vided into 4 semi-isolated housing units, allowing for piglets per unit with individual feeding arrangements Flooring consisted of an open weave rubberized mat o a perforated stainless steel grate raised 10 cm for wast collection. Each unit was covered with an inflatable 2 mil plastic canopy and fitted with 2 pair of dry-bo gloves for feeding and procedures inside the canopy Each canopy was secured and sealed with duct tape an ratchet straps to the unit. Ventilation was supplied by a electric fan maintaining sufficient positive pressure in side the canopy to keep the canopy inflated above th unit. Incoming and outgoing air to each unit was HEPA filtered. Each unit was initially sterilized using 47 aerosolized formalin, and allowed to dissipate for 2 week prior to introduction of the animals. All incoming an outgoing materials needed during the study (eg. swabs injectable medication, bleeding supplies) were passe through an air-tight stainless steel port and sterilize sing 5 % peracetic acid before entering or exiting the ort.

reparation of bioassay inoculum

he stainless steel unit served as the experimental unit; herefore, all 4 piglets in each unit received the same inredient. To assess PEDV survivability throughout the enire model period, samples from batch 4 were tested, ncluding both treated and non-treated ingredients. Rearding non-treated samples, all PCR-positive and VI-egative samples in batch 4 were tested. In regards to LA-reated and MCFA-treated ingredients, treated equivalents f non-treated samples that were VI or swine bioassay ositive, again from batch 4 samples were tested. For reparation of the inoculums, 60 g of each specific ingreient was mixed with 50 mL of sterile PBS in a 250 mL entrifuge tube, inverted 10 times to mix and vortexed for min. The suspension was then centrifuged at 5200 g for 5 min, supernatant decanted and tested by PCR prior to iglet inoculation. Each pig in the unit received 1 mL of he designated inoculum orally via syringe and observed or a 7 day period. To minimize the number of animals eeded for the study, pigs that were confirmed negative fter 7 DPI would be inoculated with a different ingredint. A negative control unit was included in the design, ith these pigs receiving sterile saline PO.

iglet testing

ollowing inoculation, the PEDV status of each group of iglets was monitored [5, 8]. On a daily basis, ARW ersonnel inspected animals for clinical signs of PED nd collected rectal swabs (Dacron swabs, Fisher Scienific, Franklin Lakes, NJ, USA) from each pig, starting ith the negative control unit. Showers were taken upon ntry to the rooms and room-specific coveralls, footwear, airnets, gloves and P95 masks (3 M, St. Paul, MN USA) ere worn. In addition, each room was ventilated indiidually and HEPA filtration for both incoming and outoing air was employed per room. If clinically affected nimals were observed, swabs of diarrhea and/or vomitng, in conjunction with the daily rectal swab were colected. Swabs were submitted to the SDSU ADRDL and ested by PCR. If PEDV was diagnosed in a specific unit, ll animals were swabbed, humanely euthanized with ntravenous sodium pentobarbital, the small intestinal racts submitted for PCR testing, units were cleaned and anitized as described and re-stocked with new piglets as eeded.

ata analysis

escriptive statistics, *T*-test and ANOVA were used to nalyze data, when applicable.

Results

Sample size

A total of 360 feed ingredient samples were used for this study.

PCR

All feed ingredient samples were PCR negative on day 0 of the study. Successful PEDV inoculation was confirmed, as all day 1 samples were PCR-positive. Results of PCR testing of treated and non-treated ingredients on 1 and 37 DPC are summarized in Table 3. The mean Ct of LA-treated samples was 24.5 (SD = 2.4) on 1 DPC and 32.5 (SD = 3.9) on 37 DPC ($p < 0.0001$). The mean Ct of MCFA-treated samples was 24.2 (SD = 4.2) on 1 DPC and 25.5 (SD = 3.7) on 37 DPC ($p = 0.25$). The mean Ct values across non-treated ingredients on day 1 was 22.9 (SD = 2.4) and 23.1 (SD = 3.5) on day 37 ($p = 0.34$). At 1 DPC, the mean Ct values of all 3 groups (non-treated, LA-treated and MCFA-treated) were not significantly different ($p = 0.14$); however, at 37 DPC, the mean Ct of LA-treated samples was significantly higher ($p < 0.0001$) than the mean Ct of MCFA-treated and non-treated samples.

Virus isolation

A summary of VI data is provided in Table 4. Viable PEDV was recovered from organic and conventional SBM, lysine and Vitamin D across all 4 batches of non-treated samples, including batch 3 representing entry to the US at the San Francisco terminal and batch 4, representing shipment to and storage in Des Moines. No other samples harbored viable virus beyond batch 2 (Beijing and Shanghai segments) including the PEDV stock virus control. Multiple samples were VI negative on 1 DPC. All negative control samples and all LA-treated or MCFA-treated ingredients were VI negative across all batches.

Swine bioassay

Samples selected for swine bioassay testing consisted of treated and non-treated ingredients from batch 4. The non-treated ingredients tested included those which were PCR- positive and VI-negative, specifically Vitamins A & E, tryptophan, D-L methionine, soybeans (organic and conventional), and choline

Table 3 Summary of PCR Ct data mean & (SD) across treated and non-treated groups on day 1 and 37 of the study

Group	Day 1 mean (SD)	Day 37 mean (SD)
Control ingredients	22.9^{a} (2.4)	23.1^{a} (3.5)
LA-treated ingredients	24.5^{a} (2.4)	32.5^{b} (3.9)
MCFA-treated ingredients	24.2^{a} (4.2)	25.5^{a} (3.7)

Values with different superscripts (a/b) are significantly different at $p < 0.05$

Table 4 Summary of mean PCR Ct and FFU/mL across all 4 batches of non-treated ingredients

Ingredient	Mean Ct/FFU titer Batch 1	Mean Ct/FFU titer Batch 2	Mean Ct/FFU titer Batch 3	Mean Ct/FFU titer Batch 4
Soybeans (organic)	20.76/5120	23.27/neg	26.42/neg	25.52/ne
Soybean meal (organic)	19.20/40,960	19.10/1920	20.10/800	22.55/60
Soybeans (conventional)	22.39/3840	24.18/40	28.86/neg	20.99/ne
Soybean meal(conventional)	19.75/7680	19.71/1920	19.76/5120	16.04/60
Lysine hydrochloride	18.54/1280	18.51/40	18.79/100	17.83/10
D-L methionine	22.17/2560	21.25/neg	25.03/neg	19.50/ne
Tryptophan	23.56/160	22.54/neg	25.30/neg	21.31/ne
Vitamin A	25.22/neg	22.66/neg	25.23/neg	26.85/ne
Vitamin D	22.28/3840	21.29/640	22.72/320	20.94/40
Vitamin E	28.54/neg	22.86/neg	26.15/neg	30.86/ne
Choline chloride	20.82/40	20.90/40	20.41/neg	20.77/ne
Rice hulls	24.73/neg	24.47/neg	25.93/neg	22.99/ne
Corn cobs	23.66/80	22.83/neg	24.68/neg	24.49/ne
Tetracycline	38/neg	38/neg	38/neg	38/neg
(−) control feed	38/neg	38/neg	38/neg	38/neg
Virus stock	17.15/245,760	18.86/30	21.19/neg	23.73/ne

Ingredient: Two 30 g replicates per ingredient
Mean Ct/FFU titer: Mean Ct value and FFU/mL across the 2 samples per ingredient

chloride. Viable PEDV was detected in piglets administered non-treated samples of choline chloride (Table 5). Affected animals displayed evidence of mild diarrhea, shed PEDV in feces and samples of small intestine were PCR and immunohistochemistry-positive at necropsy, with microscopic lesions of villous blunting, fusion and re-epithelialization [5]. All other samples were bioassay negative. In regards to treated ingredients, LA-treated and MCFA-treated samples of soybean meal (conventional and organic), lysine, vitamin D and choline chloride were tested. All piglets inoculated with the aforementioned LA-treated or MCFA-treated ingredients were determined to be non-infectious, as piglets remained clinically norma throughout the testing period and all rectal swab and in testinal samples were negative by PCR (Table 6).

Environmental data

Figure 2 provides a summary of the mean dail temperature and % RH data recorded in the environ mental chamber throughout the 37-day study period For the purpose of statistical analysis, the 37-da period was divided into 4 segments: Days 1–8, repre senting time in China, days 9–25, representing tim travelling across the Pacific, days 26–32, representin

Table 5 Summary of results of PCR (+)/VI (−) non-treated control feed ingredients from batch 4 tested by swine bioassay

Ingredient	Ct of inoculum	Clinical signs/rectal swabs	PCR testing of small intestin
Soybean-organic	25.52	negative	negative
Soybean-conventional	26.34	negative	negative
Vitamin A	26.86	negative	negative
Vitamin E	30.86	negative	negative
Rice hulls	22.94	negative	negative
Corn cobs	23.95	negative	negative
Tryptophan	21.31	negative	negative
D/L methionine	19.75	negative	negative
Choline chloride	20.79	positive	positive
(−) control	>38	negative	negative

Table 6 Summary of results of PCR (+)/VI (–) LA-treated or MCFA-treated control feed ingredients from batch 4 tested by swine bioassay

Ingredient[a]	Treatment	Ct of inoculum	Clinical signs & rectal swabs	PCR testing of small intestine
Soybean meal-conventional	LA	31.44	negative	negative
Soybean meal-organic	LA	22.38	negative	negative
Vitamin D	LA	38	negative	negative
Lysine	LA	17.83	negative	negative
Choline chloride	LA	33.70	negative	negative
Soybean meal-conventional	MCFA	23.78	negative	negative
Soybean meal-organic	MCFA	17.75	negative	negative
Vitamin D	MCFA	20.60	negative	negative
Lysine	MCFA	20.33	negative	negative
Choline chloride	MCFA	21.24	negative	negative
(-) control	Saline	38	negative	negative

[a] Ingredients were selected based on the recovery of viable PEDV in their non-treated equivalent samples

time spent in the San Francisco terminal and days 33–37, time spent during transport from California to Iowa with time in Des Moines (Table 7). In summary, mean temperature and mean % RH recorded during the San Francisco segment were significantly different ($p = 0.0004$ and $p = 0.0025$, respectively) from that recorded during the other 3 segments.

Discussion

Over the course of less than 1 year (April 2013-February 2014), several novel corona viruses have been detected in the US including the PEDV prototype strain, the PEDV S INDEL strain and the porcine deltacoronavirus [14–16]. As of this writing, the route(s) of entry of these pathogens has not been identified; however, phylogenetic

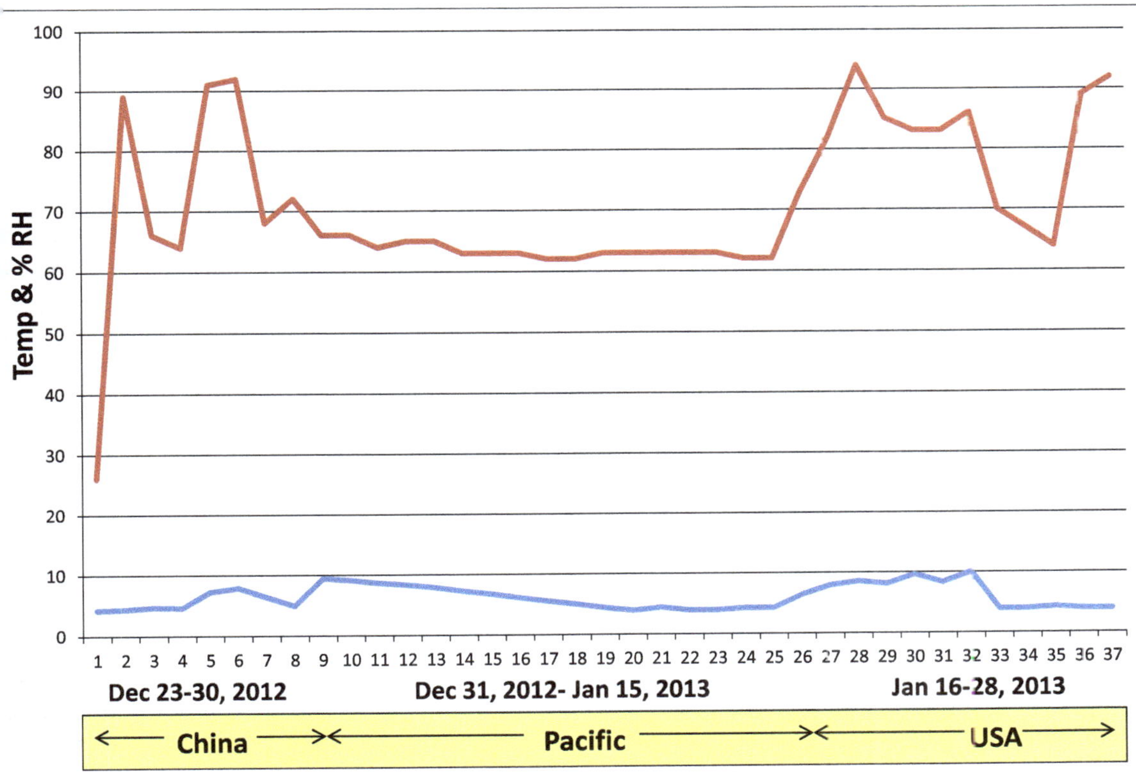

Fig. 2 Mean daily temperature and % RH recorded during the 37-day study period. This figure depicts the summary of the environmental conditions recorded during the simulated period of December 23, 2012 to January 28, 2013

Table 7 Descriptive summary of temperature and % RH data per the 4 segments of the 37-day study period

Temp C0	Segment 1 (China)	Segment 2 (Pacific)	Segment 3 (SF)	Segment 4 (DSM
	1–8 DPC	9–25 DPC	26–32 DPC	33–37 DPC
Mean	5.5	6.0	8.4	3.9
95 % CI	4.3–6.7	5.2–6.8	7.1–9.6	2.5–5.4
SD	1.4	2.0	1.2	.13
Median	4.8	5.5	8.3	3.9
Range	4.2–7.8	3.9–9.4	6.3–10	3.9–4.2
% RH	Segment 1 (China)	Segment 2 (Pacific)	Segment 3 (SF)	Segment 4 (DSM
	1–8 DPC	9–25 DPC	26–32 DPC	33–37 DPC
Mean	71	63	84	76
95 % CI	63–79	58–69	75–92	66–87
SD	21.6	1.3	6.2	13.1
Median	70	63	83	70
Range	26–92	62–66	73–94	64–92

analyses support the possibility of a Chinese origin [11, 14–16]. Since the initial detection of PEDV in the US, feed has been proposed as a possible route of entry and widespread, rapid distribution throughout the country; however, objective data supporting this hypothesis were lacking. Therefore, the objectives of this study were to develop a model to evaluate the transboundary risk of PEDV-contaminated swine feed ingredients and test the effect of two mitigation strategies during a simulated transport event from China to the US. This approach allowed us to design a study to successfully simulate the introduction of PEDV into the US in feed ingredients; the first such objective data of its kind.

The central component of the study was the development of a model to accurately represent the conditions of a trans-oceanic shipping event to determine whether the virus could actually survive the process. Key components of the model were the selection of the proper ingredients, the calculation of an accurate timetable, and the simulation of representative environmental conditions to challenge virus viability. In regards to ingredient selection, we utilized the US Government Harmonized Tariff Schedule to include products regularly imported to the US from China, 5 of which ended up harboring viable PEDV throughout the 37-day period: vitamin D, lysine hydrochloride, choline chloride, organic and conventional soybean meal. It was interesting to note that viable virus was once again recovered from 3 ingredients, (conventional soybean meal, lysine and choline chloride). This was similar to our previous report [10], despite the fact that the 2 studies were conducted under very different environmental conditions and that laboratory personnel were blinded to sample identity/origin in both studies. This level of repeatability strengthens the conclusions drawn from both studies, thereby increasing the significance of these specific ingredients as potentia transboundary risks.

Besides the consistency of the results, these ingredi ents were interesting for several other reasons. I regards to soybean meal, it was surprising to learn of th large quantity of soy products imported to the US fron China, as the US is a major producer/exporter of soy beans and soybean meal. Using Google to search fo sources of both organic and conventional soy product from China, we identified multiple soybean and soybea meal manufacturers in the eastern region of the countr supplying product for agricultural use in bags, totes containers or bulk quantities, including products desig nated as "organic", targeted specifically for organic live stock feeding. Therefore, these data, in combinatio with our previous work demonstrating extended PED survival in soybean meal in cold climates [10] sugges that soy-based ingredients could be considered a signifi cant transboundary risk for pathogen transmission, in cluding the organic variety. Another ingredient whic harbored viable virus throughout the 37-day transpor period was lysine hydrochloride, a similar finding to tha reported in the 30-day wintertime study [10]. Lysine i an interesting ingredient as the volume imported to th US from China is large (particularly in 2013) whic could enhance the significance of this ingredient as a po tential risk factor for transboundary spread of PEDV. Fi nally, this study brought forth new information on th risk of PEDV survival in vitamins, specifically vitamin D During the early stages of the PED epidemic in 2013, vi tamins and trace minerals were proposed as a route o viral entry, based on the volume of product importe from China. While viable PEDV was not recovered fron previously tested vitamin/trace mineral mixes [10], i was speculated that this may have been due to th otentially caustic effect of the minerals on the virus. herefore, we decided to investigate vitamins individu-lly, and while vitamin A and E did not support virus, esults were different with vitamin D. Finally, as in the revious study [10], choline chloride again proved cap-ble of harboring viable PEDV over time, thereby raising s significance as a possible transboundary risk factor.

Along with ingredient selection, the second key com-onent of the model was the calculation of the shipping imetable in order to truly represent this journey. Using earates.com, we developed an accurate estimate of time equired to move from the various cities and ports vithin the model. It did not, however, include time in ort for preparation for shipping or clearance of cus-oms. Therefore, a 7-day period of time was added at the oint of each port to better represent reality (T. Schmitt, PC Inc., personal communication, 2015), increasing he calculated timetable from 23 to 37 days. This modifi-ation further challenged the viability of the virus, hereby strengthening the model.

Finally, perhaps the most novel component of the nodel was the development of the environmental curve vhich included actual temperature and % RH data from cean containers travelling from Asia to the US [12]. his interesting project was carried out by the technical taff of the Xerox Company and involved the use of data oggers placed inside the actual containers, collecting eal time temperature and % RH data as they traveled round the world. As one of the datasets involved a hipping event from Asia to the US in the months of December and January, we used this information as the enterpiece of our model and were able to reproduce he consistent trans-Pacific temperatures and % RH de-cribed in their publication along with the greater vari-bility observed on land. Combining this with historical ata from the various cities and ports using Weather Jnderground, we were able to develop a representative emperature and % RH curve, allowing us to program he environmental chamber accordingly (Fig. 2). One in-eresting observation was the rapid reduction in stock irus titer observed from the initial titer used to inocu-ate batch 1 (mean titer = 245,760 FFU) to that detected days later in batch 2 (mean titer = 30 FFU) with the ventual loss of viability (batch 3) in the stock virus con-rol, despite storage in MEM, an ideal medium for virus torage. This observation indicates that the environmen-al conditions used in the study were rigorous, thereby hallenging virus survival. This was most likely due to he warmer temperatures and high % RH present in the nodel, conditions quite unlike the winter time project vhere long-term PEDV stock virus survival was ob-erved [10]. We insured that ingredients would be ex-osed to the effect of the % RH by adding the holes in he sides of each container model. It also suggests the need for a supportive matrix to maintain viability in the container during shipment and that under the correct conditions, PEDVis highly susceptible to environmental pressures if left unprotected in its respective shipping container. Finally, the fact that viable PEDV was recov-ered from only 5 of 14 ingredients suggests that individ-ual ingredient chemistry may provide a protective effect, potentially shielding virus from the environment and allowing it to survive and this may be particularly true of the meal form of soy versus the intact bean. In contrast, the high alkalinity of feed grade tetracycline (pH 13) ap-parently degraded the RNA immediately post-contamination, resulting in PCR-negative readings in all 4 batches.

In an effort to assess the potential for chemical mitiga-tion of ingredient risk, two interventions, the liquid anti-microbial SalCURB® and the medium chain fatty acid blend were included in the design. While we had vali-dated the LA in previous studies [8, 10], this was our first opportunity to assess the MCFA option. While the effect of the LA on PEDV RNA degradation over the course of the study was significantly different than the response to MCFA, both products appeared to have equivalent effect on virus viability. This outcome sup-ports the validity of chemical mitigation as a means to reduce the risk of PEDV in feed ingredients stored under conditions modeling the trans-oceanic voyage, as well as provides options for treatment.

In addition to an improved understanding of risks and mitigation, other strengths of the study included an ex-perimental design where the only variables in the study were the individual ingredients, and the presence or ab-sence of the treatment. Specifically, we inoculated equal amounts of each ingredient with an equivalent quantity of virus in an attempt to mimic published viral loads as-sociated with field cases of PEDV in feed. All ingredients were stored in identical models of shipping containers, exposed to the same environment and tested in a single laboratory, involving consistent, trained personnel and validated assays for the detection of PEDV. We orga-nized samples in a manner to prevent cross-contamination by insuring that the individual sample storage containers were never opened from the time of PEDV inoculation until testing occurred at the labora-tory. While this may have resulted in some variability of the PCR assay since a new batch was submitted each time, the fact that our negative control samples remained free of contamination throughout the entire project validated these protocols. Finally, we used mul-tiple metrics (PCR, VI and bioassay) to document viral load across a total of 360 samples, exceeding our previ-ous work.

However, as with all studies there were both strengths and limitations. For example, we were limited to 14 ingredients primarily due to cost; however, the decision to use similar ingredients across the 2 studies enhanced replication and confidence in the data. While we were limited in the number of replicates, each batch contained 2 replicates/ingredient/batch; resulting in 8 replicates per ingredient. Furthermore, these results were derived from gram quantities of feed and may not directly equate to the vast quantity of tonnage used in actual swine production or feed manufacturing facilities. The bioassay protocol, while helpful at identifying ingredients containing low levels of virus was costly and difficult to carry out. As we evaluated only one shipping route over a defined period of time under a specific set of environmental conditions, this does not allow for extrapolation of results across other climates, other routes or over longer periods of time. Finally, as this was an experiment and did not take place in China, we could not provide proof on how the contamination of ingredients could actually take place. However, from our experiences in the US, we could speculate that contamination of feed could take place through the inclusion of contaminated ingredients or through contact with the virus in the environment, either at the farm or at the mill [6, 10]. As PEDV dispersion throughout the mill setting appears to be widespread, contact with ingredients within a milling storage facility seems logical [17].

In closing, under the conditions of this study, we provided the first proof of concept data indicating that a subset of contaminated feed ingredients could successfully transport live PEDV into the US using a novel transboundary shipping model. These are the first objective data suggesting that feed ingredients could potentially serve as vehicles for pathogen transfer between countries, as well as providing a plausible explanation regarding how PEDV was introduced to the US in 2013. This study also provides insight on how the onset of organic farming could serve to elevate risk of pathogen introduction into the US, secondary to the entry of organic soy products. This study also introduces a model which could enhance further transboundary research efforts, possibly employing surrogate viruses (bovine viral diarrhea virus for swine fever virus or Seneca Valley virus for foot-and-mouth disease virus) to test feed-related risks for other foreign animal diseases, further the investigation of the risk of organic ingredients, along with the continuing validation of mitigation strategies. With this information, it is hoped that veterinarians, feed industry experts and government officials will work together to develop a comprehensive plan of ingredient management to reduce global risk. It is time for discussions on how to adequately treat feed, how to increase biosecurity at the port level, as well as where to purchase biosecure ingredients, with the end result being a lowered incidence of feed-related disease transmission around the world.

Conclusions

These results indicate the ability of PEDV to survive i specific feed ingredients under modeled condition simulating shipment from China to the US. This is th first proof of concept suggesting that contaminated fee ingredients could serve as transboundary risk factors fo PEDV, along with the identification of effective mitiga tion options.

Abbreviations

PEDV: porcine epidemic diarrhea virus; PED: porcine epidemic diarrhea; Ct: Cycle threshold; PCR: polymerase chain reaction; ARW: Animal Resource Wing; MEM: minimal essential media; SBM: soybean meal; LA: liquid antimicrobial.

Competing interests

The authors declare no competing or conflicting interests associated with this study.

Authors' contributions

SD: Developed study, co-wrote paper. CN: Developed study, provided swine nutrition expertise, reviewed paper. TC: Conducted molecular diagnostics, co-wrote paper. AS: Provided virological expertise at the laboratory level, co-wrote paper. JCH: Provided critical review and revising of paper. EN: Provided virological expertise at the laboratory level, co-wrote paper. CJ & RC: Provided MCFA product, resources, co-wrote paper. GP: Analyzed the US government Harmonized Tariff Schedule website, reviewed paper. GS: Developed study, reviewed paper, mentored project. All authors read and approved the final manuscript.

Acknowledgements

The authors would like to recognize Dr. Michele Mucciante and the Animal Resource Wing team for their significant contributions to the success of this study. The authors would also like to thank Kemin Industries, APC Inc and the National Pork Board for providing the technical expertise, funding and in-kind resources necessary to complete this project.

Author details

[1]Pipestone Applied Research, Pipestone Veterinary Services, 1300 Box188 Hwy 75 S, Pipestone, MN 56164, USA. [2]Animal Disease Research and Diagnostic Laboratory, South Dakota State University, Brookings, SD, USA. [3]Department of Grain Science, Kansas State University, Manhattan, KS, USA. [4]Center for Animal Health and Food Safety, University of Minnesota, St. Paul, MN, USA.

References

1. Saif LJ, Pensaert MB, Sestak K, Yeo S, Jung K. Coronaviruses. In: Zimmerman JJ, Karriker LA, Ramierez A, Schwartz KJ, Stevenson GW, editors. Diseases of Swine. 10th ed. Ames: Wiley and Sons; 2012. p. 501–24.
2. Chen Q, Ganwu L, Stasko J, Thomas JT, Stensland WR, Pillatzki AE, Gauger PC, Schwartz KJ, Madson D, Yoon KJ, Stevenson GW, Burrough ER, Harmon KM, Main RG, Zhang J. Isolation and characterization of Porcine Epidemic Diarrhea Viruses associated with the 2013 disease outbreak among swine in the United States. J Clin Microbiol. 2014;52:234–43.
3. American Association of Swine Practitioners, National Pork Producers Council and USDA Center for Epidemiology and Animal Health. PEDV Investigation 2013. http://www.aasv.org. Accessed 22 July 2015.
4. Goyal S. Interventions to control PEDV in feed and feed ingredients. http://www.pork.org/pedv-2014-research/pedv-feed. (2014). Accessed 23 March 2015.

Dee S, Clement T, Schelkopf A, Nerem J, Knudsen D, Hennings J, Nelson E. An evaluation of contaminated complete feed as a vehicle for porcine epidemic diarrhea virus infection of naïve pigs following consumption via natural feeding behavior: Proof of concept. BMC Vet Res. 2014;10:176.
Pascik J, Berhane Y, Ojkic D, Maxie G, Embury-Hyatt C, Swekla K, Handel K, Fairles J, Alexandersen S. Investigation into the role of potentially contaminated feed as a source of the first-detected outbreaks of porcine epidemic diarrhea in Canada. Transbound Emerg Dis. 2014;61:397–410.
Schumacher L, Woodworth JC, Zhang J, Gauger PC, Chen Q, Welch M, Salzebrenner H, Thomas J, Main R, Dritz S, Cochrane R, Jones C. Determining the minimum infectious dose of PEDV in a feed matrix. Proceedings of the 2015 Midwest Animal Science Conference Des Moines, IA, USA, Abstract. 2015;160.
Dee S, Neill C, Clement T, Hennings J, Nelson E. An evaluation of a liquid antimicrobial (SalCURB®) for reducing the risk of porcine epidemic diarrhea virus infection of naïve pigs during consumption of contaminated feed. BMC Vet Res. 2014;10:220.
Cochrane R. Evaluation of chemical mitigation of PEDV in feed and ingredients. ADSA-ASAS Midwest Meeting, Abstract. 2015;11670.
0. Dee SA, Neill C, Clement T, Singrey A, Christopher-Hennings J, Nelson E. An evaluation of PEDV survival in individual feed ingredients in the presence or absence of a liquid antimicrobial. Porcine Health Management. 2015;1:9.
1. Huang YW, Dickerman A, Pineyro P, Long L, Fang L, Kiehne R, Opressnig T, Meng XJ. Origin, evolution and genotyping of emergent porcine epidemic diarrhea virus strains in the United States. mBio. 2013;4:00737–13.
2. Leinberger D. Temperature and humidity in ocean containers. Technical report: Xerox Corporation; 2006. http://www.ista.org/pages/resources/TempRH.php.
3. Okda F, Liu X, Singrey A, Clement T, Christopher-Hennings J, Nelson EA, Lawson S. Development of an indirect ELISA, blocking ELISA, fluorescent microsphere immunoassay and fluorescent focus neutralization assay for serological evaluation of exposure to North American strains of porcine epidemic diarrhea virus. BMC Vet Res. 2015;11:180.
4. Wang L, Byrum B, Zhang Y. Detection and genetic characterization of deltacoronavirus in pigs Ohio US. Emerg Infect Dis. 2014;20:1227–30.
5. Vlasova A, Marthaler D, Wang Q, Culhane M, Rossow K, Rovia A, Collins J and Saif L. Distinct characteristics and complex evolution of porcine epidemic diarrhea virus strains in North America: May 2013-February 2014. Emerg Infect Dis. 2014;20:1620–8.
6. Wang L, Byrum B, Zhang Y. New variant of porcine epidemic diarrhea virus, United States. Emerg Infect Dis. 2014;20:917–9.
7. Schumacher LL, Cochrane RA, Evans CE, Kalivada JR, Woodworth JC, Stark CE, Jones CK, Main RG, Zhang J, Dritz SS, Gauger PC. Evaluating the effect of manufacturing porcine epidemic virus diarrhea virus-contaminated feed and subsequent feed mill environmental surface contamination. Kansas Agricultural Experiment Station Research Report. 2015, Vol 1, Issue 7.

12

Immunogenicity evaluation of inactivated virus and purified proteins of porcine circovirus type 2 in mice

Xiaohui Liu†, Ting Ouyang†, Teng Ma, Hongsheng Ouyang, Daxin Pang and Linzhu Ren*

Abstract

Background: Vaccination is considered as an effective and economical way to against PCV2 infection. However, some of commercial available vaccines are based on inactivated viruses, while the others are based on purified protein of PCV2. In the present study, we aimed to compare the immunogenicity of inactivated virus and purified proteins of porcine circovirus type 2 in mice.

Results: The results showed that positive antiserum titers were significantly increased after second, third and fourth immunization using inactivated PCV2 or purified proteins as coating antigen. Moreover, the inactivated PCV2 induced significantly higher levels of PCV2-specific antibodies than that of PCV2 subunit proteins. After PCV2 wild strain challenged, the average daily gain was comparable with that of mice in the mock group, and the sera from both inactivated PCV2-immunized animals and subunit protein Cap+ORF3 + Rep immunized animals had significantly higher neutralizing antibody titers than that of the PBS group. As expected, the neutralizing antibody in the inactivated PCV2 group was significantly higher than that of the subunit protein group. These results indicated that positive antiserum induced by the inactivated PCV2 had a better reactivity and specificity than that of the positive antiserum induced by the purified proteins.

Conclusions: The results in the present study demonstrated inactivated PCV2 is more effective than PCV2 subunit proteins in stimulating immune response to against PCV2 infection.

Keywords: Porcine circovirus type 2 (PCV2), Inactivated, Subunit, Immunogenicity, Mice, Vaccine

Background

Porcine circovirus 2 (PCV2) is the causative agent of porcine circovirus diseases and porcine circovirus-associated diseases (PCVD/PCVAD), including a number of different syndromes and diseases in pigs, such as post-weaning multi-systemic wasting syndrome (PMWS), porcine respiratory disease complex (PRDC), reproductive failure, granulomatous enteritis, necrotizing lymphadenitis, exudative epidermitis and congenital tremor, which are widely present in every major swine farm [1–3].

To date, the exact mechanisms of PCVD/PCVAD are currently unknown. Although several commercial vaccines based on PCV2a are effective in protecting pigs against a challenge with PCV2a, they cannot protect pigs against the PCV2b genotype that is prevalent worldwid or against other PCV2 genotypes [4, 5]. Therefore, stud ies focused on an effective vaccine are still urgent an important for PCV2 infection.

Based on current knowledge, many documents wer reported either based on inactivated PCV2 or PCV subunit proteins [6–9]. However, few studies were re ported to compare the efficiency of inactivated PCV and PCV2 subunit proteins. Previously, we expresse and purified Rep, ORF3, and different fragments o PCV2 Cap protein [6, 7]. In the present study, we aime to compare the immunogenicity of inactivated virus an purified proteins of PCV2 in mice. The results of th present study may be useful for production of PCV vaccine.

* Correspondence: renlz@jlu.edu.cn
†Equal contributors
Jilin Provincial Key Laboratory of Animal Embryo Engineering, College of Animal Sciences, Jilin University, Changchun, Jilin 130062, China

Methods

thics statement

ll animal experiments were prospectively planned and all rocedures were carried out under an ethical approval ranted by the Animal Care and Ethics Committee of Jilin Jniversity (Changchun, China). The Animal Ethics Committee approval number was LSXK2018051.

'iruses and proteins

'he titer of PCV2 strain CC1 [10] on PK-15 cell was 10^9 CID_{50}/mL. PCV2 strain CC1 was inactivated by 0.4% f formaldehyde (*v*/v) for 72 h at 37 °C.

PCV2 Cap, Rep and ORF3 proteins were prepared and urified according to the protocols described previously 6, 7]. Briefly, the ΔCap17–233 with truncated version of he Cap gene lacking the 5′-end 48 nt encoding the N-erminal 16 amino acid residues was amplified and sub-loned into the expression vector pET28b (+) (Novagene, Germany) to generate recombinant expression plasmids ET28b-ΔCap17–233. The ORF3 and Rep genes were mplified and subcloned into the expression vector pET-8c (+) (Novagene, Germany) to generate recombinant xpression plasmids, pET-28c-ORF3 and pET-28c-Rep, espectively. The plasmids were transformed into *E. oli* BL21 (DE3) competent cells and expressed with PTG (1.0 mmol/L) induction. Proteins were purified sing HisPur™ Ni-NTA Resin (Thermo scientific) ccording to the manufacturer's instruction and stored t 4 °C for use within one week or at – 80 °C for use fter a longer time.

nimal immunization

pecific pathogen-free (SPF) BALB/c mice were purchased rom the Laboratory Animal Center, Norman Bethune Iealth Science Center of Jilin University (Changchun, China). Mice were acclimatized at an environment with a emperature of 24–26 and humidity of 60% for 7 days be-ore experiment.

To compare the immunogenicity of inactivated virus and urified proteins, thirty female BABL/C mice, 5 weeks old, vere randomly divided into six groups (5 mice per group), ncluding inactivated virus immunized group (7 log10 CID_{50}/mL, A), Cap+ORF3 immunized group (mol/mol = :1, B), Cap+Rep immunized group (mol/mol = 1:1, C), ORF3 + Rep immunized group (mol/mol = 1:1, D), Cap ORF3 + Rep immunized group (mol/mol = 1:1:1, E), and 'BS group (control group), and housed in separate isolation ooms. Preimmune serum was collected prior to nmunization. The inactivated virus (100 μL) or purified roteins (100 μg) were emulsified as a 1:1 (*v*/v) mixture vith a complete Freund's adjuvant (Sigma). Mice were mmunized subcutaneously with 200 μL of the purified pro-eins or the inactivated virus. Then, the mice were injected ubcutaneously with 200 μL of the proteins or the inactivated virus mixed with incomplete Freund's adjuvant (Sigma) two week, four weeks and six weeks later, respectively. One week after the fourth immunization, the mice were euthanized by cervical dislocation and the sera were harvested for antibody analyses. The sera were collected and stored in aliquots at – 20 °C.

To further demonstrate whether the inactivated virus and purified proteins induce a sufficiently protective immune response against PCV2, thirty female BABL/C mice, 5 weeks old, were randomly divided into three groups (10 mice per group), including inactivated virus immunized group (9 log10 $TCID_{50}$/mL, A), Cap+ORF3 + Rep immunized group (mol/mol = 1:1:1, B), and negative control group (PBS), and housed in separate isolation rooms. Preimmune serum was collected prior to immunization. The inactivated virus (100 μL) or purified proteins (100 μg, Cap:Rep:ORF3 = 34:43:23) were emulsified as a 1:1 (*v*/v) mixture with a complete Freund's adjuvant (Sigma). Mice were immunized subcutaneously with 200 μL of the purified proteins or inactivated virus. Then, the mice were injected subcutaneously with 200 μL of the proteins or the inactivated virus mixed with incomplete Freund's adjuvant (Sigma) two week, four weeks and six weeks later, respectively. 72 h after each immunization, the sera of five mice per group were harvested. Two weeks following fourth immunization, all the mice were infected with 200 μL of PCV2 at 7 log10 $TCID_{50}$/mL or 200 μL of PBS by intramuscular injection, respectively. All mice were observed three times daily for changes in physical appearance and deaths (if any) for up to 14 days post virus exposure. Generally, mice were weighed every other day to determine the average weight change of the group and were observed for clinical signs of distress. Fourteen days post infection, mice were euthanized by cervical dislocation and the sera were collected and stored in aliquots at – 20 °C.

Assay of mice blood antibody levels

Antibody levels in mice blood was measured by ELISA. Briefly, ELISA plates (Costar) were coated with 100 μL of PCV2 or purified protein, which was diluted to a final concentration of 2 μg/mL in coating buffer (PH = 9.6), at 4 °C overnight and then washed with PBS containing 0. 05% Tween 20 (PBST, PH = 7.4) for three times. Unspecific binding of the antibodies was avoided by blocking with 100 μL of 0.5% BSA for 30 min at room temperature. After washing three times with PBST, 100 μL of appropriately diluted serum in PBST containing 0.5% BSA was added and incubated for 30 min at 37 °C. After washing three times with PBST, the bound antibodies were incubated with 100 μL of goat anti-mouse IgG (1:1000). After incubation for 1 h at room temperature and three PBST washes, 100 μL of TMB

(Sigma) was added to each well and the mixture was incubated for 15 min at room temperature. The reaction was stopped by adding 100 μL of 1 N sulfuric acid to the mixture, and the optical density at 450 nm was measured (Bio-RAD microplate reader).

Virus neutralization test (VNT)

Neutralization assay was performed to assess the ability of the serum samples to neutralize the PCV2 according to the protocol described by Jin [11]. Briefly, serum samples were heat inactivated at 56 °C for 30 min, followed by serial dilution in 2-fold increments in Dulbecco's modified Eagle medium (DMEM) supplemented with 2% of fetal bovine serum (FBS), and mixed 1:1 with 200 $TCID_{50}$ of PCV2 strain CC1 for 2 h at 37 °C. Thereafter, 100 μL of serum-virus mixture was added to 50% confluency of PK-15 cells and incubated for 1 h at 37 °C. After incubation, the serum-virus mixture was removed, and the cells were washed with PBS for three times and further incubated in DMEM supplemented with 2% of FBS at 37 °C and 5% CO_2. After incubation for 72 h, an indirect fluorescence assay (IFA) was performed as previously described by Yang [12].

Statistical analysis

Statistical significance was calculated using one-way or two-way analysis of variance (ANOVA), followed by the Bonferroni multiple comparison test. Statistical analysis was performed using GraphPad Prism software, version 5 (GraphPad Software, SanDiego, CA). The results were statistically significant at $p < 0.05$. For each separate set of assays, at least 3 independent experiments were evaluated. The results are expressed as the mean ± standard deviation (SD).

Results

Inactivated PCV2 is more effective than four PCV2 subunit proteins in stimulating immune response

To compare immunogenicity, inactivated PCV2 and four different combinations of PCV subunit proteins (different combinations of Cap+ORF3, Cap+Rep, ORF3 + Rep, and Cap+ORF3 + Rep) were used as antigens to raise antiserum, respectively. After four immunizations, the antisera were collected and detected by ELISA using PCV2 as coating antigen. The results showed that the inactivated PCV2 induced significantly higher levels of PCV2-specific antibodies than that of the PCV2 subunit proteins, indicating the inactivated PCV2 was more effective than the PCV2 subunit proteins in stimulating immune response (Table 1). Furthermore, PCV2 subunit protein Cap+ORF3 + Rep showed a better immunogenicity than the other subunit proteins, whereas antibodies were undetectable in the mock groups. Therefore, the inactivated PCV2 and the subunit protein Cap+ORF3 + Rep were selected in the following studies.

To compare serum antibody level after immunization in mice, 200 uL of sera were obtained from 5 mice of each group by needle puncture of tail tip vein 72 h after each immunization, followed by ELISA. The results of ELISA showed that positive antiserum titers were significantly increased after second, third and fourth immunization using inactivated PCV2 (Fig. 1) or purified proteins (Fig. 2) as coating antigen. Furthermore the antiserum developed from the inactivated PCV2 was significantly higher than that of the purified proteins group when inactivated PCV2 was used as coating antigen (Fig. 1). Moreover, when purified proteins Cap +Rep (1:1) was used as coating antigen, the antisera developed from both inactivated PCV2 and purified proteins were significantly higher than that of the control (PBS) group (Fig. 2). These results indicated that positive antiserum induced by the inactivated PCV2 had a better reactivity and specificity than that of the purified proteins.

Inactivated PCV2 induced more effective immunity than purified subunit proteins against PCV2

To elucidate whether the inactivated PCV2 and purified protein were effective in protecting mice against PCV2, the mice were infected with 200 μL of PCV2 at 7 log10 $TCID_{50}$/mL by intramuscular injection 14 days after the fourth immunization. The results showed that average daily gain had no significant difference between the groups as well as in each group

Table 1 ELISA results (Mean ± SD) of different groups in stimulating immune response

Dilution of Antiserum	Inactivated virus	Cap+ORF3	Cap+Rep	ORF3 + Rep	Cap+ORF3 + Rep	Negative Serum	PBS
1/200	1.1430 ± 0.0463	0.1437 ± 0.0161	0.1033 ± 0.0062	0.0633 ± 0.0045	0.2972 ± 0.0683	0.0649 ± 0.0047	0.0516 ± 0.000
1/400	1.1476 ± 0.0423	0.1985 ± 0.0557	0.0802 ± 0.0101	0.0554 ± 0.0021	0.1666 ± 0.0431	0.0509 ± 0.0046	0.0558 ± 0.001
1/800	1.1624 ± 0.0955	0.1712 ± 0.0440	0.0628 ± 0.0037	0.0565 ± 0.0017	0.1132 ± 0.0225	0.0514 ± 0.0012	0.0556 ± 0.001
1/1600	1.1033 ± 0.0981	0.1146 ± 0.0231	0.0649 ± 0.0054	0.0565 ± 0.0023	0.0550 ± 0.0012	0.0504 ± 0.0016	0.0575 ± 0.002
1/3200	1.0049 ± 0.1002	0.0802 ± 0.0104	0.0561 ± 0.0016	0.0511 ± 0.0010	0.0512 ± 0.0016	0.0517 ± 0.0009	0.0558 ± 0.001
1/6400	0.8501 ± 0.0854	0.0634 ± 0.0042	0.0536 ± 0.0011	0.0524 ± 0.0007	0.0541 ± 0.0012	0.0532 ± 0.0014	0.0536 ± 0.001
1/12800	0.7245 ± 0.0916	0.0567 ± 0.0017	0.0531 ± 0.0007	0.0543 ± 0.0005	0.0557 ± 0.0003	0.0526 ± 0.0006	0.0562 ± 0.001

Note:Detection limits were underlined. *Positive, Sample/negative serum ≥2

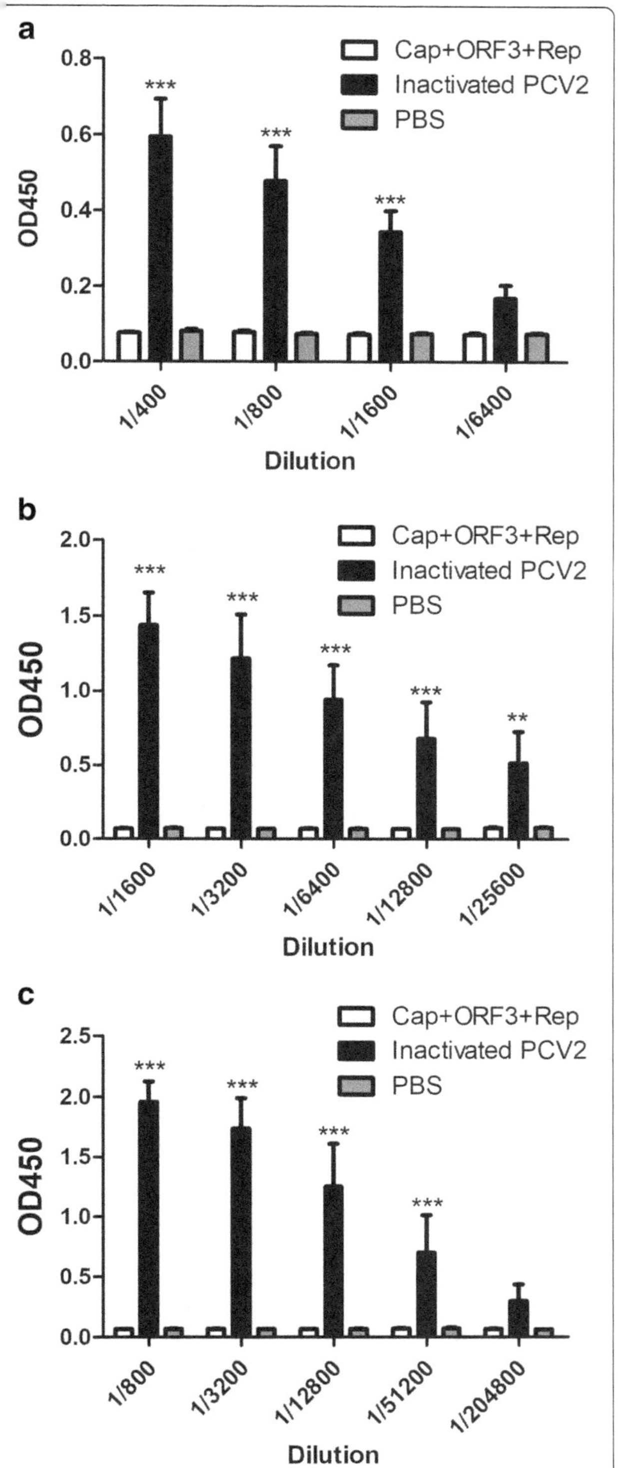

Fig. 1 Serum antibody level after different immunizations in mice. Inactivated PCV2 and subunit protein Cap+ORF3 + Rep were used as antigens to raise antiserum, respectively. After each immunization, the antisera were collected as described in the Materials and methods section. ELISA was performed using PCV2 as coating antigen. (**a**) Second immune; (**b**) Third immune; (**c**) Fourth immune

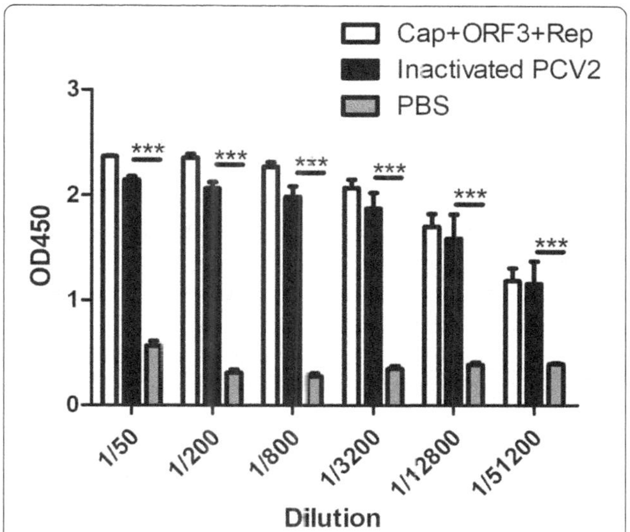

Fig. 2 Serum antibody level after fourth immunization using purified proteins (Cap + Rep, 1 1) as antigen. Inactivated PCV2 and subunit protein Cap+ORF3 + Rep were used as antigens to raise antiserum, respectively. After fourth immunization, the antisera were collected and analyzed

and the weight gain was not altered by immunization in mice (Fig. 3).

The antisera from each group were collected and detected by ELISA using inactivated PCV2, Cap protein and Rep protein as coating antigen, respectively. The results demonstrated that serum antibody developed from the inactivated PCV2 showed high levels using inactivated PCV2, Cap protein or Rep protein

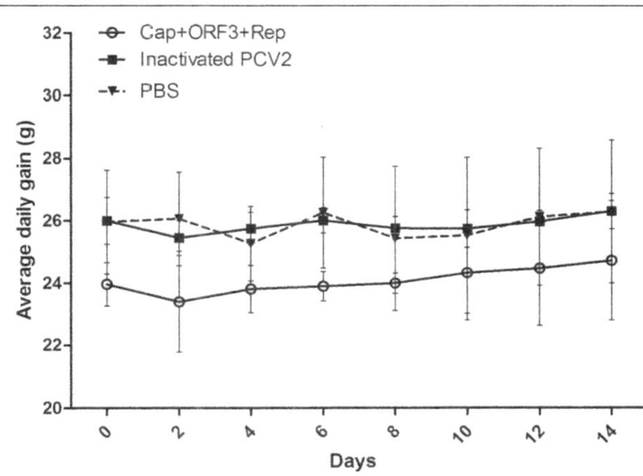

Fig. 3 Average daily gain. Thirty female BABL/C mice, 5 weeks old, were randomly divided into three groups and immunized subcutaneously with 200 μL of the purified proteins or inactivated virus. Two weeks following fourth immunization, all the mice were infected with 200 μL of PCV2 at 7 log10 $TCID_{50}$/mL or 100 μL of PBS by intramuscular injection, respectively. All mice were observed three times daily for changes in physical appearance and deaths (if any) for up to 14 days post virus exposure. Generally, mice were weighed every other day to determine the average weight gain of the group

as coating antigen, respectively (Fig. 4). Furthermore, serum antibody developed from the subunit protein Cap+ORF3 + Rep showed high levels using Cap protein or Rep protein as coating antigen (Figs. 4b and c).

To assess the ability of the serum samples to neutralize the PCV2, neutralization assay was performed and evaluated using IFA. The results showed that the sera from both inactivated PCV2-immunized animals and subunit protein Cap+ORF3 + Rep immunized animals had significantly higher neutralizing antibody titers than that of PBS group (Fig. 5). These results indicated that the inactivated PCV2 and subunit protein Cap +ORF3 + Rep were effective in inducing PCV2-neutralizing antibody responses in mice. Moreover, the neutralizing antibody in the inactivated PCV2 group was significantly higher than that of the subunit protein group. Therefore, these results indicated that immune effect of the inactivated PCV2 was better than the PCV2 subunit protein Cap+ORF3 + Rep in the present study.

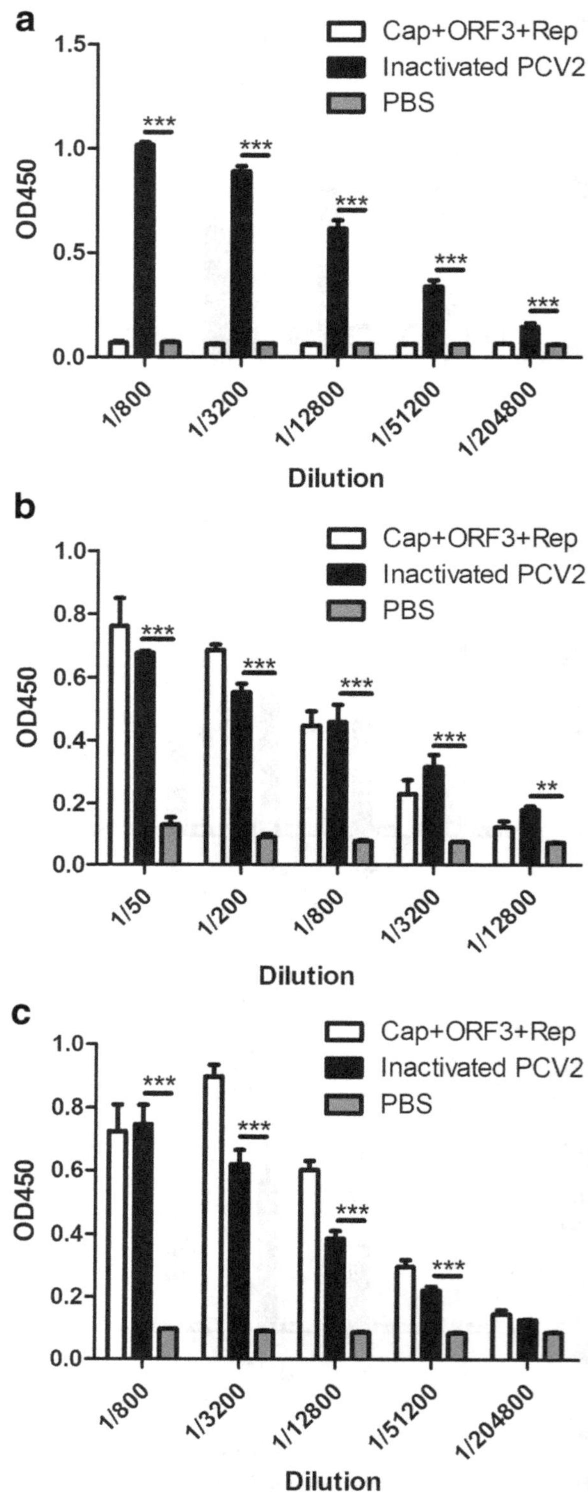

Fig. 4 ELISA results of different groups used as coating antigen. a Inactivated PCV2 as coating antigen; **b** Cap protein as coating antigen; **c** Rep protein as coating antigen

Discussions

The PCV2 genome has eleven open reading frames (ORFs), ORF1 to ORF11 [3]. ORF1 of PCV2 is highly conserved and encodes viral DNA replication-associated proteins, and ORF2 encodes the relatively variable structural protein Cap. Currently, both Rep and Cap are considered as significant immunogenic proteins of PCV2 that play important roles in cell-mediated immunity to constrain PCV2 replication and prevent the progression of PCV2 infection toward PCVD/PCVAD [13–15]. It was reported that PCV2-inoculation induced a cellular immunity against Cap protein as well as Rep protein in pigs [14, 15]. There are eight replication-associated proteins encoded by *ORF1* gene, including two major products (designated Rep and Rep0) and six minor products (designated Rep3a, Rep3b, Rep3c, NS515, NS672, and NS0) [13]. Rep proteins likely contribute to viral pathogenicity in vivo [16]. It was reported that the Rep can not only interact with cellular filament protein and transcriptional regulator c-myc, but also can interact with Cap protein [17], indicating Rep proteins are important in PCV2 infection and pathogenicity. Additionally, Rep protein, especially N-terminus of Rep (RepN), is conserved and immunogenic [18]. However, the N-glycosylation 23–25 aa, 256–258 aa mutation of Rep protein reduced virus replication, but 286–288 aa mutation can enhance virus replication in PK-15 cells [19]. Previously, we found that the reactivity of the antiserum of Rep protein in PCV2 infected cells was significantly better than that of ORF3 [7]. The possible reason was that different native forms encoded by the viral *ORF1* gene in the PCV2-infected cells might enhance the binding affinity of the polyclonal antibody and the

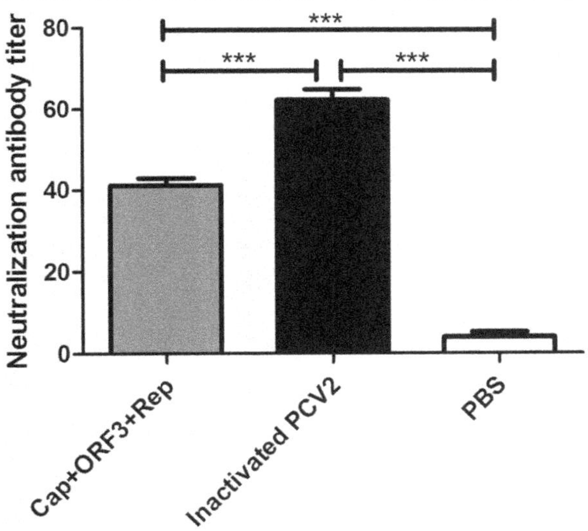

Fig. 5 Neutralizing assay of the immunized sera. Serum samples were heat inactivated at 56 °C for 30 min, followed by serial dilution in 2-fold increments in Dulbecco's modified Eagle medium (DMEM) supplemented with 2% of fetal bovine serum (FBS), and mixed 1:1 with 100 $TCID_{50}$ of PCV2 strain CC1 for 2 h at 37 °C. Thereafter, 100 μL of serum-virus mixture was added to 50% confluency of PK-15 cells and incubated for 1 h at 37 °C. After incubation, the serum-virus mixture was removed, and the cells were washed with PBS for three times and further incubated in DMEM supplemented with 2% of FBS at 37 °C and 5% CO_2. After incubation for 72 h, an indirect fluorescence assay (IFA) was performed to assess the neutralizing activity of the immunized sera. The results represent the means ± S.D. of three replicates of each group. *P*-values were calculated using two-way analysis of variance (ANOVA), followed by the Bonferroni multiple comparison test. $^{*}p < 0.05$, $^{**}p < 0.01$, $^{***}p < 0.001$

eplication-associated proteins [7]. These results indicate hat the Rep protein is promising for PCV2 antibody nd vaccine development [7]. Moreover, many reports howed that ORF3 protein (11.9 kDa) not only involved n PCV2-induced apoptosis by activating caspase-8 and aspase-3 pathways, but also played an important role in iral pathogenesis [3, 20–23]. T lymphocyte responses to CV2 are primarily directed toward epitopes of Rep and)RF3 proteins [24]. Therefore, we propose that different ombinations of PCV2 proteins can induce immunogen-city. In this study, we compared immunogenicity of four ifferent combinations of PCV2 proteins (Cap+ORF3, ap+Rep, ORF3 + Rep, and Cap+ORF3 + Rep). The re-ults demonstrated that the subunit protein Cap+ORF3 Rep showed a better immunogenicity than the other CV2 subunit proteins. Therefore, subunit protein Cap ORF3 + Rep were selected in the following studies to ompare with inactivated PCV2.

Vaccination is considered as an effective and econom-cal way to against PCV2 infection. Some of commercial vailable vaccines are based on inactive viruses, while the others are based on purified protein of PCV2. Although subunit vaccines are safe, however, their immunogenicity is low [25]. Therefore, it is difficult to choose an economical vaccine. To elucidate whether the inactivated PCV2 and purified protein were effective in protecting mice against PCV2, the mice were infected with PCV2 by intramuscular injection 14 days after the fourth immunization. As expected, the average daily gain was comparable with that of mice in the mock group, and the inactivated PCV2 and the purified protein Cap +ORF3 + Rep can significantly induced PCV2-neutralizing antibody in serum. However, serum antibody developed from the inactivated PCV2 showed higher levels using inactivated PCV2, Cap protein or Rep protein as coating antigen, respectively. Furthermore, the neutralizing antibody in the inactivated PCV2 group was significantly higher than that of the subunit protein group. These results demonstrated that the inactivated virus can induce superior immune responses than that of subunit viral proteins, which were consistent with the results reported by the other groups [26]. The results of the present study indicated that inactivated PCV2 is more effective than purified proteins against PCV2.

Adjuvant is crucial for efficacy of vaccines. In this study, the most commonly used adjuvant, Freund's adjuvant, was used. The results showed that high levels of specific antibodies were induced in mice, indicating both antigens and adjuvant were effective. There are different classes of adjuvants that can push immune response in different directions, including inorganic compounds, mineral oil, bacterial products, and cytokines, etc. [27, 28]. However, each adjuvant has its advantages and disadvantages. It was reported that GM-CSF as an adjuvant with PCV2 subunit vaccines markedly increases specific humoral immune response [25]. Previously, we found that immunological reactions were significantly increased in HMGCR-inhibited cells and mice [29, 30], and IL-2 can enhance PCV2 infection in vitro *and* in vivo [12, 31]. Thus, we hypothesis that IL-2 used as an adjuvant, combined with downregulated HMGCR, can induce stronger immune response in vivo. Further studies are in progress to test this hypothesis.

Conclusions

In conclusion, the positive antiserum of inactivated PCV2 had a better reactivity and specificity compared with that of the purified proteins. The inactivated PCV2 can induce better immune response to protect mice against PCV2 infection than that of the PCV2 subunit proteins used in this study. The results in the present study may be useful for production of PCV2 vaccine.

Abbreviations

ORF: Open reading frame; PCV2: Porcine circovirus 2; PCVD/PCVAD: Porcine circovirus diseases and porcine circovirus-associated diseases; PMWS: Post-weaning multi-systemic wasting syndrome; PPV: Porcine parvovirus; PRDC: Porcine respiratory disease complex; PRRSV: Porcine reproductive and respiratory syndrome virus; SIV: Swine influenza virus; SPF: Specific pathogen-free; TCID: Tissue culture infective dose.

Funding

This work was financially supported by the National Key Research and Development Program of China (No. 2017YFD0500103), the National Natural Science Foundation of China (No. 31772747 and 31272385), the Program for JLU Science and Technology Innovative Research Team (JLUSTIRT, No. 2017TD-28), the Fundamental Research Funds for the Central Universities, the Graduate Innovation Fund of Jilin University, the Program for Changjiang Scholars and the University Innovative Research Team (No. IRT1248).

Authors' contributions

LXH, OYT and MT performed the laboratory tests and drafted the manuscript. OYHS, PDX and RLZ conceived the study and participated in its design. RLZ and OYHS participated in the data analysis and results interpretation. All authors critically read and contributed to the manuscript, approving its final version.

Competing interests

The authors declare that they have no competing interests.

References

1. Segales J. Porcine circovirus type 2 (PCV2) infections: clinical signs, pathology and laboratory diagnosis. Virus Res. 2012;164(1–2):10–9.
2. Finsterbusch T, Mankertz A. Porcine circoviruses–small but powerful. Virus Res. 2009;143(2):177–83.
3. Ren L, Chen X, Ouyang H. Interactions of porcine circovirus 2 with its hosts. Virus Genes. 2016;52(4):437–44.
4. Meng XJ. Porcine circovirus type 2 (PCV2): pathogenesis and interaction with the immune system. Annu Rev Anim Biosci. 2013;1:43–64.
5. Afghah Z, Webb B, Meng XJ, Ramamoorthy S. Ten years of PCV2 vaccines and vaccination: is eradication a possibility? Vet Microbiol. 2017;206:21–8.
6. Chen F, Yang X, Pang D, Peng Z, Dong M, Liu X, Ouyang H, Ren L. Expression, purification and antibody preparation using different constructs of PCV2 capsid protein. Int J Biol Macromol. 2014;67:289–94.
7. Peng Z, Ma T, Pang D, Su D, Chen F, Chen X, Guo N, Ouyang T, Ouyang H, Ren L. Expression, purification and antibody preparation of PCV2 rep and ORF3 proteins. Int J Biol Macromol. 2016;86:277–81.
8. Li D, Du Q, Wu B, Li J, Chang L, Zhao X, Huang Y, Tong D. Immunogenicity of adenovirus vaccines expressing the PCV2 capsid protein in pigs. Vaccine. 2017;35(36):4722–9.
9. Zhang G, Jia P, Cheng G, Jiao S, Ren L, Ji S, Hu T, Liu H, Du Y. Enhanced immune response to inactivated porcine circovirus type 2 (PCV2) vaccine by conjugation of chitosan oligosaccharides. Carbohydr Polym. 2017;166:64–72.
10. Yang X, Chen F, Cao Y, Pang D, Ouyang H, Ren L. Complete genome sequence of porcine circovirus 2b strain CC1. J Virol. 2012;86(17):9536.
11. Jin J, Park C, Cho SH, Chung J. The level of decoy epitope in PCV2 vaccine affects the neutralizing activity of sera in the immunized animals. Biochem Bioph Res Co. 2018;496(3):846–51.
12. Yang X, Chen F, Cao Y, Pang D, Ouyang H, Ren L. Comparative analysis of different methods to enhance porcine circovirus 2 replication. J Virol Methods. 2013;187(2):368–71.
13. Lv QZ, Guo KK, Zhang YM. Current understanding of genomic DNA of porcine circovirus type 2. Virus Genes. 2014;49(1):1–10.
14. Fort M, Sibila M, Nofrarias M, Perez-Martin E, Olvera A, Mateu E, Segales J. Porcine circovirus type 2 (PCV2) cap and rep proteins are involved in the development of cell-mediated immunity upon PCV2 infection. Vet Immunol Immunopathol. 2010;137(3–4):226–34.
15. Fort M, Sibila M, Nofrarias M, Perez-Martin E, Olvera A, Mateu E, Segales J. Evaluation of cell-mediated immune responses against porcine circovirus type 2 (PCV2) cap and rep proteins after vaccination with a commercial PCV2 sub-unit vaccine. Vet Immunol Immunopathol. 2012;150(1–2):128–32.
16. Hua T, Wang X, Bai J, Zhang L, Liu J, Jiang P. Attenuation of porcine circovirus type-2b by replacement with the rep gene of porcine circovirus type-1. Virus Res. 2013;173(2):270–9.
17. Timmusk S, Fossum C, Berg M. Porcine circovirus type 2 replicase binds the capsid protein and an intermediate filament-like protein. J Gen Virol. 2006; 87(Pt 11):3215–23.
18. Meng T, Jia Q, Liu S, Karuppannan AK, Chang CC, Kwang J. Characterization and epitope mapping of monoclonal antibodies recognizing N-terminus of rep of porcine circovirus type 2. J Virol Methods. 2010;165(2):222–9.
19. Shi J, Peng Z, Fu F, Xu S, Xu S, Cong X, Yuan X, Yu J, Wu J, Sun W, et al. Mutant rep protein of the porcine circovirus type 2 N-glycosylation:23-25aa 256-258aa mutation reduced virus replication but 286-288aa mutation enhanced virus replication in PK-15 cells. Vet Microbiol. 2015;177(3–4):370–
20. Liu J, Chen I, Kwang J. Characterization of a previously unidentified viral protein in porcine circovirus type 2-infected cells and its role in virus-induced apoptosis. J Virol. 2005;79(13):8262–74.
21. Liu J, Chen I, Du Q, Chua H, Kwang J. The ORF3 protein of porcine circovirus type 2 is involved in viral pathogenesis in vivo. J Virol. 2006;80(10 5065–73.
22. He JL, Dai D, Zhou N, Zhou JY. Analysis of putative ORF3 gene within porcine circovirus type 2. Hybridoma (Larchmt). 2012;31(3):180–7.
23. Choi CY, Rho SB, Kim HS, Han J, Bae J, Lee SJ, Jung WW, Chun T.The ORF3 protein of porcine circovirus type 2 promotes secretion of IL-6 and IL-8 in porcine epithelial cells by facilitating proteasomal degradation of regulator of G protein signalling 16 through physical interactionJ Gen Virol.2015;96(Pt 5):1098-108.
24. Stevenson LS, Gilpin DF, Douglas A, McNeilly F, McNair I, Adair BM, Allan GM. T lymphocyte epitope mapping of porcine circovirus type 2. Viral Immunol. 2007;20(3):389–98.
25. Zhang H, Qian P, Peng B, Shi L, Chen H, Li X. A novel subunit vaccine co-expressing GM-CSF and PCV2b cap protein enhances protective immunity against porcine circovirus type 2 in piglets. Vaccine. 2015;33(21):2449–56.
26. Stoel M, Pool J, de Vries-Idema J, Zaaraoui-Boutahar F, Bijl M, Andeweg AC, Wilschut J, Huckriede A. Innate responses induced by whole inactivated virus or subunit influenza vaccines in cultured dendritic cells correlate with immune responses in vivo. PLoS One. 2015;10(5):e0125228.
27. Johnson AG. Molecular adjuvants and immunomodulators: new approache to immunization. Clin Microbiol Rev. 1994;7(3):277–89.
28. Mbow ML, De Gregorio E, Valiante NM, Rappuoli R. New adjuvants for human vaccines. Curr Opin Immunol. 2010;22(3):411–6.
29. Yang X, Ouyang H, Chen F, Ma T, Dong M, Wang F, Pang D, Peng Z, Ren L. Inhibition of 3-hydroxy-3-methylglutaryl-coenzyme a reductase increases the expression of interferon-responsive genes. Clin Exp Pharmacol Physiol. 2014;41(12):950–5.
30. Yang X, Ma T, Ouyang H, Chen F, Peng Z, Li C, Ma Y, Chen X, Li B, Pang D, et al. Effect of atovastatin treatment on porcine circovirus 2 infection in BALB/c mice. Clin Exp Pharmacol Physiol. 2015;42(8):817–21.
31. Ma T, Ouyang T, Ouyang H, Chen F, Peng Z, Chen X, Pang D, Ren L. Porcine circovirus 2 proliferation can be enhanced by stably expressing porcine IL-2 gene in PK-15 cell. Virus Res. 2017;227:143–9.

13

Rope-based oral fluid sampling for early detection of classical swine fever in domestic pigs at group level

laas Dietze*, Anna Tucakov, Tatjana Engel, Sabine Wirtz, Klaus Depner, Anja Globig, Robert Kammerer nd Susan Mouchantat

Abstract

Background: Non-invasive sampling techniques based on the analysis of oral fluid specimen have gained substantial importance in the field of swine herd management. Methodological advances have a focus on endemic viral diseases in commercial pig production. More recently, these approaches have been adapted to non-invasive sampling of wild boar for transboundary animal disease detection for which these effective population level sampling methods have not been available. In this study, a rope-in-a-bait based oral fluid sampling technique was tested to detect classical swine fever virus nucleic acid shedding from experimentally infected domestic pigs.

Results: Separated in two groups treated identically, the course of the infection was slightly differing in terms of onset of the clinical signs and levels of viral ribonucleic acid detection in the blood and oral fluid. The technique was capable of detecting classical swine fever virus nucleic acid as of day 7 post infection coinciding with the first detection in conventional oropharyngeal swab samples from some individual animals. Except for day 7 post infection in the "slower onset group", the chances of classical swine fever virus nucleic acid detection in ropes were identical or higher as compared to the individual sampling.

Conclusions: With the provided evidence, non-invasive oral fluid sampling at group level can be considered as additional cost-effective detection tool in classical swine fever prevention and control strategies. The proposed methodology is of particular use in production systems with reduced access to veterinary services such as backyard or scavenging pig production where it can be integrated in feeding or baiting practices.

Keywords: Non-invasive, Rope-in-a-bait, Surveillance, Hog cholera, Group level, Backyard pig production

ackground

arly field detection of transboundary animal diseases TADs) remains a key challenge within prevention and ontrol efforts in the veterinary field. To overcome the hortage of timely information on the circulation of athogens, oral fluid testing offers an opportunity to easily ollect group-level disease data [1]. Over the past years, on-invasive sampling techniques based on the collection f oral fluid specimen have gained substantial importance n the field of swine herd health management. Aggregate evel testing of oral fluid specimen has shown to be a aluable approach for increasing the efficiency and cost effectiveness of pathogen surveillance. For relevant, often endemic viral diseases affecting commercial swine production, such as porcine circovirus type 2, porcine reproductive and respiratory syndrome virus, and influenza A virus, protocols for sample collection and analysis are available [2]. However, the 2011 outbreak of foot and mouth disease (FMD) in Bulgaria, affecting mainly wildlife species, has highlighted the need for alternative surveillance methods at population level for TADs beyond the above mentioned [3]. This is in fact not only true for the wildlife sector, but also for farming structures where the access to the individual animal is limited, such as in certain backyard and scavenging production systems, where standard surveillance based on blood samples is challenging to implement.

Correspondence: klaas.dietze@fli.de
iedrich-Loeffler-Institut, Federal Research Institute for Animal Health,
dufer 10, 17493 Greifswald Insel Riems, Germany

A rope-in-a-bait sampling technique (referred to as pSWAB: "pathogen sampling of wild animals by baits") for saliva collection of wild boar (*Sus scrofa*) has been developed and tested for its suitability to timely detect FMD virus shedding of experimentally infected animals [4]. For classical swine fever (CSF), due to the unexpected mild course of the infection during the experimental study on CSF in wild boar, detailed insights into the suitability of the sampling technique for early detection could not be obtained [5] and remained therefore speculative. The approach of non-invasive sampling for TADs was later picked up by Grau et al. [6] successfully detecting the shedding of viral genome of FMDV, ASFV and CSFV in oral fluids collected by the conventional chewing rope technique from infected animals using a multiplex RTqPCR. With CSF remaining one of the most relevant TADs for the pig sector at global level with dramatic socio-economic consequences for producers and other value chain stakeholders [7], the need for additional tools to improve field level disease information in the domestic pig population remains pertinent.

The aim of the present study was therefore to verify the assumed applicability of a recently developed, wild boar adapted, oral fluid sampling method for saliva collection and early CSF virus (CSFV) nucleic acid detection in domestic pigs.

Methods

Animal experiment

Eight pigs with a body weight of approximate 25 kg were purchased from commercial breeders, randomly separated in groups of four for management reasons and kept in a high containment isolation unit. Each animal was infected with a viral dose of 10^6 tissue culture infectious dose 50% ($TCID_{50}$) of CSFV wild type Alfort/Tübingen, administered intramuscularly. Starting from day −1, all animals were examined daily until day 15 post infection (pi) following the clinical scoring scheme by Mittelholzer et al. [8], with modifications as described by Tews et al. [9]. Body temperature was measured rectal and increased temperatures above 39,5 °C were regarded as fever. The scheme allowed a structured observation of the clinical course of the infection and to determine humane end points for the individual animal. Animals developing severe clinical signs, not exceeding defined end point criteria like fever over 42 °C, massive disorders of the CNS or bloody diarrhea were assigned to get slaughtered by legitimated staff of the Friedrich-Loeffler-Institute. To comply with the biorisk regulations of the research facility the slaughter extends to all pigs that survived until the end of the study.

Sampling

For the oral fluid sample collection, eight to ten "pSWAB" sampling baits consisting of a raw cotton rope embedded in a cereal based bait matrix as described by Mouchanta et al. [5] were provided per pen on days −1, 2, 5, 7, 9, 1 and 15 pi. The "pSWABs" where distributed randoml within the pen by throwing them one-by-one over th pen barrier just avoiding the area the animals chose fo defecation. Chewed on cotton ropes were collecte from the pen flooring as found either at the same da or the next morning, incubated for one hour at roon temperature in 3 ml of medium (Eagels's minimum es sential medium) of which aliquots of 1 ml were store at −20 °C until further analysis. Blood samples were take on days following the pSWAB distribution scheme usin Monovette® EDTA KE/9 ml (Sarstedt, Numbrech Germany) and stored at −70 °C until further analysis. Con ventional oropharyngeal swab (Copan Rayon Regular Ti cat. no. 155C, Hain Lifescience GmbH, Nehren, Germany samples were taken in parallel to the blood samples whil animals were restrained. These were subsequently soake in 1 ml of medium (Eagels's minimum essential medium and incubated for one hour at room temperature, ali quoted and stored at −20 °C until further analysis.

Sample analysis

Extraction of RNA from all obtained samples was per formed using the MagAttract Virus Mini M48 Kit fo automated extraction (Qiagen GmbH, Hilden, Germany according to the manufacturer's recommendation. Spe cific CSF viral RNA detection was done through rea time reverse transcription polymerase chain reactio (RTqPCR) according to the protocol of Hoffmann et a [10]. Samples with C_q values below 40 were considere positive.

Results

All animals developed clinical CSF but with differing de grees of severity (refer to Additional file 1 for details) One animal in group 1 had to be euthanized at day 8p due to animal welfare reasons. All other animals remaine in the experiment until day 15pi.

The pSWABs distributed in the pen were found to b attractive to the animals, they chewed on the ropes ex tensively and eventually just dropped them on the pe floor where they got picked up by another animal irre spectively of visible baiting matrix still present on th rope or not. It was observed, for each distribution, tha the cotton ropes were chewed on by more than one ani mal of the group and sometimes animals chewed o more than one rope at the same time. The number rope collected per sampling date for analysis varied between and 9 per pen and represent the total number of visibl chewed ropes found. The ropes were collected manuall from the pen flooring and did have slightly differing de grees of visible contamination depending on the locatio they got dropped by the last animal chewing on it. N opes were found heavily contaminated with faeces and he subsequently obtained samples for analysis were visbly clear.

The laboratory results of the oral fluid and blood anaysis are summarized in Table 1. Within the applied samling interval, CSFV nucleic acid was detectable in the lood starting from 2dpi in 2 out of 8 animals infected, nd was evident in all animals on day 5pi. The detection n the blood lasted in all infected animals until the end f the experiment at day 15pi. The minor difference in he course of infection of the two equally treated groups described by the faster onset of positive blood samples starting from day 2pi) in combination with a first fever eak (see recorded rectal temperatures in Fig. 1) and verall lower C_q values over the course of the experiental period for animals in group 2.

An overview on the level of CSFV nucleic acid detecion in oral fluid collected at individual level compared o the group level sampling for both groups is given in ig. 2. For group 1, on day 7pi one animal was tested oubtful in the oropharyngeal swab with all collected SWABs remaining negative. Group 2 had one out of 4 nimals tested positive on day 7pi with the oropharyngeal wab. At the same time 50% of the collected pSWABs $n = 4$) tested positive. Throughout the remaining course of the experiment, CSFV specific RNA detection was always possible in all collected pSWABs, meanwhile the individual oropharyngeal testing of animals showed changing results in particular in group 1.

Discussion

Building on the experiences made for oral fluid collection at population or herd level in wild boar [4], the present study was designed to determine the applicability of this rope-in-a-bait group based oral fluid sampling method for the detection of CSFV nucleic acid shedding during the course of a field virus infection of domestic pigs under controlled conditions. In a similar approach this has been tested in wild boar by Mouchantat et al. [5] but a sound evaluation of this non-invasive sampling methodology was not possible due to an unexpected mild course of the experimental infection. The results obtained later by Grau et al. [6] showed the feasibility of using the similar conventional rope sampling technique for CSFV genome detection but leaving out the "baiting component" essential for extensive production systems or wild boar sampling. In addition, focusing on the analytical sensitivity of the multiplex RTqPCR, this study did not deliver comparative values for blood samples and the different oral fluid samples over the course of infection.

able 1 Viral RNA detection in domestic swine infected with viral doses of 10^6 $TCID_{50}$ CSFV Alfort/Tübingen

			Day post infection						
roup	Animal/sample	Sample Type	−1	2	5	7	9	12	15
	1	EDTA blood	neg	neg	**33,76**	**32,24**	**27,48**	**27,6**	**27,22**
		OP swab	neg	neg	neg	neg	neg	neg	37,03
	2	EDTA blood	neg	neg	36,26	**30,03**	**29,61**	**28,3**	**29,57**
		OP swab	neg	neg	neg	39,01	**35,7**	neg	**35,95**
	3	EDTA blood	neg	neg	36,11	**30,14**	-	-	-
		OP swab	neg	neg	neg	neg	-	-	-
	4	EDTA blood	neg	neg	**34,35**	**32,01**	**28,26**	**26,5**	**25,77**
		OP swab	neg	neg	neg	neg	neg	36,7	**31,62**
	pSWAB	saliva	neg	neg	neg	neg	1(4)	9(9)	9(9)
		average Cq of positive					**34,46**	**33,1**	**28,98**
	5	EDTA blood	neg	39,1	**27,27**	**24,18**	**21,49**	**20,1**	**19,78**
		OP swab	neg	neg	neg	neg	38	**33,2**	**31,36**
	6	EDTA blood	neg	**34,85**	**27,37**	**22,09**	**17,08**	**18,1**	**18,44**
		OP swab	neg	neg	neg	neg	**32,49**	**31,4**	**26,3**
	7	EDTA blood	neg	neg	**27,58**	**28,9**	**18,45**	**18,2**	**17,71**
		OP swab	neg	neg	neg	neg	**29,31**	**29,4**	**28,16**
	8	EDTA blood	neg	**34,4**	**27,11**	**21,3**	**17,74**	**16,9**	**16,41**
		OP swab	neg	neg	neg	**31,22**	**33,35**	**29,3**	**26,37**
	pSWAB	saliva	neg	neg	neg	4(8)	4(4)	4(4)	4(4)
		average Cq of positive				**33,82**	**30,23**	**28**	**28,74**

q values for EDTA blood, oropharyngeal (OP) swabs, pSWAB. Cq values ≥40 were considered negative, values between 36 and 40 doubtful and values <36 n bold) positive. Counts for pSWABs are number of positive (total collected). (−): animal euthanized for animal welfare reasons

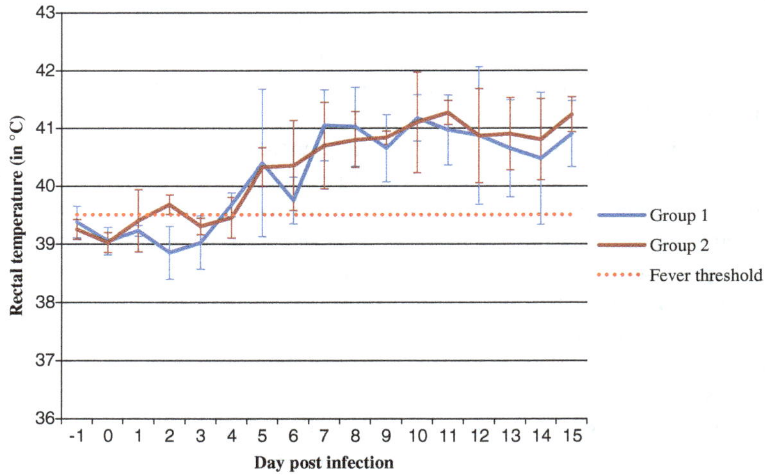

Fig. 1 Mean rectal temperatures (°C) of the animals by group

The observed onset and duration of the detection of CSFV nucleic acid in blood samples in this study confirmed the existing knowledge on longer lasting viremic periods and CSFV specific RNA detection in blood of CSFV infected pigs [11]. Oropharyngeal shedding of CSFV nucleic acid was detectable starting from day 7pi and continued over the 15 day pi observation period, although in group 1 the shedding was not detectable continuously. These results are comparable to the findings made by Kaden et al. [12] for conventional oral swab testing in CSFV infected wild boar. Comparing these results with the detection of CSFV nucleic acid using the pSWAB, hence not targeting the individual animal but a group of animals housed togethe the time window for virus genome detection is no differing.

The slightly differing course of the infection in the groups, with group 1 showing a slower onset and lowe levels of CSF viral RNA, brought up a difference in th initial detection of CSFV nucleic acid using the pSWAB With only one very weakly positive animal (oral swab Cq value close to negative cut off) in group 1 on day 7pi the group level test was not sensitive enough. Apart fron that circumstance, the group-level test showed similar o better sensitivity as the standard oropharyngeal swa

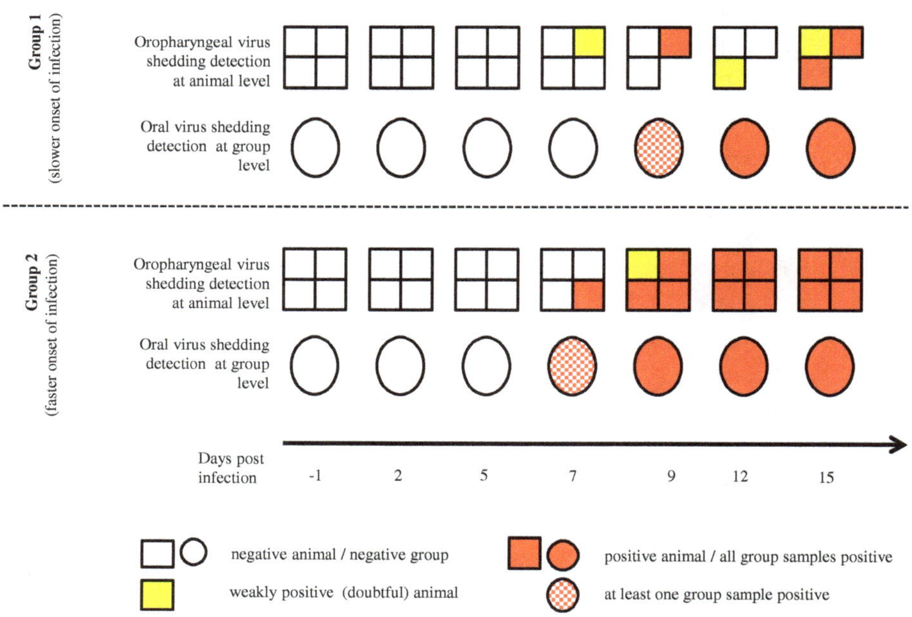

Fig. 2 Comparison of CSFV nucleic acid detection in oral fluid collected at individual level (swab) or group level (pSWAB)

ampling of individual animals (Fig. 2). The differing levels f excretion depending on the severity of the infection are n-line with findings from Weesendorp et al. [13]. The fact hat the cotton ropes where collected from the pen floorng, hence an "open environment", leaves room for potenal cross contamination from other excreta of the animals n the group. This could to some extend lead to a false atribution of CSFV genome detection to saliva. Considering he results obtained by Weesendorp et al. [13] on virus deection in different excreta over the course of a CSF infecon, this should not impact the onset of detection unless rather substantial sample dilution takes place.

With the high variability of clinical signs that can be ssociated with CSF, pathogen detection remains an ssential component of its diagnosis [14] confirming dequate field samples as an integral component of CSF surveillance that must not be compromised due o access problems. Despite the availability of good accines and robust diagnostic protocols, CSF control fforts often run into difficulties when dealing with pig opulations less accessible to the implementing veterinary ersonnel [15]. As a consequence, alternative strategies for ffective population or herd level monitoring of circulating iruses such as the pSWAB-methodology could assist in etter targeting of field interventions in settings where ampling of individual animals is challenging, despite the educed sensitivity and timeliness compared to blood ampling.

The acquired knowledge can on the one hand be useful or disease prevention strategies as well as surveillance ool within an immediate response to a CSF epidemic. On he other hand, it might be considered relevant for CSF urveillance in endemic settings. Countries with large proortions of pigs kept in disperse production systems such s free range, scavenging or certain types of backyard pig roduction tend to struggle in the collection of sound epiemiological field data on CSFV circulation. The collecion of saliva at group level with a rope-in-a-bait method an easily be integrated in baiting or feeding regimes comnonly practiced in extensive or scavenging pig production s well as in wild boar management. As the method aplied does not rely on purity of oral fluids analyzed, noderate contamination with other body fluids or faees are not likely to influence the results negatively.

However, case studies in the field will be needed to dentify realistic best practices in the timely backflow of ecovered cotton ropes to the laboratories capable of onduction CSFV nucleic acid detection in particular ooking into the suitability of oral fluid samples as samling material under these distinct field conditions. In articular, the overall environmental impact through emperature and humidity on virus genome stability will need to be evaluated when applying this method. This needs fine-tuning of the approach to specific local conditions in CSF endemic countries before considering it for larger scale implementation.

Conclusions

The importance to expand the methodologies of noninvasive sampling for the surveillance of some of the major TADs that can affect suids became once more evident in the 2011 FMD outbreak in Bulgaria [3]. For host populations with limited access to the individual animal sample acquisition will need to focus on group-level testing. It can be concluded that under experimental conditions, the described "rope-in-a-bait" sampling technique has confirmed its suitability in principle to detect circulating CSFV and can potentially lead to easier and cheaper field sample collection leading to overall more cost-effective surveillance in these specific target population.

Abbreviations

CSF: Classical swine fever; CSFV: Classical swine fever virus; FMD: Foot and mouth disease; pi: Post infection; pSWAB: Pathogen sampling of wild animals by baits; RTqPCR: Real time reverse transcription polymerase chain reaction; TADs: Transboundary animal diseases; $TCID_{50}$: Tissue culture infectious dose 50%

Acknowledgements

The authors thank Anne Leske for the excellent technical assistance as well as Kathrin Gellert, Thomas Moeritz and Matthias Jahn for the animal husbandry throughout the experiment.

IDT Biologika (Riems) GmbH & Co. KG is acknowledged for the provision of bait material.

Funding

No funding was obtained for this study.

Authors' contribution

KDi analyzed the data and drafted the manuscript. AT, TE, SW conducted the animal experiment. SM, AT conducted the laboratory work. KDe and SM, planned and supervised the study and critically revised the manuscript. AG, RK provided technical expertise throughout the study and critically revised the manuscript. All authors read and approved the final manuscript.

Competing interests

The authors declare that they do not have competing interests.

Consent for publication

Not applicable.

References

1. Prickett JR, Zimmerman JJ. The development of oral fluid-based diagnostics and applications in veterinary medicine. Anim Health Res Rev. 2010;11(02): 207–16.
2. Ramirez A, Wang C, Prickett JR, Pogranichniy R, Yoon KJ, Main R, Johnson JK, Rademacher C, Hoogland M, Hoffmann P, et al. Efficient surveillance of pig populations using oral fluids. Prev Vet Med. 2012;104(3–4):292–300.
3. Alexandrov T, Stefanov D, Kamenov P, Miteva A, Khomenko S, Sumption K, Meyer-Gerbaulet H, Depner K. Surveillance of foot-and-mouth disease (FMD) in susceptible wildlife and domestic ungulates in Southeast of Bulgaria following a FMD case in wild boar. Vet Microbiol. 2013;166(1–2):84–90.

4. Mouchantat S, Haas B, Bohle W, Globig A, Lange E, Mettenleiter TC, Depner K. Proof of principle: Non-invasive sampling for early detection of foot-and-mouth disease virus infection in wild boar using a rope-in-a-bait sampling technique. Vet Microbiol. 2014;172(1–2):329–33.
5. Mouchantat S, Globig A, Bohle W, Petrov A, Strebelow HG, Mettenleiter TC, Depner K. Novel rope-based sampling of classical swine fever shedding in a group of wild boar showing low contagiosity upon experimental infection with a classical swine fever field strain of genotype 2.3. Vet Microbiol. 2014;170(3–4):425–9.
6. Grau FR, Schroeder ME, Mulhern EL, McIntosh MT, Bounpheng MA. Detection of African swine fever, classical swine fever, and foot-and-mouth disease viruses in swine oral fluids by multiplex reverse transcription real-time polymerase chain reaction. J Vet Diagn Invest. 2015;27(2):140–9.
7. Moennig V. Introduction to classical swine fever: virus, disease and control policy. Vet Microbiol. 2000;73(2–3):93–102.
8. Mittelholzer C, Moser C, Tratschin JD, Hofmann MA. Analysis of classical swine fever virus replication kinetics allows differentiation of highly virulent from avirulent strains. Vet Microbiol. 2000;74(4):293–308.
9. Tews BA, Schurmann EM, Meyers G. Mutation of Cysteine 171 of Pestivirus E-rns RNase Prevents Homodimer Formation and Leads to Attenuation of Classical Swine Fever Virus. J Virol. 2009;83(10):4823–34.
10. Hoffmann B, Beer M, Schelp C, Schirrmeier H, Depner K. Validation of a real-time RT-PCR assay for sensitive and specific detection of classical swine fever. J Virol Methods. 2005;130(1–2):36–44.
11. Durand B, Davila S, Cariolet R, Mesplede A, Le Potier MF. Comparison of viraemia- and clinical-based estimates of within- and between-pen transmission of classical swine fever virus from three transmission experiments. Vet Microbiol. 2009;135(3–4):196–204.
12. Kaden V, Lange E, Polster U, Klopfleisch R, Teifke JP. Studies on the virulence of two field isolates of the classical swine fever virus genotype 2.3 Rostock in wild boars of different age groups. J Vet Med Ser B-Infect Dis Vet Public Health. 2004;51(5):202–8.
13. Weesendorp E, Stegeman A, Loeffen W. Dynamics of virus excretion via different routes in pigs experimentally infected with classical swine fever virus strains of high, moderate or low virulence. Vet Microbiol. 2009;133(1–2):9–22.
14. Penrith ML, Vosloo W, Mather C. Classical Swine Fever (Hog Cholera): review of aspects relevant to control. Transbound Emerg Dis. 2011;58(3):187–96.
15. Dietze K, Milicevic V, Depner K. Prospects of improved classical swine fever control in backyard pigs through oral vaccination. Berliner Und Munchener Tierarztliche Wochenschrift. 2013;126(11–12):476–80.

14

Evidence for the presence of African swine fever virus in an endemic region of Western Kenya in the absence of any reported outbreak

ian F. Thomas[1,2†], Richard P. Bishop[2†], Cynthia Onzere[2], Michael T. Mcintosh[3], Karissa A. Lemire[3], William A. de Glanville[1,2], E. Anne J. Cook[1,2] and Eric M. Fèvre[2,4*]

Abstract

Background: African swine fever (ASF), caused by African swine fever virus (ASFV), is a severe haemorrhagic disease of pigs, outbreaks of which can have a devastating impact upon commercial and small-holder pig production. Pig production in western Kenya is characterised by low-input, free-range systems practised by poor farmers keeping between two and ten pigs. These farmers are particularly vulnerable to the catastrophic loss of livestock assets experienced in an ASF outbreak. This study wished to expand our understanding of ASFV epidemiology during a period when no outbreaks were reported.

Results: Two hundred and seventy six whole blood samples were analysed using two independent conventional and real time PCR assays to detect ASFV. Despite no recorded outbreak of clinical ASF during this time, virus was detected in 90/277 samples analysed by conventional PCR and 142/209 samples analysed by qPCR. Genotyping of a sub-set of these samples indicated that the viruses associated with the positive samples were classified within genotype IX and that these strains were therefore genetically similar to the virus associated with the 2006/2007 ASF outbreaks in Kenya.

Conclusion: The detection of ASFV viral DNA in a relatively high number of pigs delivered for slaughter during a period with no reported outbreaks provides support for two hypotheses, which are not mutually exclusive: (1) that virus prevalence may be over-estimated by slaughter-slab sampling, relative to that prevailing in the wider pig population; (2) that sub-clinical, chronically infected or recovered pigs may be responsible for persistence of the virus in endemic areas.

Keywords: African swine fever virus, Epidemiology, Kenya, Slaughter house, p72 PCR, ASFV real time PCR, Genotype IX

Background

African swine fever virus (ASFV) is a highly infectious virus of the family *Asfarviridae* and is the causative agent of African swine fever (ASF) infection which may lead to mortality of up to 100 % in naïve domestic pig populations [1]. Per-acute and acute ASF present as high fever, anorexia, depression, cutaneous hyperaemia (per-acute), erythema and or areas of cutaneous cyanosis particularly of the abdomen, ears and distal extremities with sudden death within 1–7 days [2]. Low virulence strains of the virus have been reported and there is evidence from Senegal, Cameroon, Nigeria, Madagascar, Malawi, Mozambique, Zambia and possibly Angola that pigs in endemic areas may have developed resistance or that chronic or sub-clinical infections may be increasing [3–6].

ASFV has at least three distinct transmission cycles; (1) involving an argasid soft tick (genus *Ornithodoros*) and warthogs; (2) between argasid tick vector and domestic pigs

Correspondence: Eric.Fevre@liverpool.ac.uk
Equal contributors
International Livestock Research Institute, PO Box 30709, Nairobi 00100, Kenya
Institute for Infection and Global Health, University of Liverpool, Leahurst Campus, Chester High Road, Neston CH64 7TE, UK
Full list of author information is available at the end of the article

and (3) direct pig to pig transmission without the tick vector. Direct pig to pig transmission is probably the major mode of transmission across Africa in areas not adjacent to national parks [7, 8]. The role of other wild suiforms (bush pigs, wild boars and giant forest hogs) in the epidemiology of ASFV is yet to be fully understood [8]. Pig to pig transmission can occur both through contact between live pigs, fomites or ingestion of infected pork meat [4].

Pig keeping in Kenya generally occurs as a small-holder enterprise with between two and ten pigs per farm [9, 10]. The majority of pigs are kept under a free-range system [11], especially in urban and peri-urban areas [12]. In western Kenya where this study was conducted pigs kept under a free-range system travel an average of 4 km very 12 h whilst scavenging for food within a mean home range of 10,343 m^2 (range 2937–32,759 m^2) [13]. This scavenging behaviour puts these pigs at risk of acquiring multiple infectious organisms, including ASFV from the environment, neighbouring domestic pigs, or wildlife reservoirs.

There is currently no vaccine or chemotherapeutic available for ASFV and control therefore relies on preventing contact of pigs with the virus. Free-range pig production systems, as utilised in Kenya, require considerable improvements to biosecurity in order to prevent pigs coming into contact with potentially infected animals or animal products [4].

Several outbreaks of ASF have been reported in western Kenya. Prior to the instigation of this study there were two outbreaks between October 2006 and February 2007 resulting in 82 porcine deaths from Busia (formerly Western Province) and Kisumu (formerly Nyanza Province) [14], and after the completion of the present study, between December 2010 and March 2012, 163 porcine deaths were reported in Mahiakolo (formerly Western Province) and Kisumu East (formerly Nyanza Province) [15]. Outbreaks of diseases causing high mortality, such as ASF, are of high concern to poor farmers such as those in western Kenya, with the potential to catastrophically threaten their livelihoods through the rapid loss of their livestock assets [16].

Exactly how the virus persists within endemic pig populations is not known but a role has been proposed for survivor, sub-clinical and chronically infected pigs to maintain virus [17]. There is evidence that recovered animals can transmit the virus to naïve populations for up to 3 months [18] and may be persistently infected with virus for up to 6 months [18, 19]. Low virulence strains of ASFV have been reported in the Dominican Republic, Spain and Portugal, which appear to lead to chronic infections with prolonged viremia lasting several weeks to several months [20]. These chronic infections, however, have never been reported in the African continent [2].

Viral DNA has been detected in asymptomatic pigs in both south-western Kenya [21], Uganda [22] and Tanzania [23]. Genotyping suggests that the isolates associated wit this situation in Kenya are likely of low virulence (Genotype X) and of high virulence in Tanzania (Genotype II Georgia 2007). In Mozambique, populations of pigs hav been identified with high levels of circulating antibodies suggesting resistance to virulent isolates [6]. Reasons fo the apparent resistance of some pigs to potentially virulen isolates of ASFV have been suggested but are as yet un proven. Breed resistance has been proposed [23] but herit ability did not appear to be the case in Mozambique wit all offspring of apparently resistant pigs succumbing t challenge by isolates of the same genotype [6].

As western Kenya is an area where ASF is a regula occurrence, an ongoing programme of porcine samplin presented and opportunity to further investigate the epi demiology of ASFV during a period when no outbreak were reported. This study therefore aimed to investigat the presence of ASFV viral DNA in domestic pigs pre sented to slaughter during a time period with no offi cially reported outbreaks of ASF and, should any viru be found, to determine which genotype was represented

Method

Study site

This study represents a sub-study of the "People, Animal & their Zoonoses" (PAZ) project in western Kenya [24] The study site is a 45 km radius semi-circle from Busi Town and is largely representative of the Lake Victori Crescent ecosystem. It is bounded to the west by th border with Uganda, to the south by Lake Victoria and t the North by Mount Elgon. The ten divisions (the 3rd lar gest administrative unit prior to the 2013 constitution re form) with the highest pig-population and at least on registered porcine slaughter facility (slab) were purposivel selected from within the study site; each selected divisio contained over 2 % of the total pig population of the stud area. Figure 1 illustrates the larger 'PAZ' study area, th pig population density (according to the District Livestoc and Production Office 2009 figures) and the location o registered slabs.

Sample collection

Sample collection took place at slabs in the selected divi sions, which were registered at the time of sampling wit the District Veterinary Office. The pathogen of primar focus for this sampling was *Taenia solium* as previousl described [25] and the sample size (319) was calculate accordingly, using WinEpiscope 2.0 [26] with an as sumed *T. solium* prevalence of 14 % [12] with 5 % preci sion and 99 % confidence level. Our interest in ASF was solidified after the sampling frame was devised a which point a collaboration was brokered which enable testing of these samples, this unfortunately resulted in

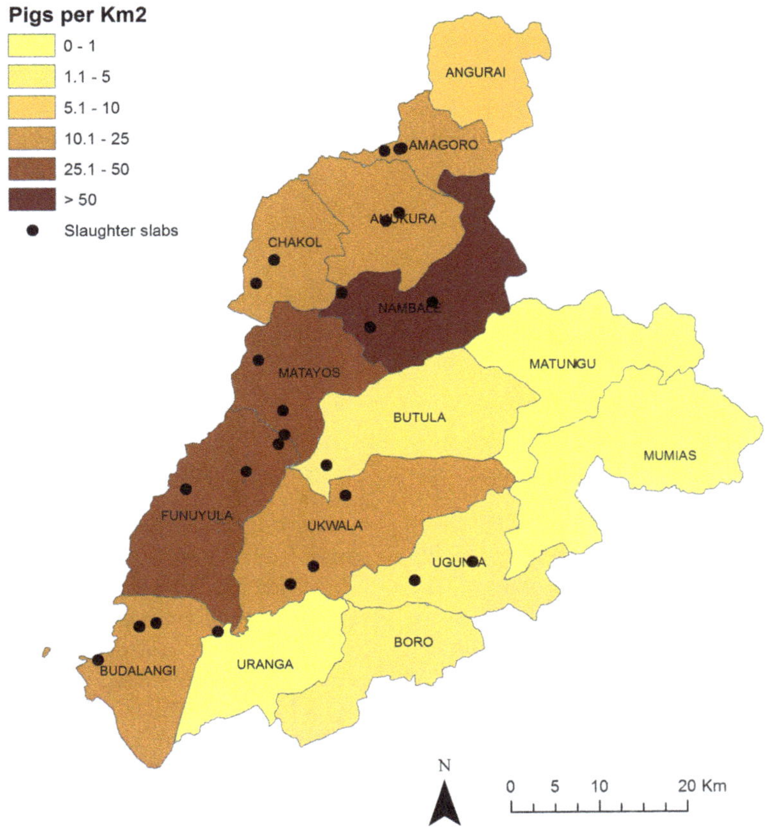

Fig. 1 Map depicting study site showing divisional pig population density and location of registered porcine slaughter facilities at time of sampling. This map was produced using ArcMap™ version 9.1 with geographical data provided by ILRI GIS unit http://www.ilri.org/gis and pig population data provided by the District Livestock and Production Office 2009 figures and overlaid with the location of slaughter facilities collected in the field using a hand held Garmin® eTrex GPS unit

lack of appropriate samples being obtained from the first 6 pigs sampled.

Twenty-six registered slabs were identified and were visited on the day of highest through-put, as identified by the meat inspector or slab owner, and all pigs being slaughtered on the day of visit were sampled. In these low-throughput slaughter slabs producing pork for local consumption, categorised as 'C' by the Kenya Meat Control Act generally 1–4 pigs are slaughtered per day, with a legal maximum of 6 pigs slaughtered on any one day [27]. Facilities were re-visited until a quota proportional to the percentage of the total pig population in that division had been fulfilled as indicated in Table 1.

All sample collection was undertaken by a small research team of one veterinarian (the lead author) and two animal health assistants according to protocols devised by the lead author. All members of the team were present for every sampling event except in the occasion of illness or unavoidable travel.

The permission of the person presenting the pig for slaughter was sought prior to sampling and the division of origin of the pig was recorded. Pigs were restrained with a pig snare behind the canine teeth, a brief visual exam was conducted and anterior vena cava blood samples were collected in BD Vacutainer® 4 ml EDTA tubes [28]. Blood samples were transported to the laboratory, on ice, where they were stored at −40 °C until transported, on dry ice, to the International Livestock Research Institute (ILRI) facility in Nairobi where they were stored at −80 °C for 2 to 7 months prior to analysis. After each slab visit the government meat inspector was called and asked if any carcass or part thereof was condemned that day for any reason.

African swine fever virus detection by conventional and real time PCR

Total DNA was extracted from each blood sample using the DNeasy Blood and Tissue kit (Qiagen, Hilden, Germany) according to the manufacturer's instructions. Negative extraction controls (NEC) consisting of sterile phosphate buffered saline (PBS) pH 7.0 were included during DNA extraction to check for contamination.

Table 1 Divisional pig population, sampling quota and number of registered porcine slaughter facilities at the time of sampling

Division	Pig population	% of total study site pig population	Quota of pigs to sample	No. of pigs sampled	No. of registered slab
Amagoro	1418	3.2	10	10	3
Amakura	3800	8.5	27	21	5
Budalangi	2640	5.9	19	19	4
Butula	1010	2.3	7	13	2
Chakol	1950	4.4	14	14	2
Funyula	8910	19.9	63	53	1
Matayos	5700	12.7	41	20	2
Nambale	14680	32.8	105	103	3
Ugunja	912	2.0	6	7	2
Ukwala	3700	8.3	27	17	3
Total	44720	100	319	277	27

Conventional PCR was performed using the ASFV diagnostic primers PPA1 and PPA2 that target the highly conserved VP72 capsid protein coding region of the ASFV genome [29]. No template controls (NTC) were included during PCR. Positive extraction and amplification controls (PEC & PAC) consisted of a known ASFV positive DNA sample extracted from an ASFV positive spleen tissue. Positive samples were identified by the presence of a discrete band of 257 base pairs (bp) after electrophoresis through a 2 % agarose gel.

DNA samples were further tested at the United States Department of Agriculture (USDA) Foreign Animal Disease Diagnostic Laboratory in Plum Island NY using a modification of the ASFV real-time PCR (qPCR) which has a diagnostic specificity of 100 % and was therefore selected as an ideal confirmatory tool [30]. Briefly, 2.5 μl DNA was amplified in 25 μl reactions containing 0.3 μM forward and reverse ASFV primers, and 0.2 μM ASFV TaqMan®FAM™-MGB probe using firstly the TaqMan® EZ-RT-PCR Kit (Applied Biosystems Foster City, CA, USA), and later repeated using the Life Technologies Path-ID Multiplex One Step PCR Kit (Thermo Fisher Scientific, Waltham, Massachusetts, USA) as the TaqMan®EZ reagents were discontinued by the manufacturer. Controls included an NEC consisting of 2.5 μl nuclease-free water, PEC and PAC consisting of 2.5 μl of DNeasy extracted DNA from the ASFV Killean III strain cultivated in primary porcine macrophages. qPCR was conducted using the Applied Biosystems 7500 fast platform (Thermo Fisher Scientific, Waltham, Massachusetts, USA) in standard mode with automatic baseline. Cycling conditions were 95 °C for 10 min denaturation and activation followed by 45 cycles of 95 °C for 10 s and 60 °C for 30 s. Positive reactions were identified when fluorescence exceeded 0.2 units prior to or at a cycle threshold (Ct) of 40. Results beyond the qPCR cut-off Ct of 40 or undetermined were considered negative or undetermined, respectively. Results with Ct < 30 wer considered as strong positives by qPCR.

In order to avoid potential cross-contamination, DNA extraction was conducted in batches of 20 including extraction controls and deep cleaning of the hood and pipettes were done using 10 % hypochlorite and 70 % ethanol between the batches. All PCR reagents were manipulated separately and ahead of sample handling. PEC and PAC, derived from known ASFV positive materia and assayed along with test samples, were manipulate only after test samples were processed and manipulate for PCR. All negative and positive PCR and qPCR controls performed as expected.

Genotyping

To identify the ASFV genotype(s) in the positive samples; genotypic analysis of 20 randomly selected positiv samples was carried out by analysis of two polymorphi loci. This included:

I. The 3′ -variable end of the *B646L* gene that encodes the major capsid protein p72 by utilization of the p72U/p72D primer set in the amplification of a 478 bp region [31].
II. The *E183L* gene that encodes the p54 ASFV protein critical in the recruitment of envelope precursors to the assembly site [32] by amplification of a 676 bp region using the PPA89/PPA722 primer set [33].

The discrete bands were directly cut and purified from the agarose gels using the gel purification kit (Qiagen Hilden, Germany) according to the manufacturer's instructions. Sequencing was then carried out using th Sanger sequencing method. Conflicts within the sequenc reads were identified using BIOEDIT [34] and contig were built using CAP3 [35] available in the Mobyle porta (http://mobyle.pasteur.fr/cgi-bin/portal.py#forms::cap3)

eference sequences corresponding to the two loci were etrieved from Genbank (http://www.ncbi.nlm.nih.gov/ enbank/) for comparison to the data obtained from anger sequencing. Multiple sequence alignments for each ocus with reference to the Genbank sequences were performed using MEGA version 6.06 [36] CLUSTAL W [37] o determine the ASFV genotype(s) associated with the ositive samples. The alignment data was transferred onto LC genomics workbench for visualization of insertion or eletion of bases (INDELS) and measurement of conser- ation (http://www.clcbio.com/products/clc-genomics- vorkbench/). Phylogenetic analysis of each locus was exe- uted using MEGA version 6.06 [36] and the evolutionary istory was inferred using the Minimum Evolution (ME) nethod [38] after application of the Neighbor-joining al- orithm in generation of the initial tree. The evolutionary istances were computed using the p-distance method nd the ME trees were searched using the Close- Jeighbor-Interchange (CNI) algorithm at a search level of . Data from both loci were resampled 1000 times using he bootstrap method [39].

tatistical analysis

s the study described here comprised 'convenience' ampling, with a sample size and strategy based upon an nrelated pathogen, we did not feel it was appropriate to tate the prevalence within this population.

esults

hree hundred and forty three pigs were sampled in his survey. All animals appeared to be asymptomatic or ASF on visual examination by the animal health ssistants and veterinarian conducting the sampling rocedure and government meat inspectors reported o sick animals. Whole blood samples were available or DNA extraction and conventional PCR from 277 igs, of which 90 samples were positive for ASFV. A ubset (207) of the 277 samples were independently ested using a modified real time PCR at the USDA. n total 152 of 207 samples tested positive by qPCR sing the Path-ID reagents, of which 23 samples rep- esented strong positives (ct values <30) (The results f the conventional and qPCR analysis are shown in able 2 and Additional file 1).

Twenty of the positive samples had their genotype equences determined. Analysis of the *B646L* gene, evealed that genotype IX was associated with the ositive samples. No INDELS were observed in these wo polymorphic loci, and the viruses were similar at oth loci to virus associated with the 2006 and 2007 SF outbreaks in Kenya [33]. The phylogenetic tree is lustrated in Figs. 2 and 3 and the Genbank accession umbers for the twenty isolates can be found in dditional file 2.

Table 2 Detection of African swine fever virus in pigs at slaughter in western Kenya detected by conventional and qPCR

Division of slaughter	No. pigs positive by conventional PCR	No. pigs positive by qPCR (Path-ID)
Amagoro	7/10	6/7
Amakura	5/21	9/17
Budalangi	4/19	11/17
Butula	2/13	2/6
Chakol	7/14	7/9
Funyula	22/53	31/40
Matayos	4/20	13/14
Nambale	30/103	64/84
Ugunja	3/7	1/4
Ukwala	6/17	8/9
Total	90/277	152/207

Discussion

This study has provided evidence for the presence of ASFV DNA in the blood of visually asymptomatic pigs presenting to slaughter within a period when there were no reported outbreaks in western Kenya. Accurate determination of prevalence in this population is limited mainly by the convenience nature of the sampling (the study design relating to a different pathogen) and the fact that only a sub-set of samples were analysed by both PCR methods. The high number of PCR positive pigs found in this study is interesting, because extensive horizontal household sampling of asymptomatic pigs on farms in the area of the current study between 2011 and 13 (>1000 animals in 600 households; R. Bishop, E. Okoth and C. Onzere, unpublished data), did not reveal PCR positive pigs.

Diagnostic specificity of the USDA ASFV qPCR, using TaqMan EZ reagents, was previously determined within the US National Animal Health Laboratory Network on US populations of domestic and feral swine (Unpublished results). Positive controls performed as expected and no false positives were observed among a negative cohort of EDTA blood samples tested from 895 domestic and 217 feral swine. Diagnostic specificity of the USDA ASFV qPCR was observed to be 100 % using a 95 % confidence interval with lower bound limits of 0.99 and 0.98 for domestic and feral swine, respectively.

ASFV viral DNA has been demonstrated by PCR previously in asymptomatic pigs at slaughter elsewhere in Kenya [40] and neighbouring Uganda [22] as well as in pigs at small holder farms in South-West Kenya [21]. This is not, a consistent finding, with another Ugandan study detecting no viral DNA despite high apparent disease incidence [41].

Genotyping of a sub-set of samples from this study revealed the virus to belong to genotype IX. This genotype

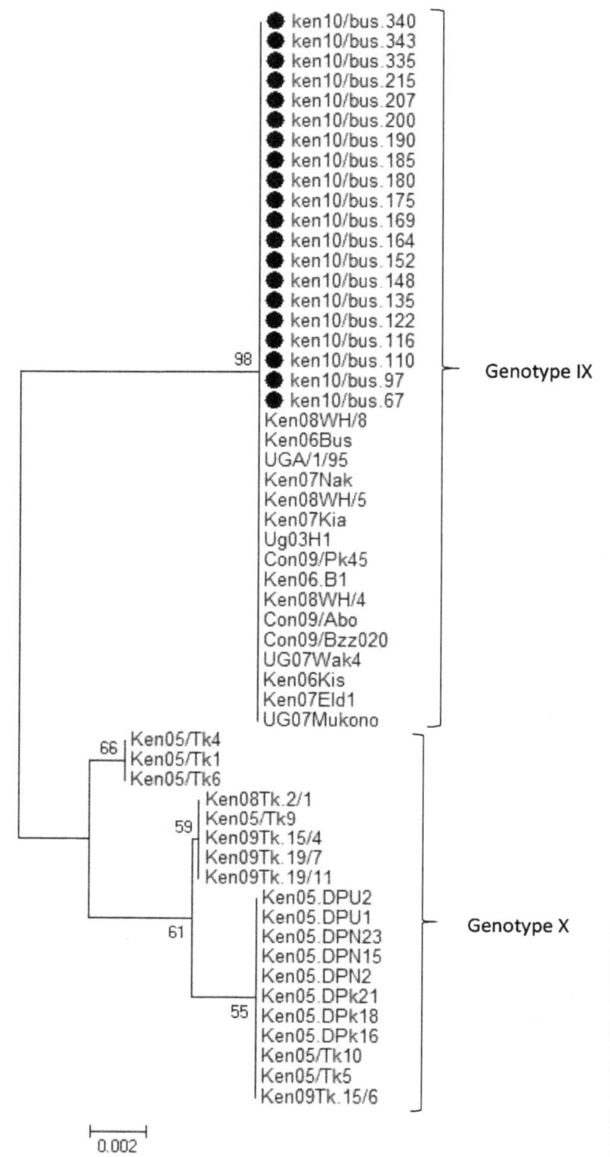

Fig. 2 Phylogenetic tree based on the 3′-variable end of the B646L gene. ● Indicates the 20 nucleotide sequences analyzed in this study in comparison to 35 reference sequences obtained from Genbank. The 20 sequences clustered within ASFV genotype IX. The evolutionary history was inferred using the Minimum Evolution (ME) method after initial application of the Neighbor-joining algorithm. The percentage of replicate trees in which the associated taxa clustered together in the bootstrap test (1000 replicates) are shown next to the branches. The tree was drawn to scale, with branch lengths in the same units as those of the evolutionary distances used to infer the phylogenetic tree. The p-distance method was used to compute evolutionary distances and the Close-Neighbor-Interchange (CNI) algorithm at a search level of 1 was used to determine the strength of the ME tree

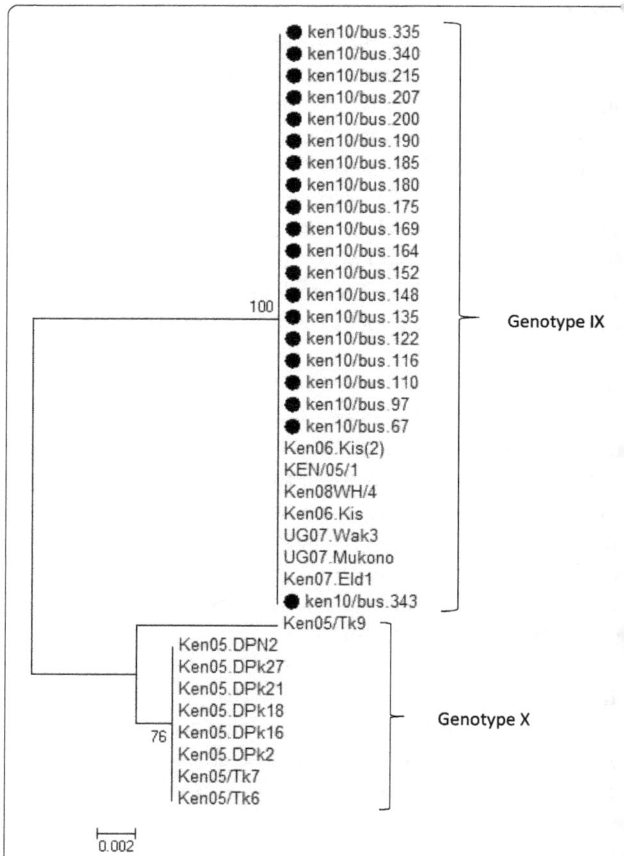

Fig. 3 Phylogenetic tree based on the full length *E183L* gene. ● Indicates the 20 sequences analyzed in this study that cluster within genotype IX in comparison to 16 reference sequences obtained from Genbank. The evolutionary history was inferred using the Minimum Evolution method after initial utilization of the Neighbor-joining algorithm. The percentage of replicate trees in which the associated taxa clustered together in the bootstrap test (1000 replicates) are shown next to the branches. The tree is drawn to scale, with branch lengths in the same units as those of the evolutionary distances used to infer the phylogenetic tree. The evolutionary distances were computed using the p-distance method and are in the units of the number of base differences per site. The ME tree was searched using the Close-Neighbour-Interchange (CNI) algorithm at a search level of 1

appears to have been involved in all outbreaks in Uganda since 1995 and Kenya since 2006, including Ugandan outbreaks in 1995, 2003 [42], 2007 [43], 21 outbreaks between 2011 and February 2013, as well as Kenyan out breaks in 2006 and 2007 [33]. This genotype was origin ally thought to be specific to domestic pigs with n evidence of involvement of a sylvatic cycle [42]. It ha since been identified in Kenyan warthogs; although, th role of the warthog in recent transmission of the virus t domestic pigs remains unclear [40].

Five months after sampling was completed (Januar 2011), two outbreaks were reported in western Keny (Mahiakolo) and neighbouring Nyanza province (Kisum East) where 163 pigs died, an apparent case fatality rate o 82.5 % according to information submitted to the Worl Animal Health Information System (WAHIS) [15].

As the last reported outbreak in Kenya prior to ampling was in 2007, and all animals sampled in this tudy appeared to be asymptomatic based on visual ıspection by the research team, the high number of CR-positive pigs found in this study suggests that irus may have been circulating within the porcine opulation without clinical signs manifesting. This is urprising as isolates of genotype IX are generally ıought to be highly virulent [33]. However, isolates f this genotype have also been detected in apparently symptomatic pigs at slaughter in Uganda [44]. Isoıtes of genotype X are generally found to be of lower irulence in experimental infection and have been lentified in asymptomatic pigs in Kenya both at laughter [40] and in the community [21].

Although these East African genotypes are similar verall in genome sequences, there are differences in the ıulti-copy 360 and 550 family genes encoded at the irus termini. Changes in the copy number and location f these genes appears to be correlated with perceived irulence of the virus isolates in pigs [45].

Antibody detection and virus isolation were not ndertaken in this study for several reasons. Antibody etection is notoriously sporadic due to the immunoıodulatory effect of the ASFV infection. Antibody etection demonstrates both past and present infecons [2] but differentiation of these situations is diffiult [46]. It is also apparent that in the case of the ast African p72 Genotypes IX and X which are gentically very close [45], the antibody response is often ifficult to detect, potentially due to the immunogeetics of the indigenous pig population [40, 43]. Likeise, antibody or low abundance of virus may hinder irus isolation, as animals were apparently asymptomtic at the time of sampling. The process of virus isotion is also difficult and lengthy as there is not a uitable cell line for diagnostic virus isolation of SFV. ASFV must be propagated in primary porcine ıacrophages for more than a month or adapted to ero cells. Neither of these approaches guarantees btaining a virus isolate. For these reasons, qPCR sureillance represents a fast, sensitive, specific and relible system for tracking ASFV epidemiology and is urrently considered the 'gold standard' for ASF genme detection [47].

The data obtained from qPCR does not indicate, hower, whether or not the virus present is infectious. Vhile PCR could be used to identify possible routes of irus shedding and transmission, the goal of this study as to determine if ASFV was present within a populaion of visually asymptomatic pigs in the field and to hen characterize the genotype of the virus.

Finding high viral loads within an apparently healthy ig population, is unusual, though not unprecedented, in the field of ASFV virology as ASF is typically associated with 90 to 100 % mortality in pigs [1] [48]. For example, a Ugandan study of over 1300 pigs, established primarily to determine the persistence of viral DNA in asymptomatic animals found only three qPCR positive animals, all of which were directly associated with ASF outbreak events on their farm of origin [41]. High viral DNA loads have, however, been identified in a small number of clinically asymptomatic pigs in Tanzania [23, 48].

A potential explanation for our results is that, although no official outbreak of ASF was reported in Kenya at the time of sampling, we could have detected diseased animals which were being slaughtered illegally. Under-reporting of ASF has been documented in neighbouring Uganda for reasons of distrust of government, poor compensation for destroyed animals and stigmatisation of afflicted farmers [49–51]. Up-to 20 % of farmers in northern Uganda reported "panic sales", or the quick removal of all animals (sick and healthy) at the onset of an ASF outbreak. They further reported that this activity was taking place clandestinely, often at night [49]. A small study of pork butchers in Busia district (Kenya) suggested that 19 % (3/16) reported buying a pig "after being approached by farmers or after an Africa Swine Fever (ASF) outbreak" [10].

The pigs sampled in this study did, appear on visual examination (by a veterinarian or animal health assistant) to be asymptomatic. It is possible therefore to hypothesis that farmers may not have explicitly sold animals due to clinical ASF, but use alternative cues to decide whether to send animals for slaughter, such as sudden in-appetence. This has been reported in the case of other diseases such as leptospirosis and brucellosis [52, 53]. There is also evidence that farmers may sell their pigs in response to rumours of ASF in their vicinity prior to the detection of sick or dying animals [54]. It would have been very interesting, but unfortunately not recorded in this study, to know which animals were sold due to active approaches by farmers' to traders or vice versa. The latter scenario being the most common in our study site [10, 55].

In Kenya, official inspection of pigs is required by law at the slaughter facility The ad-hoc arrangement of the market, in conjunction with an understaffed meat inspectorate in this situation, allows a large proportion of pork to enter the food chain without inspection [25, 56, 57]. In our study area, only 5 % (95 % CI 3–7) of pigs are subjected to ante-mortem inspection, and the slaughter of 'sick' animals has been reported in 5 % (95 % CI 3–7) of pig slaughterhouses (Cook et al. In prep.). This poorly regulated slaughter industry provides the opportunity for the unscrupulous slaughter of potentially sick animals. Hence slaughter based surveillance may over-represent disease prevalence and could explain the findings of this study. Similarly, there has been high prevalence of disease detected in market based sampling compared to community-based sampling reported in areas of Uganda endemic for trypanosomiasis in cattle [58]. These scenarios highlight the potential for markets or slaughter facilities to act as sensitive sentinels for disease and central point sampling at such facilities to provide a cost-effective method of disease detection.

Another explanation for the high rates of ASFV detection in this study is that infected pigs may have been brought into the study site for slaughter from neighbouring Uganda where outbreaks had been reported in April, July, August and November of 2010 [59]. The border between these two countries is distinctly porous, and pigs are bought and sold across the international border [10, 54]. Studies of farmers, butchers and pig traders in this area, suggest that the majority of pigs originate within 1–20 km [10], with the vast majority travelling <5 km although this pattern may be disrupted in cases of 'panic selling' [54]. This hypothesis might explain some of the PCR-positive pigs identified in the study, the spatial distribution of the positive samples, throughout the study site, does not support the theory of extensive cross-boundary incursion in the current situation.

The system of procuring pigs for the slaughterhouses and slaughter slabs in this study are very informal. For the most part, a 'scout' is sent out from the slaughterhouse to the community of villages around it to convince farmers with appropriately aged pigs to sell them for that day's slaughter. As such, all pigs slaughtered in a given facility are drawn from the farms in the immediate vicinity, and the population of pigs at slaughter differs only from those in the community by age - pigs in the community represent all age groups, those sold for slaughter represent pigs aged approximately 9–12 months old. The pork meat from these facilities is sold to local butcheries (usually owned by the same people as the slaughterhouse) for small scale sale to the local community. All pigs in this study were reported to have originated from within Kenya (See Additional file 1), and as the majority of pigs are brought to slaughter by bicycle or foot [10], we believe that only pigs being slaughtered in close proximity to the border might have originated from Uganda. We are confident that the pigs in this study represent pigs of slaughter age drawn from the community surrounding the slaughterhouses.

Our results suggest, that there is ASFV circulating within the pig population without clinical signs being detected. Several mechanisms for the persistence of virus in asymptomatic pig populations have been suggested, such as chronic or sub-clinical infections or low virulence isolates, but these do not provide sufficient explanation for the situation described in this manu script. As mentioned previously, chronic infections ar not believed to occur on the African continent, Ct value would have been expected in the range of 30–40 [18 and symptoms such as emaciation and pathologic lesion such as skin necrosis, arthritis, fibrinous pleuritis, peri carditis, pleural adhesions and necrotic pneumoni should have been observed in the animals [2].

Genetic resistance to ASFV infections has been pro posed previously but the heritability has not been prove [6]. Interestingly genomic analysis of 117 pigs included i the current study revealed that animals testing negativ for ASFV on conventional PCR at ILRI ($n = 65$) had sig nificantly ($P = <0.0001$) higher indigenous ancestry, (54 % and above) compared to those testing positive ($n = 52$ (Mujibi, Okoth, Onzere, Bishop, Fevre, Thomas, Plastow Rothschild, *In prep*).

The presence of infected pigs at abattoirs and in tur the dispersal of potentially infective meat to butcherie across the study site is of particular importance to th control of ASF. Previous studies have identified th movement of infected pigs to an abattoir and the move ment of infected pork products as being major risk fac tor for outbreaks, which appear to be distinct from th sylvatic cycle [3, 60]. Unregulated slaughter increases th risk of infected pork meat being sold, and infective ma terial being transported into un-exposed areas throug contact with fomites (including bicycles, vehicles slaughter staff clothing, and machete), or becoming pi swill. These mechanisms could lead to transmission o the virus [4, 61] and may have been instrumental for ini tiation of the outbreak which occurred soon after ou sampling period ended.

The discordance between the large number of ASFV positive pigs in this study in comparison to a communit based study in the same area suggests that slaughter sla data provides an overestimate of the overall prevalence o ASFV in the local population. This is potentially promote by anthropogenic factors, such as panic selling of poten tially diseased pigs, and implies that slaughter slab dat alone cannot be used to estimate true prevalence with clea implications for ASFV transmission dynamics modelling.

Conclusion

The detection of ASFV viral DNA in a relatively hig number of pigs delivered for slaughter during a perio with no reported outbreaks provides support for two hy potheses, which are not mutually exclusive: (1) that viru prevalence may be over-estimated by slaughter-slab sam pling, relative to that prevailing in the wider pig popula tion; (2) that sub-clinical, chronically infected o recovered pigs may be responsible for persistence of th virus in endemic areas.

dditional files

Additional file 1: Results of conventional and real-time PCR. Contains sample ID and sampling location with the results from the conventional PCR assay and the real-time PCR assays using the TaqMan® EZ-RT-PCR Kit and the Life Technologies Path-ID Multiplex One Step Kit.

Additional file 2: GenBank Accession Numbers. GenBank (http://www.ncbi.nlm.nih.gov/genbank/) Accession numbers for twenty ASFV isolates for which genotypic analysis was performed.

cknowledgements

'e would especially like to thank all members of the PAZ field and boratory teams, in particular James Akoko and Omoto Lazarus, whose onstant hard work and dedication allowed us to carry out our work. We ould also like to thank those pig farmers, traders, butchers and meat spectors who so willingly participated in this study. Authors are grateful to r. Monica Reising (USDA APHIS Center for Veterinary Biologics) and embers of the US National Animal Health Laboratory Network for etermination of diagnostic specificity, including the Center for Animal ealth and Food Safety (University of California Davis), Kansas State eterinary Diagnostic Laboratory, Minnesota Veterinary Diagnostic aboratory, Indiana Animal Disease Diagnostic Laboratory (Purdue niversity), Rollins Laboratory (North Carolina), Texas Veterinary Medical iagnostic Laboratory, and Washington Animal Disease Diagnostic aboratory (Washington State University).

unding

T & WAdG would like to acknowledge the Biotechnological and Biological ciences Research Council (BBSRC) for supporting their PhD studies through Doctoral Training Grant. EAJC thanks the Medical Research Council (MRC) r their support of her PhD studies. EMF and the People, Animals and their oonoses (PAZ) project were supported by the Wellcome Trust (085308), d this work was also supported by the Biotechnology and Biological ciences Research Council, the Department for International Development, e Economic & Social Research Council, the Medical Research Council, the atural Environment Research Council and the Defence Science & echnology Laboratory, under the Zoonoses and Emerging Livestock ystems (ZELS) programme, grant reference BB/L019019/1. qPCR assays were upported by the USDA, APHIS National Veterinary Services Laboratories as art of the animal disease diagnostic mission and by interagency greements with the USDA Agricultural Research Service and Science and echnology Directorate of the US Department of Homeland Security under ward Numbers 60-1940-7-011 and HSHQPM-13-X-00211. The University of dinburgh Innovation Initiative Grant fund is acknowledged for financially upporting the sample collection. The laboratory work at ILRI was supported y GIZ-ILRI contract number 81157484. This work received support from the GIAR Research Program on Agriculture for Nutrition and Health (A4NH), RP3.7, led by the International Food Policy Research Institute (IFPRI). We also cknowledge the CGIAR Fund Donors (http://www.cgiar.org/who-we-are/giar-fund/fund-donors-2).
e funders of this study had no role or influence over the study design, terpretation or reporting.

uthors' contribution

T designed and implemented the field study, assisted with interpretation f results and drafted the manuscript. EAC & WAD assisted with nplementation of the field study and interpretation of results. EMF upervised all aspects of the study from design to manuscript preparation. O, MM & KL undertook the laboratory analysis and interpretation of results d RB supervised the laboratory analysis and undertook interpretation of esults. All authors were involved with preparing the manuscript and pproved the final manuscript.

ompeting interests

e authors declare that they have no competing interests.

Consent for publication

Not applicable.

Ethics approval and consent to participate

Ethical approval for sample collection from animals was granted by the Animal Welfare and Ethical Review Body (AWERB) at The Roslin Institute, University of Edinburgh (approval number AWA004 Broonsvort). The Kenya Medical Research Institute ethical review board granted human ethics for the wider study of which this was part (the People, Animals and their Zoonoses project (http://www.zoonotic-diseases.org/project/paz-project/), (SC1701: human sample collection). The issue of animal ethics was deferred, by KEMRIs committee, to the ethics committee of the Roslin Institute as it was recognised as an authority internationally in the area of animal research ethics.
Sampling of privately owned domestic pigs presented to slaughter houses was carried out by trained veterinarians or animal health assistants after obtaining verbal informed consent from the persons presenting the pigs to slaughter. Blood sampling was undertaken according to the guidelines provided by the National Centre for the Replacement, Refinement and Reduction of Animals in Research (http://www.nc3rs.org.uk/bloodsamplingmicrosite/page.asp?id=346).

Author details

[1]Centre for Infection Immunity, and Evolution, Institute for Immunology and Infection Research, School of Biological Sciences, University of Edinburgh, Ashworth Labs, West Mains Rd, Edinburgh EH9 3JT, UK. [2]International Livestock Research Institute, PO Box 30709, Nairobi 00100, Kenya. [3]United States Department of Agriculture, Foreign Animal Disease Diagnostic Laboratory, National Veterinary Services Laboratories, Animal and Plant Health Inspection Services, PO Box 848, Greenport, NY 1944, USA. [4]Institute for Infection and Global Health, University of Liverpool, Leahurst Campus, Chester High Road, Neston CH64 7TE, UK.

References

1. Bengis RG, Kock RA, Fischer J. Infectious animal diseases: the wildlife/livestock interface. Rev Sci Tech Off Int Epizoot. 2002;21(1):53–66.
2. Sánchez-Vizcaíno J, Mur L, Gomez-Villamandos J, Carrasco L. An update on the epidemiology and pathology of African swine fever. J Comp Pathol. 2015;152(1):9–21.
3. Costard S, Mur L, Lubroth J, Sanchez-Vizcaino J, Pfeiffer D. Epidemiology of African swine fever virus. Virus Res. 2013;173(1):191–7.
4. Penrith M-L, Vosloo W. Review of African swine fever: transmission, spread and control: review article. J S Afr Vet Assoc. 2009;80(2):58–62.
5. Haresnape J, Lungu S, Mamu F. An updated survey of African swine fever in Malawi. Epidemiol Infect. 1987;99(03):723–32.
6. Penrith M, Thomson G, Bastos A, Phiri O, Lubisi B, Du Plessis E, et al. An investigation into natural resistance to African swine fever in domestic pigs from an endemic area in southern Africa. Rev Sci Tech. 2004;23(3):965–77.
7. Anderson EC, Hutchings GH, Mukarati N, Wilkinson PJ. African swine fever virus infection of the bushpig (Potamochoerus porcus) and its significance in the epidemiology of the disease. Vet Microbiol. 1998;62(1):1–15.
8. Jori F, Bastos AD. Role of wild suids in the epidemiology of African swine fever. Ecohealth. 2009;6(2):296–310.
9. Wabacha JK, Maribei JM, Mulei CM, Kyule MN, Zessin KH, Oluoch-Kosura W. Characterisation of smallholder pig production in Kikuyu Division, central Kenya. Prev Vet Med. 2004;63(3–4):183–95.
10. Kagira JM, Maingi N, Kanyari PWN, Githigia SM, Ng'ang'a JC, Gachohi JM. Characteristics of pig trade in low income settings in Busia District Kenya. The Tropical Veterinarian. 2009;26(2):1–9.
11. Mutua FK, Randolph TF, Arimi SM, Kitala PM, Githigia SM, Willingham AL, et al. Palpable lingual cysts, a possible indicator of porcine cysticercosis, in Teso District, Western Kenya. Journal of Swine Health and Production. 2007;15(4):206.
12. Githigia SM, Murekefu A, Otieno RO. Prevalence of porcine cysticercosis and risk factors for *Taenia solium* taeniosis in Funyula Division of Busia District Kenya. Kenya Veterinarian. 2007;29(1):37–9.

13. Thomas L, de Glanville W, Cook E, Fevre E. The spatial ecology of free-ranging domestic pigs (Sus scrofa) in western Kenya. BMC Vet Res. 2013;9(1):46.
14. OIE. African Swine Fever, Kenya. 2007. http://www.oie.int/wahis_2/public/wahid.php/Reviewreport/Review?page_refer=MapFullEventReport&reportid=5341. Accessed 20 Aug 2015.
15. OIE. African Swine Fever, Kenya. 2011. http://www.oie.int/wahis_2/public/wahid.php/Reviewreport/Review?page_refer=MapEventSummary&reportid=10307.
16. Perry B, Grace D. The impacts of livestock diseases and their control on growth and development processes that are pro-poor. Philosophical Transactions of the Royal Society B: Biological Sciences. 2009;364(1530): 2643–55.
17. Gallardo MC, de la Torre RA, Fernández-Pinero J, Iglesias I, Muñoz MJ, Arias ML. African swine fever: a global view of the current challenge. Porcine Health Management. 2015;1(1):1.
18. Gallardo C, Soler A, Nieto R, Sánchez M, Martins C, Pelayo V, et al. Experimental Transmission of African Swine Fever (ASF) Low Virulent Isolate NH/P68 by Surviving Pigs. Transbound Emerg Dis. 2015;62(6):612–22.
19. Costard S, Wieland B, de Glanville W, Jori F, Rowlands R, Vosloo W, et al. African swine fever: how can global spread be prevented? Philosophical Transactions of the Royal Society B: Biological Sciences. 2009;364(1530): 2683–96.
20. Ramiro-Ibáñez F, Ortega A, Ruiz-Gonzalvo F, Escribano JM, Alonso C. Modulation of immune cell populations and activation markers in the pathogenesis of African swine fever virus infection. Virus Res. 1997;47(1):31–40.
21. Okoth E, Gallardo C, Macharia J, Omore A, Pelayo V, Bulimo D, et al. Comparison of African swine fever virus prevalence and risk in two contrasting pig-farming systems in South-west and Central Kenya. Prev Vet Med. 2013;110(2):198–205.
22. Atuhaire DK, Afayoa M, Ochwo S, Mwesigwa S, Mwiine FN, Okuni JB, et al. Prevalence of African swine fever virus in apparently healthy domestic pigs in Uganda. BMC Vet Res. 2013;9(1):263.
23. Uttenthal Å, Braae UC, Ngowi H, Rasmussen TB, Nielsen J, Johansen MV. ASFV in Tanzania: Asymptomatic pigs harbor virus of molecular similarity to Georgia 2007. Vet Microbiol. 2013;165(1):173–6.
24. Doble L, Fèvre EM. Focusing on neglected zoonoses. Vet Rec. 2010;166(18):546.
25. Thomas LF, Harrison LJS, Toye P, de Glanville WA, Cook EAJ, Wamae CN et al. Prevalence of Taenia solium cysticercosis in pigs entering the food chain in western Kenya. Tropical Animal Health and Production. 2015:1–6.
26. Thrusfield M, Ortega C, De Blas I, Noordhuizen JP, Frankena K. WIN EPISCOPE 2.0: improved epidemiological software for veterinary medicine. Vet Rec. 2001;148(18):567.
27. Government of Kenya. Meat Control Act. 2012.
28. Muirhead MR. Blood sampling in pigs. In Pract. 1981;3(5):16–20.
29. Agüero M, Fernandez J, Romero L, Mascaraque CS, Arias M, Sanchez-Vizcaino J. Highly sensitive PCR assay for routine diagnosis of African swine fever virus in clinical samples. J Clin Microbiol. 2003;41(9):4431–4.
30. Zsak L, Borca M, Risatti G, Zsak A, French R, Lu Z, et al. Preclinical diagnosis of African swine fever in contact-exposed swine by a real-time PCR assay. J Clin Microbiol. 2005;43(1):112–9.
31. Bastos AD, Penrith M-L, Cruciere C, Edrich J, Hutchings G, Roger F, et al. Genotyping field strains of African swine fever virus by partial p72 gene characterisation. Arch Virol. 2003;148(4):693–706.
32. Rodríguez JM, García-Escudero R, Salas ML, Andrés G. African swine fever virus structural protein p54 is essential for the recruitment of envelope precursors to assembly sites. J Virol. 2004;78(8):4299–313.
33. Gallardo C, Mwaengo DM, Macharia JM, Arias M, Taracha EA, Soler A, et al. Enhanced discrimination of African swine fever virus isolates through nucleotide sequencing of the p54, p72, and pB602L (CVR) genes. Virus Genes. 2009;38(1):85–95.
34. Hall TA. BioEdit: a user-friendly biological sequence alignment editor and analysis program for Windows 95/98/NT, Nucleic acids symposium series. 1999.
35. Huang X, Madan A. CAP3: A DNA sequence assembly program. Genome Res. 1999;9(9):868–77.
36. Tamura K, Stecher G, Peterson D, Filipski A, Kumar S. MEGA6: molecular evolutionary genetics analysis version 6.0. Mol Biol Evol. 2013;30(12): 2725–9. mst197.
37. Larkin MA, Blackshields G, Brown N, Chenna R, McGettigan PA, McWilliam H, et al. Clustal W and Clustal X version 2.0. Bioinformatics. 2007;23(21):2947–8.
38. Rzhetsky A, Nei M. A simple method for estimating and testing minimum-evolution trees. Mol Biol Evol. 1992;9(5):945–67.
39. Felsenstein J. Confidence limits on phylogenies: an approach using the bootstrap. Evolution. 1985; 39(4):783–91.
40. Gallardo C, Okoth E, Pelayo V, Anchuelo R, Martín E, Simon A, et al. African swine fever viruses with two different genotypes, both of which occur in domestic pigs, are associated with ticks and adult warthogs, respectively, at a single geographical site. J Gen Virol. 2011 92(2):432–44.
41. Muhangi D, Masembe C, Emanuelson U, Boqvist S, Mayega L, Ademun RO, e al. A longitudinal survey of African swine fever in Uganda reveals high apparent disease incidence rates in domestic pigs, but absence of detectabl persistent virus infections in blood and serum. BMC Vet Res. 2015;11(1):1.
42. Lubisi BA, Bastos A, Dwarka R, Vosloo W. Molecular epidemiology of Africar swine fever in East Africa. Arch Virol. 2005;150(12):2439–52.
43. Gallardo C, Ademun AR, Nieto R, Nantima N, Arias M, Martín E, et al. Genotyping of African swine fever virus (ASFV) isolates associated with disease outbreaks in Uganda in 2007. Afr J Biotechnol. 2013;10(17):3488–97
44. Atuhaire DK, Ochwo S, Afayoa M, Mwesigwa S, Mwiine FN, Okuni JB et al. Molecular characterization of African swine fever virus in apparently health domestic pigs in Uganda. African Journal of Biotechnology. 2015;13(25): 2491–99.
45. Bishop RP, Fleischauer C, de Villiers EP, Okoth EA, Arias M, Gallardo C, et al. Comparative analysis of the complete genome sequences of Kenyan Africa swine fever virus isolates within p72 genotypes IX and X. Virus Genes. 2015 50(2):303–9.
46. Cubillos C, Gómez-Sebastian S, Moreno N, Nunez MC, Mulumba-Mfumu LK, Quembo CJ, et al. African swine fever virus serodiagnosis: A general review with a focus on the analyses of African serum samples. Virus Res. 2013; 173(1):159–67.
47. Oura C, Edwards L, Batten C. Virological diagnosis of African swine fever—comparative study of available tests. Virus Res. 2013;173(1):150–8.
48. Braae UC, Johansen MV, Ngowi H, Rasmussen TB, Nielsen J, Uttenthal Å. Detection of African swine fever virus DNA in blood samples stored on FTA cards from asymptomatic pigs in Mbeya Region, Tanzania. Transbound Emerg Dis. 2015;62(1):87–90.
49. Dione M, Akol J, Roesel K, Kungu J, Ouma E, Wieland B, et al. Risk Factors fc African Swine Fever in Smallholder Pig Production Systems in Uganda. Transbound Emerg Dis. 2015.
50. Chenais E, Boqvist S, Sternberg-Lewerin S, Emanuelson U, Ouma E, Dione M, et al. Knowledge, attitudes and practices related to African swine fever within smallholder pig production in northern Uganda. Transbound Emerg Dis. 2015.
51. Chenais E, Sternberg-Lewerin S, Boqvist S, Emanuelson U, Aliro T, Tejler E, et al. african swine fever in Uganda: qualitative evaluation of three surveillance methods with implications for other resource-poor settings. Frontiers in Veterinary. Science. 2015;2.
52. Brown P, McKenzie M, Pinnock M, McGrowder D. Environmental risk factors associated with leptospirosis among butchers and their associates in Jamaica. The international journal of occupational and environmental medicine. 2010;2(1 January).
53. Nabukenya I, Kaddu-Mulindwa D, Nasinyama GW. Survey of Brucella infection and malaria among Abattoir workers in Kampala and Mbarara Districts, Uganda. BMC Public Health. 2013;13(1):901.
54. Lichoti JK, Davies J, Kitala PM, Githigia SM, Okoth E, Maru Y, et al. Social network analysis provides insights into African swine fever epidemiology. Prev Vet Med. 2016.
55. Mutua FK, Dewey CE, Arimi SM, Schelling E, Ogara WO. Prediction of live body weight using length and girth measurements for pigs in rural Wester Kenya. Journal of swine health and production. 2011;19(1):26–33.
56. Kagira JM, Kanyari PN, Maingi N, Githigia SM, Ng'ang'a JC, Karuga JW. Characteristics of the smallholder free-range pig production system in western Kenya. Tropl Anim Health Prod. 2010;42:865–73. doi:10.1007/s11250-009-9500-y.
57. Cook EAJ. The epidemiology of zoonoes in slaughterhouse workers in western Kenya. University of Edinburgh; 2014. Available at https://www.era.lib.ed.ac.uk/handle/1842/10510.
58. Fevre E, Tilley A, Picozzi K, Fyfe J, Anderson I, Magona J, et al. Central point sampling from cattle in livestock markets in areas of human sleeping sickness. Acta Trop. 2006;97(2):229–32.
59. Kalenzi Atuhaire D, Ochwo S, Afayoa M, Norbert Mwiine F, Kokas I, Arinaitwe E et al. Epidemiological overview of African swine fever in Uganda (2001–2012). J Vet Med. 2013;2013.
60. Penrith M-L, Vosloo W, Jori F, Bastos AD. African swine fever virus eradication in Africa. Virus Res. 2013;173(1):228–46.
61. Haresnape JM. African swine fever in Malawi. Tropl Anim Health Prod. 1984 16(2):123–5.

15

ʔeassortment process after co-infection of pigs with avian H1N1 and swine H3N2 influenza viruses

inga Urbaniak[1*], Iwona Markowska-Daniel[1,2], Andrzej Kowalczyk[1,3], Krzysztof Kwit[1], Małgorzata Pomorska-Mól[1], arbara Frącek[1] and Zygmunt Pejsak[1]

Abstract

Background: The influenza A virus is highly variable, which, to some degree, is caused by the reassortment of viral genetic material. This process plays a major role in the generation of novel influenza virus strains that can emerge in a new host population. Due to the susceptibility of pigs to infections with avian, swine and human influenza viruses, they are considered intermediate hosts for the adaptation of the avian influenza virus to humans. In order to test the reassortment process in pigs, they were co-infected with H3N2 A/swine/Gent/172/2008 (Gent/08) and H1N1 A/duck/Italy/1447/2005 (Italy/05) and co-housed with a group of naïve piglets.

Results: The Gent/08 strains dominated over Italy/05, but reassortment occurred. The reassortant strains of the H1N1 subtype (12.5%) with one gene (NP or M) of swine-origin were identified in the nasal discharge of the contact-exposed piglets.

Conclusions: These results demonstrate that despite their low efficiency, genotypically and phenotypically different influenza A viruses can undergo genetic exchange during co-infection of pigs.

Keywords: Avian influenza virus, Pig, Reassortment, Swine influenza virus

ackground

'he genetic material of the influenza A virus (IAV) is ıade up of eight single-stranded, negative-sense RNA egments. Such a genomic arrangement allows the exhange of RNA segments between two or more IAVs ıat co-infect a single target cell. This process is known s reassortment. It is one of the mechanisms by which ew IAVs emerge and spread in immunologically susceptble human as well as swine populations [1, 2].

Pigs have been thought to serve as intermediate hosts n the adaptation of the avian influenza virus (AIV) to umans, and as "mixing vessels" facilitating the formaion of novel genetic IAV variants with potentially panemic properties. This assumption is based on the onfirmed ability of pigs to be infected with the swine ıfluenza virus (SIV), AIV and human influenza virus (HuIV) in natural conditions [3, 4]. Furthermore, experimental studies, which confirmed pig susceptibility to infections with the majority of the AIV subtypes emphasise the importance of pigs in the IAV ecology [5–7].

The mechanism of the exchange of genetic material between IAV strains has not been fully elucidated. It is still unclear where reassortment occurs. It may take place in the nucleus during replication, during the export of the RNA from the nucleus to the cell membrane, in the cell cytoplasm after the release of progeny RNA segments, or during progeny virion assembly [8].

Recent studies on the mechanism of IAV genome packaging suggest that the interaction of specific sequences between different RNA segments guides their selective incorporation into the virion [9–16]. Therefore, the reassortment process may be controlled by certain differences in the signals that initiate packing, required for the RNA-RNA interaction of various RNA segments. This was confirmed in the studies of Chou et al. [17]

Correspondence: kinga.urbaniak@piwet.pulawy.pl
Department of Swine Diseases, National Veterinary Research Institute, 57 artyzantów Avenue, 24-100 Puławy, Poland
ull list of author information is available at the end of the article

and Inagaki et al. [18], who showed that eight different RNA segments are always packed into one virion [17] and that segments of the same genes compete with each other in the process of virion assembly [18]. Furthermore, the individual segments are packaged in a hierarchical manner. The segments encoding PB2, PA, NP and M protein are more important than the remaining segments. Moreover, RNA segments are not transported from the nucleus individually or in packages of eight [19].

The aim of the study was to evaluate the occurrence of reassortment in piglets co-infected with two influenza viruses of different subtypes and origins. We co-infected the piglets with A/swine/Gent/172/2008 (H3N2) (Gent/08) and A/duck/Italy/1447/2005 (H1N1) (Italy/05). Additionally, healthy piglets were co-housed with the infected piglets.

Methods

Study design

For experimental purposes, twelve 6- to 8-week-old piglets were purchased from a high health status herd. They were randomly divided into two groups. Matrix gene real time reverse transcriptase PCR (RT-qPCR) and the haemaglutynation inhibition assay with four SIV subtypes: avian-like H1N1 (A/swine/Belgium/1/98), human-like H1N2 (A/swine/England/96), human-like H3N2 (A/swine/Flanders/1/98) and pdm-like H1N1 (A/swine/Poland/031951/2012), performed according to the standard procedure [20], were carried out prior to commencing the study. All tested piglets were molecularly and serologically negative for SIV. During the study, the piglets were housed in isolated units.

Two viral strains, the Gent/08 and the Italy/05, were propagated in 10-day-old embryonated chicken eggs. The third and fourth passage of the virus was used in a 1:1 mixture. A 10^9 $TCID_{50}$ IAV mixture was administered intranasally (i.n.) at a volume of 2 ml per nostril to a group of six piglets (forced-infected, FI). The remaining six naïve piglets formed the contact-exposed (CE) group and were introduced to the FI animals in the second day post infection (dpi).

Clinical measurements and sampling

During the study (10 dpi/day post contact (dpc)), the clinical signs of swine influenza (SI) were assessed daily. This included collecting swab samples and monitoring body temperature. At 4 dpi/dpc three randomly selected piglets from both groups were euthanised and necropsied. Blood samples were collected from all of the piglets before the initiation of the study and on the 14th, 21st, and 28th dpi/dpc for a serological investigation.

Swabs and tissue samples

Nasal swabs and tissue samples (of the respiratory an olfactory nasal mucosa, the trachea, the right and le apical, cardiac, diaphragmatic and accessory lobe of th lungs) were collected and prepared for extraction of vira RNA using the QIAmp Viral RNA Mini kit (Qiage Germany). The obtained samples were assessed usin the RT-qPCR method, as described below.

RT-qPCR

The sequences of primers and the probe were acquire from Hoffmann et al. [21]. A single RT-qPCR was per formed using 2 μl of the template RNA, 1× QuantiTec Probe RT-PCR Master Mix, 0.2 μl QuantiTect RT Mi (Qiagen, Germany), 0.8 μM of the forward prime 0.6 μM of each reverse primer and 0.1 μM of the prob with the addition of water free from DNase and RNas to bring the total volume to 20 μl.

All the RT-qPCR assays were performed on a Strata gene MX3005P QPCR thermocycler (Agilent Technolo gies, USA) using the following temperature profil 30 min at 50 °C, 15 min at 95 °C, 40 cycles of 10 s a 94 °C and 20 s at 60 °C. The fluorescence values (FAM were collected during the annealing step. Reactions wit a cycle threshold (Ct) value of <30 were scored positive values between 30 and 35 were scored as weak positiv and values >35 were scored negative.

Plaque purification assay

All the positive and weakly positive nasal swabs as we as the tissue samples were used in the plaque purifica tion assay to obtain single IAV isolates.

Six well plates with 100% confluent MDCK cultur were washed once with PBS. The inoculum (500 μl o the sample dilution) was applied to the wells of th plates. The infected cells were incubated at 37 °C for 1 in 4% CO_2. Then, the inoculum was removed and 3 m overlays of Eagle's MEM with an addition of 0.9% agar ose and 1 μg/ml trypsin were added. The plates wer placed inversely in a 37 °C, humidified incubator con taining 5% CO_2. The plaques were visualised 2 days pos infection. The agar was punctured where the cells wer damaged by the replicating virus. The agar fragment were suspended in 500 μl of Eagle's MEM and then 5 fold diluted. Subsequently, the diluted samples were pas saged once on MDCK cells. A cytopathic effect and RT qPCR confirmed the presence of IAV. The obtaine virus isolates were used to extract viral RNA or wer stored at −80 °C for further analysis.

Molecular characterisation

Numerous conventional reverse transcriptase PCRs (RT PCRs) (Additional file 1: Table S1) were carried out t genetically differentiate Gent/08 and Italy/05. RN amples from the plaque-purified IAVs were used. The ›rimers were selected based on the nucleotide sequence ›f parental IAV genomes using version 0.4.0 of the Pri- ıer3 Input (http://bioinfo.ut.ee/primer3-0.4.0/) and the 'rimerSelect package LaserGene DNASTAR application. 'he primers for 6 RT-PCRs were used in order to amp- fy the products of the internal IAV genes (PB2, PB1, 'A, NP, M, NS). The products were then used in the nalysis of restriction fragment length polymorphism RFLP). The remaining 4 pairs of primers were specific ɔr the Gent/08 or Italy/05 HA and NA (Additional file : Table S1). RT-PCRs were performed separately using he One Step RT-PCR Kit (Qiagen, Germany).

All the primer sets were used in a single RT-PCR as ɔllows: 2.5 µl of the template RNA, 1× OneStep RT- 'CR Buffer, 1 µl of the OneStep RT-PCR Enzyme Mix ontaining reverse transcriptase and DNA polymerase Qiagen, Germany), 0.5 mM of each of the dNTPs, 10 U ›f the RNaze inhibitor (Promega, USA) and the primers 0.5 µM of each primer) were combined and water free rom DNase and RNase was added to bring the total vol- ıme to 25 µl.

The following temperature profiles were used for all he RT-PCR runs: 30 min at 50 °C, 15 min at 95 °C, 5 cycles of 45 s at 94 °C, 45 s at 58 °C, and depending ›n the length of the amplified product, from 1.5 to min at 72 °C. The last cycle was followed by a 7-min xtension at 72 °C. After the amplification, 10 µl of the roduct was subjected to electrophoresis for 40 min at 00 mA in a 2% agarose gel stained with ethidium brom- de. The amplification products were visualised and hotographed under UV illumination using the EC3 'hemi HR 410 Imaging System (Ultra-Violet Products .td., UK).

Restriction enzymes (BamHI, NheI and EcoRI) were elected for the RFLP analysis using version 3 of Restric- ionMapper (http://www.restrictionmapper.org/).

The cleavage reaction was performed in a final volume ›f 16 µl containing 5 µl of the amplified product, 1 µl of he adequate restriction enzyme (Additional file 1: Table 2) and 1 µl of the 10× Buffer (Thermo Scientific, USA), ompleted with the water free from DNase and RNase.

The enzymes were activated for 2 h at 37 °C, then nactivated for 20 min at 65 °C (*Nhe*I, *Eco*RI) or 80 °C *Bam*HI). All the RT-PCRs and cleavage reactions were erformed using the T3 Thermocycler (Biometra, ɜermany). After cleavage, the product was subjected to lectrophoresis as described above.

equencing analysis

'he amplified RT-PCR products were sequenced in ɜenomed S.A., a DNA analysis service (Poland). The nu- leotide sequences were initially compared using the 'lustalW alignment algorithm method.

Results

Clinical signs

Apart from an increase in the rectal temperature, there were no typical clinical signs for acute SI either in the FI or the CE group of piglets.

In all the FI animals, the highest rectal temperature (40.0 °C - 40.8 °C) in individual piglets lasted from 2 to 5 dpi, with modal value at 3 dpi. A rectal temperature ≥ 40 °C was observed in three of the six FI piglets on days 2 and 3. In the CE piglets, a rectal temperature ≥ 40 °C was detected only in two piglets (peak from 3 to 4 dpc) and did not exceed 40.2 °C (data not shown).

Virus detection

In total, 56 nasal swabs and tissue samples were collected with a Ct value ≤35. Seventeen of the nasal swab samples were positive and 10 were weakly positive (Table 1). Nineteen tissue samples were positive and 10 samples were weakly positive (Table 2).

Viral shedding was confirmed for all the FI animals, but only three piglets (Nos. 3, 5 and 6) shed the virus extensively (Ct < 30). In addition, Ct values of the nasal swabs of piglets no. 3 and 6 were <30 and ranged from 1 to 4 dpi. In the CE group, viral RNA was detected in swab samples from four of the six piglets (piglets A, B, C and F). However, three of them shed the virus extensively (Ct < 30), for 2 or 4 days (from 3 to 6 dpc), depending on the animal (Fig. 1).

Seven positive and 7 weakly positive tissue samples were collected from the euthanised FI piglets. In each case, samples from trachea gave a positive or a weakly positive result. In the remaining tissues, positive or weakly positive results were obtained in 1 or 2

Table 1 RT-qPCR results for nasal swabs of the FI and the CE piglets

Dpi/ dpc	Forced-infected piglet ID						Contact-exposed piglet ID					
	1	2	3	4	5	6	A	B	C	D	E	F
0	–	–	–	–	–	–	–	–	–	–	–	–
1	–	–	++	–	–	++	+	–	–	–	–	–
2	+	–	++	+	+	++	–	–	–	–	–	–
3	+	–	++	–	++	++	–	+	++	–	–	++
4	–	–	++	-[a]	+[a]	++[a]	–	++	++	-[a]	-[a]	++[a]
5	–	–	+	×	×	×	–	++	++	×	×	×
6	–	+	+	×	×	×	–	–	++	×	×	×
7	–	–	–	×	×	×	–	–	–	×	×	×
8	–	–	–	×	×	×	–	–	–	×	×	×
9	–	–	–	×	×	×	–	–	–	×	×	×
10	–	–	–	×	×	×	–	–	–	×	×	×

Results are shown as −+ for positive sample (Ct < 30), + for weak positive sample (Ct 30–35) and - for negative sample (Ct > 35)
[a] euthanasia

Table 2 RT-qPCR results for tissue samples of the FI and the CE piglets

Tissue sample	Forced-infected piglet ID			Contact-exposed piglet ID		
	4	5	6	D	E	F
Respiratory nasal mucosa	–	++	++	–	–	++
Olfactory nasal mucosa	–	++	++	–	–	++
Trachea	+	+	++	++	+	++
Right apical and cardiac lobe	++	++	–	++	–	++
Right diaphragmatic lobe	–	+	–	++	–	++
Left apical and cardiac lobe	–	+	–	–	–	++
Left diaphragmatic lobe	–	+	+	++	+	++
Accessory lobe	–	+	–	–	+	++

Results are shown as ++ for positive sample (Ct < 30), + for weak positive sample (Ct 30–35) and - for negative sample (Ct > 35)

specimens. The samples from the upper respiratory tract as well as the right apical and cardiac lung lobe (pooled samples) showed a Ct value <30. All the samples from pig no. 5 gave a positive result (Table 2).

In the case of the CE animals, 12 positive and 3 weakly positive tissue samples were obtained. All the tested trachea and left diaphragmatic lobe samples from the CE piglets were positive or weakly positive. The lung samples representing the right apical and cardiac lobe (pooled samples), the right diaphragmatic lobe and the accessory lobe gave a positive reaction in two animals. The tissue samples of the respiratory tract from piglet F were positive (Table 2).

Plaque purification assay

Plaque-purified IAV isolates were obtained from 26 tissue samples. The arithmetic mean of the number of the isolates obtained from the samples with Ct values from 30 to 35 was 7.00 ± 5.15, and was equal to 8.11 ± 4.01 for samples with a Ct < 30. The total number of isolates obtained from the tissue homogenates was 202. On hundred thirty-one of those isolates were acquired fron tissues of the CE animals and 71 came from the tissue of the FI piglets.

Twenty-six plaque-purified IAV isolates (24 from th CE piglets, 2 from the FI piglets) were obtained from 7 nasal swab samples (6 from the CE piglets, 1 from the F animal). The arithmetic mean of the number of isolate obtained from the nasal swabs was 2.67 ± 1.37 with ex clusion the sample from piglet F from the CE group, a 10 isolates were collected from this animal.

Molecular characterisation

All 228 obtained isolates were used for the genetic char acterisation. Amplicons specific for the HA (463 bp) an the NA (241 bp) Gent/08 genes were obtained for 22 isolates (96.49%) (H3N2 isolates), including 202 fron the tissue samples and 18 from the nasal swabs. Result specific for the Italy/05 genes (HA – 314 bp, NA -

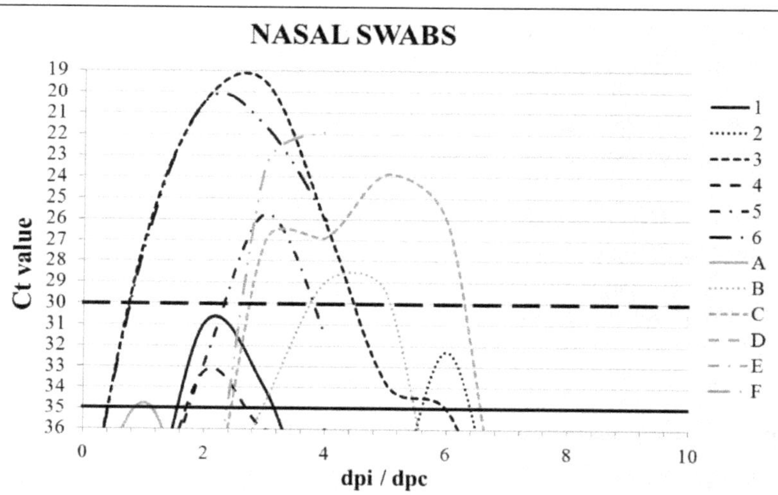

Fig. 1 Viral shedding by the FI and the CE piglets. 1–6 – FI piglets; A-F – CE piglets

27 bp) were obtained for the remaining 8 isolates H1N1 isolates) from the nasal swabs (Tables 3 and 4).

The *Bam*HI, *Nhe*I and *Eco*RI restriction enzymes were sed to differentiate six internal genes. According to the FLP analysis, the PB2, PB1, M and NS genes of all I3N2 isolates were swine-origin. Two H3N2 isolates ad one gene (PA or NP) positive for Italy/05, while the emaining H3N2 isolates had swine-origin PA and NP enes. In the case of the H1N1 isolates, all PB2, PB1, PA nd NS genes were of avian-origin. Three H1N1 isolates ad one gene (NP or M) with a Gent/08 specific cleavge pattern (Table 3).

equencing

gene fragment (RT-PCR amplification product) seuence analysis was conducted for the RNA samples seected according to the RFLP results. In total, 5 samples marked in bold in Table 3) were analysed. A mutation t the *Bam*HI cleavage site of the PA and the NP gene as identified in two H3N2 isolates positive in the RFLP or Italy/05 genes. The sequence analyses of 3 genes (M r NP) of swine-origin H1N1 isolates confirmed the FLP results.

nalysis of molecular results

ll 202 isolates obtained from the tissue samples were nfected by the H3N2 subtype. Of the 26 isolates colected from the nasal swabs, 18 were Gent/08, 5 were taly/05, and the remaining 3 were reassortants (H1N1 ubtype with one gene of swine-origin, rH1N1). All the I1N1 and 16 Gent/08 strains were obtained from swab amples from the CE animals. Two Gent/08 isolates vere from the nasal swab collected from the FI piglet o. 6 (Table 4). Each reassortant was obtained from the amples collected from different CE animals (Table 5).

iscussion

he emergence of new IAV in humans, pigs and other ost species is mostly associated with the reassortment rocess of two or more IAV strains [22–24]. This study ntended to clarify the role of pigs in this process. Our ata confirmed that pigs can be experimentally co-infected with SIV and AIV and that an exchange of RNA segments may occur.

able 3 Genetic makeup of plaque-purified IAVs based on the T-PCR and the RFLP analyses

olate	Gene origin	Gene							
		PB2	PB1	PA	HA	NP	NA	M	NS
1N1	Italy/05	8	8	8	8	6	8	7	8
	Gent/08	0	0	0	0	**2**	0	**1**	0
3N2	Italy/05	0	0	**1**	0	**1**	0	0	0
	Gent/08	220	220	219	220	219	220	220	220

esults are shown as the number of genes. Samples for sequencing shown bold

The vast majority of the isolated strains were Gent/08 (96.49%). The Italy/05 strain comprised 2.19% of the isolates, while the rH1N1 strain was confirmed in 1.32% of the isolates. All of the Italy/05 and rH1N1 strains were isolated from the nasal swabs of different CE pig.

The transmission of the Italy/05 virus in pigs confirmed in our study strongly contrasts with previous studies which showed efficient replication of this virus in pigs which was not transmitted further [5]. In our experiment, the Italy/05 could be transmitted. Moreover, our rH1N1 possessed a majority of avian-origin genes excluding the M or NP genes. It was reported that the M and NP genes have an impact on the transmission capability of IAV [25–27]. In the case of the r5 H1N1 isolates, the reassortment process may have occurred independently in two CE piglets or, presumably, in one CE or one FI piglet, which then transmitted the r5 H1N1 to naïve animals.

A study conducted in the 1990s indicated that SIV acts as a helper virus in the process of AIV replication in pigs. In that study, the animals were co-infected with SIV Sw/Hok/2/81 (H1N1) and AIV Dk/Hok/8/80 (H3N8), which showed no ability to replicate in the pig. Apart from SIVs, AIVs and rH3N1 with swine-origin NA, NP and M or NS genes were obtained [7]. The SIV used by the Japanese researchers supported the replication of the AIV, whereas in our study, SIV strongly competed with AIV. Nonetheless, in our study, the infection with Gent/08 and the clinical symptoms such as sneezing and coughing may have facilitated the transmission of Italy/05.

An antigenic shift did not occur in our study and the rH1N1 gained only one RNA segment. This could be connected with competitiveness among the used strains.

All of the rH1N1 were isolated from nasal swabs. This may suggest favourable conditions in the upper respiratory tract for the exchange of IAV RNA segments. A similar conclusion was drawn from the experimental co-infection of ferrets with A/Wyoming/03/03 (H3N2) (low virulence, high transmissivity) and A/Thailand/16/06, (avian-like H5N1) (high virulence, low transmissivity). In that study, a low reassortment (8.9%) efficiency was obtained [28], which is similar to our findings. This may be caused by phenotypic and genotypic differences of the IAVs used for co-infection.

The ability of IAV to infect different hosts largely depends on the optimal gene constellation [29]. Thus, the capacity for replication and transmission in pigs may increase in the case of reassortants that have compatible genes compared with a wholly AIV. However, without an experimental comparison we cannot assume that our rH1N1 isolates are better adapted to pigs than Italy/05.

Table 4 Plaque-purified IAVs from tissue and nasal swabs samples from the FI and the CE piglets

Virus	Forced-infected		Contact-exposed		In total
	Tissue samples	Nasal swabs	Tissue samples	Nasal swabs	
H3N2	100 (71/71)	100 (2/2)	100 (131/131)	66.67 (16/24)	96.49 (220/228
H1N1	-	-	-	20.83 (5/24)	2.19 (5/228)
rH1N1[a]	-	-	-	12.50 (3/24)	1.32 (3/228)

Results are shown as percentages, with the number of viruses/total number of viruses shown in parentheses
[a]Reassortant H1N1

In previous studies, 63 possible reassortants of the H5N1 subtypes of human seasonal A/Wyoming/3/2003 (H3N2) and avian-like A/Thailand/16/2004 (H5N1) IAVs were divided into 4 phenotypic groups based on the rescue efficiency. Strains with a similar genomic constellation to our rH1N1 were included in group 1 (r7 H5N1), while strains with good replication efficiency and marginally viable reassortants made up group 4 (r5 H5N1). The authors underlined that all of the strains in group 4 had an NP gene of mammalian-origin, but the addition of an NS gene (r5/8) or NS and M genes (r5/7/8) from the H3N2 virus significantly increased the rescue efficiency of the reassortant [30].

Another research group generated 254 reassortants of a low pathogenic AIV H5N1 subtype and a HuIV H3N2 subtype [1]. In that study, the strains with M or NP gene of mammalian-origin were included in group 1 (the M gene) and 4 (the NP gene).

Both studies [1, 30] showed that the acquisition of the M gene of mammalian-origin did not significantly affect the functionality of the AIV, while the presence of the NP gene dramatically decreased the activity of the virus. Those results differ from our findings, because 2 of the 3 obtained rH1N1 strains acquired the NP gene. This difference may result from the use of different strains of AIV. It may also be caused by better compatibility of the Gent/08 NP gene with the remaining Italy/05 RNA segments and the congruity of Gent/08 NP with other proteins, especially viral polymerase.

The acquisition of a single gene by the rH1N1 in this study did not increase the frequency of its isolation compared with Italy/05. On the other hand, the results indicate that the rH1N1 viruses have not lost the capability to replicate. Taking into consideration the results of the previous studies [30], we can assume that acquiring another gene of swine-origin could improve the replication and transmission properties of our rH1N1 and enhanc its adaptation in pigs.

The most favourable conditions for the occurrence c reassortment during co-infection in experimenta models have not been determined. Therefore, it is no clear what circumstances are needed under natural con ditions to promote the emergence of new IAV variant [8].

In order to exclude certain unfavourable reassortmen factors, such as segment mismatch, an American re search group [8] used for co-infection the H3N2 subtyp IAV strains with a different genotype. Even then, a theor etically optimal reassortment efficiency was no achieved. They found that parental strains occurre more frequently than expected, suggesting incomplet mixing of RNA segments of parental viruses in co infected cells, although this may also be related to th small differences in the input of viral particles into singl cells [8]. The authors also found that in vivo reassort ment occurred less frequently (59%) than in vitro reas sortment (88.4%) [8].

Therefore, the use of two phenotypically and genotypi cally different strains in our experiment had a significan impact on the low incidence of reassortment, mainl due to RNA segment mismatch and the competitivenes of the Gent/08 and the Italy/05 strains. The low inci dence of the reassortment was also affected by the us of an animal model.

In previous in vivo studies [31], pigs were inoculate with two SIV strains: the classical H1N1 (cSIV) and th triple reassortant H3N2. The majority (85.9%) of the ob tained isolates were reassortants. Interestingly, ther were no cSIV strains among all the isolates. This may in dicate that the cSIV strain replicates less efficiently i pigs compared to the H3N2 SIV strain and the identifie reassortants. Despite such a high percentage c

Table 5 Molecular characteristics of the obtained rH1N1

Piglet ID / Sampling day	Subtype	Molecular characterisation	Reassortar
C / 5dpc	H1N1	PB2, PB1, PA, HA, NP, NA, **M**[a], NS	r7
E / 4dpc	H1N1	PB2, PB1, PA, HA, **NP**[a], NA, M, NS	r5
F / 1dpc	H1N1	PB2, PB1, PA, HA, **NP**[a], NA, M, NS	r5

[a] genes of swine-origin

eassortants, their transmission to the CE pigs was not onfirmed [31].

The results of that study suggest that there was Italy/5 and Gent/08 reassortment in the CE piglets in our tudy. This is due to the fact that despite the use of two IV strains by the American researchers, their reassorants were not transmissible. However, as mentioned bove, the confirmed transmission of both IAVs used in ur experiment dose not exclude the possibility of reasortant transmission.

Provided there are optimal conditions for reassortnent, segment exchange is influenced by the viral trains. The functional compatibility of the synthesised roteins, the match between the sequences initiating NA segment packing to progeny virions [12] and/or he efficiency of co-infection impacts in the affinity for arious receptors [32].

The results of this study show that despite the very ow efficiency of reassortment, it can occur between geotypically and phenotypically different IAV strains in igs. This underscores the necessity for enhanced viral urveillance strategies that monitor reassortment events, s well as for experimental studies which will elucidate he the reassortment process.

Conclusions

Despite the low efficiency a reassortment between genoypically and phenotypically different influenza A virus trains can occur in pigs.

Infection with swine influenza A virus can help in the ransmission of less adapted avian influenza virus.

Additional file

Additional file 1: Table S1. Contains the names and sequences of all primers used to amplify fragments of all genes to differentiate gene segments of the Gent/08 and the Italy/05. **Table S2.** Contains the information on which gene of which strain (Italy/05 or Gent/08) is subject to restriction enzyme cleavage. It also provides the information about the size of the RT-PCR products and the fragments after the restriction enzyme digestion.

Abbreviations

IV: Avian influenza virus; CE: Contact-exposed; cSIV: Classical swine influenza rus, subtype H1N1; Ct: Cycle treshold; dpc: Day post contact; dpi: Day post fection; FI: Forced-infected; Gent/08: A/swine/Gent/172/2008 subtype 3N2; HuIV: Human influenza virus; i.n.: Intranasally; IAV: Influenza A virus; aly/05: A/duck/Italy/1447/2005 subtype H1N1; r: reassortants; FLP: Restriction fragment length polymorphism; RT-PCR: Reverse anscriptase PCR; RT-qPCR: Real time reverse transcriptase PCR; SI: Swine fluenza; SIV: Swine influenza virus

Acknowledgements

We thank prof. dr. Kristien Van Reeth, the Laboratory of Virology, Faculty of eterinary Medicine, Ghent University, Belgium and Terregino Calogero DVM, hD, the Experimental Zooprophylactic Institute in Padova, Italy for kindly roviding influenza virus strains.

Funding

This work was supported by the EU's Seventh Framework Programme (FLUPIG Project No 258084).

Authors' contributions

KU performed all molecular tests, took part in virus isolation (plaque purification), analysed and interpreted obtained data and was a major contributor in writing the manuscript. IMD helped in data analyse and writing the manuscript. AK performed sequence analyse, designed primers and choose restriction enzyme for molecular identification of used virus strains. KK and MPM performed inoculation of animals and sample collection. BF prepared inoculum and performed plaque purification. ZP, IMD, MPM and KK made substantial contributions to conception and design of animal experiment. KU, AK and BF made substantial contributions to protocols of laboratory testing and acquisition of data. All authors read and approved the final manuscript.

Consent for publication

Not applicable.

Competing interests

The authors declare that they have no competing interests.

Author details

[1]Department of Swine Diseases, National Veterinary Research Institute, 57 Partyzantów Avenue, 24-100 Puławy, Poland. [2]Present Address: Laboratory of Veterinary Epidemiology and Economics. Faculty of Veterinary Medicine, Warsaw University of Life Sciences, 159c Nowoursynowska Street, 02-776 Warsaw, Poland. [3]Present Address: Wrocław Research Centre EIT+, 147 Stabłowicka Street, 54-066 Wrocław, Poland.

References

1. Li C, Hatta M, Nidom CA, Muramoto Y, Watanabe S, Neumann G, Kawaoka Y. Reassortment between avian H5N1 and human H3N2 influenza viruses creates hybrid viruses with substantial virulence. Proc Natl Acad Sci U S A. 2010;107:4687–92.
2. Urbaniak K, Markowska-Daniel I. In vivo reassortment of influenza viruses. Acta Biochim Pol. 2014;61:427–31.
3. Nelson MI, Wentworth DE, Culhane MR, Vincent AL, Viboud C, LaPointe MP, Lin X, Holmes EC, Detmer SE. Introductions and evolution of human-origin seasonal influenza a viruses in multinational swine populations. J Virol. 2014; 88:10110–9.
4. Nelson MI, Vincent AL. Reverse zoonosis of influenza to swine: new perspectives on the human-animal interface. Trends Microbiol. 2015;23:142–53.
5. De Vleeschauwer A, Van Poucke S, Braeckmans D, Van Doorsselaere J, Van Reeth K. Efficient transmission of swine-adapted but not wholly avian influenza viruses among pigs and from pigs to ferrets. J Infect Dis. 2009;200:1884–92.
6. Hinshaw VS, Webster RG, Easterday BC, Bean WJ Jr. Replication of avian influenza a viruses in mammals. Infect Immun. 1981;34:354–61.
7. Kida H, Ito T, Yasuda J, Shimizu Y, Itakura C, Shortridge KF, Kawaoka Y, Webster RG. Potential for transmission of avian influenza viruses to pigs. J Gen Virol. 1994;75:2183–8.
8. Marshall N, Priyamvada L, Ende Z, Steel J, Lowen AC. Influenza virus reassortment occurs with high frequency in the absence of segment mismatch. PLoS Pathog. 2013; doi:10.1371/journal.ppat.1003421.
9. Fournier E, Moules V, Essere B, Paillart JC, Sirbat JD, Isel C, Cavalier A, Rolland JP, Thomas D, Lina B, Marquet R. A supramolecular assembly formed by influenza a virus genomic RNA segments. Nucleic Acids Res. 2012;40:2197–209.
10. Fujii Y, Goto H, Watanabe T, Yoshida T, Kawaoka Y. Selective incorporation of influenza virus RNA segments into virions. Proc Natl Acad Sci U S A. 2003; 100:2002–7.
11. Fujii K, Fujii Y, Noda T, Muramoto Y, Watanabe T, Takada A, Goto H, Horimoto T, Kawaoka Y. Importance of both the coding and the segment-specific noncoding regions of the influenza a virus NS segment for its efficient incorporation into virions. J Virol. 2005;79:3766–74.
12. Gao Q, Palese P. Rewiring the RNAs of influenza virus to prevent reassortment. Proc Natl Acad Sci U S A. 2009;106:15891–6.

13. Hutchinson EC, Curran MD, Read EK, Gog JR, Digard P. Mutational analysis of cis-acting RNA signals in segment 7 of influenza a virus. J Virol. 2008;82: 11869–79.
14. Marsh GA, Hatami R, Palese P. Specific residues of the influenza a virus hemagglutinin viral RNA are important for efficient packaging into budding virions. J Virol. 2007;81:9727–36.
15. Marsh GA, Rabadan R, Levine AJ, Palese P. Highly conserved regions of influenza a virus polymerase gene segments are critical for efficient viral RNA packaging. J Virol. 2008;82:2295–304.
16. Muramoto Y, Takada A, Fujii K, Noda T, Iwatsuki-Horimoto K, Watanabe S, Horimoto T, Kida H, Kawaoka Y. Hierarchy among viral RNA (vRNA) segments in their role in vRNA incorporation into influenza a virions. J Virol. 2006;80:2318–25.
17. Chou YY, Vafabakhsh R, Doganay S, Gao Q, Ha T, Palese P. One influenza virus particle packages eight unique viral RNAs as shown by FISH analysis. Proc Natl Acad Sci U S A. 2012;109:9101–6.
18. Inagaki A, Goto H, Kakugawa S, Ozawa M, Kawaoka Y. Competitive incorporation of homologous gene segments of influenza a virus into virions. J Virol. 2012;86:10200–2.
19. Gerber M, Isel C, Moules V, Marquet R. Selective packaging of the influenza a genome and consequences for genetic reassortment. Trends Microbiol. 2014;22:446–55.
20. Markowska-Daniel I, Stankevicius A. Seroprevalence of antibodies against swine influenza viruses in pigs of different age. Bull Vet Inst Pulawy. 2005;49:3–7.
21. Hoffmann B, Harder T, Lange E, Kalthoff D, Reimann I, Grund C, Oehme R, Vahlenkamp TW, Beer M. New real-time reverse transcriptase polymerase chain reactions facilitate detection and differentiation of novel A/H1N1 influenza virus in porcine and human samples. Berl Munch Tierarztl Wochenschr. 2010;123:286–92.
22. EJA S, RAM F. Host adaptation and transmission of influenza a viruses in mammals. Emerg Microbes Infect. 2014; doi:10.1038/emi.2014.9.
23. Su S, Bi Y, Wong G, Gray GC, Gao GF, Li S. Epidemiology, evolution, and recent outbreaks of avian influenza virus in China. J Virol. 2015;89:8671–6.
24. Su S, Zhou P, Fu X, Wang L, Hong M, Lu G, Sun L, Qi W, Ning Z, Jia K, Yuan Z, Wang H, Ke C, Wu J, Zhang G, Gray GC, Li S. Virological and epidemiological evidence of avian influenza virus infections among feral dogs in live poultry markets, china: a threat to human health? Clin Infect Dis. 2014;58:1644–6.
25. Chou YY, Albrecht RA, Pica N, Lowen AC, Richt JA, García-Sastre A, Palese P, Hai R. The M segment of the 2009 new pandemic H1N1 influenza virus is critical for its high transmission efficiency in the guinea pig model. J Virol. 2011;85:11235–41.
26. Ince WL, Gueye-Mbaye A, Bennink JR, Yewdell JW. Reassortment complements spontaneous mutation in influenza a virus NP and M1 genes to accelerate adaptation to a new host. J Virol. 2013;87:84330–8.
27. Campbell PJ, Danzy S, Kyriakis CS, Deymier MJ, Lowen AC, Steel J. The M segment of the 2009 pandemic influenza virus confers increased neuraminidase activity, filamentous morphology, and efficient contact transmissibility to A/Puerto Rico/8/1934-based reassortant viruses. J Virol. 2014;88:3802–14.
28. Jackson S, Van Hoeven N, Chen LM, Maines TR, Cox NJ, Katz JM, Donis RO. Reassortment between avian H5N1 and human H3N2 influenza viruses in ferrets: a public health risk assessment. J Virol. 2009;83:8131–40.
29. Shortridge KF, Zhou NN, Guan Y, Gao P, Ito T, Kawaoka Y, Kodihalli S, Krauss S, Markwell D, Murti KG, Norwood M, Senne D, Sims L, Takada A, Webster RG. Characterization of avian H5N1 influenza viruses from poultry in Hong Kong. Virology. 1998;252:331–42.
30. Chen LM, Davis CT, Zhou H, Cox NJ, Donis RO. Genetic compatibility and virulence of reassortants derived from contemporary avian H5N1 and human H3N2 influenza a viruses. PLoS Pathog. 2008; doi:10.1371/journal.ppat.1000072.
31. Ma W, Lager KM, Lekcharoensuk P, Ulery ES, Janke BH, Solórzano A, Webby RJ, García-Sastre A, Richt JA. Viral reassortment and transmission after co-infection of pigs with classical H1N1 and triple-reassortant H3N2 swine influenza viruses. J Gen Virol. 2010;91:2314–21.
32. Van Riel D, Munster VJ, De Wit E, Rimmelzwaan GF, Fouchier RA, Osterhaus AD, Kuiken T. Human and avian influenza viruses target different cells in the lower respiratory tract of humans and other mammals. Am J Pathol. 2007; 171:1215–23.

16

Development of a novel lateral flow assay for detection of African swine fever in blood

Sastre[1*], C. Gallardo[2], A. Monedero[1], T. Ruiz[1], M. Arias[2], A. Sanz[1] and P. Rueda[1]

Abstract

Background: African swine fever (ASF) is a viral infectious disease of domestic and wild suids of all breeds and ages, causing a wide range of hemorrhagic syndromes and frequently characterized by high mortality. The disease is endemic in Sub-Saharan Africa and Sardinia. Since 2007, it has also been present in different countries of Eastern Europe, where control measures have not been effective so far. The continued spread poses a serious threat to the swine industry worldwide. In the absence of vaccine, early detection of infected animals is of paramount importance for control of the outbreak, to prevent the transmission of the virus to healthy animals and subsequent spreading of the disease. Current laboratory diagnosis is mainly based on virological methods (antigen and genome detection) and serodiagnosis.

Results: In the present work, a Lateral Flow Assay (LFA) for antigen detection has been developed and evaluated. The test is based on the use of a MAb against VP72 protein of ASFV, the major viral capsid protein and highly immunogenic. First experiments using VP72 viral and recombinant protein or inactivated culture virus showed promising results with a sensitivity similar to that of a commercially available Antigen-ELISA. Moreover, these strips were tested with blood from experimentally infected pigs and field animals and the results compared with those of PCR and Antigen-ELISA. For the experimentally infected samples, there was an excellent correlation between the LFA and the ELISA, while the PCR always showed to be more sensitive (38 % positive samples by PCR versus 27 % by LFA). The LFA was demonstrated to be positive for animals with circulating virus levels exceeding 10^4 HAU. With the field samples, once again, the PCR detected more positives than either the Antigen-ELISA or LFA, although here the number of positive samples scored by the LFA exceeded the values obtained with the Antigen-ELISA, showing 60 % positivity *vs* 48 % for the ELISA. For the two groups of sera, the specificity was close to 100 % indicating that hardly any false positive samples were found.

Conclusions: The newly developed LFA allows rapid and reliable detection of ASFV, at field and laboratory level, providing a new useful tool for control programs and in situations where laboratory support and skilled personnel are limited.

Keywords: African swine fever virus, Lateral flow assay, Diagnosis

Background

African swine fever virus (ASFV) is a large, enveloped, icosahedral double-stranded DNA virus that belongs to the *Asfaviridae* family, genus *Asfivirus* [1]. ASFV was first identified in 1921 in Kenya as the cause of lethal hemorrhagic disease in domestic pigs [2]. In Europe, ASF was introduced to Portugal in 1957, and from 1960, in other countries such as Spain or Italy and the Caribbean islands, but finally eradicated. Currently, the disease is endemic in the majority of Sub-Saharan countries and Sardinia (Italy) [3, 4]. Since the introduction of ASFV into Georgia in 2007 from East Africa, several cases have been declared in Armenia, Azerbaijan and in the Russian Federation, where continued uncontrolled spreading poses a serious threat to the swine industry worldwide [5–8]. The disease again manifested itself in early 2014, when the first cases of ASF in wild boar in Lithuania and Poland were reported in areas bordering on Belarus. Since then, the ASFV has spread in Estonia, Latvia, Lithuania and Poland, mostly affecting wild boar and to a lesser extent domestic pigs [9, 10]. Presently, the disease is threatening other

*Correspondence: psastre@ingenasa.com
[1]Inmunología y Genética Aplicada S. A. (INGENASA), Madrid, Spain
Full list of author information is available at the end of the article

regions in Europe and Asia due to the potential persistent spillover of the virus to adjacent areas.

The natural hosts of ASFV are the domestic and wild suids, and soft ticks of the genus Ornithodoros. The infection of warthogs and bushpigs in Africa results in mild disease, often asymptomatic, with low viraemia titers, developing into a persistent infection in most cases [4, 11–13]. These animals act as reservoir hosts of ASFV in Africa. On the other hand, infection of domestic pigs, European wild boar, and American wild pigs leads to more acute diseases with high rates of morbidity and mortality [14].

At present, no treatment or vaccine is available to prevent ASF and the control strategy mainly relies on enforcement of sanitary measures and slaughtering of infected and exposed animals [15]. Therefore, early and specific diagnosis of the infection is urgently required for prevention, control, and eradication of the disease in affected countries. In the majority of cases, the severe nature of the epidemic disease affecting the Eastern European countries leads to mortality with high levels of viral presence in tissues and blood [16–19]. Therefore, the ASF diagnosis in the National Reference Laboratories of the affected countries should always include the detection of the virus, the antigen or the ASFV genome. The OIE-recommended tests for virus detection include virus isolation, fluorescent antibody test and both real-time and conventional PCR assays [20, 21]. However, these methods are still rather time consuming and require well-equipped laboratories and personnel, delaying the disease diagnosis in remote areas [22–25].

In the present report we describe a novel approach for detection of viral antigen by an immunochromatographic test, based on the use of a monoclonal antibody against the major viral capsid protein of ASFV, VP72. The test was first set up using semi-purified viral protein and inactivated tissue culture virus. Further studies for validation of the test were carried out using experimental and field serum samples. This novel pen-side test offers a rapid and simple assay that will allow early detection of ASFV infection, especially useful for testing wild suids in the field, and for use in small laboratories, where laboratory equipment is very simple or absent.

Methods

Monoclonal antibodies and sera

Monoclonal antibody (mAb) 18BG3, specific for th VP72 protein, was produced by Ingenasa, following th previously described protocol by other authors [26].

For this study, two groups of sera were used:

Porcine samples from ASFV experimental studies

Pigs used for experimental studies were obtained fron a local commercial farm. One hundred and fifty thre EDTA-blood samples were collected at regular interval until the end of the study, from three independen experimental infections with virulent ASFV isolate belonging to P72 genotype II, currently circulating in Eas Europe, and IX, which is present in East Africa. The number and type of experimental samples is summarized i Table 1. Animal experiments were conducted at the BSL animal facilities at INIA in accordance with EC Directiv 86/609/EEC, which regulates the accommodation an care of animals used for experimental and other scientifi purposes. The experiments were conducted as follows:

Experimental infections with ASFV Ken06. Bus isolat (Kenya 2006): four Landrace x Large White pigs were inoculated intramuscularly with 10 HAD50/ml of the ASF Ken06-Bus isolate. Two untreated pigs were maintaine in contact, housed in the same box as the inoculated animals. Inoculated and in-contact animals developed acut forms of clinical disease and were slaughtered or died as result of the infection, between 8 to 17 days post inocula tion (dpi)/ days post-exposure (dpe) [27, 28].

Experimental infection with the ASFV Ukr12/Zapo isolate (Ukraine 2012): four domestic pigs were inoculated b the intramuscular route with 10 HAD50/ml of the Ukrain ASFV Ukr12/Zapo isolate. The inoculated pigs were place in contact with two naive pigs being housed in the sam box. All the pigs developed peracute to acute form of th disease and died, or were ethically slaughtered, between and 10 dpi (for infected pigs) and 11–12 dpe (for in-contac pigs) [29].

Experimental infections with ASFV LT14/1490 isolat (Lithuania 2014): ten naive pigs were placed in contac with eight pigs experimentally inoculated by the intramuscular route with 10 HAD50/ml of the Lithuanian LT14 1490 strain. The Lithuanian ASFV strain induced an acut disease which resulted in 94,5 % mortality. Seven of th

Table 1 Description of the tested experimental samples collected from animals infected with ASFV genotype II and IX viruses

Clinical form	Virulence designation	ASFV Strain	Origin (P72 genotype)	N° PIGS examined	Days Post Infection (DPI)	N of samples tested	Reference
Acute	Virulent	Ken06.Bus	Kenya (IX)	6	0–14	23	Tignon et al., 2011 [27]
Acute	Virulent	Ukr12/Zapo	Ukraine (II)	6	0–12	19	Gallardo et al., 2013
Acute	Virulent	LT14/1490	Lithuania (II)	18	0–61	111	Gallardo et al., 2015 [18, 2
	Total samples tested					153	

ight inoculated animals, died or were euthanized due to he severity of symptoms between 7 and 9 dpi. One inocuted pig showed a delayed course of the disease, resembling the course observed in the in-contact animals, which ied or were slaughtered between 14 and 22 dpe. One inontact pig remained asymptomatic throughout the xperiment and was slaughtered at day 61 [30].

Porcine samples from field ASFV-infected areas within he EUA.

Panel of 58 field EDTA-blood samples collected during he 2014 and 2015 outbreaks in EU countries (Lithuania, oland and Estonia) were used in this study. These samples vere taken from 46 wild boar and 12 domestic pigs during he surveillance programs and were sent to INIA-CISA' by he National Reference Laboratories (NRLs) of Lithuania, oland and Estonia for confirmatory diagnosis in accordnce with the duties of INIA-CISA as EURL for ASF.

evelopment and assembly of the lateral flow device

apture reagents

Ab to VP72 protein (18BG3) was used as the test line apture reagent. The 18BG3 MAb was diluted to 1 mg/ nl in Tris/HCl 20 mM buffer at pH 7.5 containing 5 % ucrose and 0.095 % sodium azide as preservative. The nti-control protein IgG monoclonal antibody was used s the control line capture reagent. It was diluted to mg/ml in the same buffer used for the test lines. The ontrol line is essential in order to validate the test.

The test and control capture reagents were dispensed n two parallel lines on 25 × 300 mm HiFlow Plus nitroellulose membrane (HF120, Millipore) at 1 μl/cm. After rying for 5 min at 45 °C, the membranes were sealed nd stored at room temperature under dry conditions.

reparation of latex microparticle conjugates

he detector reagents consisted of 415 nm coloured arboxyl-modified latex microspheres (Estapor® Micropheres). The MAb against VP72 protein was covalently onjugated to black latex beads while blue latex particles vere covalently conjugated with the LFA control deector reagent. Previously to protein conjugation, latex articles were activated with EDC (1-ethyl-3-(3-dimethyaminopropyl) carbodiimide hydrochloride) and NHS N-Hydroxysuccinimide) and then coupled to the monolonal antibody at a surface concentration of 1 mg/m^2. inally, conjugated latex particles were diluted in Tris/ ICl 10 mM pH 8.2 and the microsphere solutions were tored at 4 °C before use.

reparation of the conjugate pad

o prepare the conjugate solution, the MAb-latex and ontrol-latex particles previously prepared were diluted at a oncentration of 0.2 % each, in a Tris/HCl 25 mM pH 9.5 uffer containing humidity preservatives and blocking agents. The mixture was dispensed onto the rayon conjugate pad. The pads were dried for 30 min at 45 °C and stored at room temperature under dry conditions.

Preparation of chromatographic strips

A master card was assembled as follows: nitrocellulose membrane, conjugated pad, sample pad and absorbent pad were pasted on a plastic backing with adhesive and covered with a protector film. The master card was then cut into strips of 4.2 mm width, which were placed individually in a plastic device. A special sample pad to retain the erythrocytes (Cytosep 1662) was used, since the test was designed to be used with blood samples.

Test procedure

The test has been designed for use with blood samples. Blood samples must be fresh or refrigerated up to 4 days at 2–8 °C and collected with an anticoagulant (EDTA, heparin, etc.). Blood samples without anticoagulant could contain micro-clots that could block the device and result in nonspecific reactions. It is also very important to ensure the devices are stored in dry conditions, to avoid any negative effect on the result. Finally, several trials in the lab have demonstrated that the test runs correctly in a range of temperatures from 15 to 37 °C (data not shown).

Twenty microliters of sample (blood) are applied to the sample pad followed by 120 μl of running buffer (Tris/ HCl pH 7.5, NaCl, casein, Tween-20 and NaN_3 as preservative). The mixture migrates through the conjugate pad and the nitrocellulose membrane by capillarity. Results are interpreted 10 minutes after adding the sample. In the presence of ASFV, the VP72 protein is captured first by the MAb-coated microparticles, forming a latex-antibody-antigen immune complex. This immune complex then reacts with the immobilized MAb on the membrane, making the black test line visible along with the blue control line. In the case of a negative test, only a blue line appears. The blue control line must appear always; otherwise, the test has to be considered invalid.

ASF virus detection

ASFV genome detection by PCR

Field and experimental samples were tested for ASFV genome detection using the OIE real-time PCR [21, 31] and the Universal Probe Library (UPL) real-time PCR [32]. The DNA was extracted from each blood sample using the High Pure PCR Template Preparation Kit (Roche Diagnostics GmbH, Roche Applied Science, Mannheim, Germany). For amplification of the ASFV genomic DNA the PCRs were carried out using undiluted and 1/10 diluted extracted DNA for each sample.

ASFV antigen detection by ELISA

Experimental and blood samples were tested for ASF antigen detection using a commercially available antigen detection ELISA, the Double Antibody Sandwich (DAS) ELISA test manufactured by INGENASA (®INGENASA-INgezim PPA DAS K2, INGENASA, Madrid, Spain). The samples were analysed undiluted and at 1/10 dilution according to the manufacturer's instructions and the results obtained were compared to those obtained using the PCR assays and the new LFA developed.

ASF virus isolation and titration

Virus isolation was assessed in PCR-positive experimental samples using a hemadsorption assay on PBMC (Peripheral blood mononuclear cells), as described in the Manual of Diagnostic Tests and Vaccines for Terrestrial Animals [21]. The plates were examined for hemadsorption over a period of 6 days. Samples were blind passaged three times. Titres were estimated using a hemadsorption assay, to monitor the end-point dilution of ASFV isolates on PBMC by the Reed and Muench method, and expressed as 50 % hemadsorbing doses per ml (HAD50/ml) per sample.

Statistical analysis

The concordance between each test was the overall percentage agreement between the results of the two assays calculated using two-by-two contingency tables. Kappa Coefficient (k) statistics were used to evaluate the significance of the level of concordance between results beyond that expected by chance, with k values of 0.81–1.00 representing almost perfect agreement, values of 0.61–0.80 substantial agreement, values of 0.41–0.60 good agreement, values of 0.21–0.40 moderate agreement, values of 0.01–0.20 slight agreement, and values of 0.00 no agreement (48). From the overall analysis of the results the final sensitivity and specificity of the new assay were calculated using the results of the UPL-PCR as a reference test for virus detection. Values measured included the number of true positives (TP), the number of true negatives (TN), the number of false positives (FP) and the number of false negatives (FN). Sensitivity was calculated as 100 × TP/(TP + FN), specificity was calculated as 100 × TN/(TN + FP).

Results

Development of the immunochromatographic assay

A monoclonal antibody, 18BG3, against the VP72 protein of ASFV, was used as the capture reagent on the test line in the LFA for ASFV detection. A specific monoclonal antibody for the control protein was used as the control line.

Since it is known that over 90 % of the virus is associated with red blood cells [33], our purpose was to adapt the test to be used not only with serum samples, but more importantly with blood samples. Therefore, a special sample pad was used in the design of the test, in order to retain the erythrocytes, allowing the free virus to move along the strip. Besides, different running buffers containing detergent were tested in order to release as much virus as possible from the erythrocytes. Different colored beads were analyzed for antibody conjugation, taking into consideration that in case of hemolized blood samples, hemoglobin would move along the strip, staining it and thus making the visualization of the test line more difficult. For this reason, black latex beads were chosen to develop the test. Moreover, different antibody concentrations for conjugation to the latex beads were also studied to determine optimal conditions. Finally, the test protocol was established as follows: after addition of the sample to the round window of the device, the running buffer is added and after ten minutes, the results must be interpreted. Appearance of a black test line and the blue control line indicates a positive result, while appearance of the control line alone indicates a negative sample (Fig. 1).

Performance of the LFA for ASFV detection

In order to test the performance of the newly developed test, first experiments were carried out using semi-purified VP72 viral protein and inactivated tissue culture virus, BA71 strain. A spike-in test was assessed in the laboratory by adding the viral semi-purified protein to blood from a healthy donor pig used as the matrix. Serial dilutions of the viral protein in blood were analyzed by LFA. The analytical sensitivity of the assay was down to 3 ng/test, comparable to that of a commercially available double antibody sandwich ELISA (INgezim® PPA DAS) with 1.9 ng/test (Fig. 2). When the test was performed using the tissue culture virus, the detection limit was down to 10^4 pfu/ml (data not shown).

Evaluation of the LFA for ASFV detection

Out of the 153 blood samples collected at different times post infection from the 30 experimentally infected pigs, the number of positives using the UPL rt-PCR was 60 (39.21 %), 57 (37.25 %) using the OIE rt-PCR and 4[illegible] (26.79 %) using the LFA. Thirteen out of the 19 samples (68.42 %) which gave a false negative result with the LFA were correlated to blood samples with rt-PCR Cycle Threshold (C_T) values above 30, mainly collected at initial stages of the infection or from in-contact animals exposed to the virulent Lithuania 2014 ASFV isolate (LT14/1490), which remained asymptomatic throughout the experimental infection (Table 2). When comparing with the virus isolation, the LFA was unable to detect the presence of ASFV antigen in blood samples with viral loads below 10^4 HAU. Good correlation was observed between the LFA and the antigen INgezim

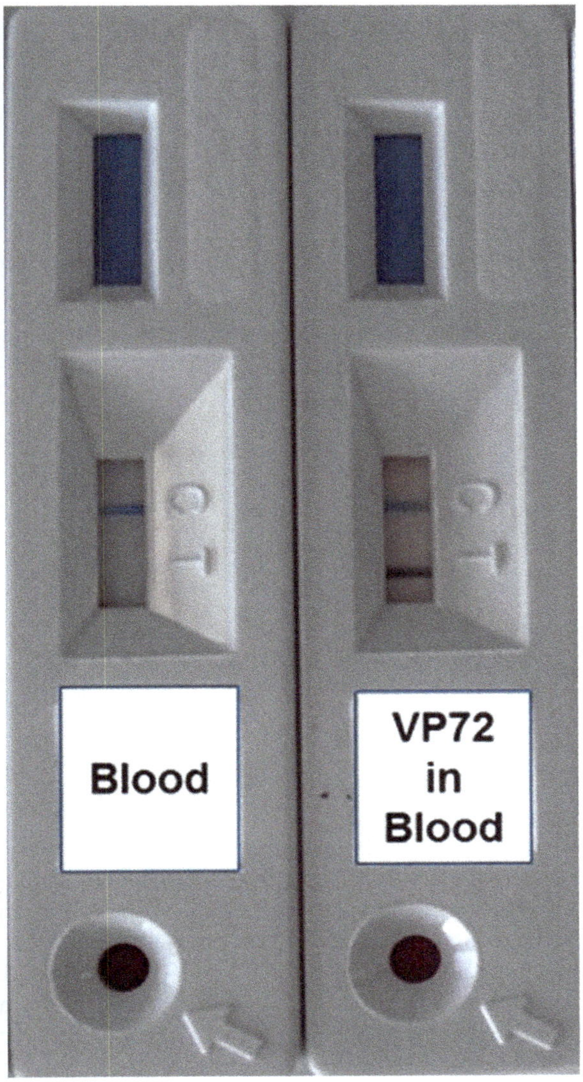

Fig. 1 Picture of the lateral flow device for ASFV detection. The left device shows a negative result using a blood sample from a healthy donor pig; where only the blue control line is detected. The right test shows a positive result by spiking the semi-purified VP72 protein in blood; in this scenario, the two lines, control line (*blue*) and test line (*black*) will appear

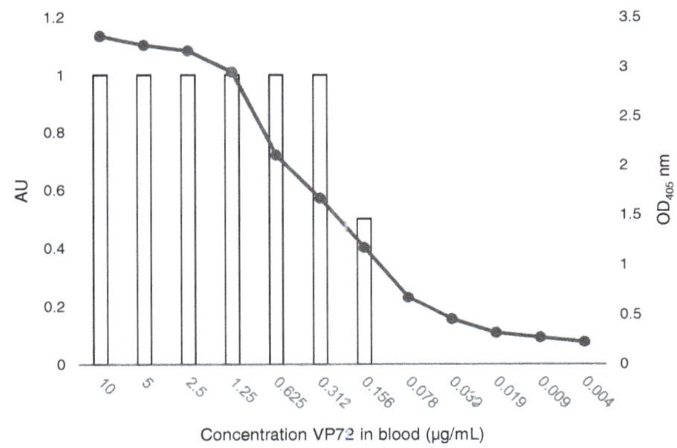

Fig. 2 Comparison of the performance of the LFA and the commercial DAS-ELISA. Serial dilutions of semi-purified VP72 protein in blood were tested by LFA and Double antibody sandwich ELISA (DAS-ELISA) and results were compared. Both assays are based on MAbs specific for VP72 protein. The detection limit of both tests was very similar (3 ng viral protein/test by LFA *vs* 1,9 ng viral protein/test in ELISA)

PA DAS ELISA with just 2 of the 41 ELISA positive amples testing negative in the LFA. Among the negative amples, two were tested as false positives by using the FA whereas only one produced a false positive when ested with the antigen-ELISA.

To evaluate the ability of the new LFA to diagnose SF during the current epidemic outbreaks in the EU ountries, 58 samples collected in 2014 and 2015, from omestic pigs (12) and wild boar (46) from affected EU ountries were included in the study. The samples were ested in parallel using the two real time PCRs, the ntigen-ELISA and the LFA. As with the results obtained using the experimental blood samples, the number of positive samples detected by the UPL-rt-PCR was 52 (89.65 %), whereas the number decreased to 51 (87.93 %) with the OIE rt-PCR, 35 (60.34 %) with the LFA and 28 (48.27 %) with the INgezim® PPA DAS ELISA assay (Table 3). Contrary to what was observed in the analysis of the experimental samples, only 7 out of the 17 (41 %) samples which resulted false negatives using the LFA displayed Ct values above 30 (Table 4).

From the results obtained in both experimental and field samples collected from animals with known infectious status and selecting the UPL-PCR as the reference method, the sensitivity and specificity of the LFA were calculated. Of the 112 ASF positive samples, there were 36 false negatives from the LFA, resulting in a sensitivity value of 67.86 %. The number of false positive samples was 2 out of 99 giving a specificity of 97.98 %. When comparing the LFA results with those obtained using the INgezim® PPA DAS ELISA assay, the Kappa values of 0.92 [CI 95 % = 0.86–0,98] showed almost perfect agreement between the two assays.

Discussion

Early diagnosis of African swine fever is essential in order to establish effective surveillance programmes and control measures to prevent the spread of ASF. Rapid, sensitive and specific assays are required by diagnostic laboratories. A positive diagnosis involves the detection and identification of ASFV-antigens, antibodies or DNA in a given sample. The development of new easy-to-handle diagnostic tools designed for non-specialized front-line laboratories with limited equipment and allowing deployment at field level, would be very helpful in improving ASF control programmes. This applies

Table 2 Description of the false negative (FN) samples using the LFA by the analysis of experimental samples collected from animals infected with ASFV genotype II and IX viruses

ASFV Strain	ID PIG	Days post infection	UPL-PCR CT value	OIE real-time PCR CT value	Virus isolation (TITER $_{HAD50/ml}$)	Ag-ELISA (INGENASA
LT14/1490	L10	13	30.88	30.39	$3,16 \times 10^3$	FN*
LT14/1490	L10	17	17.61	16.49	$6,81 \times 10^5$	POS
LT14/1490	L11	13	26.43	27.41	$3,16 \times 10^2$	FN
LT14/1490	L12	13	36.67	37.21	NEGATIVE	FN
LT14/1490	L13	3	32.73	32.47	NEGATIVE	FN
LT14/1490	L14	17	33.04	34.79	NEGATIVE	FN
LT14/1490	L15	13	25.93	24.71	$6,81 \times 10^4$	FN
LT14/1490	L15	17	18.27	16.73	$6,81E \times 10^6$	FN
LT14/1490	L16	13	32.41	32.62	NEGATIVE	FN
LT14/1490	L17	3	37.46	37.45	NEGATIVE	FN
LT14/1490	L17	7	23.14	23.07	$3,16 \times 10^5$	POS
LT14/1490	L18	17	36.95	FN	NEGATIVE	FN
LT14/1490	L18	34	38.51	FN	NEGATIVE	FN
LT14/1490	L18	38	38.46	FN	NEGATIVE	FN
LT14/1490	L2	14	34.54	33.95	3,16E + 01	FN
LT14/1490	L3	3	32	33.04	NEGATIVE	FN
LT14/1490	L4	10	31.67	31.85	3,16E + 03	FN
LT14/1490	L6	14	27.2	26.91	3,16E + 08	FN
Ken06.Bus	CC6	D10	35.34	39.63	NEGATIVE	FN

*false negative

particularly to positive results, allowing for control measures, such as restriction of animal movement, to be adopted immediately, until confirmation from official reference laboratories is received. In case of virulent strains, animals usually develop high levels of viremia, dying soon after infection. Virus, antigen or genome detection is very useful to diagnose these hyperacute/acute forms of the disease. In case of ASFV infection with moderate or low virulent strains, these usually induce high or medium viremia levels at the beginning of the infection, and high antibody titers from the second week post infection. In these cases, both virus and antibody detection must be used to obtaint a reliable diagnosis.

In the present study, a lateral flow assay for antige detection was developed and tested with blood sample from pigs inoculated experimentally with ASFV an from field infected animals. The assay was based on monoclonal antibody to the VP72 protein, which is th major capsid protein of ASFV [34, 35] and therefore a appropriate target antigen for virus detection. The dat obtained by the LFA were compared with those obtaine by both rt-PCR (UPL rt-PCR and OIE rt-PCR) and b INgezim PPA DAS. It has been recently described tha the UPL-rt-PCR is the most sensitive and trustworth method for detecting ASF, followed by the OIE-rt-PC [20]. In that study the INgezim PPA DAS was include

Table 3 Comparison between the two PCR tests, the antigen-ELISA and the LFA used to detect ASFV in field-collected blood samples from wild boar and domestic pigs during the epidemic outbreaks in EU countries

Country	Host	UPL real-time PCR		OIE real time PCR		LFA		Ag-ELISA INGENASA	
		N° positives/total	%	N° positives/total	%	N° positives/total	%	N° positives/total	%
Estonia	Wild boar	1/1	100	1/1	100	0/1	0	0/1	0
Latvia	Wild boar	1/1	100	0/1	0	0/1	0	0/1	0
Lithuania	Wild boar	20/26	76.92	20/26	76.92	9/26	34.61	8/26	34,6
	Domestic pig	11/11	100	11/11	100	10/11	90.9	6/11	90,9
Poland	Wild boar	18/18	100	18/18	100	15/18	83.3	13/18	83,3
	Domestic pig	1/1	100	1/1	100	1/1	100	1/1	100
Total		52/58	89.65	51/58	87.93	35/58	60.34	28/58	48.2

Table 4 Description of the false negative (FN) samples using the LFA by the analysis of field samples

COUNTRY	HOST	UPL-PCR CT value	OIE real-time PCR CT value	Ag-ELISA (INGENASA).
ESTONIA	WILD BOAR	21,46	23,91	FN
LATVIA	WILD BOAR	35.99	FN	FN
LITHUANIA	DOMESTIC PIG	21.29	20.62	FN
LITHUANIA	WILD BOAR	24.29	24.5	FN
LITHUANIA	WILD BOAR	34.42	38.32	FN
LITHUANIA	WILD BOAR	26.3	27.15	POS
LITHUANIA	WILD BOAR	25.44	25.91	FN
LITHUANIA	WILD BOAR	26.48	26.04	FN
LITHUANIA	WILD BOAR	32.97	31.02	FN
LITHUANIA	WILD BOAR	21.36	19.01	FN
LITHUANIA	WILD BOAR	34.9	35.28	FN
LITHUANIA	WILD BOAR	32.81	32.11	FN
LITHUANIA	WILD BOAR	34.73	39.95	FN
LITHUANIA	WILD BOAR	34.51	34.36	FN
POLAND	WILD BOAR	25.44	25.03	POS
POLAND	WILD BOAR	24.27	24.59	FN
POLAND	WILD BOAR	27.03	27.94	FN

In grey are labelled false negative samples with Ct > 30 by using the UPL-real time PCR

for comparison purposes, showing a good-to-moderate agreement with the UPL-rt-PCR (k = 0.67 [95 % CI, 0.58 to 0.76]). The data analyzed in the present work showed that the sensitivity of the LFA was lower than that obtained by either rt-PCR, as was expected, detecting 68 and 72 % of the positive samples from experimentally infected animals, in comparison with UPL-rt-PCR and OIE-rt-PCR, respectively. Besides, more than 50 % of the false negative results by LFA corresponded to samples with C_T values higher than 30, obtained from second week of infection and onwards, and therefore with low viral loads. Nevertheless, when compared to the results of the antigen-ELISA, only two false negative samples were detected by LFA. It is important to take into account that these two techniques are detecting viral antigen, while the rt-PCRs detect viral genome, and therefore being more sensitive. In any case, the specificity of the newly developed test was very close to 100 %, indicating a low percentage of false positive results, which is crucial in order to avoid unnecessary states of alarm and consequent expenses.

In a similar way, when the field samples were analyzed by the LFA, 67 % of positivity was found in comparison with the reference technique, UPL-rt-PCR. However, in this case, the majority of the false negative results did not show Ct values above 30. This discrepancy could be due to the quality of the sample, since these field samples came mostly from carcasses of animals found dead or hunted. This aspect is critical in the analysis of the samples by LFA, affecting the result even if the viral loads are high enough to be detected by this method.

Although PCR is the technique most frequently used for viral detection, it is a laborious technique, which requires good training to avoid contamination and therefore false positive results. Besides, samples need to be transported quickly to the corresponding laboratory in order to obtain a result. Although LFA is less sensitive than rt-PCR tests, this novel pen-side test offers some advantages and benefits, especially in field scenarios: it is a rapid, economic and simple-to-use diagnostic tool, since it does not require any kind of instrumentation and the result is interpreted at a glance and with very high specificity. Furthermore, the test has been designed to be used with blood, thus making sample processing easy and feasible. All these features make these devices very suitable for field application or basic laboratories, especially in countries where laboratory infrastructure is deficient or even absent. Further validation is currently ongoing in different countries in Europe, Asia and Africa. Field validation is particularly crucial before these tests can be used as front-line diagnostic assays. This should include samples not only from domestic pigs, but also wild boar.

Conclusion

In conclusion, the newly developed LFA allows the detection of ASFV with viral loads from 10^4 HAU, corresponding to days 4–7 depending on the virulence of the viral strain and depending on the condition of the sample. This is a very valuable tool accompanying the antibody detection tests (including pen-side tests) in any scenario. It will assist especially local veterinary services, where in many cases first evidence of the disease is based only on clinical symptoms.

Acknowledgements

The research was funded by the EU, Seventh Research Framework Program FP7-KBBE-2207-2013 under grant number n° 311931 (ASFORCE).

Authors' contributions

PS, PR and AS designed the study. PS, TR and AM performed the immunological experiments. CG and MA designed and performed the animal experiments. PS, PR, CG and MA drafted the manuscript. All authors read and approved the final manuscript.

Competing interest

The authors declare that they have no competing interests.

Consent for publication

Not applicable.

Author details

[1]Inmunología y Genética Aplicada S. A. (INGENASA), Madrid, Spain. [2]European Union Reference Laboratory for ASF (EURL), Centro de Investigación en Sanidad Animal, INIA, Madrid, Spain.

References

1. Dixon LK, Alonso C, Escribano JM, Martins C, Revilla Y, Salas MLHT. Asfaviridae. In: Virus Taxonomy. 2011.
2. Montgomery RE. A form of swine fever occurring in British East Africa (Kenya Colony). J Comp Pathol. 1921;34:159–91.
3. Mur L, Atzeni M, Martinez-Lopez B, Feliziani F, Rolesu S, Sanchez-Vizcaino JM. Thirty-five-year presence of African swine fever in Sardinia: history, evolution and risk factors for disease maintenance. Transbound Emerg Dis. 2016;63(2):e165–77.

4. Penrith ML, Vosloo W. Review of African swine fever: transmission, spread and control. J S Afr Vet Assoc. 2009;80(2):58–62.
5. Oganesyan AS, Petrova ON, Korennoy FI, Bardina NS, Gogin AE, Dudnikov SA. African swine fever in the Russian Federation: spatio-temporal analysis and epidemiological overview. Virus Res. 2013;173(1):204–11.
6. Sanchez-Vizcaino JM, Mur L, Martinez-Lopez B. African swine fever (ASF): five years around Europe. Vet Microbiol. 2013;165(1–2):45–50.
7. Rowlands RJ, Michaud V, Heath L, Hutchings G, Oura C, Vosloo W, Dwarka R, Onashvili T, Albina E, Dixon LK. African swine fever virus isolate, Georgia, 2007. Emerg Infect Dis. 2008;14(12):1870–4.
8. Food and Agriculture Organization, United Nations, 2013: African swine fever in the Russian Federation: risk factors for Europe and beyond. EMPRES (Emerging prevention system) Watch. 2013;28.
9. Gallardo C, Fernandez-Pinero J, Pelayo V, Gazaev I, Markowska-Daniel I, Pridotkas G, Nieto R, Fernandez-Pacheco P, Bokhan S, Nevolko O, et al. Genetic variation among African swine fever genotype II viruses, eastern and central Europe. Emerg Infect Dis. 2014;20(9):1544–7.
10. European Food Safety Authority (EFSAE) Journal: African swine Fever. 2015; doi:10.2903/j.efsa.2015.4163
11. Anderson EC, Hutchings GH, Mukarati N, Wilkinson PJ. African swine fever virus infection of the bushpig (Potamochoerus porcus) and its significance in the epidemiology of the disease. Vet Microbiol. 1998;62(1):1–15.
12. Boinas FS, Wilson AJ, Hutchings GH, Martins C, Dixon LJ. The persistence of African swine fever virus in field-infected Ornithodoros erraticus during the ASF endemic period in Portugal. PLoS One. 2011;6(5), e20383.
13. Thomson GR. The epidemiology of African swine fever: the role of free-living hosts in Africa. Onderstepoort J Vet Res. 1985;52(3):201–9.
14. Sanchez-Vizcaino JM, Mur L, Gomez-Villamandos JC, Carrasco L. An update on the epidemiology and pathology of African swine fever. J Comp Pathol. 2015;152(1):9–21.
15. Sanchez-Vizcaino JM. African swine fever. Diseases of Swine, vol. Chapter 13. 9th Ed. Ames: Blackwell Publishing; 2006.
16. Guinat C, Reis AL, Netherton CL, Goatley L, Pfeiffer DU, Dixon L. Dynamics of African swine fever virus shedding and excretion in domestic pigs infected by intramuscular inoculation and contact transmission. Vet Res. 2014;45:93.
17. Pietschmann J, Guinat C, Beer M, Pronin V, Tauscher K, Petrov A, Keil G, Blome S. Course and transmission characteristics of oral low-dose infection of domestic pigs and European wild boar with a Caucasian African swine fever virus isolate. Arch Virol. 2015;160(7):1657–67.
18. Gallardo C, Soler A, Nieto R, Sanchez MA, Martins C, Pelayo V, Carrascosa A, Revilla Y, Simon A, Briones V, et al. Experimental transmission of African Swine Fever (ASF) Low virulent isolate NH/P68 by surviving pigs. Transbound Emerg Dis. 2015;62(6):612–22.
19. Gabriel C, Blome S, Malogolovkin A, Parilov S, Kolbasov D, Teifke JP, Beer M. Characterization of African swine fever virus Caucasus isolate in European wild boars. Emerg Infect Dis. 2011;17(12):2342–5.
20. Gallardo C, Nieto R, Soler A, Pelayo V, Fernandez-Pinero J, Markowska-Daniel I, Pridotkas G, Nurmoja I, Granta R, Simon A, et al. Assessment of African swine fever diagnostic techniques as a response to the epidemic outbreaks in eastern european union countries: How to improve surveillance and control programs. J Clin Microbiol. 2015;53(8):2555–65.
21. World Organisation for Animal Health (OIE). African swine fever. In: Manual of Diagnostic Tests and Vaccines for Terrestrial Animals. 2012;2:2.8.1.
22. Aguero M, Fernandez J, Romero L, Sanchez Mascaraque C, Arias M, Sanchez-Vizcaino JM. Highly sensitive PCR assay for routine diagnosis of African swine fever virus in clinical samples. J Clin Microbiol. 2003;41(9):4431–4.
23. Oura CA, Edwards L, Batten CA. Virological diagnosis of African swine fever–comparative study of available tests. Virus Res. 2013;173(1):150–8.
24. Pastor MJ, Arias M, Escribano JM. Comparison of two antigens for use in an enzyme-linked immunosorbent assay to detect African swine fever antibody. Am J Vet Res. 1990;51(10):1540–3.
25. Zsak L, Borca MV, Risatti GR, Zsak A, French RA, Lu Z, Kutish GF, Neilan JG, Callahan JD, Nelson WM, et al. Preclinical diagnosis of African swine fever in contact-exposed swine by a real-time PCR assay. J Clin Microbiol. 2005;43(1):112–9.
26. Sanz A, Garcia-Barreno B, Nogal ML, Vinuela E, Enjuanes L. Monoclonal antibodies specific for African swine fever virus proteins. J Virol. 1985;54(1):199–206.
27. Tignon M, Gallardo C, Iscaro C, Hutet E, Van der Stede Y, Kolbasov D, De Mia GM, Le Potier MF, Bishop RP, Arias M, et al. Development and inter-laboratory validation study of an improved new real-time PCR assay with internal control for detection and laboratory diagnosis of African swine fever virus. J Virol Methods. 2011;178(1–2):161–70.
28. Bishop RP, Fleischauer C, de Villiers EP, Okoth EA, Arias M, Gallardo C, Upton C. Comparative analysis of the complete genome sequences of Kenyan African swine fever virus isolates within p72 genotypes IX and X. Virus Genes. 2015;50(2):303–9.
29. Gallardo C. Biological and molecular characterization of ASFV isolated in Ukraine, 2012. Personal communication at the ANNUAL MEETING OF THE European Union REFERENCE LABORATORY FOR AFRICAN SWINE FEVER, Brussels, Belgium, 3rd June 2013. 2012.
30. Gallardo C, Soler A, Nieto R, Cano C, Pelayo V, Sanchez MA, Pridotkas G, Fernandez-Pinero J, Briones V, Arias M. Experimental infection of domestic pigs with African swine fever virus Lithuania 2014 genotype II field isolate. Transbound Emerg Dis. 2015. doi:10.1111/tbed.12346.
31. King DP, Reid SM, Hutchings GH, Grierson SS, Wilkinson PJ, Dixon LK, Bastos AD, Drew TW. Development of a TaqMan PCR assay with internal amplification control for the detection of African swine fever virus. J Virol Methods. 2003;107(1):53–61.
32. Fernandez-Pinero J, Gallardo C, Elizalde M, Robles A, Gomez C, Bishop R, Heath L, Couacy-Hymann E, Fasina FO, Pelayo V, et al. Molecular diagnosis of African Swine Fever by a new real-time PCR using universal probe library. Transbound Emerg Dis. 2013;60(1):48–58.
33. Blome S, Gabriel C, Beer M. Pathogenesis of African swine fever in domestic pigs and European wild boar. Virus Res. 2013;173(1):122–30.
34. Garcia-Escudero R, Andres G, Almazan F, Vinuela E. Inducible gene expression from African swine fever virus recombinants: analysis of the major capsid protein p72. J Virol. 1998;72(4):3185–95.
35. Gomez-Puertas P, Rodriguez F, Oviedo JM, Ramiro-Ibanez F, Ruiz-Gonzalvo F, Alonso C, Escribano JM. Neutralizing antibodies to different proteins of African swine fever virus inhibit both virus attachment and internalization. J Virol. 1996;70(8):5689–94.

Geographic distribution and molecular analysis of porcine reproductive and respiratory syndrome viruses circulating in swine farms in the Republic of Korea between 2013 and 2016

Hyeonjeong Kang[1,2], Ji Eun Yu[1], Ji-Eun Shin[1], Areum Kang[3], Won-Il Kim[3], Changhee Lee[2], Jienny Lee[1], In-Soo Cho[1], Se-Eun Choe[1] and Sang-Ho Cha[1,4*]

Abstract

Background: Porcine reproductive and respiratory syndrome virus (PRRSV) causes devastating disease characterized by reproductive failure and respiratory problems in the swine industry. To understand the recent prevalence and genetic diversity of field PRRSVs in the Republic of Korea, open reading frames (ORFs) 5 and 7 of PRRSV field isolates from 631 PRRS-affected swine farms nationwide in 2013–2016 were analyzed along with 200 Korean field viruses isolated in 2003–2010, and 113 foreign field and vaccine strains.

Results: Korean swine farms were widely infected with PRRSVs of a single type (38.4 and 37.4% for Type 1 and Type 2 PRRSV, respectively) or both types (24.2%) with up to approximately 83% nucleotide sequence similarity to prototype PRRSVs (Lelystad or VR2332). Phylogenetic analysis based on the ORF5 nucleotide sequence revealed that Korean Type 1 field isolates were classified as subgroups A, B, and C under subtype 1, while Korean Type 2 field isolates were classified as lineages 1 and 5 as well as three Korean lineages (kor A, B, and C) with the highest infection prevalence in subgroup A (50.5%) and lineage 5 (15.3%) for Type 1 and Type 2 PRRSV, respectively, among ORF5-positive farms. In particular, the lineages kor B and C were identified as novel lineages in this study, and lineage kor B comprised only the field viruses isolated from Gyeongnam Province in 2014–2015, establishing regionally unique genetic characteristics. It has also recently been confirmed that commercialized vaccine-like viruses (subgroup C) of Type 1 PRRSV and NADC30-like viruses of Type 2 PRRSV (lineage 1) are spreading rapidly in Korean swine farms. The Korean field viruses were also expected to be antigenically variable as shown in the high diversity of neutralizing epitopes and N-glycosylation sites.

Conclusions: This up-to-date information regarding recent field PRRSVs should be taken into consideration when creating strategies for the application of PRRS control measures, including vaccination in the field.

Keywords: Porcine reproductive and respiratory syndrome virus (PRRSV), Genetic diversity, Open reading frame 5 (ORF5) sequence, Phylogenetic analysis

* Correspondence: virusmania@korea.kr
[1]Viral Disease Division, Animal and Plant Quarantine Agency, Gimcheon 39660, Republic of Korea
[4]Present address: PRRS research Laboratory, Viral Diseases Division, Animal and Plant Quarantine Agency, Gimcheon 39660, Republic of Korea
Full list of author information is available at the end of the article

Background

Porcine reproductive and respiratory syndrome virus (PRRSV) is one of the most common and economically significant infectious diseases in the pig industry worldwide [1, 2]. This virus causes clinical disease characterized by reproductive failure in pregnant sows and acute respiratory illness in growing pigs, causing increased preweaning mortality [3, 4]. PRRSV is a small-enveloped, single-stranded, non-segmented, and positive-sense RNA virus that is a member of the genus *Arterivirus* in the family Arteriviridae and order Nidovirales [5–7] he PRRSV genome is approximately 15 kb in size, composed of a 5′-untranslated region (UTR), 10 open reading frames (ORFs), designated ORF1a, ORF1b, ORF2a, ORF2b, and ORF3–7 including ORF5a, and a 3′-UTR [8–11]. ORF1a and ORF1b encode replication-related polymerase proteins that can be autoproteolytically cleaved into at least 16 nonstructural proteins (NSPs) [12–16]. ORFs 2a through 7 encode the following viral structural proteins: six envelope-associated proteins (GP2a, E, GP3, GP4, GP5, and M) and the nucleocapsid (N) protein [11, 17–19]. ORF5 encodes the major viral envelope protein GP5. As the most variable structural gene of PRRSV, GP5 plays an important role in viral assembly, infectivity, and the induction of neutralizing antibodies [20–23]. Owing to its high degree of genetic diversity, the ORF5 sequence has been used for diagnostic identification and classification of PRRS field viruses [4, 24–26].

PRRSV is divided into two major genotypes: Type 1 (European type) and Type 2 (North American type) PRRSV. Lelystad and VR2332 are considered reference strains of Type 1 and Type 2 PRRSV, respectively [27]. Type 1 and Type 2 PRRSV exhibit approximately 60% genomic sequence identity, and 20% nucleotide sequence variability within each genotype [28, 29]. Owing to the emergence of highly diverse field viruses, global phylogeny using the ORF5 sequence is characterized by many groups (subtypes 1–4 for Type 1 PRRSV and lineages 1–9 for Type 2 PRRSV) within each of the genotypes, composed of genetically and geographically distinct PRRSVs [30, 31].

Previous studies have also reported the genetic diversity and phylogeny of PRRSVs circulating in the Republic of Korea [32–34]. Type 2 PRRSV has infected swine farms since the mid-1980s [35], while Type 1 PRRSV has spread rapidly since its first detection in 2005 [33]. However, there has been no study regarding the current prevalence and genetic characteristics of PRRSV in PRRS-affected swine farms nationwide. Recent surveys among swine farmers in the Republic of Korea revealed that over 50% of swine farms have suffered from PRRS, which has been recognized as the most economically important disease in this industry. Combined with the introduction of new modified live vaccines into swine farms over the past three years, the active circulation of field viruses has increased concern regarding the establishment of novel genetic components, and the emergence of antigenic or virulent variants. The following study was conducted to investigate the prevalence, genetic characteristics, and phylogeny of Korean field PRRSVs in recent years (2013–2016).

Methods

Study design

Clinical samples (lung tissues and sera) submitted to diagnostic labs (Animal and Plant Quarantine Agency and Jeonbuk National University) were collected from pigs (mostly older than 4 weeks old) with poor growth and respiratory illness between 2013 and 2016. All samples were tested by multiplex reverse transcription polymerase chain reaction (RT-PCR) for amplification of ORF7 with primers designed to detect Type 1 and Type 2 PRRSV simultaneously. Virus isolation using ORF7 positive samples was attempted in the MARC-145 cell line and porcine alveolar macrophages (PAMs). Selected viral isolates were sequenced for ORF5, and further subjected to genetic analysis and compared with Korean field viruses isolated in 2003–2010, commercial vaccine strains (DV of Porcilis® PRRS, VP-046 of UNISTRAIN® PRRS, Ingelvac PRRS MLV of Ingelvac PRRS® MLV, and P129 of Fostera PRRS) commonly used in the Republic of Korea, PRRSV prototype strains (VR2332 and Lelystad), and field isolates previously reported from other countries.

Sample collection

A total of 631 clinical samples (lung tissues and sera) were obtained from swine farms located in provinces nationwide: Gyeonggi ($n = 107$), Chungbuk ($n = 9$), Chungnam ($n = 27$), Jeonbuk ($n = 69$), Jeonnam ($n = 35$), Gyeongbuk ($n = 61$), Gyeongnam ($n = 307$), Gangwon ($n = 1$), and Jeju ($n = 15$) in 2013–2016. The lung tissues were homogenized in Dulbecco's minimum essential medium (20% *w*/*v*) and filtered (0.45-μm filter). The lung homogenates and sera were stored at – 70 °C until use.

RT-PCR

Total RNA was extracted from the lung homogenates and sera using the RNeasy mini kit (Qiagen, Hilden, Germany), in accordance with the manufacturer's instructions. To detect and differentiate between Type 1 and Type 2 PRRSV, samples were first subjected to multiplex RT-PCR using genotype-specific ORF7 primers (Table 1) and a OneStep RT-PCR kit (Qiagen), which can simultaneously amplify PCR products of 39 and 433 base pairs (bp) for Type 1 and Type 2 PRRSV, respectively. The ORF7-positive sera were further subjected to RT-PCR for ORF5 amplification. The ORF5 genes of PRRSV were amplified with two pairs of primers

able 1 Primer sequences for amplification of ORF5 and ORF7

ype	Primer			Product (bp)
		Position	Sequence	
	Forward	14,653–14,671 (ORF7)	5′-ATGGCCAGCCAGTCAATCA-3′	ORF7 (398)
	Reverse	15,030-15,050 (3′NCR)	5′-TCGCCCTAATTGAATAGGTGA-3′	
	Forward	13,444–13,461 (ORF4)	5′-AATGAGGTGGGCYACAACC-3′	ORF5 (754)
	Reverse	15,030–15,050 (ORF6)	5′-GCGTGACACCTTAAGGGC-3′	
	Forward	14,933–14,951 (ORF7)	5′-ATGGCCAGCCAGTCAATCA-3′	ORF7 (433)
	Reverse	15,346–15,365 (3′NCR)	5′-TCGCCCTAATTGAATAGGTGA-3′	
	Forward	13,759–13,778 (ORF4)	5′-CCATTCTGGTGGCAATTTGA-3′	ORF5 (716)
	Reverse	14,455–14,474 (ORF6)	5′-GGCATATATCATCACTGGCG-3′	

33] for Type 1 and Type 2 PRRSV (Table 1), generating CR products of 754 and 716 bp, respectively. The amplication reaction consisted of 2.5 μl of 5× RT-PCR buffer including 2.5 mM $MgCl_2$), 0.2 mM dNTPs, 0.2 μM of ach primer, 0.5 μl of the enzyme mix, and 5 μl of RNA xtract in a final volume of 25 μl. RT-PCR was performed y reverse transcription for 30 min at 50 °C, termination f reverse transcription for 15 min at 95 °C, followed by 5 cycles of 20 s at 94 °C, 20 s at 55 °C, 30 s at 72 °C, and final extension of 10 min at 72 °C in a C1000 Thermal Cycler (Bio-Rad, Hercules, CA, USA). The RT-PCR amplions were analyzed using 1% agarose gel electrophoresis.

ucleotide (NT) and amino acid (AA) sequences and hylogenetic tree analysis

mplified ORF5 products ($n = 542$) were purified using he QIAquick Gel Extraction Kit (Qiagen) and sequenced (Macrogen, Seoul, Korea). Multiple sequence lignment was initially carried out and homology of the NT and AA sequences among the PRRSV isolates was etermined with CLC Main Workbench ver. 7.0.3. ORF5 equences were subjected to analysis of neutralizing epiopes (NEs), putative N-glycosylation sites (Asn-Xaa-Ser/Thr), and phylogenetic trees compared with those of Koean field viruses ($n = 200$) isolated between 2003 and 2010, field isolates of foreign countries ($n = 109$), including PRRSV prototype strains (VR2332 and Lelystad), and accine strains ($n = 4$) used in the Republic of Korea, vailable in the GenBank database. The phylogenetic tree was constructed using MEGA6 software with the eighbor-joining method and bootstrap values were alculated on 1000 replicates.

esults

revalence of PRRSVs in the Republic of Korea from 2013 o 2016

Among the 631 clinical samples subjected to ORF7 RT-PCR, 38.4% (242/631) were positive for Type 1 PRRSV, 7.4% (236/631) were positive for Type 2 PRRSV, and 4.2% (153/631) were positive for both PRRSV genotypes (Fig. 1). In terms of geographical prevalence by genotype, Type 1 was more prevalent in Gyeonggi and Jeonbuk Provinces, while Type 2 mainly infected in Gyeongbuk Province. Both genotypes were almost equivalently present in the remainder of the provinces.

Phylogenetic analysis and sequence homology

Phylogenetic analysis based on global PRRSV phylogeny [30, 31] indicated that all of the Korean isolates ($n = 542$) from 2003 to 2016 analyzed in this study were classified into pan-European subtype 1 for Type 1 PRRSV, and lineages 1, 4, and 5 and three Korean lineages (lineage kor A, B, and C) for Type 2 PRRSV. Regarding the recent Korean Type 1 field viruses ($n = 295$) isolated in 2013–2016, all of the isolates were classified into subgroups A ($n = 274$), B ($n = 1$), and C ($n = 20$) under subtype 1 (Fig. 2a) with infection prevalence rates of 50.5% (274/542), 0.18% (1/542), and 3.69% (20/542) among ORF5-positive farms, respectively. The recent Korean isolates of subgroup A were grouped with 77 Korean field viruses, two Korean reference strains (E38 and KNU-07) isolated in 2005–2009, and a Spanish strain, CRESA11. One isolate of subgroup B was grouped with four Korean field viruses isolated in 2005–2009, a Thai isolate (03RB1), and 12 European reference strains. Subgroup C was formed with only 20 recent Korean isolates, Lelystad, two vaccine strains (DV and VP-046), and 13 European reference strains. Meanwhile, subtypes 2, 3, and 4 were formed with only Eastern European reference strains. NT (AA) sequence similarity to Lelystad was 84.9–89.8% (82.2–91.6%), 85.9% (85.6%), and 93.9–98.4% (90.1–96.5%) in subgroups A, B, and C of field viruses isolated in 2013–2016, respectively. Meanwhile, NT (AA) sequence similarity rates to Lelystad were 87.8–90.9% (85.1–91.6%) and 85.8–86.9% (85.2–89.1%) for subgroups A and B of field viruses isolated in 2005–2009, respectively. In terms of sequence similarity to vaccine strains, NT (AA) sequence similarity to DV was similar to Lelystad for field viruses isolated in 2013–2016 as well as in 2005–2009. NT (AA) sequence similarity to VP-046 was 84.2–88.9% (81.7–92.6%), 85.5%

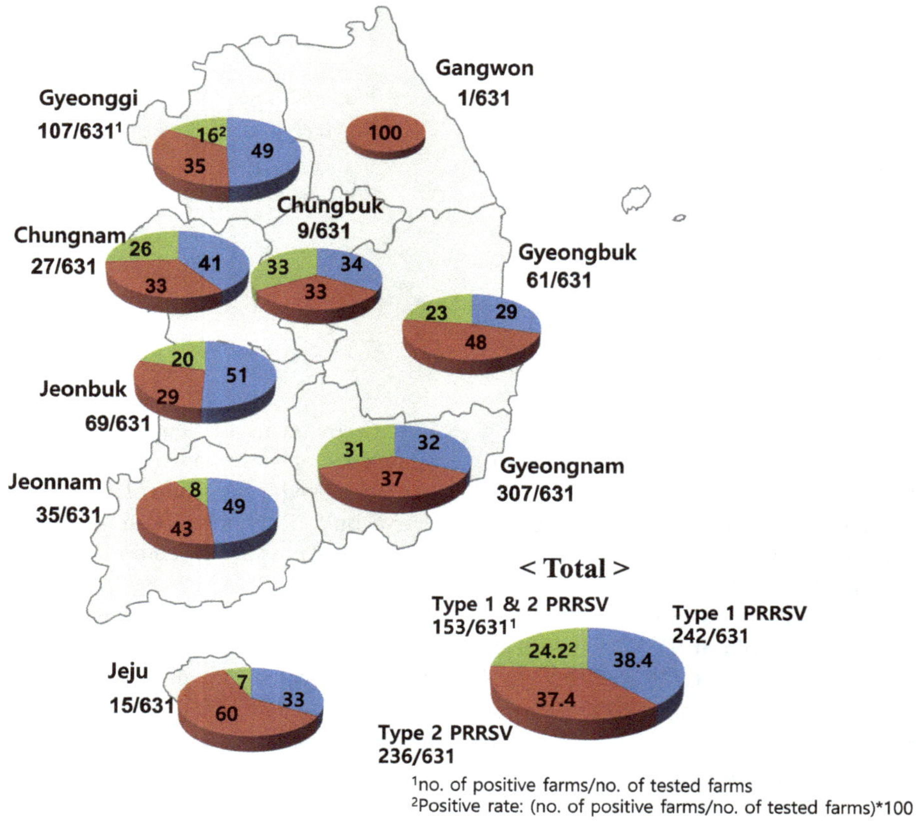

Fig. 1 Geographic distribution of Korean field viruses infected in 631 swine farms with respect to single (Type 1 or Type 2 PRRSV) and co-infection (Type 1 & 2 PRRSV)

(86.1%), and 93.7–99.8% (90.6–99.5%) in subgroups A, B, and C of field viruses isolated in 2013–2016, while 86.8–89.8% (85.6–91.1%), and 85.5–87.5% (85.2–88.6%) in subgroups A and B of field viruses isolated in 2005–2009, respectively (Table 2A).

The Korean Type 2 field viruses (n = 247) isolated in 2013–2016 were classified into five different lineages: lineage 1 (n = 9), lineage 5 (n = 83), lineage kor A (n = 33), lineage kor B (n = 72), and lineage kor C (n = 50) (Fig. 2b), with infection prevalence rates of 1.66% (9/542), 15.3% (83/542), 6.08% (33/542), 13.2% (72/542), and 9.22% (50/542) among ORF5-positive farms, respectively. The recent isolates of lineage 1 were grouped with highly virulent viruses of the United States (NADC30 virus, MN184, etc.) and China (Fig. 1c). The recent isolates of lineage 5 were grouped with 57 Korean viruses, three Korean reference strains (CA-1, PL97-1, and LMY) isolated in 2005–2009 [36], and VR2332, Ingelvac PRRS MLV, and so on. Meanwhile, three Korean lineages (kor A, B, and C) formed their own group separate from PRRSVs isolated from foreign countries. Importantly, lineage kor B was grouped only with recent field viruses isolated in 2014–2016, while lineages kor A and C included 24 and 32 field viruses isolated in 2003–2010, respectively [32, 36]. NT (AA sequence similarity rates to VR2332 were 82.3–86.9% (81.7–87.6%), 87.6–99.3% (85.6–99.0%), 85.1–89.1% (82.1–87.6%), 85.7–89.1% (83.6–90.1%), and 85.2–86.4% (83.6–86.1%) for lineages 1 and 5 and lineages kor A, B and C of field viruses isolated in 2013–2016, respectively. Meanwhile, NT (AA) sequence similarity rates to VR2332 were 88.9% (88.1%), 88.9–99.5% (88.1–99.0%), 87.6–89.6% (82.6–88.6%), and 84.7–87.1% (84.1–88.6%) for lineages and 5 and kor A and C of field viruses isolated in 2003–2010, respectively. Regarding sequence similarity to vaccine strains, NT (AA) sequence similarity to Ingelvac PRRS MLV was highly similar to VR2332 fo field viruses isolated in 2013–2016 as well as in 2003–2010. NT (AA) sequence similarity to P129 was 85.2–86.6% (84.6–86.6%), 86.7–91.7% (84.6–91.5%), 85.6–89.2% (85.1–90.1%), 86.1–89.1% (85.1–89.1%), and 82.6–86.9% (81.6–87.6%) in lineages 1 and 5 and kor A, B, and C o field viruses isolated in 2013–2016, while 89.7% (89.1%), 88.2–91.9% (88.1–92.5%), 87.2–90.2% (86.1–93.0%), and 85.4–88.1% (84.1–89.1%) in lineages 4 and 5 and kor A and C of field viruses isolated in 2003–2010, respectively (Table 2B).

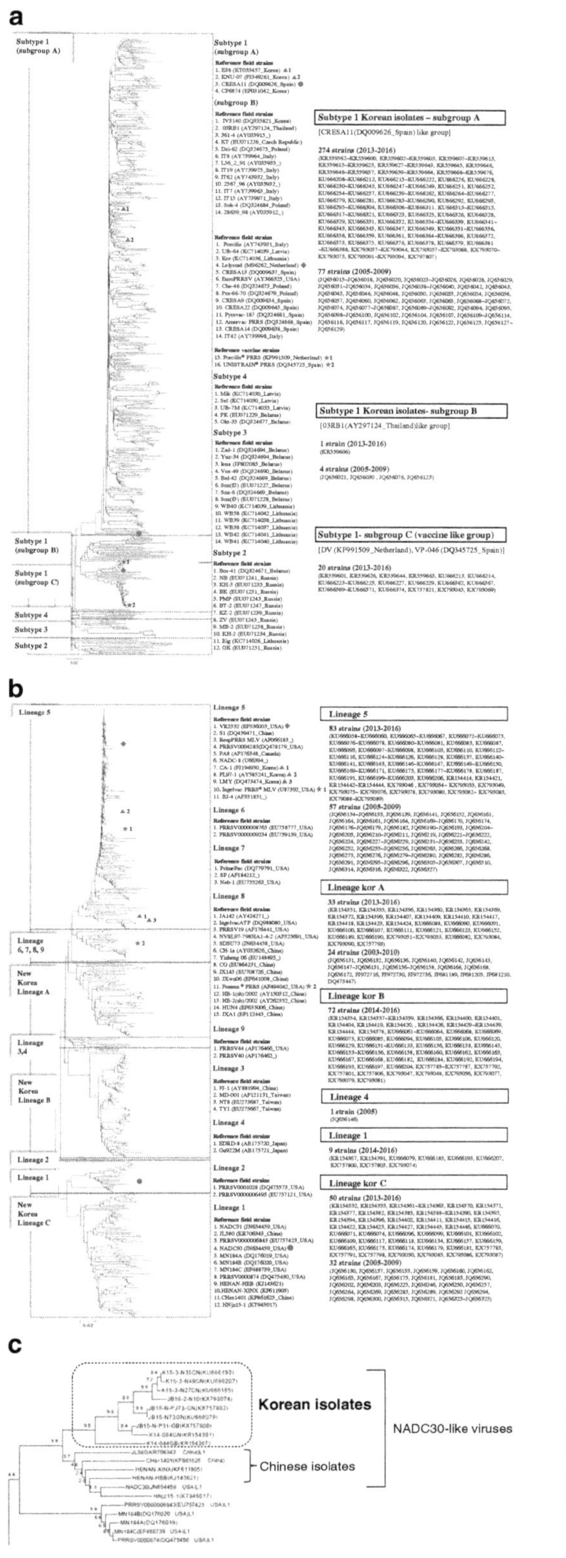

Fig. 2 Phylogenetic analysis using ORF5 nucleotide sequences of Type 1 (**a**) and Type 2 PRRS (**b**) field isolates obtained from this study and the GenBank database The tree was constructed by maximum-likelihood method and the grouping was referred from the previous studies [30, 31, 56]. Prototype viruses of each type, vaccine viruses used in Korean swine farms and Korean reference strains were marked with ◆, ★ and ▲, respectively. CRESA11 was marked with ●. A group of NADC30-like viruses was magnified in (**c**)

NEs and N-glycosylation sites of ORF5 amino acid sequences

NT sequence deletions or additions in the ORF5 sequence were not observed in the Korean isolates. Korean Type 1 PRRSV showed 7 and 25 different AA sequences of NEs (residues 29–35) [23] for field viruses isolated in 2005–2009 and 2013–2016, respectively. For Type 2 PRRSV, 12 and 23 different AA sequences in NEs (residues 37–45) [37] were observed for Korean field viruses isolated in 2003–2010 and 2013–2016, respectively. NEs (WSFADGN for DV or Lelystad, WSFVDGN for VP-046, SHLQLIYNL for Ingelvac PRRS MLV, or VR2332 and SHFQLIYNL for P129) of vaccine or PRRSV prototype strains (VR2332 and Lelystad) were compared with those of field isolates (Table 3). NEs of vaccine or PRRSV prototype strains were observed in 91.4% (74/81) and 80.0% (236/295) of Type 1 PRRSV field isolates of 2005–2009 and 2013–2016, and 67.5% (77/114) and 61.1% (151/247) of Type 2 PRRSV field isolates of 2003–2010 and 2013–2016, respectively. The NE (WSFADGN) of DV or Lelystad appeared as a main epitope in subgroups A, B, and C for all Korean Type 1 PRRS isolates, while the NE (SHLQLIYNL) of Ingelvac PRRS MLV or VR2332 was observed as the primary epitope of all Type 2 PRRSV lineages except for kor A and B of field isolates of 2013–2016, in which the NE (SHFQLIYNL) of P129 was the primary epitope. Regarding the pattern of N-glycosylation (number and sites of N-glycosylation), putative N-glycosylation sites were found at residues 37, 46, and 53 among the majority of Type 1 PRRS field isolates, resulting in 37-46-53 as the main N-glycosylation pattern throughout all subgroups in 2005–2016. In contrast, even if the putative N-glycosylation sites were highly conserved at residues 44 and 51 for Type 2 PRRS field isolates, the N-glycosylation pattern was significantly variable regardless of isolation year and lineage: 4–5 sites (residues 30, 33, 34, 44, 51, and 59) for lineage 1, 3–5 sites (residues 30, 32–35, 43, 44, 50, and 51) for lineage 5, 2–4 sites (residues 32–35, 44, and 51) for lineage kor A, 2–4 sites (residues 32–35, 43, 44, 50, and 51) for lineage kor B, and 2–5 sites (residues 30, 32–35, 44, and 51) for lineage kor C. Although the N-glycosylation pattern of Ingelvac PRRS MLV (30-33-44-51) was identified as the main pattern in lineages 1 and 5 of field viruses isolated in 2003–2010, novel N-glycosylation patterns appeared highly dominant overall. The N-glycosylation pattern (34-44-51)

Table 2 ORF5 nucleotide (NT) and amino acid (AA) sequence similarity of subtype 1/subgroups of type 1 PRRSV (A) and lineages of type 2 PRRSV (B) to prototypes/vaccine strains

Type	Isolated year	Subtype /Lineage	Sequence similarity		
			prototype	Vaccine strain	
			Lelystad virus	DV (Porcilis® PRRS)	VP-046 (UNISTRAIN® PRRS
(A)					
1	2005-2009	subtype 1-A	87.8-90.9 (86.1-91.6)[a]	87.6-91.1 (86.1-91.6)	86.8-89.8 (85.6-91.1)
		subtype 1-B	85.8-86.9 (85.2-89.1)	85.3-86.8 (84.2-88.1)	85.5-87.5 (85.2-88.6)
	2013-2016	subtype 1-A	84.9-89.8 (82.2-91.6)	85.0-89.6 (82.2-90.6)	84.2-88.9 (81.7-92.6)
		subtype 1-B	86.0 (85.6)	85.5 (84.7)	85.5 (86.1)
		subtype 1-C	93.9-98.4 (90.1-96.5)	93-4-99.5 (89.6-98.5)	93.7-99.8 (90.6-99.5)
Type	Isolated year	Subtype /Lineage	Sequence similarity		
			prototype	Vaccine strain	
			VR2332	Ingelvac PRRS MLV (Ingelvac® PRRS MLV)	P129 (Fostera® PRRS)
(B)					
2	2003-2010	lineage 4	88.9 (88.1) [b]	88.9 (88.6)	89.7 (89.1)
		lineage 5	88.9-99.5 (88.1-99.0)	89.9-99.8 (87.6-99.5)	88.2-91.9 (88.1-92.5)
		lineage kor A	87.6-89.6 (82.6-88.6)	86.7-89.7 (84.1-91.5)	87.2-90.2 (86.1-93.0)
		lineage kor C	84.7-87.1 (84.1-88.6)	84.7-87.1 (83.6-88.1)	85.4-88.1 (84.1-89.1)
	2013-2016	lineage 1	82.3-86.9 (81.7-87.6)	84.9-86.1 (83.1-85.6)	85.2-86.6 (84.6-86.6)
		lineage 5	87.6-99.3 (85.6-99.0)	87.9-99.7 (87.1-99.5)	86.7-91.7 (84.6-91.5)
		lineage kor A	85.1-89.1 (82.1-87.6)	85.4-88.7 (82.6-88.1)	85.6-89.2 (85.1-90.1)
		lineage kor B	85.7-89.1 (83.6-90.1)	85.7-89.1 (83.1-89.6)	86.1-89.1 (85.1-89.1)
		lineage kor C	85.2-86.4 (83.6-86.1)	83.6-87.6 (81.2-87.1)	82.6-86.9 (81.6-87.6)

[a]NT and AA sequence similarity to Type 1 PRRSV prototypes (Lelystad) and vaccine strains (DV and VP-046). Parenthesis indicates AA sequence similarity
[b]NT and AA sequence similarity to Type 2 PRRSV prototypes (VR2332) and vaccine strains (Ingelvac PRRS MLV, P129). Parenthesis indicates AA sequence similarity

of VR2332 was identified in all lineages of Korean field viruses isolated in 2003–2016, while the N-glycosylation pattern (46-53) of Lelystad was not identified in all field isolates. Many of the AA changes were observed in hypervariable regions of Korean Type 1 (residues 99–106) and Type 2 (residues 32–39 and 57–61) field viruses isolated in 2013–2016 (Fig. 3).

Discussion

In this study, the recent geographic prevalence and genetic characteristics of Korean PRRSVs were investigated using field isolates circulating in swine farms nationwide. RT-PCR of 631 clinical samples (farms) revealed that 38. 4% (242/631) were infected by Type 1 PRRSV, 37.4% (236/631) were infected by Type 2 PRRSV, and 24.2% (153/631) were simultaneously infected by both Type 1 and Type 2 PRRSV. When compared with a previous report [38], in which the single infection rates of Type 1 or Type 2 PRRSV and co-infection of both types in swine farms were 29.4, 54.4, and 16.2%, respectively, it was noted that Type 1 PRRSV has become highly prevalent in the 10 years following its first isolation in 2005. In addition, the increased number of farms infected with both Type 1 and Type 2 PRRSV suggested that effective control against PRRS in the Republic of Korea migh have to be implemented with the use of control measures against both genotypes.

All of the Korean Type 1 PRRS viruses were classifie into the subgroups A, B, and C of subtype 1, consisten with a previous report [34]. The majority of the Korea Type 1 PRRS isolates (274 isolates from 2013 to 201 and 77 isolates from 2005 to 2009) belonged to subgroup A, showing close relatedness with a Spanis strain, CRESA11. Subgroup B viruses (one isolate fron 2013 to 2016 and four isolates from 2005 to 2009) wer grouped with a Thai strain (03RB1) and pan-Europea strains. Subgroup C viruses (20 isolates from 2013 t 2016) were grouped with Type 1 PRRS live vaccin strains (DV and VP-046) and other pan-Europea strains. Lee et al. [39] first reported that a Korean isolat was grouped with DV. However, it is not possible t define genetic relatedness between the field isolate an the vaccine strain due to the lack of sequence information. Subgroup C viruses (5 DV- and 15 VP-046-lik strains) isolated in this study showed a phylogeneti closeness to the vaccine strains with greater than 99 NT sequence similarity without geographical predominance. Therefore, it has been suggested that the vaccine

Table 3 Diverse neutralizing epitopes and putative N-glycosylation sties on GP5 of Korean field PRRSVs isolated in 2003–2016 and commercial vaccine strains

Type	Vaccine strain/ Isolated year	Subgroup /Lineage	AA sequence of neutralizing epitopes	AA position for putative N-glycosylation sites
1	DV	subgroup C	WSFADGN	37-46-53
	VP-046	subgroup A	WSFVDGN	35-46-53
	2005-2009	subgroup A	WSFADGN(71)[a], WSFVDGN(1), WSFADGS(3), WSFASGN(1), WSFADCN(1)	37-46-53(75), 37-53(2)
		subgroup B	WSFADGN(2), WSFANGN(1), WSFVDGS(1)	37-46-53(3), 37-53(1)
	2013-2016	subgroup A	WSFADGN(214), WSFAYGN(1), WSFVDGN(5), WSFADGT(7), WSFADGS(11), WSSADGR(1), WSFADGK(2), WSFANGN(1), WSFADGD(2), WSSADGS(3), WPFADGN(4), WSSADGN(5), CSFAAGS(4), WSSADGE(1), WSFADGA(1), WSFADAN(1), WPFAAGS(3), WSFAGGN(2), WSFAEGN(1), WSSANGS(1), LSFVDCN(1), WPFAEGN(1), YSSANGN(1), LSYADGS(1)	37-46-53 (252), 37-53 (12), 35-46-53 (2), 33-37-46-53 (1), 37-46-53-61(2), 37-38-46-53(2), 46-53(1), 36-46-53(1), 46 (1)
		subgroup B	WSFANGN(1)	37-46-53(1)
		subgroup C	WSFADGN(15), WSFVDGN(1), WSFVDGS(2), WSFADGS(1), WSFANGN(1)	37-46-53(14), 35-46-53(4), 37-53(2)
2	IngelvacPRRS MLV	lineage 5	SHLQLIYNL	30-33-44-51
	P129	lineage 8	SHFQLIYNL	32-44-51
	2003-2010	lineage 4	SHLQLIYNL	30-33-44-51
		lineage 5	SHLQLIYNL(43), SNLQLIYNL(11), SKFQLIYNL(1), XNLQLIYNL(1), SNLQSIYNL(1)	30-33-44-51(17), 34-44-51(17), 32-33-44-51(7), 33-34-44-51(3), 32-44-51(2), 30-35-44-51(1), 30-33-43-50(1), 30-33-34-44-51(4), 30-34-44-51(3), 30-34-35-44-51(1), 33-44-51(1)
		lineage kor A	SHFQLIYNL(9), SHLQLIYNL(1), SKFQLIYNL(1), SKIQLIYNL(2), SHIQLIYNL(1), SKLQSIYKL(1), SNLQLIYNL(2), SNFQLIYNL(4), SKLQLIYNL(3)	32-44-51(5), 33-44-51(5), 33-51(1), 32-33-44-51(3), 32-43-50(1), 35-43-50(1), 33-43-50(3), 30-33-44-51(1), 34-44-51(2), 33-34-44-51(1), 30-35-44-51(1)
		lineage kor C	SHLQLIYNL(24), SHLQSIYNL(8)	30-34-44-51(13), 34-44-51(3), 30-44-51(1), 30-33-44-51(2), 33-34-44-51(5), 30-33-34-44-51(4), 30-35-44-51(2), 33-44-51(2)
	2013-2016	lineage 1	SHLQLIYNL(9)	30-33-34-44-51(4), 30-34-44-51(1), 34-44-51-59(2), 33-34-44-51(1), 30-33-44-51(1)
		lineage 5	SHLQLIYNL(77), SKFQLIYNL(2), SNLQLIYNL(3), SRLQSIYNL(1)	30-33-44-51(48), 32-35-44-51(1), 33-34-44-51(4), 30-33-34-44-51(10), 34-44-51(7), 30-33-43-50(2), 30-44-51(2), 30-35-44-51(4), 32-33-44-51(3), 33-44-51(2)
		lineage kor A	SHFQLIYNL(14), SHLQLIYNL(2), SKFQLIYNL(2), SNLQLIYNL(1), SYSQLIYNL(4), SYSQSIYDL(1), SYSQSIYNL(1), SKLQLIYNL(4), SKLQLIYNM(1), SNFQLIYNL(2), SHIQLIYNL(1)	34-44-51(17), 33-44-51(3), 32-33-44-51(6), 32-44-51(3), 32-35-44-51(2), 33-34-44-51(1), 32-51 (1)
		lineage kor B	SNLQLIYNL(47), SHLQLIYNL(2), STLQLIYNL(12), STSQLIYNL(1), SKLQLIYNL(7), SNPQLIYNL(1), SKLQLIYDL(1),SHLQSIYNL(1)	34-44-51(39), 34-43-50(2), 34-35-44-51(6), 33-44-51(4), 34-51(1), 33-44-51(1), 32-44-51(8), 33-43-50(1), 33-34-44-51(9), 32-33-44-51(1)
		lineage kor C	SHLQLIYNL(38), SHLQLIYKM(1), SHLQSIYNL(4), SHSQLIYNL(1), SHFQSIYNL(1), SHLQLIYDL(1), SQLQLIYNL(3), SHLQLIYKL(1)	30-33-44-51(8), 30-35-44-51(6), 34-44-51(5), 30-34-44-51 (4), 32-35-44-51(1), 32-33-44-51(2), 33-51(1), 30-34-35-44-51 (4), 33-34-44-51(2), 35-51(1), 34-35-44-51(3), 33-44-51 (6), 30-33-51(1), 30-33-34-44-51(5), 35-44-51(1)

[a]Main neutralizing epitope and pattern of N-glycosylation site at each subgroup or lineage were underlined

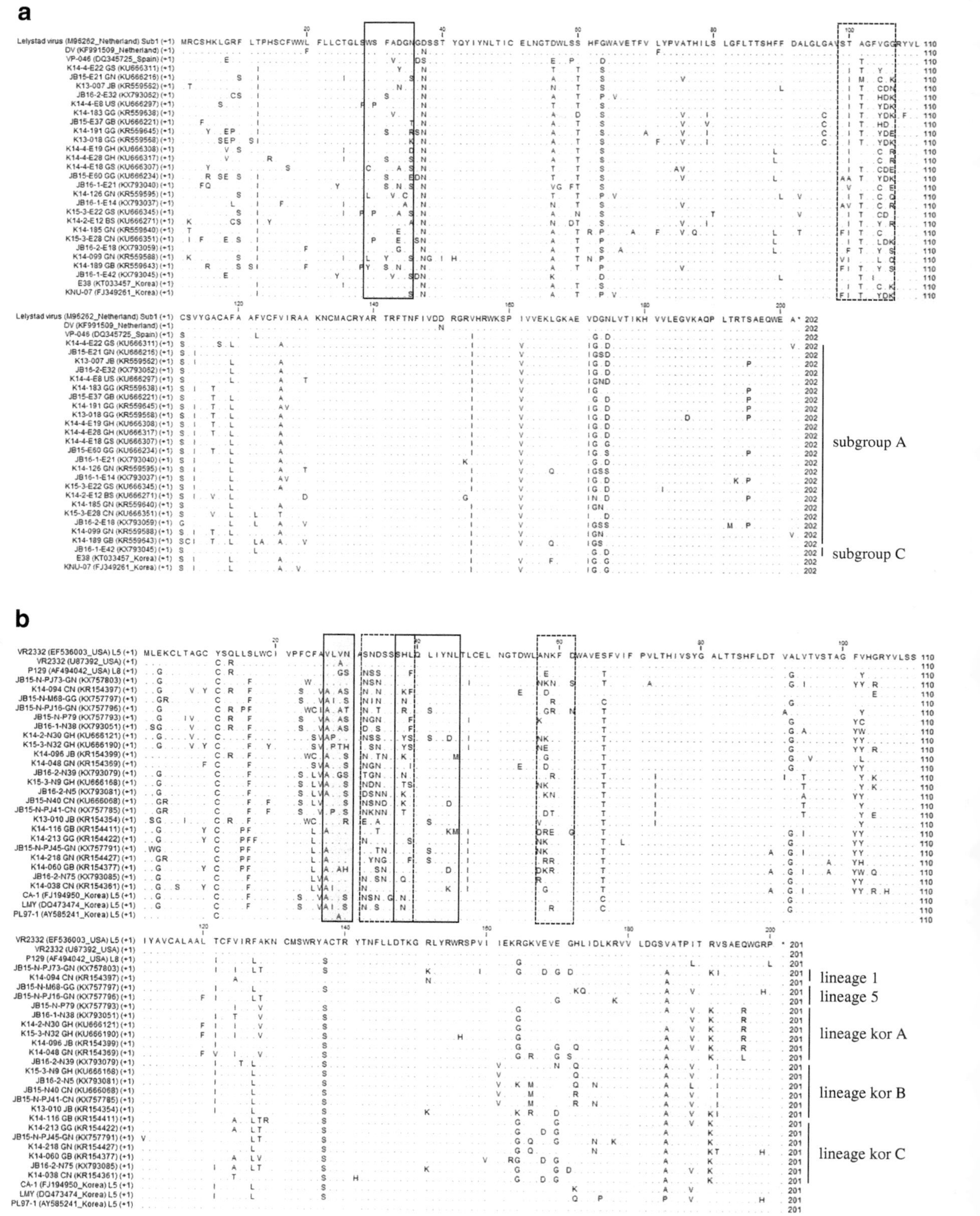

Fig. 3 (See legend on next page.)

(See figure on previous page.)
Fig. 3 Multiple alignment of ORF5 amino acid sequences of representative isolates in each subgroup (Type 1 PRRSV) (**a**) and lineage (Type 2 PRRSV) (**b**). The representative isolates were selected based on main amino acid sequence of neutralizing epitope of Type 1 PRRSV (residues 29–35) [23] and Type 2 PRRSV (residues 37–45) [37]. The solid line box and gray color box represent neutralizing epitope and decoy epiotpe (residues 27–31) [57], respectively. The dot-line box indicates hypervariable regions [58]

ke viruses originated from the Type 1 PRRS live accines commercialized in 2014 and would become ighly prevalent over time in the Republic of Korea.

Korean Type 2 PRRS viruses have been divided into neages 1, 4, and 5, as well as the Korean lineages kor , B, and C based on global PRRSV phylogeny [30]. The najority of the Korean Type 2 PRRS field isolates elonged to lineage 5 and the Korean lineages. Lineage 5 iruses were grouped with VR2332-like viruses genetically close to the Ingelvac PRRS MLV vaccine virus, which has been used commercially since 1996. The neage also included Korean reference field strains, L97-1 [40], LMY [32, 33], and CA-1 [41]. Regarding he emergence of novel Korean lineages, lineages kor B nd C were first classified in this study, while lineage kor was first reported as a Korean lineage in a previous tudy of field isolates of 2010 [36]. Lineages kor A and C vere observed to include field viruses isolated in 2005–009 and 2013–2016, which indicated that these groups ave developed genetic components geographically disnct from those in foreign countries for longer than 0 years. Meanwhile, lineage kor B comprised only ecent isolates that originated from Gyeongnam Province between 2014 and 2016, suggesting that this group nay have recently established regionally unique genetic roperties within the Republic of Korea.

Nine viruses of lineage 1 isolated between 2014 and 015 were closely related to NADC30, with 92.3–94.9% JT sequence similarity to NADC30, which was one of he representative virulent strains along with MN184 nd SDSU73 in the United States [42]. Chinese JADC30-like viruses (HNjz15, JL580, HENAN-HEB, IENAN-XINX, and CHsx140) were also reported to ause obvious clinical symptoms in pigs with virulence omparable to that of NADC30 [43–45]. It should be oted that the circulation of NADC30-like viruses in the Republic of Korea has not been previously reported. lthough the virulence of NADC30-like viruses is nown to be less than that of highly pathogenic PRRS iruses [43], there is a strong need to define the viruence of recent NADC30-like isolates in pigs in Korean arms. There are two possible explanations for the recent mergence of NADC30-like viruses. First, the NADC30-ke viruses may have recently been introduced by the mportation of breeding pigs, likely as Chinese JADC30-like viruses [45]. Second, it has been assumed hat NADC30 was introduced 7–10 years ago, circulated a particular environment (e.g., with wild boars as hosts) based on an estimated mutational change rate (0.78% per year) of ORF5 NTs identified in previous studies [24, 46], and was recently transmitted to domestic swine farms in various ways (e.g., wild boar farming).

The NEs and N-glycosylation patterns of GP5 were highly variable, and novel epitopes and N-glycosylation patterns continuously emerged and disappeared in the field viruses, although this was more apparent in field viruses isolated in 2013–2016 than in 2003–2010 (Table 3). As expected, NEs of vaccine strains or PRRSV prototype strains existed in the majority of field isolates (82.2 and 61.0% for Type 1 and Type 2 PRRSV, respectively) without a preference for a certain subgroup or lineage. In particular, NEs of DV (or Lelystad) (WSFADGN) and Ingelvac PRRS MLV (or VR2332) (SHLQLIYNL) were maintained in approximately 80.4 and 54.6% of field isolates, respectively. It has been speculated that the dominance of the two NEs might be due to extensive vaccination using vaccine strains (Ingelvac PRRS MLV and DV) that originated from PRRSV prototype strains. Nevertheless, it has been noted that the emergence of novel NEs has been significantly expedited over time in PRRSV field isolates (8.6% of 2005–2009 field isolates vs. 20.3% of 2013–2016 field isolates for Type 1 PRRSV; 31.8% of 2005–2009 field isolates vs. 42.3% of 2013–2016 field isolates for Type 2 PRRSV). Regarding the N-glycosylation pattern, it was interesting to note that N-glycosylation sites were highly diverse and changeable in Korean Type 2 PRRS field isolates, while being conserved in Korean Type 1 PRRS field isolates. NEs and the N-glycosylation pattern are closely associated with virus propagation, neutralization, and immunological protection [47–51]. Therefore, it has been suggested that the strong preference for mutation of NEs and the N-glycosylation pattern, particularly in Type 2 PRRSV, might be associated with limited protective efficacy of PRRS vaccination against heterologous viruses in the field, as shown in previous studies [52–54].

Type 2 vaccine-like viruses have become highly prevalent since the first use of Ingelvac PRRS MLV in 1996 [32]. In this study, lineage 5, including the Type 2 vaccine strain and vaccine-like viruses, showed the highest prevalence (15.3%) in the field. Likewise, the recent prevalence of subgroup C, including Type 1 vaccine-like viruses, is low (3.69%). However, extensive use of Type 1 live vaccines may result in a dramatically increased prevalence of Type 1 vaccine-like viruses and/or isolation of field viruses sharing a genomic part of Type 1 live vaccine strains in the near future, caused by genetic evolution mechanisms of PRRSV, random point mutations, and homologous recombination [55]. To minimize the circulation of live vaccine strains in the field, we may have to strengthen swine farm bio-security to prevent contamination of live vaccine strains among swine farms vaccinated with live vaccines. At the same time, limited use of live vaccines may be recommended in young pigs (3–8 weeks old) or pregnant gilts/sows of PRRS-affected farms.

Conclusions

This study suggests that PRRS viruses in the Republic of Korea have recently developed genetic characteristics geographically distinct from currently prevalent global PRRS viruses or commercial vaccine strains. Therefore, further study will be required to evaluate how the established genetic characteristics have affected PRRS outbreaks in domestic swine farms, which will provide important information for the implementation of control and preventive measures in swine farms.

Abbreviations

AA: Amino Acid; NE: Neutralizing epitope; NT: Nucleotide; ORF: Open Reading Frame; PRRSV: Porcine reproductive and respiratory syndrome virus

Acknowledgements

We would like to thank our funding sources.

Funding

This work was funded by grant (project no.: QIA I-1541780-2012-14-03) from the Animal and Plant Quarantine Agency (APQA), Ministry of Agriculture, Food and Rural Affairs, Republic of Korea as well as by grant (313005-3 and 315029-3) from the Technology Development Program for Bio-industry, Ministry of Food, Agriculture, Forestry and Fisheries, Republic of Korea.

Authors' contributions

HJK, JEY and JES conducted the experiments and produced data. ARK, WIK, CHL, JL, ISC and SEC provided field samples and worked for analysis of the data. CSH designed and supervised the study. HJK and CSH wrote the manuscript. All authors contributed to the final editing and approval of the manuscript.

Competing interests

The authors declare that they have no competing interests.

Author details

[1]Viral Disease Division, Animal and Plant Quarantine Agency, Gimcheon 39660, Republic of Korea. [2]Animal Virology Laboratory, School of Life Sciences, Kyungpook National University, Daegu 41566, Republic of Korea. [3]College of Veterinary Medicine, Jeonbuk National University, Iksan 54596, Republic of Korea. [4]Present address: PRRS research Laboratory, Viral Diseases Division, Animal and Plant Quarantine Agency, Gimcheon 39660, Republic o Korea.

References

1. Holtkamp DJ, Kliebenstein JB, Neumann E, Zimmerman JJ, Rotto H, Yoder TK, Wang C, Yeske P, Mowrer CL, Haley CA. Assessment of the economic impact of porcine reproductive and respiratory syndrome virus on United States pork producers. J Swine Health Prod. 2013;21(2):72.
2. Neumann EJ, Kliebenstein JB, Johnson CD, Mabry JW, Bush EJ, Seitzinger AH, Green AL, Zimmerman JJ. Assessment of the economi impact of porcine reproductive and respiratory syndrome on swine production in the United States. J Am Vet Med Assoc. 2005;227(3): 385–92.
3. Keffaber K. Reproductive failure of unknown aetiology. AASP Newslett. 1989;1:1–10.
4. Andreyev VG, Wesley RD, Mengeling WL, Vorwald AC, Lager KM. Genetic variation and phylogenetic relationships of 22 porcine reproductive and respiratory syndrome virus (PRRSV) field strains based on sequence analysis of open reading frame 5. Arch Virol. 1997;142(5):993–1001.
5. Cavanagh D. Nidovirales: a new order comprising Coronaviridae and Arteriviridae. Arch Virol. 1997;142(3):629–33.
6. Fauquet CM, Mayo MA, Maniloff J, Desselberger U, Ball LA. Virus taxonomy classification and nomenclature of viruses. In: Fauquet CM, Mayo MA, Maniloff J, Desselberger U, Ball LA, editors. 8th ICTV report of the international committee on taxonomy of viruses. London: Elsevier/Academ Press; 2005. p. 1259.
7. Spaan WJM, Brian D, Cavanagh D, de Groot RJ, Enjuanes L, Gorbalenya AE, Holmes KV, Masters PS, Rottier PJ, Taguchi F, Talbot P. Family coronaviridae In: Fauquet CM, Mayo MA, Maniloff J, Desselberg U, Ball LA, editors. Virus taxonomy: eighth report of the international committee on taxonomy of viruses. London: Elsevier Academic Press; 2005. p. 947–64.
8. Firth AE, Zevenhoven-Dobbe JC, Wills NM, Go YY, Balasuriya UB, Atkins JF, Snijder EJ, Posthuma CC. Discovery of a small arterivirus gene that overlaps the GP5 coding sequence and is important for virus production. J. Gen. Virol. 2011;92(Pt 5):1097–106.
9. Johnson CR, Griggs TF, Gnanandarajah J, Murtaugh MP. Novel structura protein in porcine reproductive and respiratory syndrome virus encoded by an alternative ORF5 present in all arteriviruses. J Gen Virol 2011;92(Pt 5):1107–16.
10. Snijder EJ, Meulenberg JJ. The molecular biology of arteriviruses. J. Gen. Virol. 1998;79(Pt 5):961–79.
11. Wu WH, Fang Y, Farwell R, Steffen-Bien M, Rowland RR, Christopher-Hennings J, Nelson EA. A 10-kDa structural protein of porcine reproductive and respiratory syndrome virus encoded by ORF2b. Virology. 2001;287(1):183–91.
12. Bautista EM, Faaberg KS, Mickelson D, McGruder ED. Functional properties of the predicted helicase of porcine reproductive and respiratory syndrome virus. Virology. 2002;298(2):258–70.
13. Fang Y, Snijder EJ. The PRRSV replicase: exploring the multifunctionality of an intriguing set of nonstructural proteins. Virus Res. 2010;154(1-2):61–76.
14. Fang Y, Treffers EE, Li Y, Tas A, Sun Z, van der Meer Y, de Ru AH, van Veele PA, Atkins JF, Snijder EJ, Firth AE. Efficient −2 frameshifting by mammalian ribosomes to synthesize an additional arterivirus protein. Proc Natl Acad Sc U S A. 2012;109(43):E2920–8.
15. Snijder EJ, Spaan WJM. Arteriviruses In Knipe DM, Howley PM, Griffin DE, Lamb RA, Martin MA, Roizman B and Straus SE (eds). Fields virology, 5th ed. Philadelphia: Lippincott Williams and Wilkins Publishers; 2007. pp.1337-1355
16. van Aken D, Zevenhoven-Dobbe J, Gorbalenya AE, Snijder EJ. Proteolytic maturation of replicase polyprotein pp1a by the nsp4 main proteinase is essential for equine arteritis virus replication and includes internal cleavage of nsp7. J Gen Virol. 2006;87(Pt 12):3473–82.
17. Doan DN, Dokland T. Structure of the nucleocapsid protein of porcine reproductive and respiratory syndrome virus. Structure. 2003;11(11):1445–51
18. Meulenberg JJ, van Nieuwstadt AP, van Essen-Zandbergen A, Bos-de Ruijte JN, Langeveld JP, Meloen RH. Localization and fine mapping of antigenic sites on the nucleocapsid protein N of porcine reproductive and respirator syndrome virus with monoclonal antibodies. Virology. 1998;252(1):106–14.

9. Wootton S, Yoo D, Rogan D. Full-length sequence of a Canadian porcine reproductive and respiratory syndrome virus (PRRSV) isolate. Arch Virol. 2000;145(11):2297–323.

0. Dea S, Gagnon CA, Mardassi H, Pirzadeh B, Rogan D. Current knowledge on the structural proteins of porcine reproductive and respiratory syndrome (PRRS) virus: comparison of the north American and European isolates. Arch Virol. 2000;145(4):659–88.

1. Pirzadeh B, Gagnon CA, Dea S. Genomic and antigenic variations of porcine reproductive and respiratory syndrome virus major envelope GP5 glycoprotein. Can J Vet Res. 1998;62(3):170–7.

2. Wissink EH, Kroese MV, van Wijk HA, Rijsewijk FA, Meulenberg JJ, Rottier PJ. Envelope protein requirements for the assembly of infectious virions of porcine reproductive and respiratory syndrome virus. J Virol. 2005;79(19):12495–506.

3. Wissink EH, van Wijk HA, Kroese MV, Weiland E, Meulenberg JJ, Rottier PJ, van Rijn PA. The major envelope protein, GP5, of a European porcine reproductive and respiratory syndrome virus contains a neutralization epitope in its N-terminal ectodomain. J. Gen. Virol. 2003;84(Pt 6):1535–43.

4. Cha SH, Chang CC, Yoon KJ. Instability of the restriction fragment length polymorphism pattern of open reading frame 5 of porcine reproductive and respiratory syndrome virus during sequential pig-to-pig passages. J Clin Microbiol. 2004;42(10):4462–7.

5. Dee, S.A., Torremorell, M., Rossow, K., Mahlum, C., Otake, S., Faaberg, K., 2001. Identification of genetically diverse sequences (ORF 5) of porcine reproductive and respiratory syndrome virus in a swine herd. Can.J.Vet.Res. 65(4), 254-260.

6. Kapur V, Elam MR, Pawlovich TM, Murtaugh MP. Genetic variation in porcine reproductive and respiratory syndrome virus isolates in the midwestern United States. J. Gen. Virol. 1996;77(Pt 6):1271–6.

7. Kuhn JH, Lauck M, Bailey AL, Shchetinin AM, Vishnevskaya TV, Bao Y, Ng TF, LeBreton M, Schneider BS, Gillis A, Tamoufe U, Diffo Jle D, Takuo JM, Kondov NO, Coffey LL, Wolfe ND, Delwart E, Clawson AN, Postnikova E, Bollinger L, Lackemeyer MG, Radoshitzky SR, Palacios G, Wada J, Shevtsova ZV, Jahrling PB, Lapin BA, Deriabin PG, Dunowska M, Alkhovsky SV, Rogers J, Friedrich TC, O'Connor DH, Goldberg TL. Reorganization and expansion of the nidoviral family Arteriviridae. Arch Virol. 2016;161(3):755–68.

8. Kim WI, Yoon KJ. Molecular assessment of the role of envelope-associated structural proteins in cross neutralization among different PRRS viruses. Virus Genes. 2008;37(3):380–91.

9. Meng XJ. Heterogeneity of porcine reproductive and respiratory syndrome virus: implications for current vaccine efficacy and future vaccine development. Vet Microbiol. 2000;74(4):309–29.

0. Shi M, Lam TT, Hon CC, Hui RK, Faaberg KS, Wennblom T, Murtaugh MP, Stadejek T, Leung FC. Molecular epidemiology of PRRSV: a phylogenetic perspective. Virus Res. 2010;154(1-2):7–17.

1. Shi M, Lam TT, Hon CC, Murtaugh MP, Davies PR, Hui RK, Li J, Wong LT, Yip CW, Jiang JW, Leung FC. Phylogeny-based evolutionary, demographical, and geographical dissection of north American type 2 porcine reproductive and respiratory syndrome viruses. J Virol. 2010;84(17):8700–11.

2. Cha SH, Choi EJ, Park JH, Yoon SR, Song JY, Kwon JH, Song HJ, Yoon KJ. Molecular characterization of recent Korean porcine reproductive and respiratory syndrome (PRRS) viruses and comparison to other Asian PRRS viruses. Vet Microbiol. 2006;117(2-4):248–57.

3. Choi EJ, Lee CH, Song JY, Song HJ, Park CK, Kim B, Shin YK. Genetic diversity of porcine reproductive and respiratory syndrome virus in Korea. J Vet Sci. 2013;14(2):115–24.

4. Kim SH, Roh IS, Choi EJ, Lee C, Lee CH, Lee KH, Lee KK, Song YK, Lee OS, Park CK. A molecular analysis of European porcine reproductive and respiratory syndrome virus isolated in South Korea. Vet Microbiol. 2010; 143(2-4):394–400.

5. Shin J-H, Kang Y-B, Kim Y-J, et al. Sero-epidemiological studies on porcine reproductive and respiratorysyndrome in Korea. I. Detection of indirect fluorescent antibodies. RDA J Agri Sci. 1993;35:572–6.

5. Kim HK, Nguyen VG, Kim IO, Park JH, Park SJ, Rho SM, Han JY, Park BK. Epidemiologic and phylogenetic characteristics of porcine reproductive and respiratory syndrome viruses in conventional swine farms of Jeju Island as a candidate region for PRRSV eradication. Transbound Emerg Dis. 2012;59(1):62–71.

7. Larochelle R, D'Allaire S, Magar R. Molecular epidemiology of porcine reproductive and respiratory syndrome virus (PRRSV) in Quebec. Virus Res. 2003;96:3–14.

8. Lee C, Kim H, Kang B, Yeom M, Han S, Moon H, Park S, Kim H, Song D, Park B. Prevalence and phylogenetic analysis of the isolated type I porcine reproductive and respiratory syndrome virus from 2007 to 2008 in Korea. Virus Genes. 2010;40(2):225–30.

39. Lee JA, Lee NH, Lee JB, Park SY, Song CS, Choi IS, Lee SW. Genetic diversity of the Korean field strains of porcine reproductive and respiratory syndrome virus. Infect Genet Evol. 2016;40:288–94.

40. Kang SY, Yun SI, Park HS, Park CK, Choi HS, Lee YM. Molecular characterization of PL97-1, the first Korean isolate of the porcine reproductive and respiratory syndrome virus. Virus Res. 2004;104(2):165–79.

41. Koo HN, Oh JM, Lee JK, Choi JY, Lee KS, Roh JY, Je YH, Jin BR, Yoo SS, Kim JS, Kim YI, Yoon IJ, Woo SD. Molecular characterization of ORFs 2 to 7 of Korean porcine reproductive and respiratory syndrome virus (CA) and its protein expression by recombinant baculoviruses. J Microbiol. 2008;46(6):709–19.

42. Brockmeier SL, Loving CL, Vorwald AC, Kehrli ME Jr, Baker RB, Nicholson TL, Lager KM, Miller LC, Faaberg KS. Genomic sequence and virulence comparison of four type 2 porcine reproductive and respiratory syndrome virus strains. Virus Res. 2012;169(1):212–21.

43. Sun Z, Wang J, Bai X, Ji G, Yan H, Li Y, Wang Y, Tan F, Xiao Y, Li X, Tian K. Pathogenicity comparison between highly pathogenic and NADC30-like porcine reproductive and respiratory syndrome virus. Arch Virol. 2016;161(8):2257–61.

44. Zhao K, Ye C, Chang XB, Jiang CG, Wang SJ, Cai XH, Tong GZ, Tian ZJ, Shi M, An TQ. Importation and recombination are responsible for the latest emergence of highly pathogenic porcine reproductive and respiratory syndrome virus in China. J Virol. 2015;89(20):10712–6.

45. Zhou L, Wang Z, Ding Y, Ge X, Guo X, Yang H. NADC30-like strain of porcine reproductive and respiratory syndrome virus. China Emerg infect Dis. 2015;21(12):2256–7.

46. Chang CC, Yoon KJ, Zimmerman JJ, Harmon KM, Dixon PM, Dvorak CM, Murtaugh MP. Evolution of porcine reproductive and respiratory syndrome virus during sequential passages in pigs. J Virol. 2002;76(10):4750–63.

47. Ansari IH, Kwon B, Osorio FA, Pattnaik AK. Influence of N-linked glycosylation of porcine reproductive and respiratory syndrome virus GP5 on virus infectivity, antigenicity, and ability to induce neutralizing antibodies. J Virol. 2006;80(8):3994–4004.

48. Das PB, Vu HL, Dinh PX, Cooney JL, Kwon B, Osorio FA, Pattnaik AK. Glycosylation of minor envelope glycoproteins of porcine reproductive and respiratory syndrome virus in infectious virus recovery, receptor interaction, and immune response. Virology. 2011;410(2):385–94.

49. Delputte PL, Nauwynck HJ. Porcine arterivirus infection of alveolar macrophages is mediated by sialic acid on the virus. J Virol. 2004;78(15):8094–101.

50. Faaberg KS, Hocker JD, Erdman MM, Harris DL, Nelson EA, Torremorell M, Plagemann PG. Neutralizing antibody responses of pigs infected with natural GP5 N-glycan mutants of porcine reproductive and respiratory syndrome virus. Viral Immunol. 2006;19(2):294–304.

51. Li J, Tao S, Orlando R, Murtaugh MP. N-glycosylation profiling of porcine reproductive and respiratory syndrome virus envelope glycoprotein 5. Virology. 2015;478:86–98.

52. Hu J, Zhang C. Porcine reproductive and respiratory syndrome virus vaccines: current status and strategies to a universal vaccine. Transbound EmergDis. 2014;61(2):109–20.

53. Kim T, Park C, Choi K, Jeong J, Kang I, Park SJ, Chae C. Comparison of two commercial type 1 porcine reproductive and respiratory syndrome virus (PRRSV) modified live vaccines against heterologous type 1 and type 2 PRRSV challenge in growing pigs. Clin Vaccine Immunol. 2015;22(6):631–40.

54. Labarque G, Reeth KV, Nauwynck H, Drexler C, Van Gucht S, Pensaert M. Impact of genetic diversity of European-type porcine reproductive and respiratory syndrome virus strains on vaccine efficacy. Vaccine. 2004;22(31-32):4183–90.

55. Liu D, Zhou R, Zhang J, Zhou L, Jiang Q, Guo X, Ge X, Yang H. Recombination analyses between two strains of porcine reproductive and respiratory syndrome virus in vivo. Virus Res. 2010;155:473–86.

56. Stadejek T, Oleksiewicz MB, Scherbakov AV, Timina AM, Krabbe JS, Chabros K, Potapchuk D. Definition of subtypes in the European genotype of porcine reproductive and respiratory syndrome virus : nucleocapsid characteristics and geographical distribution in Europe. Arch Virol. 2008;153:1479–88.

57. Ostrowski M, Galeota JA, Jar AM, Platt KB, Osorio FA, Lopez OJ. Identification of neutralizing and nonneutralizing epitopes in the porcine reproductive and respiratory syndrome virus GP5 ectodomain. J Virol. 2002;76:4241–50.

58. Key KF, Hagshenas G, Guenette DK, Swenson SL, Toth TE, Meng XJ. Genetic variation and phylogenetic analyses the ORF5 gene of acute porcine reproductive and respiratory syndrome virus isolates. Vet Microbiol. 2001;83:249–63.

18

Expression, purification, crystallization and preliminary X-ray diffraction analysis of swine leukocyte antigen 2 complexed with a CTL epitope AS64 derived from Asia1 serotype of foot-and-mouth disease virus

Feng-shan Gao[1*†], Lei Feng[1†], Ping Jiang[1†], Zi-bin Li[2], Hua Gao[1], Xiao-xin Zhai[1], Zong-hui Zhang[1] and Xiao Hu[1]

Abstract

Background: Currently, the structural characteristics of the swine major histocompatibility complex (MHC) class I molecule, also named swine leukocyte antigen class I (SLA-I) molecule need to be further clarified.

Results: A complex of SLA-I constituted by an SLA-2*HB01 molecule with swine β_2-microglobulin and a cytotoxic T lymphocyte (CTL) epitope FMDV-AS64 (ALLRSATYY) derived from VP1 protein (residues 64–72) of Asia 1 serotype of foot-and-mouth disease virus (FMDV) was expressed, refolded, purified and crystallized. By preliminary X-ray diffraction analysis, it was shown that the diffraction resolution of the crystal was 2.4 Å and the space group belonged to $P2_12_12_1$ with unit cell parameters a = 48.37, b = 97.75, c = 166.163 Å.

Conclusion: This research will be in favor of illuminating the structural characteristics of an SLA-2 molecule associated with a CTL epitope derived from Asia1 serotype of FMDV.

Keywords: Swine leukocyte antigen 2, Crystal structure, Foot-and-mouth disease virus, Asia 1 serotype

Background

Class I of major histocompatibility complex (MHC) molecules are membrane-surface proteins, which are mainly responsible for binding and presenting endogenous antigenic peptides degraded from proteins coded by virus genome in target cells [1] or autoantigen [2]. These endogenous antigenic peptides usually constituted by 8–10 residues in length are derived from endogenous antigens degraded by cellular proteasome [3, 4]. When a peptide is complexed and correctly refolded with MHC class I molecule in the antigen presenting cells (APCs), it will be presented to the membrane surface of the APCs to intrigue the cytotoxic T lymphocytes (CTLs). On this occasion, the peptide is defined as a CTL epitope [5]. Once CTLs are activated by the CTL epitopes, CTLs will recognize the epitopes and then kill the infected cells [6]. Therefore, the expressed MHC class I molecules on membrane of APC should contain three components: a polymorphic heavy chain (α chain) of class I, a monomorphic light chain of β_2-microglobulin (β_2m) noncovalently linking the α3 domain of the heavy chain and an epitope bound in a groove formed by the α1 and α2 domains of the heavy chain [7]. Analysis of structural characteristics of MHC class I is necessary so that the mechanism of antigen presentation associated with MHC class I molecule will be explored.

MHC class I genes in pigs (*Sus scrofa* domestica) located in the 7p1.1 band of the short arm of chromosome 7 are also named as swine leukocyte antigen class I (SLA-I) [8]. There are three constitutively expressed classical and polymorphic SLA-I genes in the genome, namely SLA-1, SLA-2 and SLA-3 [9]. Among them, SLA-2 is different

* Correspondence: gfsh0626@126.com
†Feng-shan Gao, Lei Feng and Ping Jiang contributed equally to this work.
[1]Department of Bioengineering, |College of Life Science and Technology, Dalian University, Xuefu street 10, Dalian, Liaoning 116622, People's Republic of China
Full list of author information is available at the end of the article

rom SLA-1 and SLA-3 in the N-terminal of their coding egions as previously described [10]. The swine β$_2$m sβ$_2$m) is monomorphic and noncovalently links with he heavy chain of the SLA-I molecules, which bind viral or an auto CTL epitope. Foot-and-mouth disease irus (FMDV) is a great danger to cloven-hoofed animals ncluding pigs, because it can cause animals to develop an cute, febrile, and highly contagious infectious disease 11]. In FMDV, there are seven serotypes named as A, O, C, Asia1, SAT1, SAT2, and SAT3. However, none of them ave mutual cross-immunity [12, 13]. Among them, the sia1 serotype often occurs in Asian countries as previ-usly reported [14, 15]. Therefore, to further epitope accine development, more CTL epitopes and their nteractions with SLA-I should be investigated. Re-ently, crystal data of the SLA-1, SLA-2 and SLA-3 had een announced, and a few CTL epitopes derived from wine-origin influenza virus, O serotype of FMDV, Ebola irus and respiratory syndrome virus (PRRSV) were also iscovered [16–19]. However, crystal of SLA-2 associated vith CTL epitope derived from Asia1 serotype of FMDV emains elusive.

In this article, we introduce the expression, refolding, urification, crystallization and preliminary X-ray diffrac-ion analysis of SLA-2*HB01 with an AS64 CTL epitope erived from the Aisa1 serotype of FMDV.

Methods

xpression and isolation of the proteins of SLA-2*HB01 nd sβ$_2$m

To construct the expression system of the SLA-2 haplo-ype HB01 allele (GenBank accession No. AB602431) oding for 275 amino acids in extracellular domain, a air of primers was designed as shown in Table 1. The PCR product was recovered and cloned into pMD®19-T imple vector as previously described [10, 19]. After

Table 2 Crystallizing condition

Method	Sitting-drop vapor diffusion
Temperature (°C)	4
Protein concentration (mg/mL)	15
Buffer composition of protein solution	50 mM NaCl, 20 mM Tris–HCl pH 8.0
Composition of reservoir solution	0.1 M BIS-TRIS pH 6.5, 0.2 M Ammonium acetate, 25% (*w/v*) PEG 3350
Volume and ratio of drop	1 μL protein solution mixed with 1 μL reservoir solution
Volume of reservoir (μL)	120

identification by digestion with *Nde* I and *Xho* I and followed by sequencing, the interest of SLA-2*HB01 was further cloned into the pET21a (+) vector. The recom-binant pET21a (+) containing the sβ$_2$m had been done in our laboratory previously [19]. The two recombinant SLA-2*HB01 and sβ$_2$m plasmids were induced to ex-press in BL21 (Rosetta) *Escherichia coli* strain. The in-clusion bodies were extracted as follows [17, 19]: In 2 L Luria–Bertani medium (LB), the SLA-2*HB01 and sβ$_2$m expression strains were inoculated and incubated at 180 rpm for 3–4 h in a shaking incubator at 37 °C until the OD_{600} value reached 0.5–0.6. Then, a final concentration of 1 mM isopropyl-β-D-thiogalactopyranoside (IPTG) was used in the medium to induce the interest of pro-teins to express in same cultivating environment as above. After 5 h, the bacteria were collected and cooled at 4 °C for 30 min. Then the bacteria were cen-trifugated for 15 min at 6000 rpm at 4 °C to collect pellets followed by washing them for three times with a solution buffer consisting of 50 mM Tris–HCl, 100 mM NaCl, 10 mM EDTA, 0.5% (*v/v*) Triton X-100, 1 mM DTT. In the end, a guanidinium chloride

able 1 SLA-2*HB01-AS64-sβ$_2$m complex information

ource organism	*Sus scrofa*
NA source	Plasmid DNA
pper primer	GGAATTCCATATGGGCCCGCATTCCCTGAGCTATTCTTAC
ower primer	AGTCTCGAGTTAGTCCCATCTCAGGGTGAGGGGCTCCTGC
loning vector	pMD®19-T simple
xpression vector	pET21a (+)
xpression host	*E. coli* (Rosetta)
omplete amino-acid sequence of the construct produced	GPHSLSYSYTAVSRPDRGDSRFFIVGYVDDTQFVRFDSDAPNAKMEPRAQWIQ QEGQEYWDRETQISKETAQNYRVDLNTLRGYYNQSEAGSRTIQRVYGCYLGPD GLLLRGYRQDAYDGADYIALNEDLRSWTAADMAAQITKRKWEWNEAEGERSYL QGRCVEWLQKYLVMGKDTLQRAEPPKTHVTRHPSSDLGVTLRCWALGFYPKEISLS WQREGQDQSQDMELVETRPSGDGTFQKWAALVVPPGEEQSYTCHVQHEGLQEPLTL RW**ALLRSATYY***VARPPKVQVYSRHPAENGKPNYLNCYVSGFHPPQIEIDLLKNGEKMN AEQSDLSFSKDWSFYLLVHTEFTPNAVDQYSCRVKHVTLDKPKIVKWDRDH*

he restriction-enzyme cleavage sites are underlined in the upper and lower primers. The normal font, bold and italics of residues expressed by the vector are om the heavy chain of SLA-2*HB01, AS64 and the light chain of sβ$_2$m in the amino-acid sequences, respectively

buffer [6 M guanidinium chloride, 100 mM NaCl, 10 mM EDTA, 50 mM Tris–HCl pH 8.0, 10% (v/v) glycerine, 10 mM DTT] was used to dissolve the isolated inclusion body proteins to a final concentration of 30 mg/mL.

Refolding and purification of the SLA-2*HB01-AS64-sβ_2m complex

The refolded SLA-I (SLA-2*HB01-AS64-sβ_2m) complex wa carried out as described previously [6] with improvemen

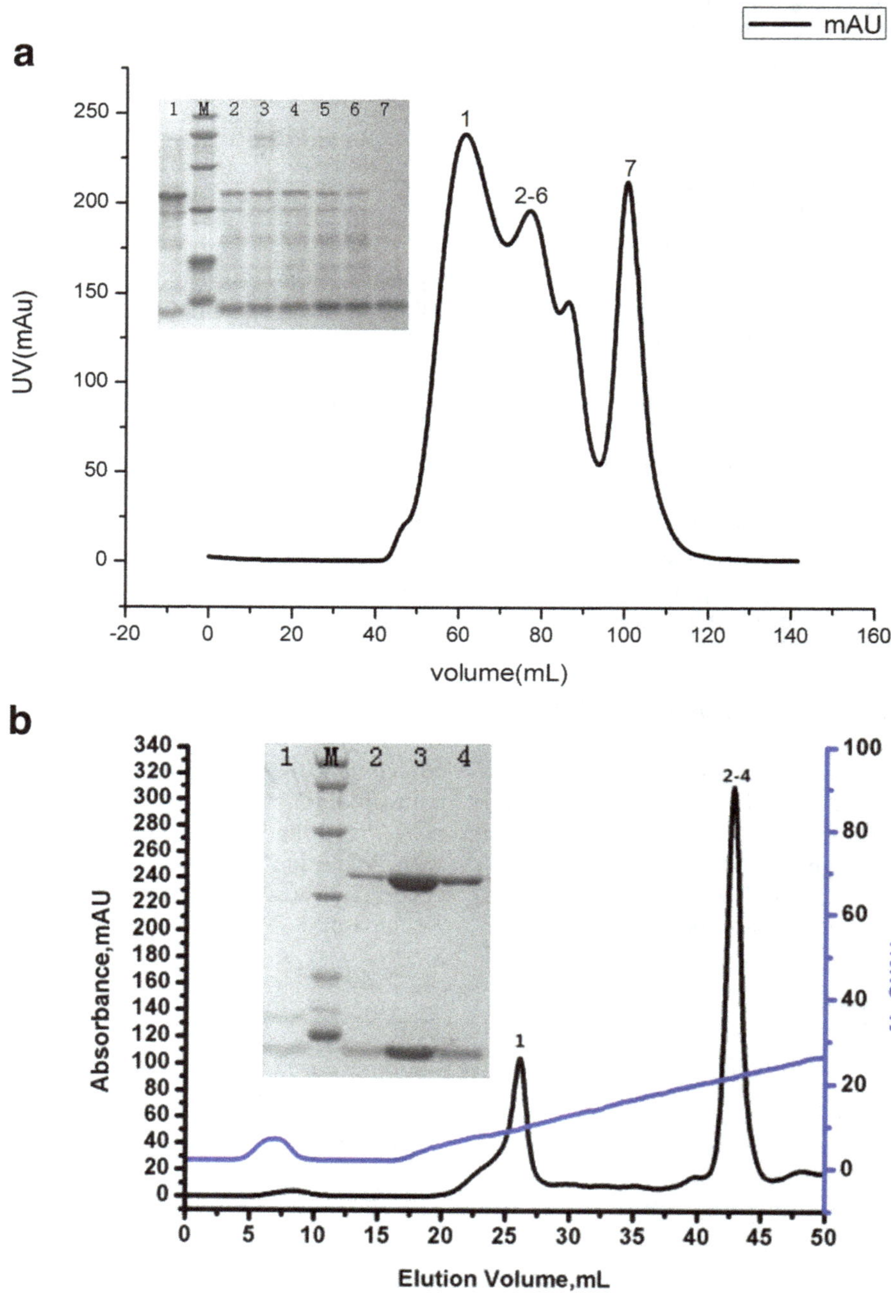

Fig. 1 Purification of the refolded SLA-2*HB01-AS64-sβ_2m by FPLC Superdex 200 16/60 Hi-Load gel-filtration and anion-exchange chromatography Resource Q (GE Healthcare). **a** Gel-filtration profile of the refolded SLA-2*HB01-AS64-sβ_2m products. Peak 1 represents aggregated heavy chains of SLA-2*HB01, peaks 2–6 represent correctly refolded SLA-2*HB01-AS64-sβ_2m complex (~ 44 kDa) and peak 7 represents surplus sβ_2m. Inset: SDS–PAGE gel detection (15%) for peaks 1, 2–6 and 7. M, the low molecular-weight protein ladder (kDa) with 97.1, 66.3, 43.0, 31.0, 20.1 and 14.4. **b** Further purification of the refolded SLA-2*HB01-AS64-sβ_2m by anion-exchange chromatography Resource Q. Peak 1 contains aggregated light chain of sβ_2m, peaks 2–4 represent the refolded SLA-2*HB01-AS64-sβ_2m products, which was eluted with a NaCl concentration of 21.5–26.5%. Inset: SDS-PAGE gel detection (15%) for peaks 1 and 2–4. M, the low molecular-weight protein ladder (kDa) with 97.1, 66.3, 43.0, 31.0, 20.1 and 14.4

recommended by Feng et al. [19]. Firstly, the epitope AS64 (ALLRSATYY) derived from the VP1 protein residues 64–72 of Asia1 FMDV was firstly dissolved in dimethyl sulfoxide (DMSO) and then diluted in water. The inclusion body proteins of SLA-2*HB01 and sβ_2m were renatured and refolded with the AS64 epitope according to a 1:1:3 molar ratio by using the gradual dilution method in a refolding buffer (100 mM Tris pH 8.0, 400 mM L-Arg HCl, 2 mM EDTA, 5 mM GSH, 0.5 mM GSSH, 0.5 mM PMSF) at 4 °C. After refolding for 24 h, the soluble SLA-2*HB01-AS64-sβ_2m complex was further concentrated and purified by chromatography separation on a Superdex 200 16/60 HiLoad size-exclusion column (GE Healthcare) followed by an anion-exchange chromatography Resource Q (GE Healthcare). SLA-2*HB01-AS64-sβ_2m complex information is shown in Table 1.

Crystallizing the SLA-2*HB01-AS64-sβ_2m complex

The final purified SLA-2*HB01-AS64-sβ_2m complex proteins (~ 44 kDa) were further dialyzed against a crystallizing buffer (50 mM NaCl, 20 mM Tris–HCl pH 8.0) overnight at 4 °C and then concentrated to 15 mg/mL. Crystallizing assays were tried with Index and Crystal Screen kit (Hampton Research) at 4 °C and 18 °C by using the sitting-drop vapor diffusion method as previously described [19, 20]. Two protein solution drops each with 1 μl (at 7.5 and 15 mg/mL) and 1 μL of reservoir crystallizing buffer were placed and mixed together over a well containing 120 μL reservoir solution using an MRC Maxi plate (HR3–179, Hampton Research). Crystals of SLA-2*HB01-AS64-sβ_2m were obtained at 14th day by using a protein concentration of 15 mg/mL in the Index solution No. 79 (0.2 M Ammonium acetate, 25% *w/v* PEG 3350, 0.1 M BIS-TRIS pH 6.5) at 4 °C. Crystallizing condition is shown in Table 2.

Data collection and processing

The SLA-2*HB01-AS64-sβ_2m crystal was firstly soaked in reservoir solution supplemented with 17% (*v/v*) glycerol as a cryoprotectant for several seconds and then flash-cooled in a nitrogen stream at − 173 °C [21]. Data collection was carried out using an ADSC Q315 CCD detector at a wavelength of 1.00000 Å. By using beam line BL17U of the Shanghai Synchrotron Radiation Facility (Shanghai, China), the crystal was collected to 2.4 Å resolution. The raw data was indexed, integrated, corrected for absorption, scaled and merged using HKL-2000 [22].

Results

After purification to homogeneity by Superdex 200 16/60 HiLoad size-exclusion chromatography, it was shown that the heavy chain of SLA-2*HB01 was successfully refolded together with the light chain of sβ_2m and the CTL epitope of AS64. The yield of the SLA-2*HB01-AS64-sβ_2m complex is about 10%. It was shown four peaks in the chromatographic elution profile (Fig. 1a). The peak 1 should be aggregated heavy chains of SLA-2*HB01. The peaks 2–6 detected in lanes 2 to 6 with SDS-PAGE should be the refolded SLA-2*HB01-AS64-sβ_2m complex (44 kDa). The peak 7 detected in lane 7 with SDS-PAGE should be surplus sβ_2m (see inset in Fig. 1a). Another peak between peak 2–6 and peak 7, not shown in SDS-PAGE detection, should be some degraded proteins according to our previous practice. The refolded SLA-2*HB01-AS64-sβ_2m complex was further purified by an anion-exchange chromatography Resource Q with a NaCl elution concentration of 21.5–26.5%. It was shown two peaks for the further purified complex (Fig. 1b). The peak 1 detected in lane 1 with SDS-PAGE contains free sβ_2m. The peaks 2–4 detected in lanes 2 to 4 with SDS-PAGE contain two bands at the expected molecular weights of SLA-2*HB01 heavy chain (32 kDa) and sβ_2m light chain (12 kDa) (see inset in Fig. 1b).

The purified SLA-2*HB01-AS64-sβ_2m was concentrated to 15 mg/mL for crystal screening. Crystals occurred after 7 days in the Index solution No. 79 at 4 °C and then they were harvested at 14th d (Fig. 2). After preliminary X-ray diffraction analysis, it was shown that the diffraction resolution of the SLA-2*HB01-AS64-sβ_2m crystal used for data collection was 2.4 Å. The space group of the crystal belongs to $P2_12_12_1$. The unit-cell parameters of the crystal were shown as a = 48.37, b = 97.75, c = 166.163 Å (Fig. 3). The crystal has a solvent content of 61.9%. Data-collection and processing statistics are summarized in Table 3.

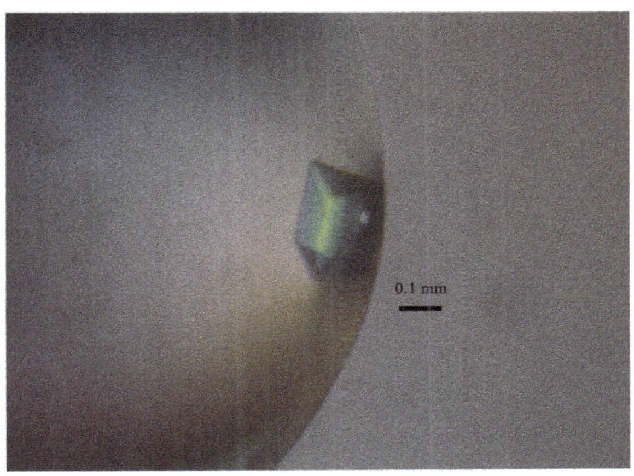

Fig. 2 Picture of the SLA-2*HB01-AS64-sβ2m crystal growing in the Index solution No. 79 at 4 °C

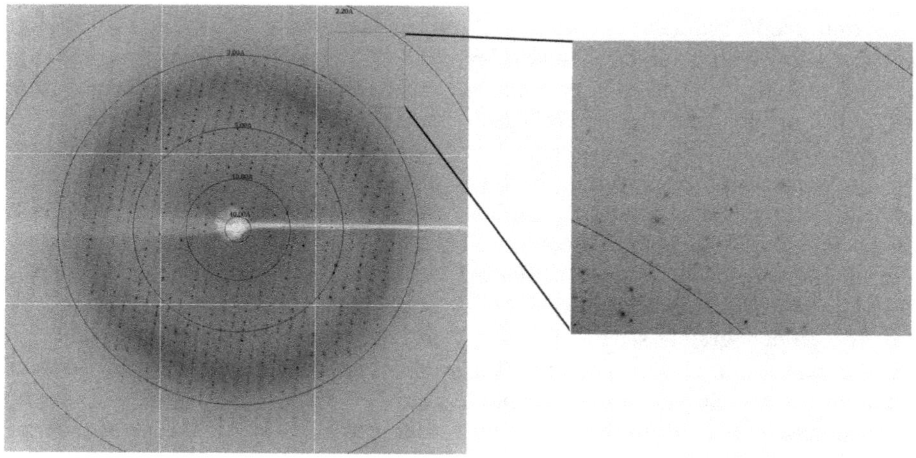

Fig. 3 Diffraction pattern of the SLA-2*HB01-AS64-sβ_2m complex. Spots corresponding to diffraction to high resolution are highlighted in the box

Discussion

Previously, we reported a multiple amino-acid sequence alignment between SLA-2*HB01 and other known MHC class I alleles in swine, human and mouse [10]. Based on human HLA-A2 crystal data, the structure of SLA-2*HB01 was predicted by using homology modeling. We noticed SLA-2*HB01 preserved some key functional sites of HLA-A2 and H-2, which indicated that SLA-2*HB01 should be crucial in binding and presenting antigenic peptides [23, 24]. In addition, SLA-2*HB01 has 85.0–93.9, 86.2–97.0 and 83.3–88.6% sequence identity to other SLA-1, SLA-2 and SLA-3 alleles, respectively. Comprehensive analysis of SLA-2*HB01, it should be a novel allele o SLA-2 with specific genetic characteristics [10].

In this work, the crystal of the SLA-2*HB01 molecul complexed with swine β_2m and a CTL epitope AS64 de rived from the Asia1 serotype of FMDV was reported. I seems the space group type of SLA-2*HB01-AS64-sβ_2m crystal is consistent with that of SLA-1 crystal but quit different from that of SLA-3 crystal, which indicates th structure of SLA-2 might be more similar to that o SLA-1 [17, 18]. Recently, a crystal of SLA-2*HB01 com plex associated with an Hu64 CTL epitope derived fron O serotype of FMDV was reported. It was shown tha the two crystals were similar in space group type, bu different in unit-cell parameters [19]. To learn about th elaborate structural characteristics of SLA-2, espe cially the special characteristics that differ from SLA- and SLA-3, the 3-dimentional structure of the SLA- complex associated more CTL epitopes derived fron swine-origin virus is required to be revealed as soo as possible.

Table 3 X-ray diffraction data and processing statistics. Values in parentheses are for the highest resolution shell

Diffraction source	BL17U, SSRF
Wavelength (Å)	1.00000
Temperature (°C)	−173
Detector	ADSC Q315 CCD
Crystal-to-detector distance (mm)	350.00
Space group	$P2_12_12_1$
Unit-cell parameters (Å)	a = 48.37, b = 97.75, c = 166.16
Resolution range (Å)	50.0–2.40 (2.40–2.49) [a]
Total No. of reflections	222,792
No. of unique reflections	31,827
Completeness (%)	99.2
Average $I/\sigma(I)$	21.8
R_{merge} [b] (%)	7.8 (31.8)
Redundancy	7.0 (7.1)

[a]Values in parentheses refer to statistics in the outermost resolution shell
[b]$R_{merge} = \Sigma_{hkl}\Sigma_i \mid I_i - \langle I\rangle \mid / \Sigma_{hkl}\Sigma_i I_i$, where I_i is the observed intensity and $\langle I\rangle$ is the average intensity of multiple observations of symmetry related reflections

Conclusions

The research data will be used to further elucidate th 3-dimentional structure of the SLA-2 molecules and de sign more refined viral epitopes.

Abbreviations

APCs: Antigen presenting cells; CTL: Cytotoxic T lymphocyte antigen; DMSO: Dimethyl sulfoxide; FMDV: Foot-and-mouth disease virus; IPTG: Isopropyl-β-D-thiogalactopyranoside; LB: Luria–Bertani medium; MHC: Major histocompatibility complex; SLA: Swine leukocyte antigen

Acknowledgments

We thank Professor George F. Gao (Institute of Microbiology, Chinese Academy of Sciences) for providing experimental condition.

unding

his work was supported in part by a grant from the National Natural cience Foundation of China (31672525), a grant from the National Natural cience Foundation of China (31172304), and a grant from the Liaoning ducation Bureau Key Laboratory Project (LZ2015003).

uthors' contributions

SG designed, wrote, revised and submitted the manuscript. LF and PJ ontributed to conduct the work, analysis and interpretation of results. ZBL, G, XXZ and ZHZ contributed to the data collection and analysis. XH ontributed to the manuscript revision. All authors read and approved the nal manuscript.

onsent for publication

ot applicable

ompeting interests

he authors declare that they have no competing interests.

uthor details

Department of Bioengineering, |College of Life Science and Technology, alian University, Xuefu street 10, Dalian, Liaoning 116622, People's Republic f China. [2]Department of Microbiology and Immunology, College of eterinary Medicine, China Agricultural University, Beijing 100094, People's epublic of China.

eferences

Lu X, Gibbs JS, Hickman HD, David A, Dolan BP, Jin Y, Kranz DM, Bennink JR, Yewdell JW, Varma R. Endogenous viral antigen processing generates peptide-specific MHC class I cell-surface clusters. Proc Natl Acad Sci U S A. 2012;109(38):15407–12.

Weidanz JA, Piazza P, Hickman-Miller H, Woodburn D, Nguyen T, Wahl A, Neethling F, Chiriva-Internati M, Rinaldo CR, Hildebrand WH. Development and implementation of a direct detection, quantitation and validation system for class I MHC self-peptide epitopes. J Immunol Methods. 2007; 318(1–2):47–58.

Vigneron N, Ferrari V, Stroobant V, Abi Habib J, Van den Eynde BJ. Peptide splicing by the proteasome. J Biol Chem. 2017;292(51):21170–9.

Wolf BJ, Princiotta MF. Viral and bacterial minigene products are presented by MHC class I molecules with similar efficiencies. Mol Immunol. 2011;48(4): 463–71.

Klein J, Satta Y, O'HUigin C, Takahata N. The molecular descent of the major histocompatibility complex. Annu Rev Immunol. 1993;11:269–95.

Garboczi DN, Ghosh P, Utz U, Fan QR, Biddison WE, Wiley DC. Structure of the complex between human T-cell receptor, viral peptide and HLA-A2. Nature. 1996;384(6605):134–41.

Bjorkman PJ, Saper MA, Samraoui B, Bennett WS, Strominger JL, Wiley DC. Structure of the human class I histocompatibility antigen, HLA-A2. J Immunol. 2005;174(1):6–19.

Smith TP, Rohrer GA, Alexander LJ, Troyer DL, Kirby-Dobbels KR, Janzen MA, Cornwell DL, Louis CF, Schook LB, Beattie CW. Directed integration of the physical and genetic linkage maps of swine chromosome 7 reveals that the SLA spans the centromere. Genome Res. 1995;5(3):259–71.

Ando A, Kawata H, Shigenari A, Anzai T, Ota M, Katsuyama Y, Sada M, Goto R, Takeshima SN, Aida Y, et al. Genetic polymorphism of the swine major histocompatibility complex (SLA) class I genes, SLA-1, −2 and −3. Immunogenetics. 2003;55(9):583–93.

0. Gao FS, Bai J, Gong XJ, Zhang XH, Zhang WJ, Guo D, Zhang S. Analyzing the genetic characteristics and function of the swine leukocyte antigen 2 gene in a Chinese inbreed of pigs. Microbiol Immunol. 2012;56(3):208–15.

1. Salguero FJ, Sanchez-Martin MA, Diaz-San Segundo F, de Avila A, Sevilla N. Foot-and-mouth disease virus (FMDV) causes an acute disease that can be lethal for adult laboratory mice. Virology. 2005;332(1):384–96.

12. Tully DC, Fares MA. Unravelling selection shifts among foot-and-mouth disease virus (FMDV) serotypes. Evo Bioinformatics Online. 2006;2:211–25.

13. Yang J, Leen EN, Maree FF, Curry S. Crystal structure of the 3C protease from southern African territories type 2 foot-and-mouth disease virus. PeerJ. 2016;4:e1964.

14. Baba Sheikh MO Rashid PMA, Marouf AS, Raheem ZH, Janga SC. Phylogenic analysis of serotype Asia1 foot-and-mouth disease virus from Sulaimani/Iraq using VP1 protein: heterogeneity with vaccine strain As1/Shamir/89. Iran J Vet Res. 2017;18(3):212–5.

15. Subramaniam S, Mohapatra JK, Sharma GK, Das B, Dash BB, Sanyal A, Pattnaik B. Phylogeny and genetic diversity of foot and mouth disease virus serotype Asia1 in India during 1964-2012. Vet Microbiol. 2013 167(3–4):280–8.

16. Pan X, Qi J, Zhang N, Li Q, Yin C, Chen R, Gao F, Xia C. Complex assembly, crystallization and preliminary X-ray crystallographic studies of the swine major histocompatibility complex molecule SLA-1*1502. Acta Crystallogr Sect F Struct Bio Cryst Commun. 2011;67(Pt 5):568–71.

17. Zhang N, Qi J, Feng S, Gao F, Liu J, Pan X, Chen R, Li Q, Chen Z, Li X, et al. Crystal structure of swine major histocompatibility complex class I SLA-1 0401 and identification of 2009 pandemic swine-origin influenza a H1N1 virus cytotoxic T lymphocyte epitope peptides. J Virol. 2011;85(22):11709–24.

18. Fan S, Wu Y, Wang S, Wang Z, Jiang B, Liu Y, Liang R, Zhou W, Zhang N, Xia C. Structural and biochemical analyses of swine major histocompatibility complex class I complexes and prediction of the epitope map of important influenza a virus strains. J Virol. 2016;90(15):6625–41.

19. Feng L, Sun MW Jiang P, Li ZB, Gao H, Zhai XX, Han Y, Zhang ZH, Gao FS. Purification, crystallization and preliminary X-ray crystallographic studies of swine MHC class I complexed with an FMDV CTL epitope Hu64. Res Vet Sci. 2018;119:205–8.

20. Chen Z, Zhang N, Qi J, Chen R, Dijkstra JM, Li X, Wang Z, Wang J, Wu Y, Xia C. The structure of the MHC class I molecule of bony fishes provides insights into the conserved nature of the antigen-presenting system. J Immunol. 2017;199(10):3668–78.

21. Parkin SH, H. J Appl Crystallogr. 1998;31:945–53.

22. Otwinowski Z, Minor W. Processing of X-ray diffraction data collected in oscillation mode Methods Enzymol 1997;276:307–26.

23. Gao FS, Bai J, Zhang Q, Xu CB, Li Y. Construction of multiple recombinant SLA-I proteins by linking heavy chains and light chains in vitro and analyzing their secondary and 3-dimensional structures. Gene. 2012;502(2): 147–53.

24. Gao FS, Zhai XX, Jiang P, Zhang Q, Gao H, Li ZB, Han Y, Yang J, Zhang ZH. Identification of two novel foot-and-mouth disease virus cytotoxic T lymphocyte epitopes that can bind six SLA-I proteins. Gene. 2018;653:91–101.

The influence of experimental inflammation and axotomy on leucine enkephalin (leuENK) distribution in intramural nervous structures of the porcine descending colon

Slawomir Gonkowski*, Krystyna Makowska and Jaroslaw Calka

Abstract

Background: The enteric nervous system (ENS), located in the intestinal wall and characterized by considerable independence from the central nervous system, consists of millions of cells. Enteric neurons control the majority of functions of the gastrointestinal tract using a wide range of substances, which are neuromediators and/or neuromodulators. One of them is leucine–enkephalin (leuENK), which belongs to the endogenous opioid family. It is known that opioids in the gastrointestinal tract have various functions, including visceral pain conduction, intestinal motility and secretion and immune processes, but many aspects of distribution and function of leuENK in the ENS, especially during pathological states, remain unknown.

Results: During this experiment, the distribution of leuENK – like immunoreactive (leuENK-LI) nervous structures using the immunofluorescence technique were studied in the porcine colon in physiological conditions, during chemically-induced inflammation and after axotomy. The study included the circular muscle layer, myenteric (MP), outer submucous (OSP) and inner submucous plexus (ISP) and the mucosal layer. In control animals, the number of leuENK-LI neurons amounted to 4.86 ± 0.17%, 2.86 ± 0.28% and 1.07 ± 0.08% in the MP, OSP and ISP, respectively. Generally, both pathological stimuli caused an increase in the number of detected leuENK-LI cells, but the intensity of the observed changes depended on the factor studied and part of the ENS. The percentage of leuENK-LI perikarya amounted to 11.48 ± 0.96%, 8.71 ± 0.13% and 9.40 ± 0.76% during colitis, and 6.90 ± 0.52% 8.46 ± 12% and 4.48 ± 0.44% after axotomy in MP, OSP and ISP, respectively. Both processes also resulted in an increase in the number of leuENK-LI nerves in the circular muscle layer, whereas changes were less visible in the mucosa during inflammation and axotomy did not change the number of leuENK-LI mucosal fibers.

Conclusions: LeuENK in the ENS takes part in intestinal regulatory processes not only in physiological conditions, but also under pathological factors. The observed changes are probably connected with the participation of leuENK in sensory and motor innervation and the neuroprotective effects of this substance. Differences in the number of leuENK-LI neurons during inflammation and after axotomy may suggest that the exact functions of leuENK probably depend on the type of pathological factor acting on the intestine.

Keywords: Leucine-enkephalin (leuENK), Enteric nervous system (ENS), Inflammation, Axotomy, Colon, Pig

* Correspondence: slawomir.gonkowski@uwm.edu.pl
Department of Clinical Physiology, Faculty of Veterinary Medicine, University of Warmia and Mazury, Oczapowski Str, 13 Olsztyn, Poland

Background

It is well-known that neural control of all functions of the gastrointestinal (GI) tract is performed by both extrinsic innervation [1–4] and the enteric nervous system (ENS) [5, 6]. Localization of extrinsic neurons supplying the stomach and intestine depend on the innervated regionof the GI tract. These neurons may be located in prevertebral sympathetic ganglia, sympathetic chain, dorsal root ganglia, sensory and parasympathetic ganglia of vagal nerve, as well as in parasympathetic nuclei of sacral spinal cord [1, 2, 4, 6]. In turn, the ENS is situated in the wall of the GI tract. It is composed of a large number of neurons, which are characterized by considerable independence from the central nervous system and, for this reason, it has also been called the "second" or "intestinal" brain [7]. The structure of the ENS depends on the species studied and the regionof the GI tract. In porcine, large intestine enteric neurons are grouped into three separate ganglionated plexuses, which are interconnected with a dense network of nerves (Fig. 1). There are three types of these plexuses: myenteric plexus (MP) – located between the longitudinal and circular muscles, outer submucous plexus (OSP) – immediately adjacent to internal side of the circular muscle layer and inner submucous plexus (ISP) – positioned between muscularis mucosa and lamina propria [5, 8]. Neuronal cells within the above-mentioned plexuses belong to various functional classes, play different functions and show the presence of a broad range of active substances which, importantly, can play various roles as neuromediators and/or neuromodulators [6].

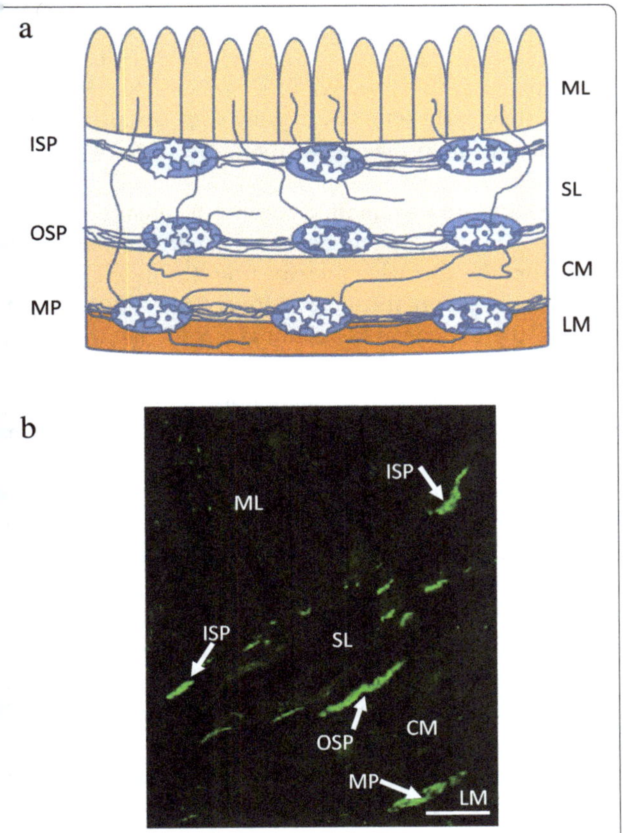

Fig. 1 The organization of the enteric nervous system (ENS) in the porcine descending colon. **a** the scheme; **b** the view under florescent microscope, where nervous structures are labelled with directed towards protein gene product 9.5 (PGP 9.5) used as panneronal marker. LM – longitudinal muscle layer; CM – circular muscle layer; submucosal layer; ML – mucosal layer; MP – myenteric plexus; OSP – outer submucous plexus; ISP – inner submucous plexus. Bar 100 μm

It should be pointed out that the ENS plays a key role in the regulation of intestinal functions not only in physiological conditions, but also during various pathological states. This fact may be expressed by structural, functional or chemical changes within enteric neurons, which may be a result of adaptive responses to operating factors. Till now, such changes in the ENS have been observed under physiological changes, such as development, aging or diet modification, but they are more visible during pathological processes, including intestinal and systemic diseases or nerve injury [8–11].

One of the many active substances occurring within enteric neurons is leucine-enkephalin (leuENK) which, along with methionine-enkephalin, is an endogenous opioid. These substances are pentapeptides derived from a precursor (proenkephalin) and described for the first time within the porcine brain in the 1970s [12]. Later investigations found that leuENK may also arise from α-neo-endorphin, dynorphin A or dynorphin B, which derived from prodynorphin [13]. Enkephalins, like as exogenous opioids (e.g. morphine) act via a different type of G-protein coupled receptors, including δ-opioid, κ-opioid and μ-opioid receptors [14, 15]. Although the main action of enkephalins is a mechanism connected with analgesia, previous studies have shown that these substances are also involved in other physiological processes, such as regulation of respiratory [16], urinary [17] or circulatory [18] systems.

To date, enkephalins have been described within the GI tract in various mammals species, including humans, in both the ENS and intestinal mucosal enterochromaffin cells [15, 19–21] as well as in the extrinsic innervation of intestine [1, 2]. Even so, the exact roles of opioids within the digestive system are not entirely clarified, although it is known that these substances mainly take part in reducing visceral pain [14]. Other functions of opioids within the GI tract include participation in intestinal immune processes, as well as inhibition of intestinal motility and secretion [14, 22, 23]. The inhibitory effects of enkephalins mentioned above cause an increase in food transit time in the GI tract and may contribute to constipation [14]. In addition, some previous studies have described changes in the number of enteric neurons immunoreactive to enkephalins under pathological factors, which suggests the participation of these substances in adaptive or neuroprotective processes within the intestine [1, 2, 21]. Nonetheless, many questions connected with the functions of leuENK in the ENS during pathological processes are not clear, especially in the GI tract of the pig, which is increasingly becoming an optimal laboratory animal due to well-established anatomical, biochemical and physiological resemblances to humans [24, 25]. These similarities primarily concern the organization of the ENS [26], which makes the pig a perfect animal model for experiments on changes in enteric neurons under various pathological factors.

The aim of the present investigation was to describe, for the first time, the influence of selected pathological factors, including experimental inflammation and axotomy on leucine enkephalin-like immunoreactive (leuENK-LI) enteric neurons in the porcine descending colon. It should be pointed out that the selection of this fragment of the GI tract as a subject of the present study was also not accidental, since various pathological processes often develop within the large intestine both in human and animals [8, 27–30].

Methods

Experimental animals

The present experiment was performed on 20 immature sows of the Large White Polish breed at the age of 8 weeks (about 18 kg body weight) bought on the commercial farm of pig production in Bałcyny (Poland). Animals were kept in normal laboratory conditions in the animal quarters of Faculty of Veterinary Medicine, University of Warmia and Mazury, Olsztyn (Poland) with feeding typical for this species and age of animal. The pigs were maintained in the pens (5 animals in each pen) with an area of about 4 m^2. All experimental procedures, as well as number of experimental animals were consistent with the instructions and agreements of the Local Ethical Committee in Olsztyn (Poland), with special attention paid to minimizing any stress reaction during and after surgery (agreement numbers: 90/2007 from 20 November 2007 and 85/2008 from 17 December 2008). Animals during unloading after the transport were randomly (without any determined method) divided into four groups, each of which consisted of five pigs located in separate pens. Then the assignment of animals from each pen to the particular procedures were performed by drawing lots. Experimental groups were as follows: control (C group) – without any experimental procedures, control 1 (C1) – animals subjected to "sham" operations, inflammatory (I group) - pigs with chemically-induced colitis and axotomy (A group), where animals were subjected to the cutting of specific nerves (see below).

After five-day adaptive period the experiment was started. The sows from C1, I and A groups were subjected to median laparotomy performed under general anaesthe sia, which consisted of premedication with Stressn (Janssen, Belgium, 75 µl/kg of body weight, give intramuscularly) 15 min. Before the administration of th main aesthetic – sodium thiopental (Thiopental, Sandoz Kundl-Rakúsko, Austria; 20 mg/kg of body weight, give intravenously) prior to the surgery. Chemically-induce inflammation and axotomy were made using the method previously described by Gonkowski et al. [31]. Accordin to these methods, the animals of group I were injecte with 80 µl of 10% formalin solution in saline (microinjec tions of 5–8 µl) into the wall of the descending colon (to depth of 0,2–0,5 mm) in an area, where nerves from th inferior mesenteric ganglia supply the gut. Surgery o animals of group A consisted of the bilateral transectio of caudal colonic nerves connecting to the inferior mesen teric ganglion with the descending colon (Fig. 2). Animal of group C1 were subjected to "sham" operations, whic were aimed at exclusion of surgical manipulations on th enteric nervous system. Pigs of group C1were injected i the same manner as group I, but a pure saline solutio was used instead of formalin. After 5 days, all animal were anaesthetized in the same way as described abov and euthanized by an overdose of sodium thiopental an immediately perfused transcardially with freshly prepare 4% buffered paraformaldehyde (pH 7.4).

Double-labelling immunofluorescence technique

Segments of the descending colon (approximately 2 cm long) from the area where nerves from the inferior mesen teric ganglia supply the colon were collected from all pig used in the experiment. Inflammation in the animals o group I was confirmed by a histopathological examinatio which was made at the Laboratory of Histopatholog (Faculty of Veterinary Medicine, University of Warmi and Mazury, Olsztyn, Poland). Immediately after collec tion, colonic fragments were post-fixed by immersion wit 4% buffered paraformaldehyde (pH 7.4) for 20 min an rinsed in phosphate buffer (0.1 M, pH 7.4, at 4 °C) for days with the exchange of buffer every day. Th tissues were then put into 18% phosphate-buffere sucrose (at 4 °C) for 2 weeks. Finally, they were frozen a -22 °C. After freezing samples were coded and since the the assessors did know which samples belonged to whic experimental group. Coding of samples was performed t avoid any bias in the evaluation of colonic fragments. The tissues were cut perpendicular to the lumen of the colo into 14-µm-thick sections using microtome (Microm, HM 525, Walldorf, Germany) and fixed on glass slides.

The fragments of colon were subjected to standar double-labelling immunofluorescence, which has bee described previously by Gonkowski et al. [31, 32] During the present study, the combination of two kind of primary antisera were used: mouse monoclona

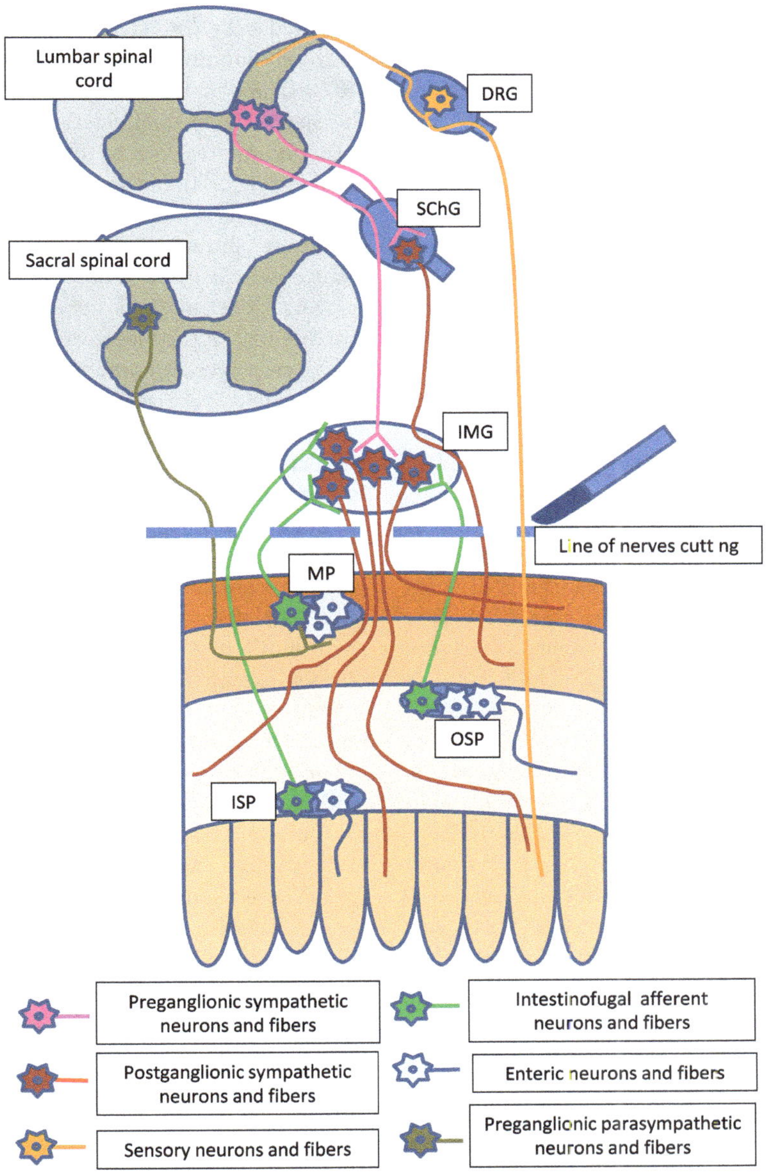

Fig. 2 Different types of nerve fibers, which were interrupted during the cutting of caudal colonic nerves DRG – dorsal root ganglion; SChG - sympathetic chain ganglion; IMG – inferior mesenteric ganglion; MP – myenteric ganglion; OSP – outer submucous ganglion; ISP – inner submucous ganglion

ntibody directed towards protein gene-product 9.5 PGP 9.5, Biogenesis, UK, working dilution 1:2000, sed here as a pan-neuronal marker) and rabbit olyclonal anti – leucine-enkephalin antibody (leuENK, bcam, UK, working dilution 1:1000). The primary ntisera mentioned above were visualized by a combination of species-specific secondary antibodies, i.e. Alexa luor 488 donkey anti-mouse IgG and Alexa fluor 546 onkey anti-rabbit IgG (both from Invitrogen, Carlsbad, CA, USA, working dilution 1:1000).

Standard control probes were made to test the specificity of primary antibodies. These included pre-absorption, omission and replacement of primary antibodies by non–immune sera. The pre-absorption test consisted of incubation (for 18 h at 37 °C) of primary antibodies in working dilutions with the appropriate antigen. Antibodies directed towards PGP 9.5 were pre-incubated with native human protein gene product 9.5 (AbD Serotec, UK), and anti-leuENK antibody with synthetic human leucine-enkephalin peptide (Abcam, UK). The concentration of each antigen was 20 µg per 1 ml of diluted antibody. This procedure, as well as omission and replacement of primary antisera by non-immune sera, completely eliminated specific stainings.

Counting the nerve structures and statistical analysis

To delimit the percentage of enteric neurons immunoreactive to leuENK, at least 600 PGP-9.5- positive cells in a particular enteric plexus (MP, OSP and ISP) of each studied animal were examined for leuENK-like immunoreactivity. Double-labelled perikarya (only neurons with clearly visible nucleus) were evaluated using an Olympus BX51 microscope equipped with epi-fluorescence and appropriate filter sets. The obtained results were pooled and presented as mean ± SEM. To prevent double counting of leuENK-LI neurons, the sections were located at least 100 µm apart.

For semi-quantitative evaluation of the density of leuENK-LI nerves within the enteric ganglia, an arbitrary scale was used, where (–) indicated the absence of studied fibers, (+) - single fibers, (++) - rare fibers, (+++) – dense network of fibers and (++++) depicted a very dense meshwork of fibers studied.

In turn, denotation of the density of intramuscular and intramucosal nerves immunoreactive to leuENK was based on counting all leuENK-LI nerve fibers *per* microscopic observation field (0.55 mm^2). Nerves were counted in four sections per animal (in 5 fields per section) and the obtained data were pooled and presented as a mean. It should be pointed out that the nerves in the intestine can form very small bundles and it is not always possible to count exact numbers of fibers in fibre bundles. Therefore the present study includes only fibers that could have been counted.

All pictures were captured by a digital camera connected to a PC. Statistical analysis was carried out with an Anova test (Graphpad Prism v. 2.0; GraphPad Software Inc., San Diego, CA, USA). The differences were considered statistically significant at $p \leq 0.05$. No statistical power calculation was conducted prior to the study, and the determination of the size of animal experimental groups was based on data available in the previous studies, where the number of five animals in the case of pigs during neuro-immunofluorescence investigations are commonly accepted.

Results

During the present investigation, leuENK-positive nervous structures were observed within the descending colon in animals of all experimental groups and their number clearly depended on both the pathological factor studied and the part of the ENS (Table 1).

Under physiological conditions, a relatively small number of leuENK-LI neurons was noted in all "kinds" of enteric plexuses (Table 1). The percentage of such neuronal cells (in relation to number of all PGP 9.5-LI neurons) amounted to 4.86 ± 0.17%, 2.86 ± 0.28% and 1.07 ± 0.08% in MP, OSP and ISP, respectively. Regarding the view of individual enteric ganglia, only single neuronal cells immunoreactive to leuENK were noted in control animals (Fig. 3. I), but the majority of ganglia did not show the presence of leuENK-LI neurons (Figs. 4.I and 5.I). Moreover, intraganglionic leuENK-positive nerve fibers were observed in all kinds of enteric ganglia. The dense network (+++) of these nerves were encountered in OSP, whereas in MP they were rare (++), and in ISP only single (+) nerve processes immunoreactive to leuENK were noted (Table 1). A relatively dense network of clearly visible LeuENK-positive nerves (Fig. 6.Ia) was also observed in the circular muscle layer (15.30 ± 0.77 nerves/observation field). In turn, only single, thin and delicate leuENK-LI nerves were noted in the mucosal layer (Fig. 6.Ib).

Statistically significant differences were not observed between control and "sham" operated animals, but both pathological states studied changed the immunoreactivity to leuENK. These changes are generally expressed by an increase in the number of leuENK-positive neuronal structures, but their intensity depended on the pathological factor acting on the intestine (Table 1).

The highest percentage of neurons immunoreactive to leuENK were found within the myenteric plexus during the inflammatory process (Fig. 3.II), where the number of these cells increased by above 6.5 percentage points (pp). These changes were accompanied by an increase in the density of leuENK-LI intraganglionic nerve fibers. In animals suffering from inflammation, two "kinds" of myenteric ganglia were observed. One of them was characterized by the presence of leuENK-LI cells and a not very dense network of fibers immunoreactive to this peptide (Fig. 3.II). In the other MP, only very dense intraganglionic leuENK-LI nerves were visible, without leuENK-positive neurons (Fig. $3.II_1$). Axotomy also caused an increase in the number of leuENK-LI neurons and intraganglionic fibers in the MP (Fig. 3.III), but these changes were less visible.

The pathological states studied caused an increase in the percentage of leuENK- positive neuronal cells located in OSP (Fig. 4). Contrary to MP, the differences between inflammation and axotomy were not observed. Both investigated states produced an increase in the number of leuENK-LI neurons by about 5.5 pp. (Table 1). These changes in OSP were accompanied by a decrease in the density of intraganglionic nerve fibers immunoreactive to leuENK (Fig. 4).

An increase in the leuENK-positive neuron number was also noted in the ISP (Fig. 5). As with myenteric plexus, more visible modifications were observed during the inflammatory process, where the percentage of leuENK-LI

'able 1 Leucine-enkephalin – like immunoreactive nervous structures in the porcine descending colon

owel part		No. of animal	C Group	C1Group	I Group	A Group
ML[1]		1	16.40	14.60	30.80	23.30
		2	17.15	17.15	28.90	26.20
		3	13.80	12.85	32.60	24.15
		4	13.15	14.50	29.05	23.15
		5	16.00	14.40	32.75	26.80
		average	15.30 ± 0.77[a]	14.70 ± 0.69[a]	30.82 ± 0.83[b]	24.72 ± 0.75[c]
1P	CB[2]	1	5.06	5.13	9.25	6.12
		2	5.23	5.15	12.06	8.63
		3	4.53	3.80	9.92	6.10
		4	4.38	4.30	11.44	7.60
		5	5.10	5.62	14.73	6.05
		average	4.86 ± 0.17[a]	4,80 ± 0.33[a]	11.48 ± 0.96[b]	6,90 ± 0.52[c]
	NF[3]	average	++	++	++++	+++
)SP	CB[2]	1	1.90	1.58	8.70	8.26
		2	3.05	3.38	8.76	8.68
		3	2.80	3.58	9.15	8.46
		4	2.90	1.38	8.60	8.15
		5	3.64	3.93	8.35	8.75
		average	2.86 ± 0.28[a]	2.77 ± 0.53[a]	8.71 ± 0.13[b]	8.46±12[b]
	NF[3]	average	+++	+++	+	+
;P	CB[2]	1	0.84	0.58	7.52	3.48
		2	1.27	1.02	11.94	5.92
		3	1.07	0.60	9.61	4.64
		4	1.20	0.86	8.20	3.60
		5	0.98	1.34	9.73	4.76
		average	1.07 ± 0.08[a]	0.88 ± 0.14[a]	9.40 ± 0.76[b]	4.48 ± 0.44[c]
	NF[3]	average	+	+	+	+
/ML[1]		1	0.85	1.20	3.00	0.85
		2	1.30	1.00	4.45	1.30
		3	1.15	1.30	4.20	1.20
		4	1.45	2.00	2.80	1.15
		5	1.50	1.15	3.65	1.95
		average	1.25 ± 0.12[a]	1.33 ± 0.17[a]	3.62 ± 0.32[b]	1.29 ± 0.18[a]

group control animals, *C1group* "sham" operated animals, *I group* pigs suffering from inflammation, *A group* animals after axotomy

ML circular muscle layer, *MP* myenteric plexus, *OSP* outer submucous plexus, *ISP* inner submucous plexus, *S/ML* submucosal/mucosal layer, *CB* cell bodies, *NF* erve fibers

Average number of nerve profiles per area studied (mean ± SEM)

Relative frequency of particular neuronal subclasses is presented as % (mean ± SEM) of all neurons counted within the ganglia stained for PGP 9.5

The density of intraganglionic nerve fibers positive for leuENK is presented in arbitrary units

tatistically significant data ($p \leq 0.05$) between C group and group C1, I and A in the number of leuENK-LI nervous structures within particular part of the colon are narked by different letters and not significant data are marked by the same letters

ells grew nine-fold in relation to control animals and mounted to 9.40 ± 0.76% of all neurons immunoreactive o PGP 9.5. This was the clearest change of all parts of the ENS studied. Axotomy also caused an increase in the number of cells immunoreactive to leuENK, but changes were less visible (Table 1). Contrary to the number of leuENK-positive neurons, the density of leuENK-LI intraganglionic nerves in the ISP was not changed during the pathological factors studied (Table 1).

Both inflammation and axotomy caused an increase in the density of leuENK-positive nerve fibers in the circular muscle layer (Fig. 6.I). In this case, as in the MP and

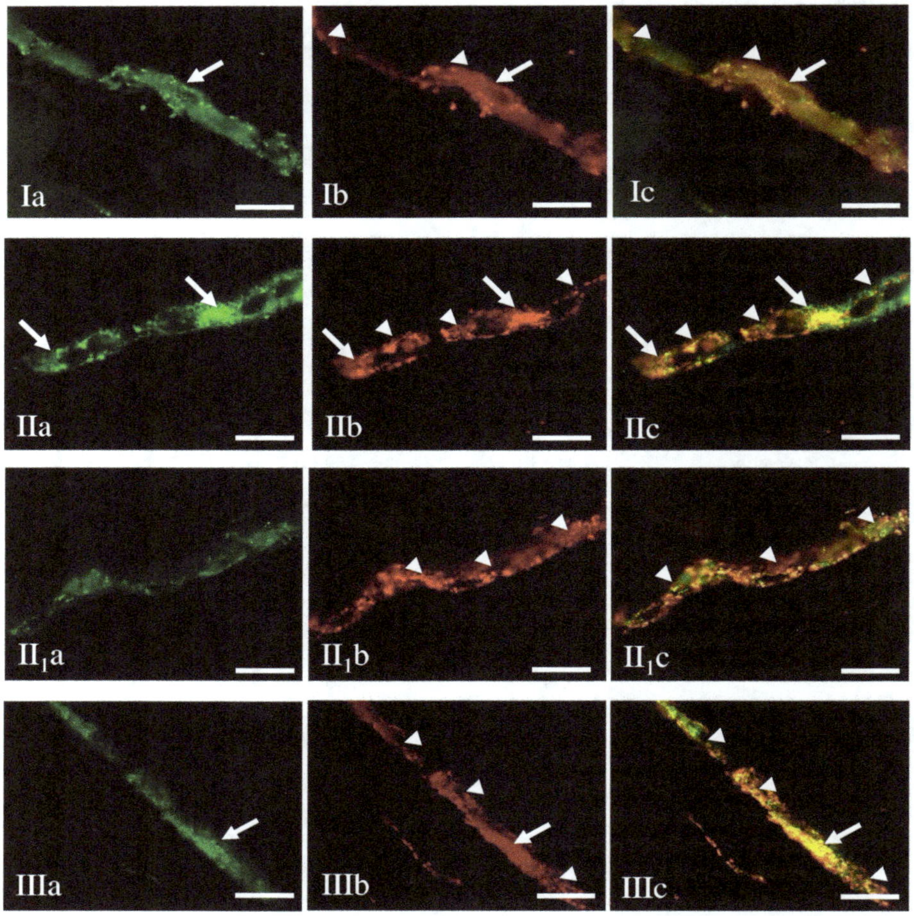

Fig. 3 Myenteric plexus of the porcine descending colon under physiological conditions (I), during inflammation (II, II_1) and after axotomy (III) immunostained for PGP 9.5 (a) and leuENK (b). The right column of the pictures (c) shows the overlap of both stainings. Co-localisation of both antigens is indicated with arrows (perikarya) and arrow heads (nerve fibers). Bar, 20 μm

ISP, more visible changes were observed during inflammatory process, where the number of fibers immunoreactive to leuENK was doubled versus control animals (Table 1). In contrast, the number of leuENK-positive nerves localized in the mucosal layer only increased during inflammation, whereas axotomy did not change their number (Fig. 6.II, Table 1).

Discussion

During the present investigation, leuENK-positive nerve structures have been observed in all parts of the ENS studied, as well as in intramuscular and intramucosal nerve fibers. These structures under physiological conditions (in spite of nerves within circular muscle layer) were rather limited. This is in agreement with the majority of previous studies, where the presence of leuENK has been described both in the ENS and extrinsic innervation of the GI tract in various mammal species, including humans [15, 19, 21]. The results obtained during the present study show that distribution of leuENK-positive nervous structures in the descending colon of the pig and other studied species are similar. In the pig (like in rats, guinea pigs or cats) such structures were first observed in the myenteric plexus and the circular muscle layer, whereas in the mucosa and submucosal enteric ganglia they are rather rare [20, 33, 34]. Particular similarities in the distribution of leuENK-positive nervous structures in the intestinal wall may also be observed between humans [15, 35, 36] and pigs (this study). This suggests that relatively well-known resemblances in the ENS organization of both these species [26] also apply to the distribution of leuENK.

Moreover, it should be pointed out that there are some discrepancies in the localization of porcine enteric neurons immunoreactive to leuENK in the light of previous studies. For example, in the stomach, some investigations have noted the absence of this peptide in the ENS [37], other authors have described relatively numerous leuENK-LI neurons, especially in the MP [38]. The reason for these discrepancies remains unclear, although they

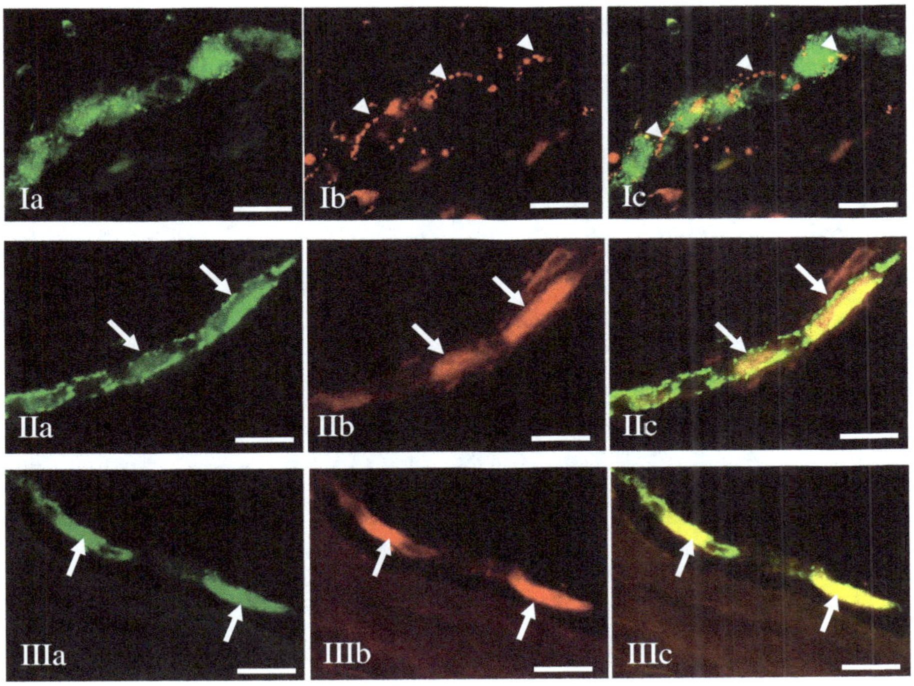

Fig. 4 Outer submucous plexus of the porcine descending colon under physiological conditions (I), during inflammation (II) and after axotomy (III) immunostained for PGP 9.5 (a) and leuENK (b). The right column of the pictures (c) shows the overlap of both stainings. Co-localisation of both antigens is indicated with arrows (perikarya) and arrow heads (nerve fibers). Bar, 20 μm

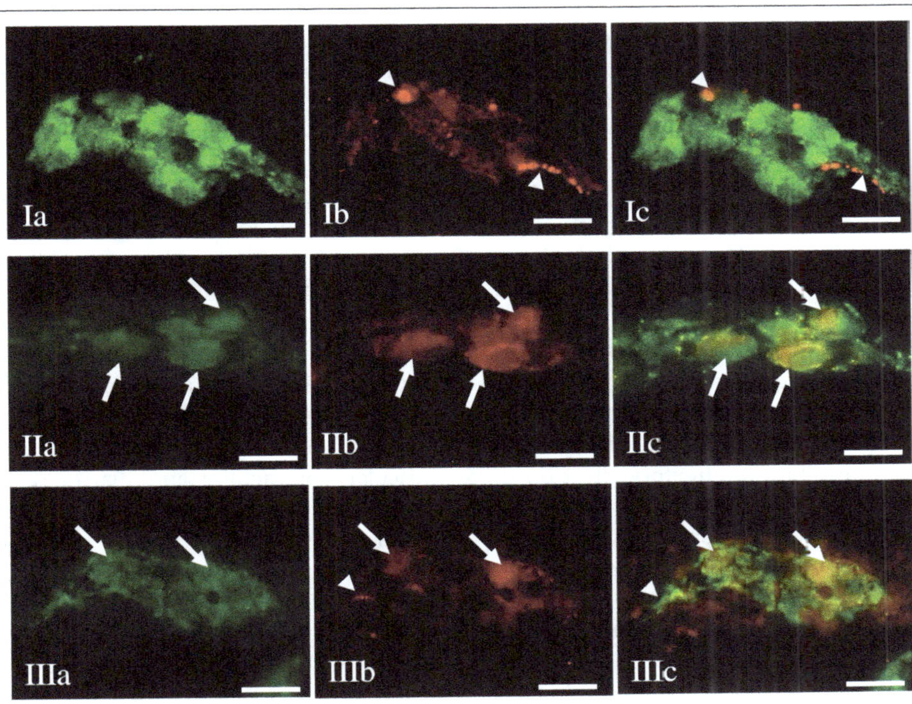

Fig. 5 Inner submucous plexus of the porcine descending colon under physiological conditions (I), during inflammation (II) and after axotomy (III) immunostained for PGP 9.5 (a) and leuENK (b). The right column of the pictures (c) shows the overlap of both stainings. Co-localisation of both antigens is indicated with arrows (perikarya) and arrow heads (nerve fibers). Bar, 20 μm

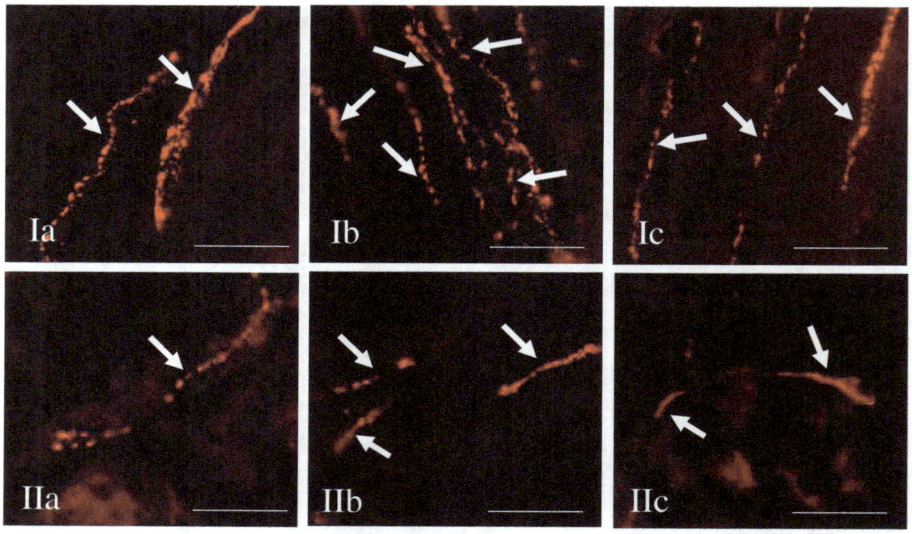

Fig. 6 Distribution pattern of nerve fibers (arrows) immunostained for leuENK in the circular muscle layer (I) and mucosal layer (II) of porcine descending colon under physiological conditions (a), during inflammation (b) and after axotomy (c). Bar, 20 μm

strongly suggest that enteric neurons can change leuENK expression under various physiological factors, such as nutritional differences, farming factors and/or environmental bacterial flora, which in all probability is associated with some currently unknown functions of opioids within the ENS.

Till now, opioids (including leuENK) in the digestive tract have been described as factors affecting the nociception, intestinal immune functions, motility and secretion [14] and their exact roles depends on both the type of opioid and receptors class. Opioid receptors, belonging to G-protein coupled receptors, have been described in the central and peripheral nervous structures, including the enteric nervous system [39–41] and three kinds of them (δ-opioid, κ-opioid and μ-opioid receptors) can participate in the regulation of gastrointestinal physiology. Previous studies showed that each class of opioid receptors has its preferred ligand and regulates specific processes. κ-opioid receptors, which bind mainly with dynorphin and μ-opioid receptors (their ligand is β-endorphin), are primarily responsible for visceral antinociception [14, 41]. In turn, δ-opioid receptors, preferred ligands of which are enkephalins, first of all exhibit an inhibitory effect on the intestinal motility, causing an increase in the transit time of digestive tract content [14]. Moreover, previous studies have described other gastrointestinal functions of opioids, such as suppression of intestinal secretion, participation in immune processes and protective roles during inflammation [14].

During the present study, both chemically-induced inflammation and axotomy caused changes in the number of leuENK-positive colonic nerve structures, and the influence of inflammatory processes has been more visible. The differences in leuENK-like immunoreactivity have probably been connected with roles of opioids in intestinal immune functions. It is known that these substances, as well as their receptors, are present in macrophages, monocytes and some classes of lymphocytes and take part in mechanisms connected with cytokines production and T-cells proliferation [14, 42]. Another reason for the observed changes may be the participation of enkephalins in sensory stimuli conduction and anti-nociceptive mechanisms, which has been described within both the central nervous system and the enteric neurons [43–45].

Moreover, it is well-established that opioids can reduce the activity of intestinal muscles by various mechanisms such as a reduction in the release of stimulating neurotransmitters, changes in the excitability of enteric neurons and/or neuromodulatory effects on intestinal motoneurons [14, 41, 46]. Enkephalins, acting through δ-opioid receptors, which are located mainly in the myenteric plexus of the ENS, are also a major factor reducing intestinal motility [14]. It is possible that changes observed during inflammation, where an often excessive increase of muscular contractility and diarrhoea are present, may result from compensatory activity of enteric neurons. In this case, the increase of leuENK expression would have to be aimed at peristalsis inhibition and return to physiological conditions. This assumption is all the more probable that the most numerous leuENK-LI nervous structures have been noted during the inflammatory process in the muscular plexus and circular muscle layer. Since enkephalins are also known as inhibitors of intestinal secretions, the mechanisms of changes noted in the ISP could be similar to those mentioned above.

Changes in leuENK-like immunoreactivity observed in animals suffering from inflammation may also result from the participation of opioids in mechanisms connected with typical symptoms of gastrointestinal diseases, including nausea and emesis [14] and/or from neuroprotective actions of these substances. Previous studies have shown that synthetic agonists of δ-opioid receptors may prolong the cell life of many organs, such as heart, lung or kidney [47, 48], as well as have a neuroprotective influence on neuronal cells in various regions of the brain [49–51] and spinal cord [52]. It is not yet known whether endogenous or synthetic enkephalins can prolong the life of neurons supplying the GI tract in the pig, but the results obtained during the present study, as well as previous investigations on extrinsic innervation of porcine digestive tract [2, 53, 54], where pathological factors also caused an increase in leuENK-like immunoreactivity strongly suggest this fact, because it is well-established that injury to neurons causes an increase in the expression of active substances which promote the regeneration of injured cells [55].

During the present study, changes in the number of leuENK-LI nervous structures after axotomy have been less visible than during inflammation. The cutting of nerves connecting the inferior mesenteric ganglia with the descending colon caused the destruction of various types of nerves (Fig. 2). The majority of these were postganglionic sympathetic nerves, axons of neurons located predominantly in the inferior mesenteric ganglia as well as in the sympathetic chain. Other nerves derived from afferent sensory cells located in dorsal root ganglia, parasympathetic preganglionic neurons in sacral spinal cord or intestinofugal afferent (also named "viscerofugal") neurons (IFANs). IFANs, belonging to the ENS, are situated in the wall of intestine, in all kinds of enteric plexuses, send axons to prevertebral sympathetic ganglia, including coeliac ganglion, cranial mesenteric ganglion or inferior mesenteric ganglion (depending on the segment of the GI tract) and take part in intestino – intestinal reflexes without the participation of the central nervous system [56–58]. Thus, changes in leuENK-like immunoreactivity noted after axotomy may result from compensative activity of enteric neurons after the destruction of colonic extrinsic innervation or neuroprotective processes in IFANs, which is more likely in light of the relatively well-known neuroprotective effects of enkephalins, which were discussed above.

It should be pointed out that the mechanisms of changes observed during the present investigation may be variable. They can arise from an increase in leuENK synthesis in enteric neurons or modifications in intraneuronal transport of this substance from the cell body to nerve endings. In the case of fluctuations in leuENK synthesis, the changes may be due to different types of changes during transcription, translation or post-translational processes.

Conclusions

The present study shows that leuENK-positive nervous structures are present in the porcine descending colon and their distribution is similar to other species, especially to humans, which suggests the possibility of using the pig as a model animal in investigations of this peptide in the human ENS. Moreover, leuENK-like immunoreactivity in the porcine ENS undergoes fluctuations during chemically-induced inflammation and after axotomy. The increase in the number of leuENK-LI neurons and nerves can suggest neuroprotective roles of the described substance within the ENS. The present results are the first step toward exploitation of synthetic enkephalins as a medicine, not only during colitis, which has been suggested by previous studies [45], but also after intestinal innervation damage.

On the other hand, the observed changes clearly depended on both the part of the ENS and the type of factor studied.

This is prob-ably caused by different roles of leuENK in intestinal innervation, according to the type of acting pathological stimulus. These roles are still not fully explained and require further study.

Abbreviations

A group: Animals after axotomy; C group: Control group; C1 group: "Sham" operated animals; ENS: Enteric nervous system; GI tract: Gastrointestinal tract; I group: Inflammatory group; ISP: Inner submucous plexus; leuENK: Leucine enkephalin; MP: Myenteric plexus; OSP: Outer submucous plexus; Pp: Percentage point; SEM: Standard error of the mean

Funding

Publication was supported by the grant No 15.610.003-300 (statutory research) of University of Warmia and Mazury in Olsztyn (Poland) and KNOW (Leading National Research Centre) Scientific Consortium "Healthy animal – Safe Food", decision of Ministry of Science and Higher Educiation, No. 05-1/KNOW 2/2015.

Authors' contributions

SG is the originator and main performer of experiment as well as the major contributor in writing the manuscript. KM takes part in the statistical analysis of data creation of figures. JC checked the manuscript linguistically and grammatically. All authors read and approved the final manuscript.

Competing interests

The authors declare that they have no competing interests.

References

1. Wojtkiewicz J, Rowniak M, Gonkowski S, Crayton R, Majewski M, Robak A, Bialkowska J, Barczewska M. Proliferative enteropathy (PE)-induced changes in the calbindin-immunoreactive (CB-IR) neurons of inferior mesenteric ganglion supplying the descending colon in the pig. J Mol Neurosci. 2012;48:757–65.
2. Wojtkiewicz J, Rowniak M, Crayton R, Gonkowski S, Robak A, Zalecki M, Majewski M, Klimaschewski L. Axotomy-induced changes in the chemical coding pattern of Colon projecting Calbindin-positive neurons in the inferior mesenteric ganglia of the pig. J Mol Neurosci. 2013;51:99–108.
3. Chen BN, Sharrad DF, Hibberd TJ, Zagorodnyuk VP, Costa M, Brookes SJ. Neurochemical characterization of extrinsic nerves in myenteric ganglia of the Guinea pig distal colon. J Comp Neurol. 2015;523:742–56.
4. Rytel L, Calka J. Acetylsalicylic acid-induced changes in the chemical coding of extrinsic sensory neurons supplying the prepyloric area of the porcine stomach. Neurosci Lett. 2016;23:218–24.
5. Gonkowski S, Substance P. As a neuronal factor in the enteric nervous system of the porcine descending colon in physiological conditions and during selected pathogenic processes. Biofactors. 2013;39:542–51.
6. Furness JB, Callaghan BP, Rivera LR, Cho HJ. The enteric nervous system and gastrointestinal innervation: integrated local and central control. Adv Exp Med Biol. 2014;817:39–71.
7. Avetisyan M, Schill EM, Heuckeroth RO. Building a second brain in the bowel. J Clin Invest. 2015;125:899–907.
8. Gonkowski S, Burlinski P, Calka J. Proliferative enteropathy (PE) – induced changes in galanin – like immunoreactivity in the enteric nervous system of the porcine distal colon. Acta Vet-Beogr. 2009;59:321–30.
9. Saffrey MJ. Ageing of the enteric nervous system. Mech Ageing Dev. 2004;125:899–906.
10. Di Giancamillo A, Vitari F, Bosi G, Savoini G, Domeneghini C. The chemical code of porcine enteric neurons and the number of enteric glial cells are altered by dietary probiotics. Neurogastroenterol Motil. 2010;22:e271–8.
11. Vasina V, Barbara G, Talamonti L, Stanghellini V, Corinaldesi R, Tonini M, De Ponti F, De Giorgio R. Enteric neuroplasticity evoked by inflammation. Auton Neurosci. 2006;126-127:264–72.
12. Hughes J, Smith TW, Kosterlitz HW, Fothergill LA, Morgan BA, Morris HR. Identification of two related pentapeptides from the brain with potent opiate agonist activity. Nature. 1975;258:577–9.
13. Dores RM, Lecaudé S, Bauer D, Danielson PB. Analyzing the evolution of the opioid/orphanin gene family. Mass Spectrom Rev. 2002;21:220–43.
14. De Schepper HU, Cremonini F, Park MI, Camilleri M. Opioids and the gut: pharmacology and current clinical experience. Neurogastroenterol Motil. 2004;16:383–94.
15. Brehmer A, Lindig TM, Schro F, Neuhuber W, Ditterich D, Rexer M, Rupprecht H. Morphology of enkephalin-immunoreactive myenteric neurons in the human gut. Histochem Cell Biol. 2005;123:131–8.
16. Greer JJ, Carter J, Al-Zubaidy EZ. Opioid depression of respiration in neonatal rats. J Physiol. 1995;485:845–55.
17. Klarskov P. Enkephalin inhibits presynaptically the contractility of urinary tract smooth muscle. Br J Urol. 1987;59:31–5.
18. Feldman PD, Parveen N, Sezen S. Cardiovascular effects of Leu-enkephalin in the nucleus tractus solitarius of the rat. Brain Res. 1996;709:331–6.
19. Herbrecht F, Bagnol D, Cucumel F, Julé Y, Cupo A. Biochemical characterization and quantification of enkephalins in brain, prevertebral ganglia and digestive tract: a comparative study on cats, Guinea-pigs and rats. Regul Pept. 1995;57:85–95.
20. Bagnol D, Henry M, Cupo A, Julé Y. Distribution of enkephalin-like immunoreactivity in the cat digestive tract. J Auton Nerv Syst. 1997;64:1–11.
21. Wojtkiewicz J, Równiak M, Crayton R, Majewski M, Gonkowski S. Chemical coding of zinc-enriched neurons in the intramural ganglia of the porcine jejunum. Cell Tissue Res. 2012;350:215–23.
22. Puig MM, Pol O. Peripheral effects of opioids in a model of chronic intestinal inflammation in mice. J Pharmacol Exp Ther. 1998;287:1068–75.
23. Pol O, Palacio JR, Puig MM. The expression of delta- and kappa-opioid receptor is enhanced during intestinal inflammation in mice. J Pharmacol Exp Ther. 2003;306:455–62.
24. Litten-Brown JC, Corson AM, Clarke L. Porcine models for the metabolic syndrome, digestive and bone disorders: a general overview. Animal. 2010;4:899–920.
25. Verma N, Rettenmeier AW, Schmitz-Spanke S. Recent advances in the use of Sus scrofa (pig) as a model system for proteomic studies. Proteomics. 2011;11:776–93.
26. Brown DR, Timmermans JP. Lessons from the porcine enteric nervous system. Neurogastroenterol Motil. 2004;16(Suppl 1):50–4.
27. Kosugi I, Tada T, Tsutsui Y, Sato Y, Mitsui T, Itazu I. Giant inflammatory polyposis of the descending colon associated with a Crohn's disease-like colitis. Pathol Int. 2002;52:318–21.
28. Gonkowski S, Burlinski P, Szwajca P, Calka J. Changes in cocaine- and amphetamine – regulated transcript – like immunoreactive (CART-LI) nerve structures of the porcine descending colon during proliferative enteropathy. Bull Vet Inst Pulawy. 2012;56:199–203.
29. Rychlik A, Gonkowski S, Nowicki M, Calka J. Cocaine- and amphetamine-regulated transcript immunoreactive nerve fibres in the mucosal layer of the canine gastrointestinal tract under physiological conditions and in inflammatory bowel disease. Vet Med Czech. 2015;60:361–7.
30. Kinugasa T, Akagi Y. Status of colitis-associated cancer in ulcerative colitis. World J Gastrointest Oncol. 2016;8:351–7.
31. Gonkowski S, Burliński P, Skobowiat C, Majewski M, Całka J. Inflammation- and Axotomy-induced changes in galanin-like immunoreactive (GAL-LI) nerve structures in the porcine descending colon. Acta Vet Hung. 2010;58:91–103.
32. Gonkowski S, Rychlik A, Nowicki M, Nieradka R, Bulc M, Calka J. A population of nesfatin 1-like immunoreactive (LI) cells in the mucosal layer of the canine digestive tract. Res Vet Sci. 2012;93:1119–21.
33. Schultzberg M, Hökfelt T, Nilsson G, Terenius L, Rehfeld JF, Brown M, Elde R, Goldstein M, Said S. Distribution of peptide- and catecholamine-containing neurons in the gastro-intestinal tract of rat and Guinea-pig: immunochemical studies with antisera to substance P, enkephalins, somatostatin, gastrin, cholecystokinin, neurotensin and dopamine b-hydroxylase. Neuroscience. 1980;5:689–744.
34. Furness JB, Costa M, Miller RJ. Distribution and projections of nerves with enkephalin-like immunoreactivity in the Guinea-pig small intestine. Neuroscience. 1983;8:653–64.
35. Keast JR, Furness JB, Costa M. Distribution of certain peptide-containing nerve fibres and endocrine cells in the gastrointestinal mucosa in five mammalian species. J Comp Neurol. 1985;236:403–22.
36. Wattchow DA, Furness JB, Costa M. Distribution and coexistence of peptides in nerve fibers of the external muscle of the human gastrointestinal tract. Gastroenterology. 1988;95:32–41.
37. Kaleczyc J, Klimczuk M, Franke-Radowiecka A, Sienkiewicz W, Majewski M, Łakomy M. The distribution and chemical coding of intramural neurons supplying the porcine stomach - the study on normal pigs and on animals suffering from swine dysentery. Anat Histol Embryol. 2007;36:186–93.
38. Rekawek W, Sobiech P, Gonkowski S, Zarczyńska K, Snarska A, Wasniewski T, Wojtkiewicz J. Distribution and chemical coding patterns of cocaine- and amphetamine-regulated transcript-like immunoreactive (CART-LI) neurons in the enteric nervous system of the porcine stomach cardia. Pol J Vet Sci. 2015;18:515–22.
39. Simon EJ. Opioid receptors and endogenous opioid peptides. Med Res Rev. 1991;11:357–74.
40. Minami M, Satoh M. Molecular biology of the opioid receptors: structures, functions and distributions. Neurosci Res. 1995;23:121–45.
41. Sternini C, Patierno S, Selmer IS, Kirchgessner A. The opioid system in the gastrointestinal tract. Neurogastroenterol Motil. 2004;16(Suppl. 2):3–16.
42. Stein C. The control of pain in peripheral tissue by opioids. N Engl J Med. 1995;332:1685–90.
43. Skinner K, Basbaum AI, Fields HL. Cholecystokinin and enkephalin in brain stem pain modulating circuits. Neuroreport. 1997;8:2995–8.
44. Cabot PJ, Carter L, Schäfer M, Stein C. Methionine-enkephalin-and Dynorphin A-release from immune cells and control of inflammatory pain. Pain. 2001;93:207–12.
45. Sobczak M, Pilarczyk A, Jonakowski M, Jarmuż A, Sałaga M, Lipkowski AW, Fichna J. Anti-inflammatory and antinociceptive action of the dimeric enkephalin peptide biphalin in the mouse model of colitis: new potential treatment of abdominal pain associated with inflammatory bowel diseases. Peptides. 2014;60:102–6.
46. Holzer P. Opioid receptors in the gastrointestinal tract. Regul Pept. 2009;155:11–7.

7. Wu G, Zhang F, Salley RK, Diana JN, Su TP, Chien S. Delta opioid extends hypothermic preservation time of the lung. J Thorac Cardiovasc Surg. 1996;111:259–67.
8. Su TP. Delta opioid peptide [d-Ala (2), d-Leu (5)] enkephalin promotes cell sur-vival. J Biomed Sci. 2000;7:195–9.
9. Zhang J, Gibney GT, Zhao P, Xia Y. Neuroprotective role of delta-opioid receptors in cortical neurons. Am J Phys Cell Phys. 2002;282:C1225–34.
0. Borlongan CV, Wang Y, Su TP. Delta opioid peptide (d-ala 2, d-Leu 5) enkephalin: linking hibernation and neuroprotection. Front Biosci. 2004;9:3392–8.
1. Iwata M, Inoue S, Kawaguchi M, Nakamura M, Konishi N, Furuya H. Effects of delta-opioid receptor stimulation and inhibition on hippocampal survival in a rat model of forebrain ischaemia. Br J Anaesth. 2007;99:538–46.
2. Liu H, Chen B, Zhang Y, Qiu Y, Xia Y, Li S, Yao J. Protective effect of delta opioid agonist [D-Ala2, D-Leu5] enkephalin on spinal cord ischemia reperfusion injury by regional perfusion into abdominal aorta in rabbits. Neurosci Lett. 2015;584:1–6.
3. Palus K, Całka J. Alterations of neurochemical expression of the coeliac-superior mesenteric ganglion complex (CSMG) neurons supplying the prepyloric region of the porcine stomach following partial stomach resection. J Chem Neuroanat. 2016;72:25–33.
4. Palus K, Całka J. The influence of prolonged acetylsalicylic acid supplementation-induced gastritis on the neurochemistry of the sympathetic neurons supplying prepyloric region of the porcine stomach. PLoS One. 2015;10:e0143661.
5. Arciszewski MB, Ekblad E. Effects of vasoactive intestinal petide and galanin on survival of cultured porcine myenteric neurons. Regul Pept. 2005;125:185–92.
6. Luckensmeyer GB, Keast JR. Immunohistochemical characterisation of viscerofugal neurons projecting to the inferior mesenteric and major pelvic ganglia in the male rat. J Auton Nerv Syst. 1996;61:6–16.
7. Furness JB. Types of neurons in the enteric nervous system. J Auton Nerv Syst. 2000;81:87–96.
8. Ermilov LG, Miller SM, Schmalz PF, Hanani M, Lennon VA, Szurszewski JH. Morphological characteristics and immunohistochemical detection of nicotinic acetylcholine receptors on intestinofugal afferent neurones in Guinea-pig colon. Neurogastroenterol Motil. 2003;15:289–98.

20

Complete genomic characteristics and pathogenic analysis of the newly emerged classical swine fever virus in China

Hongliang Zhang[1†], Chaoliang Leng[2†], Zhijun Tian[1†], Chunxiao Liu[1], Jiazeng Chen[1], Yun Bai[1], Zhen Li[1], Lirun Xiang[1], Hongyue Zhai[2], Qian Wang[1], Jinmei Peng[1], Tongqing An[1], Yunchao Kan[2], Lunguang Yao[2], Xufu Yang[4], Xuehui Cai[1] and Guangzhi Tong[3*]

Abstract

Background: Classical swine fever (CSF) is one of the most devastating and highly contagious viral diseases in the world. Since late 2014, outbreaks of a new sub-genotype 2.1d CSF virus (CSFV) had caused substantial economic losses in numbers of C-strain vaccinated swine farms in China. The objective of the present study was to explore the genomic characteristics and pathogenicity of the newly emerged CSFV isolates in China during 2014–2015.

Results: All the new 8 CSFV isolates belonged to genetic sub-genotype 2.1d. Some genomic variations or deletions were found in the UTRs and E2 of these new isolates. In addition, the pathogenicity of HLJ1 was less than Shimen, suggesting the HLJ1 of sub-genotype 2.1d may be a moderated pathogenic isolate and the C-strain vaccine can supply complete protection.

Conclusions: The new CSFV isolates with unique genomic characteristics and moderate pathogenicity can be epidemic in many large-scale C-strain vaccinated swine farms. This study provides the information should be merited special attention on establishing prevention and control policies for CSF.

Keywords: Swine, Classical swine fever virus, Sub-genotype 2.1d, Molecular characteristics, Pathogenicity

Background

Classical swine fever virus (CSFV), the etiological agent of classical swine fever (CSF), is a single-strand, positive-sense RNA virus that belongs to the genus *Pestivirus* of the family *Flaviviridae* [1]. CSFV has a genome of about 12.3 kb comprising a single long open reading frame (ORF) coding for a polyprotein of 3, 898 amino acids flanked by two non-coding regions at the 5′ and 3′ untranslated region (UTR) [2]. The polyprotein undergoes proteolysis to produce four structural proteins (C, E^{rns}, E1, and E2) and eight non-structural proteins (N^{pro}, P7, NS2, NS3, NS4A, NS4B, NS5A, and NS5B) [3, 4].

Based on E2 and partial NS5B genes, CSFV isolates were originally classified into two genotypes and five sub-genotypes [5]. To date, CSFV have been divided into three groups with three or four subgroups (1.1, 1.2, 1.3; 2.1, 2.2, 2.3; and 3.1, 3.2, 3.3, 3.4) [6]. Sub-genotype 2.1 has been further divided into 2.1a and 2.1b groups [7, 8]. And Gong et al. reported that current CSFV sub-genotype 2.1 virus isolates in the world could be divided into 10 sub-genotypes (2.1a–2.1j) [9]. In mainland China, four sub-genotypes (1.1, 2.1, 2.2, and 2.3) of CSFV were identified, all of which contributed to CSFV outbreaks [10]. Shen et al. reported that subgroup 1.1 CSFV isolates circulated in some distinct region of south China [11]. However, sub-genotype 2.1b has become predominant within the last decade [12–14]. In recent years, sub-genotype 2.1c and 1.4 were defined [15, 16]. Recently, we confirmed a new sub-genotype 2.1d of CSFV [17]. And then the newly emerged CSFV isolates of China in 2014–2015 were also characterized by our laboratory. In the present study, the complete genomes of 8 newly emerged CSFV isolates in China in

* Correspondence: lenghan1223@126.com
[†]Hongliang Zhang, Chaoliang Leng and Zhijun Tian contributed equally to this work.
[3]Shanghai Veterinary Research Institute, Chinese Academy of Agricultural Sciences, No. 518, Ziyue Road, Minhang District, Shanghai 200241, China
Full list of author information is available at the end of the article

2014–2015 were sequenced and analyzed. Moreover, the pathogenicity of one of these isolates, HLJ1, was evaluated.

Methods

Clinical samples, virus isolation and virus strains

More than 20 Clinical samples of lung, lymphatic, and spleen tissue were collected from pigs suspected to have CSFV infections in Shandong, Jiangsu, Hebei, Jilin and Heilongjiang provinces of China between October 2014 and August 2015.

Swine testicular (ST) cells were used for CSFV propagation and titration in RPMI Medium 1640 (Gibco, USA) supplemented with 10% heat-inactivated fetal bovine serum (FBS) (Invitrogen), 0.1 mg/ml streptomycin and 100 U/ml antibiotic penicillin. Clinical tissues (Lungs) were homogenized using TissuLyser II (Qiagen, Germany) and centrifuged 10, 000×g for 10 min. The supernatant was filtered through a 0.45-μm filter and transferred to ST cells monolayer. The cells were incubated at 37 °C for 1 h. Then prepared medium was added with 6 ml in volume and the cells were incubated for another 72 h. The cultures were harvested and then stored at − 80 °C as viral stocks. CSFV adaptation in ST cells was conducted for at least 15 passages, and some normally co-infected porcine pathogens, including porcine reproductive and respiratory syndrome virus (PRRSV), pseudorabies virus (PRV), porcine circovirus type 2 (PCV2) and mycoplasma were detected in the viral stocks.

The cultures of the third passage of CSFV HLJ1 in ST cells were quantified and used for challenge virus. The CSFV Shimen strain, a highly virulent strain isolated in China in 1945, were also used as a reference challenge virus in the present study.

Primer design and RT-PCR

Six pairs of primers based on the published known sequence of CSFV Zj0801 (GenBank accession no. FJ529205) were designed for PCR analysis (Table 1). The cultures were prepared for reverse transcription PCR (RT-PCR) using an RNA extraction QIAamp viral RNA Mini Kit (Qiagen, Germany). RT-PCR was conducted as previously reported [17].

Genome cloning and sequencing

Genome cloning and sequencing was conducted as previously reported [17]. Briefly, RT-PCR products were analyzed by using 1% agarose gel electrophoresis, and the target fragments were excised from gels for purification using a Gel Extraction Kit (OMEGA, USA). The purified PCR products were then cloned into a pMD18-T vector (TaKaRa Dalian, China) and sequenced by Comate Bioscience (Jilin, China).

Table 1 Primers used for the amplification of the full-length CSFV

Fragment	Primer sequence (5'-3') [a]	Position in genome[a]	Product size (bp)[a]
CSFV-A	GTATACGAGGTTAGTTCATTCTCGT GATTACCAGAGAAAGCAACAAGAAT	1-2047	2047
CSFV-B	GATAATAGGCCCCGGTAAATTTGAC TTTCCTTACAGGTCCCTCGCTAGAG	2023–3313	1291
CSFV-C	AAATGAGACGGGTTACACGGTA CATCCCGTAGATCTCTTCACCTCCA	3124–4771	1648
CSFV-D	CATAGATGAAATAGCTGGCGGGACC TAGTGCTCTGCCAGCCTCCACAGTG	4564–7171	2608
CSFV-E	TCTGCTGATATCAGAGGAGCTG GCTTACCCAGACTTAATGTTTCTAG	6866–9668	2803
CSFV-F	GCCCTATGTAAGGTCGACACCGCTC GGGCCGTTAGGAAATTACCTTAGTC	9572–12,296	2725

[a]The sequence of primer sequence, position in genome and product size with respect to the CSFV Zj0801 (accession no. FJ529205) genome

Phylogenetic analysis

The 8 new CSFV isolates and 44 reference CSFV strains (Tables 2 and 3), based on the full of genome, were used for construction of phylogenetic tree (Fig. 1). The phylogenetic tree was constructed using MEGA 5.1 with the maximum likelihood method based on 1000 bootstraps [18]. Multiple sequence alignments were generated using MUSCLE and MEGA software [19].

Nucleotides and amino acid analysis

The complete genome sequences and deduced amino acid sequences of the 8 new isolates were analyzed and their homologies with other 8 representative CSFV strains were compared using the Clustal W method of Lasergene (Version 7.1) (DNASTAR Inc., Madison, WI, USA) (Table 4).

To explore the genetic variations of the 8 new isolates, the nucleotide sequences of the 5'UTR and the 3'UTR and the amino acid sequences of E2 were fully analyzed by CLC Sequence Viewer 8.0, together with another 23 CSFV isolates from China and other countries.

Table 2 Information of 8 newly emerged sub-genotype 2.1d CSFVs

No.	Isolates	Sample	Time	Area
1	SDLS1410	Lung	2014.10	Shandong
2	SDSG1410	Lung	2014.10	Shandong
3	JSZL1412	Serum	2014.12	Jiangsu
4	HB150309	Lung	2015.03	Hebei
5	JL150418	Lung	2015.04	Jilin
6	NK150425	Lung	2015.04	Heilongjiang
7	SDZC1506C1	Lung	2015.05	Shandong
8	HLJ1	Lung	2015.03	Heilongjiang

Table 3 The reference CSFVs used in this study

No.	Virus strain	Year	Origin	Genotype	Accession no.
1	Alfort 187	2010	Switzerland	1.1	X87939
2	Alfort A19	1997	France	1.1	U90951
3	Brescia	1998	Switzerland	1.1	AF091661
4	C-ZJ-2008	2008	China	1.1	HM175885
5	GZ-2009	2009	China	1.1	HQ380231
6	HCLV	1999	China	1.1	AF091507
7	HVRI	2006	China	1.1	AY805221
8	JL1(06)	2006	China	1.1	EU497410
9	Koslov	2010	Germany	1.1	HM237795
10	NG79–11	2014	India	1.1	KC503764
11	Shimen	1999	China	1.1	AF092448
12	VB-131	2014	India	1.1	KM262189
13	Bresciax 90	1990	Netherlands	1.2	M31768
14	RUCSFPLUM	2001	USA	1.2	AY578688
15	CSF0277	1997	Germany	2.1	JQ411566
16	96TD	2005	China	2.1a	AY554397
17	Paderborn	2001	Denmark	2.1a	AY072924
18	SXCDK	2009	China	2.1a	GQ923951
19	0406-CH	2005	China	2.1b	AY568569
20	CSF1048	2009	Germany	2.1b	HQ148063
21	GXWZ02	2003	China	2.1b	AY367767
22	HEBZ	2009	China	2.1b	GU592790
23	HuN23–2013	2013	China	2.1b	KP233071
24	SXYL2006	2006	China	2.1b	GQ122383
25	YC11WB	2011	Korea	2.1b	KC149990
26	GXF29/2013	2013	China	2.1c	KP233070
27	HNLY-2011	2011	China	2.1c	JX262391
28	HNSD-2012	2012	China	2.1c	JX218094
29	Heb52010	2010	China	2.1d	JQ268754
30	HLJZZ2014	2014	China	2.1d	KU375260
31	PC11WB	2011	Korea	2.1d	KC149991
32	Zj0801	2008	China	2.1d	FJ529205
33	39	2001	China	2.2	AF407339
34	LAL-290	2012	India	2.2	KC851953
35	Alfort/Tuebingen	1989	Germany	2.3	J04358
36	Borken	2006	Germany	2.3	GU233731
37	Euskirchen	2005	Germany	2.3	GU233732
38	Hennef	2009	Germany	2.3	GU233733
39	Jambul	2007	Bulgaria	2.3	HQ148062
40	Novska	2002	Croatia	2.3	HQ148061
41	Roesrath	2009	Germany	2.3	GU233734
42	Sp01	2001	Spain	2.3	FJ265020
43	Uelzen	2004	Germany	2.3	GU324242
44	JJ9811	1998	Korea	3.2	KF669877
45	P97	2006	–	3.4	L49347
46	TWN	1994	China	3.4	AY646427

Experimental CSFV inoculation of SPF piglets

A total of 10 five-week-old specific pathogen-free (SPF) Bama piglets were obtained from the Experimental Animal Center of the Harbin Veterinary Research Institute, and were randomly divided into three groups (A, B, and C) and maintained in individual biosafety rooms. The piglets in group A ($n = 3$) were inoculated intramuscularly (2 ml) with Shimen strain at a dose of $1 \times 10^{7.0}$ copies. The piglets in group B ($n = 3$) were inoculated with the new CSFV HLJ1 strain with the same method and dose as group A. The piglets in group C ($n = 4$) were mock infected with 2 ml RPMI Medium 1640. Clinical symptoms were observed daily throughout the study, and rectal temperatures were recorded daily before feeding. Blood samples were collected at 0, 7, 14, 21, 28, 31 and 35 days post inoculation (DPI). All remaining pigs were euthanized on 35 DPI. Tissue samples were obtained from the hearts, livers, spleens, lungs, kidney, lymph nodes, tonsils, small intestines, bladders and stomach for virus detection by RT-PCR, and histopathological or immunohistochemistry (IHC) examination. To determine the level of virulence of the new CSFV HLJ1 strain, the clinical scoring (CS) system was used as described previously [20].

Histopathological examination and IHC

Tissue samples were subjected to histopathological and IHC examination as previously described [21, 22]. Briefly, tissue samples were fixed in 10% neural buffered formalin for 48 h, embedded in paraffin wax and sectioned. Thin sections with 4-μm thickness stained with hematoxylin and eosin (H–E staining) for histopathological examinations. 4-μm sections were treated with 3% hydrogen peroxide in PBS for 20 min followed by washes in PBS and digestion with 0.05% protease (protease XIV; Sigma) for 5 min at 37 °C. Then washes with PBS, sections were incubated in blocking solutions with 8% skim milk for 40 min at room temperature. After washes with PBS, sections were incubated for 2 h at 4 °C with rabbit antiserum against CSFV (saved by our laboratory) diluted 1:200 in PBS. Then washes with PBS, sections were incubated with anti-rabbit IgG-peroxidase antibody produced in goat (Sigma) diluted 1:400 in PBS for 40 min at room temperature.

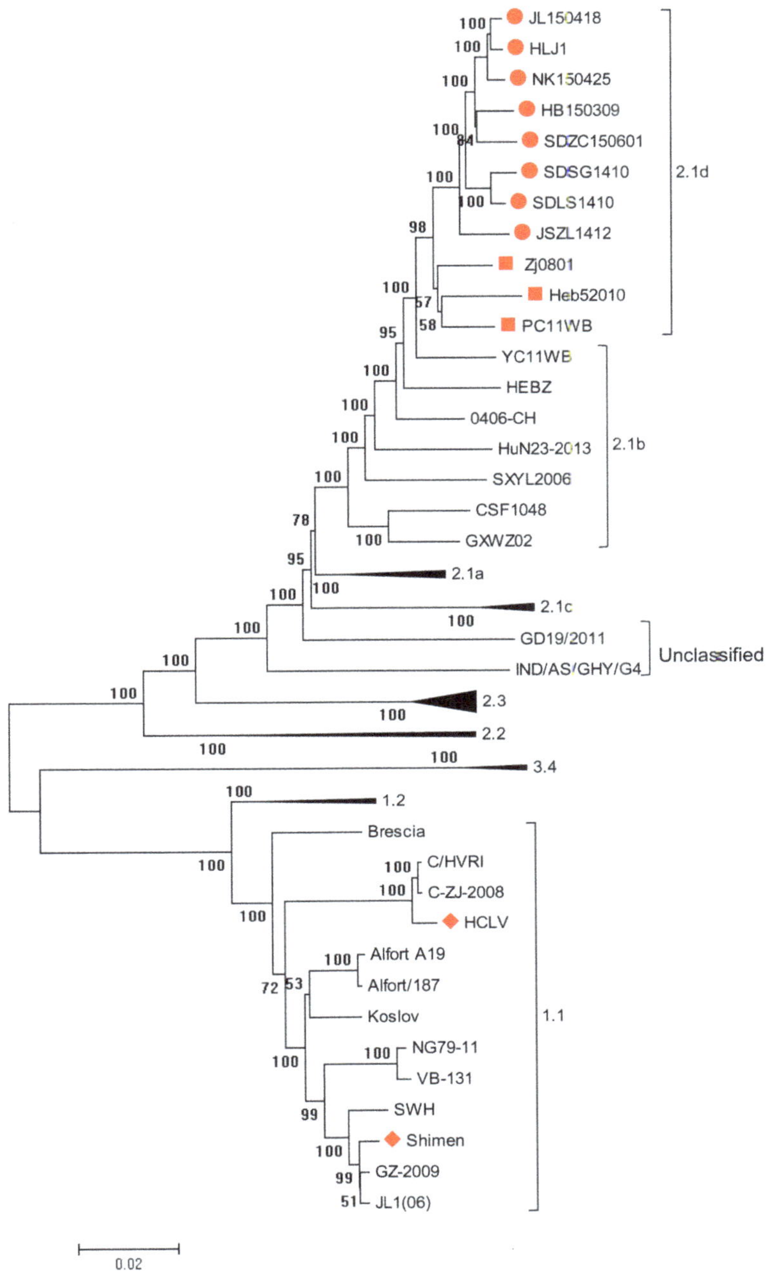

Fig. 1 Phylogenetic analysis of the 8 new isolates and 44 reference strains based on the complete CSFV genomes. The 8 new CSFV isolates and 3 reference strains were located in a branch belonging to 2.1d sub-genotype, labeled by ● and ■, respectively. The Shimen strain and its attenuated live vaccine strain, HCLV, were located in another branch belonging to 1.1 sub-genotype, labeled by ◆

Results

Virus isolation and genome sequencing

8 new CSFV isolates named HLJ1, SDSG1410, SDLS1410, JSZL1412, HB150309, JL150418, NK150425 and SDZC150601, from 5 provinces (Shandong, Jiangsu, Hebei, Jilin and Heilongjiang) in China, were acquired and sequenced (Table 2). And their complete genome sequences were 12,295, 12,295, 12,296, 12,297, 12,295, 12,295, 12,295 and 12,294 nucleotides in length, respectively.

Phylogenetic analysis

A total of 8 new CSFV isolates and 44 reference strains, based on the full genome, were used to construct phylogenetic tree (Fig. 1). CSFV isolates were divided into genotype 1, 2 and 3. Genotype 2 isolates were further

Table 4 Detailed comparison of the full-length genomes of the 8 newly emerged sub-genotype 2.1d CSFVs to other CSFV representative isolates (%)

	Shimen (1.1)	Paderborn (2.1a)	HEBZ (2.1b)	HNSD-2012 (2.1c)	Zj0801 (2.1d)	CSFV39 (2.2)	Alfort (2.3)	TWN (3.4)
Nucleotides								
5'UTR	91.4–92.2	96.5–97.3	95.4–96.2	94.4–95.2	97.0–98.7	91.6–92.5	93.3–94.1	90.3–91.9
N^{pro}	87.1–88.1	94.0–94.8	94.2–95.4	92.1–92.7	96.8–98.0	88.3–89.1	88.3–88.9	84.1–85.3
C	84.5–86.2	94.3–95.3	93.3–94.6	90.2–92.3	95.6–97.3	89.6–90.9	89.9–91.2	83.2–84.8
E^{rns}	84.1–85.3	93.2–94.6	96.5–97.1	92.1–93.1	97.7–98.2	89.4–89.7	89.6–90.5	82.4–8.4
E1	84.4–85.3	93.8–94.7	96.4–97.3	91.3–92.1	97.6–98.5	90.3–91.5	88.4–89.6	81.4–82.1
E2	83.5–84.3	93.5–94.3	95.5–96.5	90.1–91.0	96.6–97.1	87.0–87.5	86.9–87.8	82.0–82.4
P7	79.7–81.6	90.8–93.2	95.2–97.1	91.8–94.2	95.7–98.6	87.4–89.4	88.4–90.3	82.6–85.5
NS2	82.6–83.4	92.9–93.4	96.2–96.6	91.8–92.3	96.9–97.5	89.1–89.6	88.5–89.1	80.2–81.0
NS3	86.4–87.0	94.6–95.1	95.7–96.1	92.8–93.6	97.1–97.4	90.3–91.0	90.8–91.7	85.4–86.1
NS4A	86.2–87.8	94.7–96.3	94.2–95.8	91.0–92.6	97.9–98.9	87.8–89.4	87.8–89.4	82.5–94.1
NS4B	85.8–86.5	92.8–93.6	95.0–95.8	90.1–91.1	96.6–97.8	89.3–90.0	88.4–89.1	83.1–84.1
NS5A	83.7–84.3	93.6–94.0	96.2–96.7	90.7–91.3	97.0–97.3	83.8–84.3	90.6–90.9	82.5–82.9
NS5B	84.7–85.3	94.9–95.3	95.8–96.4	92.5–93.2	97.5–97.8	85.2–85.7	89.5–89.9	83.4–83.7
3'UTR	84.1–85.0	93.8–95.1	94.7–96.0	93.8–95.6	97.3–98.7	83.6–84.4	92.9–94.2	82.6–84.0
Complete	85.0–85.3	94.1–94.4	95.9–96.2	91.9–92.3	97.2–97.5	87.9–88.2	89.6–89.9	83.4–83.7
Amino acid								
N^{pro}	91.7–92.9	94.6–95.8	95.8–97.0	94.6–95.8	96.4–97.6	91.7–92.9	92.3–92.9	90.5–91.7
C	92.9–94.9	93.9–97.0	94.9–97.0	91.9–94.9	96.0–98.0	91.9–96.0	92.9–94.9	88.9–90.9
E^{rns}	89.0–89.9	96.9–97.8	97.4–98.2	96.9–97.8	98.7–99.6	94.3–95.2	95.6–96.0	90.3–91.2
E1	92.8–93.8	97.4–98.5	96.9–97.9	94.9–95.9	99.5–100.0	96.9–97.9	96.4–97.4	88.7–90.3
E2	90.1–91.2	95.4–96.5	96.2–97.6	94.9–95.7	97.1–98.1	90.9–92.0	91.4–92.5	89.0–90.1
P7	88.4–89.9	95.7–98.6	92.8–95.7	94.2–97.1	95.7–98.6	94.2–95.7	94.2–95.7	91.3–94.2
NS2	89.7–90.6	95.6–96.3	97.4–98.0	95.8–96.3	97.2–98.0	94.7–95.2	93.4–94.1	86.9–87.7
NS3	97.7–98.5	98.7–99.6	98.4–99.1	98.1–98.8	98.1–98.8	97.9–98.7	98.4–99.1	97.8–98.7
NS4A[a]	98.4	100.0	98.4	95.2	100.0	96.8	100.0	95.2
NS4B	95.1–96.3	97.4–98.6	97.7–98.6	98.3–99.4	98.3–98.8	96.5–97.1	97.4–98.6	93.7–94.8
NS5A	87.5–89.0	95.6–96.6	96.2–97.4	93.2–94.8	96.4–97.2	87.1–88.0	93.2–94.0	86.3–87.3
NS5B	92.3–93.2	97.5–98.2	97.6–98.3	97.3–98.0	98.0–98.7	93.0–93.9	96.2–97.2	89.8–90.9

[a]The amino acid homology of NS4A protein of the 8 new isolates between each other was 100%

divided into sub-genotype 2.1, 2.2, and 2.3, and sub-genotype 2.1 isolates could be further subdivided into 2.1a, 2.1b, 2.1c, and 2.1d, which were consistent with the classification results based on E2 and partial NS5B gene [17]. Phylogenetic tree also showed that the 8 new isolates and 3 reference CSFVs (Zj0801, Heb52010 and PC11W) belong to sub-genotype 2.1d. The virulent Shimen strain and its attenuated live vaccine strain HCLV belong to sub-genotype 1.1.

Analysis of full-length genomic sequences

The complete nucleotide sequences of the 8 new CSFV isolates were compared with 8 representative CSFV isolates, including Shimen, Paderborn, HEBZ, HNSD-20, Zj0801, CSFV39, Alfort and TWN (Table 4). Results indicated that the 8 new isolates shared 97.2–97.5% homology with 2.1d isolate Zj0801, the most closely related strain. Other representative CSFV strains similar to the new isolates were included 2.1a isolate Paderborn and 2.1c isolate HNSD-2012, which shared 94.1–94.4% and 91.9–92.3% homology, respectively. In addition, they shared only 83.4–89.9% homology with 1.1 isolate Shimen, 2.2 isolate CSFV39, 2.3 isolate Alfort or 3.4 isolate TWN. Taken together, these results indicate that all these isolates belong to sub-genotype 2.1d, which was consistent with the result of phylogenetic analysis.

To further examine the genomic variation of the 8 isolates, their genomic characteristics were analyzed in detail. Compared with the representative isolates, the 5'UTRs of the new isolates were the most conserved regions in the genomes, which exhibited 94.4–98.7% homology with 2.1 isolates Paderborn, HEBZ, HNSD-2012 or Zj0801, 93.3–94.1% homology with 2.3 isolate Alfort, 91.6–92.5% homology with 2.2 isolate CSFV39 and 90.3–92.2% homology with 1.1 isolate Shimen or 3.4 isolate TWN. In addition, the amino acid identities of NS3, NS4A and NS4B between the new isolates and representative isolates were higher than other regions of the CSFV genome, and the homologies were 97.7–99.6%, 95.2–100% and 93.7–99.4%, respectively. The detailed identities of the three isolates and eight other representative strain isolates are summarized in Table 4.

Sequence analysis of UTRs

Compared with sub-genotype 1.1 isolates, the 5'UTRs of the new isolates had a nucleotide A deletion at position 49 (A^{49}), which was similar to most of the 2.1 isolates (Fig. 2). In addition, the 5'UTRs of the 6 new isolates (SDSG1410, HB150309, JL150418, NK150425, SDZC150601 and HLJ1) had two continuous nucleotide A deletions at positions 357–358 compared with 2.3 isolate Broken (GU233731), while other 2 new isolates (SDLS1410 and JSZL1412) show only one nucleotide A deletion at these positions (Fig. 2). And most of the CSFV isolates shared the characteristic of the two continuous deletions at these positions (Fig. 2).

Compared with the vaccine strain HCLV, the 3'UTRs of all the 8 new isolates had 12 continuous nucleotide deletions (TTTTTCTTTTTT) at positions 63–74, which were similar to most of the CSFV isolates (Fig. 2). However, among the 23 reference CSFV isolates, the CSFV-PK15C-5NG79–11 (KC503764) strain had 7 nucleotide deletions (CTTTTTT), and the CSFV/IVRI/VB-131 (KM262189) strain had 9 nucleotide deletions (TTCTTTTTT). The other two strains, RUCSFPLUM (AY578688) and Rovac (KJ873238), had 11 nucleotide deletions (TTTTTCTTTTTT) at these positions (Fig. 2). In addition, compared with 1.1 isolates, the 3'UTRs of most 2.1 isolates, including the 8 new isolates, had two discontinuous nucleotide T deletions at positions 182 and 210, respectively (Fig. 2)

Amino acid analysis of E2

The E2 amino acid sequences of the 8 new isolates and 23 reference isolates were compared and analyzed (Fig. 3). And some unique molecular characteristics were found for the new isolates, including the amino acid R at

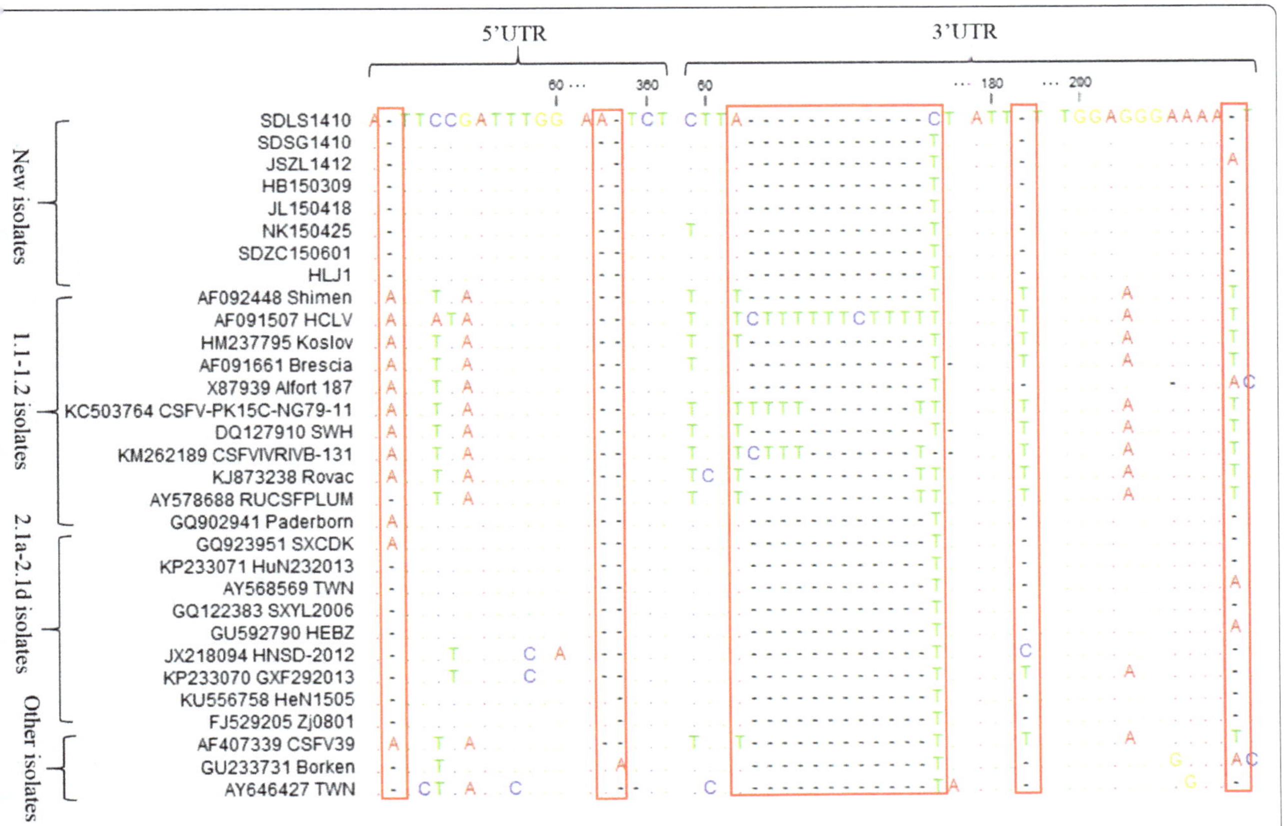

Fig. 2 Sequence alignments of 5'UTR and 3'UTR of the 8 new CSFV isolates and 23 reference isolates. Some mutation or deletion regions of these isolates are indicated by red boxes (□) and described in detail in the text

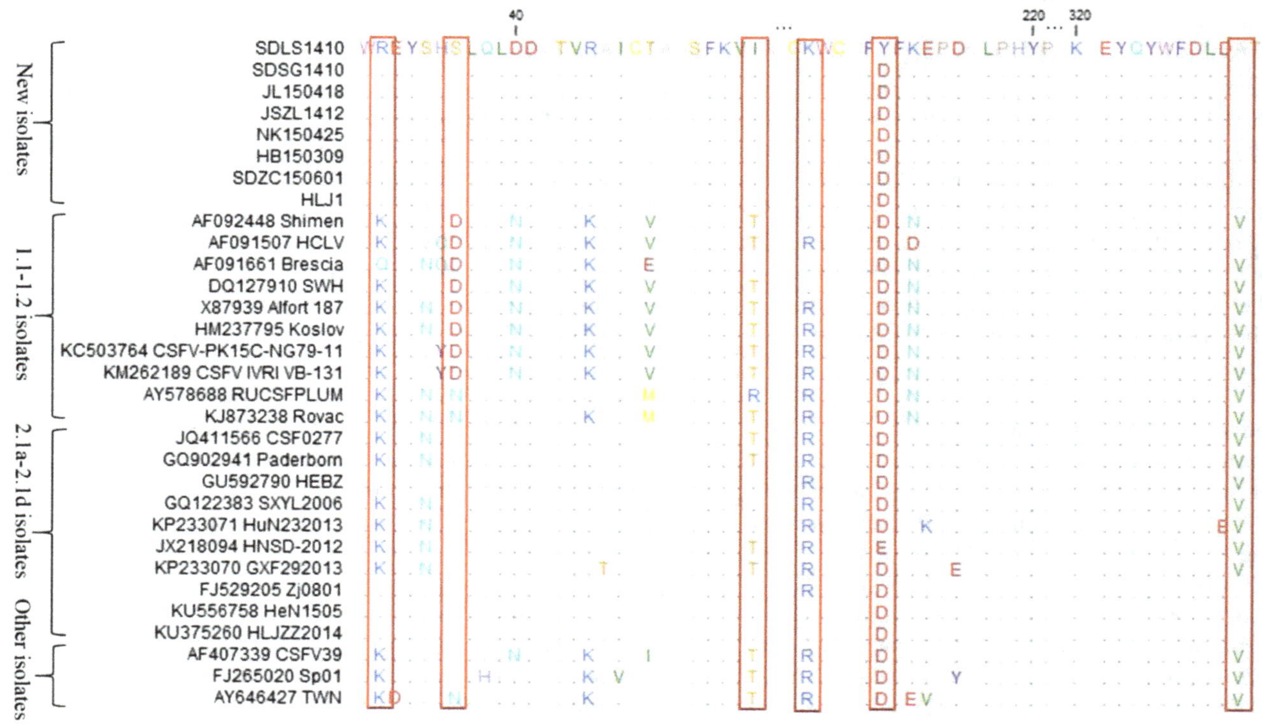

Fig. 3 Amino acid sequence alignments of E2 genes of the 8 new CSFV isolates and 23 reference isolates. The special mutation positions of these isolates are indicated by red boxes (☐) and described in detail in the text

position 31 (R^{31}), I^{56}, K^{205} and A^{331}. And these molecular characteristics were consistent with 2.1d isolates and some 2.1b isolates. In addition, the two new isolates, SDLS1410 and SDSG1410, were S^{36}, different from all other isolates. Similarly, at position 210, the SDLS1410 was amino acid Y, and all other sub-genotype isolates were amino acid D (Fig. 3).

Experimental CSFV inoculation of SPF piglets

The piglets in groups A and B displayed obvious clinical signs, including fever, anorexia and diarrhea, reddening of the conjunctiva and ocular discharge, shivering, and lethargy. In addition, the onset of fever was significantly sooner in group A (Shimen inoculation) than in group B (HLJ1 inoculation) (Fig. 4a). Furthermore, 3/3 piglets in group A died and 2/3 piglets in group B died at 11 DPI (Fig. 4b). The piglets in group C showed no clinical signs throughout the experiment. Based on the CS system, each pig was judged daily after experimental inoculation. The peak CS value of Shimen-infected and HLJ1-infected pigs were determined to be 25–26 and 12–14, respectively, indicating that the HLJ1 strain was moderately virulent (5<peak CS ≤15) (Fig. 4c). The groups A and B piglets showed lesions typical of CSF, such as necrosis in the tonsils, hemorrhaging in the lymph nodes, splenic infarcts and pint hemorrhaging in almost all of the organs (Fig. 5a1-a3 and b1-b3). Histopathology revealed lymphocyte decrease accompanied by partial lymphoid follicle atrophy in tonsils, interstitial pneumonia, and inflammatory lymphohistiocytic infiltrates in the kidney and liver, necrosis of white pulp and lymphocyte depletion in the spleen and varied degrees of hyperemia and hemorrhage in most tissues (Fig. 5a4-a6 and b4-b6). In addition, the immunoreactivity was observed in the crypt of tonsil of the piglets in groups A and B (Fig. 5a7 and b7). Virus detection of different tissues and serum samples showed that all samples of piglets in groups A and B were positive, while samples of piglets in group C were negative (data not shown).

Discussion

CSF is one of the most devastating and highly contagious viral diseases that has caused huge economic losses to pig farms and remains a lingering problem in many parts of the world [23]. Since nationwide vaccinations were implemented, large CSF outbreaks have been rare. However, no regions have been declared free of CSF, and there is still a long way to go to control and ultimately eradicate CSF in China [24]. Four CSFV sub-genotypes, 1.1, 2.1, 2.2, and 2.3, have been identified in mainland China [10]. And a new sub-genotype 2.1d was emerged in China recently [15]. Since late 2014, a

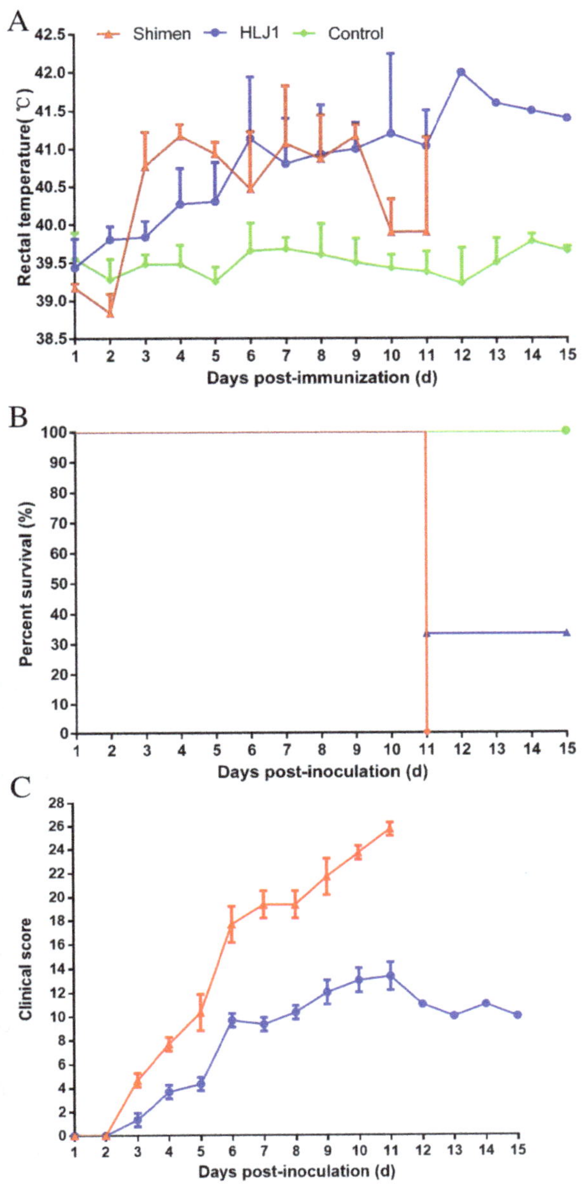

Fig. 4 Rectal temperatures (**a**), mortality rates (**b**) and clinical scores (**c**) of piglets inoculated with CSFV Shimen and HLJ1. Mean temperatures ± standard deviations (error bars) are shown (group **a**, $n = 3$; group **b**, $n = 3$ and group **c**, $n = 4$). Rectal temperatures > 40.5 °C were defined as fever

ew sub-genotype 2.1d isolates were emerged and identified in China [17, 25]. In the present study, we first reported 8 newly emerged CSFV isolates in China in 2014–2015.

The 5'UTR, partial E2 (190 nt), and partial NS5B (409 nt) gene sequences have been widely used for classification of CSFV isolates [26, 27]. Postel et al. reported that the full-length E2 gene sequence provides better resolution for phylogenetic analysis [28]. And identification of sub-genotypes 2.1c and 2.1d was based on the full-length E2 gene sequence [15, 17]. Some labs reported that the whole genome sequence of CSFV could provide more reliable classification criterion [29, 30]. In the present study, the phylogenetic tree was constructed based on the complete genomes. And 8 new isolates were classified into 2.1d sub-genotype (Fig. 1), which was consistent with the results that the phylogenetic tree was constructed based on the full-length E2 gene or partial NS5B gene (data not shown). Interestingly, the 2.1d isolates were located in a relatively concentrated branch close to 2.1b isolates (Fig. 1). The reason may be that sub-genotype 2.1b isolates have become predominant within the last decade in China and the new 2.1d isolates are found to possibly diverge from 2.1b isolates [12–14, 31].

The complete genomic sequences of the 8 new CSFV isolates were compared with other representative CSFV isolates (Table 4). The results indicated that the 8 isolates shared the highest nucleotide homology with Zj0801, the representative strain of sub-genotype 2.1d. And these new isolates also showed high homology with the sub-genotype 2.1b isolate, HEBZ. These results were consistent with the result of phylogenetic analysis. In addition, we also found that the 5'UTRs of the 8 isolates were the most conserved regions in the genomes. And NS3, NS4A and NS4B proteins were more conserved than other regions in the CSFV genome.

The 5'UTR and 3'UTR have been documented to be crucial regulatory elements in the CSFV genome [32]. Sequence alignment showed that the 5'UTRs of the 8 new isolates had the same nucleotide deletions at positions 44 compared with 1.1 isolates (Fig. 2). However, compared with 2.3 isolate Broken, the 6 new isolates (SDSG1410, HB150309, JL150418, NK150425, SDZC150601 and HLJ1) had two continuous nucleotide A deletions at positions 357–358, which was identical to most of the reference CSFV isolates. And other 2 new isolates (SDLS1410 and JSZL1412) show only one nucleotide A deletion at these positions (Fig. 2). Whether the deletions affect the structural characteristics of the 5'UTRs requires experimental confirmation. However, CSFV virulence may vary according to the number and shape of the pseudoknot loop in the secondary structure of 5'UTR and its positional direction in three-dimensional space [29, 33]. Thus, the two groups isolates may have different virulence characteristics.

The 3'UTR is the region with the most variation in the CSFV genome. And the poly-T deletion in the 3'UTR is an important virulence factor and becomes an attenuated-symptom phenotype of CSFV [34]. In the present study, we found that all the 8 new isolates had the poly-T deletion region compared to the vaccine strain HCLV (Fig. 2). We conclude that these isolates

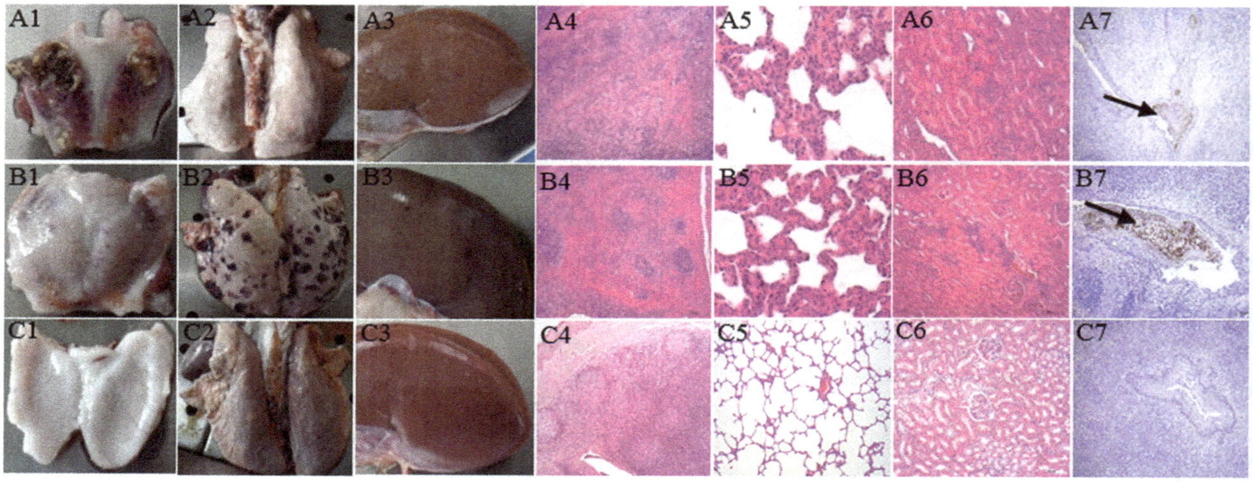

Fig. 5 Gross and histological lesions of tonsils, lungs and kidneys of piglets in different groups. Piglets infected with Shimen (**a**1-**a**3) or HLJ1 (**b**1-**b**3) showed obvious necrosis, hemorrhaging or hemorrhagic spots than mock-infected (**c**1-**c**3) piglets. Histopathology of tonsils, lungs and kidneys of Shimen- (**a**4-**a**6), HLJ1-infected (**b**4-**b**6) piglets manifested partial lymphoid follicle atrophy, interstitial pneumonia or lymph histiocytic infiltrates than control (**c**4-**c**6). Viral antigen of CSFV was detected in the tonsils of piglets in Shimen- or HLJ1-infected groups by means of IHC staining (**a**7, **b**7). The tonsils of piglets in control group were negative for CSFV (C7). Original magnification, × 200

were virulent wild CSFV strains with similar virulence. In addition, we also found several previous reported isolates, including CSFV-PK15C-NG79–11, CSFV/IVRI/VB-131, RUCSFPLUM and Rovac, with different deletions in this region, which suggested the differences in the pathogenicity of these strains. Recently, a unique poly-T tract was discovered in the 3'UTR of the CSFV Pinar del Rio strain compared with all other CSFV isolates [35]. And whether this novel insertion affect the pathogenicity of the virus remains unknown. In addition, many studies reported that NS3, NS5A and NS5B of CSFV can interact with 3'UTR to regulate viral RNA synthesis and replication [36–38]. In this study, we also found the 3'UTRs of the 8 new isolates and most sub-genotype 2.1 isolates had two discontinuous nucleotide deletions compared with those of 1.1 isolates (Fig. 2). Whether nucleotide deletions in the 3'UTR affect the interactions with other proteins requires further research.

The E2 protein is the most antigenic protein of CSFV and is involved in virus neutralization [39]. Four antigenic domains, A (86–176 amino acids), B (1–83 amino acids), C (1–110 amino acids), and D (86–110 amino acids), have been mapped on E2 [40]. And domain A has been subdivided into A1, A2, and A3 [40]. In the present study, we found several unique amino acid substitutions for the new isolates on these domains and other regions (Fig. 3). However, the influence of these substitutions on the structure and function of E2 requires further study. In addition, the six cysteines at positions 4, 48, 103, 129, 139, and 167, which were essential for binding by monoclonal antibodies of the four domains, showed no variation in the E2 proteins of these isolates [40]. Furthermore, the potential N-glycosylation sites in the E2 proteins of the 8 isolates were consistent with previous isolates.

The CSFV genotype 1 isolates, such as shimen, showed high pathogenicity, and the Chinese lapinized attenuated vaccine (C-strain) was acquired through the attenuation of the strain, while the genotype 2 or 3 isolates revealed moderate or low virulence [41, 42]. However Floegel-Niesmann et al. reported that two CSFV isolates CSF0277 and CSF0849, belonged to sub-genotype 2.1 had been characterized as moderately and highly virulent strains, respectively [43]. In the present study, the pathogenicity of the new HLJ1 isolate which belonged to sub-genotype 2.1d was assessed. Results of animal experiments indicated that the pathogenicity of HLJ1 was less than Shimen (Figs. 4 and Fig. 5), and was similar to HLJZZ2014, a sub-genotype 2.1d isolate with moderate virulence identified recently [44]. In recent years, the C-strain vaccine was widely used to prevent CSFV infection in China. And this vaccine can supply complete protection against the HLJ1 challenging in the lab (data not shown). However, the new sub-genotype 2.1d CSFV isolates could also be epidemic in many immunized pig farms, which was worth of vigilant. The deeper reasons such as immunization program, vaccine quality, interference by other pathogens and so on, need further study.

Conclusion

The complete genomes of 8 new CSFV isolates were fully analyzed in the present study. We found that the 8 isolates all belonged to genetic subgroup 2.1d. And some genomic variations or deletions were found in the UTR nd E2. Furthermore, we found that the pathogenicity of he new HLJ1 isolate was less than Shimen. And the ub-genotype 2.1d isolates could be classified into the SFV strains with moderate virulence. In any case, the pidemic of these isolates should be focus on monitoring nd the information of the present study should be considered when establishing control and vaccine strategies or CSF.

bbreviations

SF: Classical swine fever; CSFV: Classical swine fever virus; DPI: Days post noculation; FBS: Fetal bovine serum; ORF: Open reading frame; SPF: Specific athogen-free; ST: Swine testicular; UTR: Untranslated region

cknowledgements

Ve thank Fei Xiao, Shouping Hu and Xijun He (Pathology laboratory, Harbin eterinary Research Institute, CAAS) for doing the IHC.

unding

he National Key R&D Program (2016YFD0500100) and the National Natural cience Foundation of China (31502097), the Scientific and Technological roject of Henan Province (182102110240) and the Foundation of Nanyang ormal University (15082) supported this study.

uthors' contributions

LZ, CLL, XFY, XHC, ZJT and GZT conceived and designed the experiment. LZ, CXL, JZC, YB, ZL, LRX and HYZ performed the experiment. HLZ, CLL, W, JMP, TQA, YCK and LGY performed analysis and prepared the manuscript. ll authors read and approved the final manuscript.

ompeting interests

he authors declare that they have no competing interests.

uthor details

State Key Laboratory of Veterinary Biotechnology, Harbin Veterinary esearch Institute, Chinese Academy of Agricultural Sciences, Harbin 150001, hina. [2]Henan Key Laboratory of Insect Biology in Funiu Mountain, Henan rovincial Engineering Laboratory of Insects Bio-reactor, hina-UK-NYNU-RRes Joint Laboratory of Insect Biology, Nanyang Normal niversity, Nanyang 473061, China. [3]Shanghai Veterinary Research Institute, hinese Academy of Agricultural Sciences, No. 518, Ziyue Road, Minhang istrict, Shanghai 200241, China. [4]North Guangdong Collaborative Innovation nd Development Center of Pig Farming and Disease Control, Shaoguan niversity, Shaoguan 512005, China.

eferences

- Becher P, Avalos Ramirez R, Orlich M, Cedillo Rosales S, Konig M, Schweizer M, Stalder H, et al. Genetic and antigenic characterization of novel pestivirus genotypes: implications for classification. Virology. 2003;311:96–104.
- Wu HX, Wang JF, Zhang CY, Fu LZ, Pan ZS, Wang N, et al. Attenuated lapinized chinese strain of classical swine fever virus: complete nucleotide sequence and character of 3'-noncoding region. Virus Genes. 2001;23:69–76.
- Meyers G, Thiel HJ. Molecular characterization of pestiviruses. Adv Virus Res. 1996;47:53–118.
- Thiel HJ, Stark R, Weiland E, Rumenapf T, Meyers G. Hog cholera virus: molecular composition of virions from a pestivirus. J Virol. 1991;65:4705–12.
- Lowings P, Ibata G, Needham J, Paton D. Classical swine fever virus diversity and evolution. J Gen Virol. 1996;77(Pt 6):1311–21.
- Paton DJ, McGoldrick A, Greiser-Wilke I, Parchariyanon S, Song JY, Liou PP, et al. Genetic typing of classical swine fever virus. Vet Microbiol. 2000;73:137–57.

7. Deng MC, Huang CC, Huang TS, Chang CY, Lin YJ, Chien MS, et al. Phylogenetic analysis of classical swine fever virus isolated from Taiwan. Vet Microbiol. 2005;106:187–93.
8. Pan CH, Jong MH, Huang TS, Liu HF, Lin SY, Lai SS. Phylogenetic analysis of classical swine fever virus in Taiwan. Arch Virol. 2005;150:1101–19.
9. Gong W, Wu J, Lu Z, Zhang L, Qin S, Chen F, et al. Genetic diversity of subgenotype 2.1 isolates of classical swine fever virus. Infect Genet Evol. 2016;41:218–26.
10. Tu C, Lu Z, Li H, Yu X, Liu X, Li Y, et al. Phylogenetic comparison of classical swine fever virus in China. Virus Res. 2001;81:29–37.
11. Shen H, Pei J, Bai J, Zhao M, Ju C, Yi L, et al. Genetic diversity and positive selection analysis of classical swine fever virus isolates in South China. Virus Genes. 2011;43:234–42.
12. Chen N, Hu H, Zhang Z, Shuai J, Jiang L, Fang W. Genetic diversity of the envelope glycoprotein E2 of classical swine fever virus: recent isolates branched away from historical and vaccine strains. Vet Microbiol. 2008;127:286–99.
13. Chen N, Tong C, Li D, Wan J, Yuan X, Li X, et al. Antigenic analysis of classical swine fever virus E2 glycoprotein using pig antibodies identifies residues contributing to antigenic variation of the vaccine C-strain and group 2 strains circulating in China. Virol J. 2010;7:378.
14. Leng CL, Zhang HL, Kan YC, Yao LG, Li ML, Zhai HY, et al. Characterisation of newly emerged isolates of classical swine fever virus in China, 2014-2015. J Vet Res. 2017;61:9.
15. Jiang DL, Gong WJ, Li RC, Liu GH, Hu YF, Ge M, et al. Phylogenetic analysis using E2 gene of classical swine fever virus reveals a new subgenotype in China. Infect Genet Evol. 2013;17:231–8.
16. Postel A, Schmeiser S, Perera CL, Rodriguez LJ, Frias-Lepoureau MT, Becher P. Classical swine fever virus isolates from Cuba form a new subgenotype 1. 4. Vet Microbiol. 2013;161:334–8.
17. Zhang H, Leng C, Feng L, Zhai H, Chen J, Liu C, et al. A new subgenotype 2. 1d isolates of classical swine fever virus in China, 2014. Infect Genet Evol. 2015;34:94–105.
18. Tamura K, Peterson D, Peterson N, Stecher G, Nei M, Kumar S. MEGA5: molecular evolutionary genetics analysis using maximum likelihood, evolutionary distance, and maximum parsimony methods. Mol Biol Evol. 2011;28:2731–9.
19. Edgar RC. MUSCLE: a multiple sequence alignment method with reduced time and space Complexity. BMC bioinformatics. 2004;5:113.
20. Mittelholzer C, Moser C, Tratschin JD, Hofmann MA. Analysis of classical swine fever virus replication kinetics allows differentiation of highly virulent from avirulent strains. Vet Microbiol. 2000;74:293–308.
21. Ferrari M, Gualandi GL, Corradi A, Monaci C, Romanelli MG, Tosi G, et al. Experimental infection of pigs with a thymidine kinase negative strain of pseudorabies virus. Comp Immunol Microbiol Infect Dis. 1998;21:291–303.
22. Sur JH, Cooper VL, Galeota JA, Hesse RA, Doster AR, Osorio FA. In vivo detection of porcine reproductive and respiratory syndrome virus RNA by in situ hybridization at different times postinfection. J Clin Microbiol. 1996;34:2280–6.
23. Edwards S, Fukusho A, Lefevre PC, Lipowski A, Pejsak Z, Roehe P, et al. Classical swine fever: the global situation. Vet Microbiol. 2000;73:103–19.
24. Luo Y, Li S, Sun Y, Qiu HJ. Classical swine fever in China: a minireview. Vet Microbiol. 2014;172:1–6.
25. Hu D, Lv L, Gu J, Chen T, Xiao Y, Liu S. Genetic diversity and positive selection analysis of classical swine fever virus envelope protein gene E2 in East China under C-strain vaccination. Front Microbiol. 2016;7:85.
26. Blacksell SD, Khounsy S, Boyle DB, Greiser-Wilke I, Gleeson LJ, Westbury HA, et al. Phylogenetic analysis of the E2 gene of classical swine fever viruses from Lao PDR. Virus Res. 2004;104:87–92.
27. Sarma DK, Mishra N, Vilcek S, Rajukumar K, Behera SP, Nema RK, et al. Phylogenetic analysis of recent classical swine fever virus (CSFV) isolates from Assam, India. Comp Immunol Microbiol Infect Dis. 2011;34:11–5.
28. Postel A, Schmeiser S, Bernau J, Meindl-Boehmer A, Pridotkas G, Dirbakova Z, et al. Improved strategy for phylogenetic analysis of classical swine fever virus based on full-length E2 encoding sequences. Vet Res. 2012;43:50.
29. Li X, Xu Z, He Y, Yao Q, Zhang K, Jin M, et al. Genome comparison of a novel classical swine fever virus isolated in China in 2004 with other CSFV strains. Virus Genes. 2006;33:133–42.
30. Shen HY, Wang JY, Dong XY, Zhao MQ, Kang Y, Li YG, et al. Genome and molecular characterization of a CSFV strain isolated from a CSF outbreak in South China. Intervirology. 2013;56:122–33.
31. Luo TR, Liao SH, Wu XS, Feng L, Yuan ZX, Li H, et al. Phylogenetic analysis of the E2 gene of classical swine fever virus from the Guangxi Province of southern China. Virus Genes. 2011;42:347–54.

32. Hsu WL, Chen CL, Huang SW, Wu CC, Chen IH, Nadar M, et al. The untranslated regions of classic swine fever virus RNA trigger apoptosis. PLoS One. 2014;9:e88863.
33. Fletcher SP, Jackson RJ. Pestivirus internal ribosome entry site (IRES) structure and function: elements in the 5′ untranslated region important for IRES function. J Virol. 2002;76:5024–33.
34. Wang Y, Wang Q, Lu X, Zhang C, Fan X, Pan Z, et al. 12-nt insertion in 3′ untranslated region leads to attenuation of classic swine fever virus and protects host against lethal challenge. Virology. 2008;374:390–8.
35. Coronado L, Liniger M, Munoz-Gonzalez S, Postel A, Perez LJ, Perez-Simo M, et al. Novel poly-uridine insertion in the 3′UTR and E2 amino acid substitutions in a low virulent classical swine fever virus. Vet Microbiol. 2017; 201:103–12.
36. Chen Y, Xiao J, Xiao J, Sheng C, Wang J, Jia L, et al. Classical swine fever virus NS5A regulates viral RNA replication through binding to NS5B and 3′UTR. Virology. 2012;432:376–88.
37. Li S, Feng S, Wang JH, He WR, Qin HY, Dong H, et al. eEF1A interacts with the NS5A protein and inhibits the growth of classical swine fever virus. Viruses. 2015;7:4563–81.
38. Sheng C, Chen Y, Xiao J, Xiao J, Wang J, Li G, et al. Classical swine fever virus NS5A protein interacts with 3′-untranslated region and regulates viral RNA synthesis. Virus Res. 2012;163:636–43.
39. Risatti GR, Borca MV, Kutish GF, Lu Z, Holinka LG, French RA, et al. The E2 glycoprotein of classical swine fever virus is a virulence determinant in swine. J Virol. 2005;79:3787–96.
40. van Rijn PA, Miedema GK, Wensvoort G, van Gennip HG, Moormann RJ. Antigenic structure of envelope glycoprotein E1 of hog cholera virus. J Virol. 1994;68:3934–42.
41. Dong XN, Chen YH. Marker vaccine strategies and candidate CSFV marker vaccines. Vaccine. 2007;25:205–30.
42. Leifer I, Hoeper D, Blome S, Beer M, Ruggli N. Clustering of classical swine fever virus isolates by codon pair bias. BMC Res notes. 2011;4:521.
43. Floegel-Niesmann G, Blome S, Gerss-Dulmer H, Bunzenthal C, Moennig V. Virulence of classical swine fever virus isolates from Europe and other areas during 1996 until 2007. Vet Microbiol. 2009;139:165–9.
44. Luo Y, Ji S, Liu Y, Lei JL, Xia SL, Wang Y. Isolation and characterization of a moderately virulent classical swine fever virus emerging in China. Transbound Emerg Dis. 2017;64:1848–57.

Changes in alpha-amylase activity, concentration and isoforms in pigs after an experimental acute stress model

María Dolores Contreras-Aguilar[1], Damián Escribano[2], Silvia Martínez-Subiela[1], Silvia Martínez-Miró[3], Jose Joaquín Cerón[1] and Fernando Tecles[1*]

Abstract

Background: Salivary alpha-amylase (sAA) is considered a non-invasive biomarker of acute stress that can be evaluated by changes in activity and concentration, and also by changes in its isoforms, although this last way of evaluation has never been used in veterinary medicine. This research evaluated the changes of sAA by three different ways in which sAA can be evaluated in an experimental acute stress model in six pigs based in a technique of temporarily restraining. These ways of evaluation were 1) activity by a spectrophotometric assay, 2) concentration by a fluorometric assay, and 3) isoforms of the enzyme by a Western blot.

Results: Although salivary cortisol significantly increased due to the stimulus of stress and all the pigs manifested signs of stress by high-pitched vocalization, sAA activity showed an increase of different degree in the six pigs after the stress stimulus, while sAA concentration showed decreases in four of the six pigs. sAA activity did not correlate with sAA concentration or salivary cortisol, and a low correlation was observed between sAA concentration and salivary cortisol ($r = 0.48$, $p = 0.003$). The inter-individual variability was higher in sAA activity than in sAA concentration and salivary cortisol. Finally, three possible isoforms of sAA at 154–160 kDa, 65–66 kDa and 59–60 kDa were observed that showed different dynamics after the stress induction.

Conclusions: Although this pilot study's results should be taken with caution due to the low sample size, it reveals a different behavior between sAA activity and concentration in pig after an acute stressful stimulus leading to evident external signs of stress by high-pitched vocalization, and opens a new field for the evaluation of possible selected isoforms of sAA as potential biomarkers of stress.

Keywords: Biomarkers, Isoforms, Salivary alpha-amylase, Stress, Swine

Background

Nowadays there is an interest in improving the stress evaluation in highly productive indoor-housed pigs since stress can induce behavioral, physiological and immunological alterations leading to a reduction of animal welfare and health [1]. The stress can be evaluated by direct behavioral observations, for example using behavior scoring systems [2–4] or by recording high-pitched vocalizations [5, 6]. However, it can be also objectively assessed by biomarkers that can reflect the pathophysiological responses to stress [7]. Currently there is a growing interest in the use of saliva as a sample for measurement of stress biomarkers [8–11] because saliva is easily obtained and non-invasively compared to blood [12]. Salivary alpha-amylase (sAA) has been proposed as a biomarker for assessing acute psychological stress in humans due to sympathetic activation [13, 14]. In addition, sAA has been also measured in pig as a sympathetic nervous system (SNS) marker [15], whereas cortisol has been measured to assess activation

Correspondence: ftecles@um.es
Interdisciplinary Laboratory of Clinical Analysis (Interlab-UMU), Veterinary School, Campus of Excellence Mare Nostrum, University of Murcia, 30100, Espinardo, Murcia, Spain
Full list of author information is available at the end of the article

of hypothalamic–pituitary–adrenocortical (HPA) axis [7, 16]. In addition to pigs, sAA has been studied in other animal species such as bonobos and other simians [17], horses [10], sheep [18] and dogs [19].

sAA can be evaluated by its enzymatic activity, although a high inter-individual variability in response to stress has been reported in pigs [15], as well in humans [13] and horses [10]. Quantification is another way to evaluate sAA, showing a lower inter-individual variability, as described in horses [10] and humans [20]. Lastly, sAA isoforms and its possible changes after a sAA stimulation have been evaluated in humans [21, 22]. Despite the interest and use of this enzyme, to the authors` knowledge there are no studies comparing the different ways in which the sAA response against a stressor could be assessed: activity, concentration and changes in isoforms.

The aim of this research was to evaluate the individual changes of sAA in an experimental acute stress model in pig, consisting of a nasal snare immobilization [23], by the three different ways in which sAA can be evaluated: (1) measurement of activity with a spectrophotometric assay, (2) measurement of concentration with a time-resolved immunofluorometric assay (TR-IFMA), and (3) the study of the possible changes in isoforms by western blot (WB). In addition, the sAA results were compared to those obtained with salivary cortisol.

Methods

Animals and experimental acute stress model

For this study, male crossbreed pigs (Duroc × (Landrace × Large White) in the mid-fattening period (mean age = 104.8 ± 10.0 days, mean body weight = 78.3 ± 6.3 Kg) from the high sanitary/health-status farm unit of the University of Murcia (Spain) were used. All animals were subjected to a clinical examination prior to the study and no clinical signs of disease were detected. The pigs had access to a nutritionally balanced diet (commercial dry diets based in a corn-soybean meal with 15.5% of crude protein -CP-; 0.79% Ileal digestible Lys, %; and 13.5 MJ of metabolizable energy per kg -ME/kg-) and water ad libitum (from nipple drinkers) under general commercial housing and husbandry conditions conforming to the European Union Guidelines (Directive 2010/63/EU1). Each pen had an area of 1.139m^2 per animal, being in concordance to the legislation (Council Directive 2001/88/CE). The temperature in the pens was kept between a minimum of 18.0 °C and a maximum of 19.5 °C. The Murcia University Ethics Committee with the number CEEA 288/2017 approved this study.

The stressful situation consisted of a technique of temporarily restraining pigs commonly used in veterinary practice which has been demonstrated to produce a high stress to pigs [7, 23]. Six pigs were subjected to an immobilization for at least 1 min with a nasal snare or loop following the procedure described in the literature [15, 23]. Salivary samples were taken the day before the experiment took place, which was considered as basal time (Tb). On the other hand, the same day of the experiment samples were taken 5 min before restrain (T-5), for the first 30 s while the nasal snare immobilization was performed (T + 0A), for the second 30 s during immobilization (T + 0B), just after immobilization (T + 0C) and 15 min later (T + 15). The saliva collection at each time lasted 1 min, except for T + 0A and T + 0B. The sampling times were selected to evaluate the possible short-term changes in sAA. The observer responsible for sampling individually recorded if high-pitched vocalizations were present or absent during the restraint period. All animal were sampled between 9:00 to 12:00 a.m. to avoid circadian influences [24, 25], by the same person, when animals were in repose, avoiding the race and from pigs housed at different rooms to avoid suggestion; in order to homogenize the experimental conditions for all animals.

Salivary sampling

Saliva samples were collected by introducing a small sponge around the mouth and it was placed in a collection device (Salivette, Sarstedt, Aktiengesellschaft & Co, Nümbrecht, Germany), as reported before [23]. Samples were then stored in ice until arrival at the processing laboratory, where devices were centrifuged at *3.000×g* for 10 min at 4 °C. Saliva was transferred into 1.5 mL tubes and stored at – 80 °C until analysis.

Alpha-amylase enzymatic assay

sAA activity was measured in an automatic analyzer (Olympus UA600, Olympus Diagnostica GmbH) by a colorimetric commercial kit (Alpha-Amylase, Beckman Coulter Inc.) following the International Medicine (IFCC) method [26]. This spectrophotometric assay uses 4,6-ethylidene(G7)-p nitrophenol(G1)-alpha-D- maltoheptaoside (G7PNP) as a substrate of the enzyme. The intermediate product of substrate hydrolysis reacts with a-glucosidase, giving p-nitrophenol as the final product of the reaction. The rate of p-nitrophenol formation was directly proportional to the alpha-amylase activity of the sample and was determined by measuring the absorbance at 405 nm. This kit was previously validated for pigs by Fuentes et al. [15], with a intra- and inter-assay coefficients of variation (CV) lower than 10%, and a limit of detection of 11.65 U/L.

Time-resolved immunofluorometric assay

sAA concentration was measured by a time-resolved immunofluorometric assay (TR-IFMA). The assay consisted of a non-competitive indirect sandwich method based on anti-human sAA polyclonal antibody biotin-labeled as a capture reagent and the anti-human-sAA polyclonal antibody Eu^{3+}–chelates labeled as a detector. Streptavidin-coated plates (Streptavidin Microtitration Strips, DELFIA, PerkinElmer, Turku, Finland) were used for the development of this assay. The anti-human sAA polyclonal antibody used was produced by the authors according to standard protocols [27] and using as immunogen human sAA purified in the researchers' laboratory according to the procedures of Peng et al. [28].

The fluorometric assay was validated prior to use for sample measurement. Three saliva samples with a low, medium and high sAA mean concentration (10.7, 30.0 and 65.2 ng/mL, respectively) were measured five times in a single run and in five different days for the determination of intra- and inter-assay precision, respectively. The mean CV was 6.8% ± 0.8% for intra-assay, and 7.4% ± 2.3% for inter-assay. Linearity under dilution of two saliva samples yielded Pearson correlation coefficients of $r = 0.989 \pm 0.006$ (mean ± SD). The limit of detection and the lower limit of quantification calculated were 1.4 ng/mL and 18.14 ng/mL, respectively.

Western blot

WB was performed in the saliva collected at Tb, T + 0A, T + 0B and T + 0C of three pigs that showed different sAA activity response: pig 1 that showed the highest difference of sAA activity levels, pig 3 that showed intermediate differences and pig 5 that showed the lowest difference in sAA activity along the times. Saliva from pigs diluted to obtain an amount of 1 ng of sAA and 10 µg of purified human sAA (ab 77875, Abcam, Cambridge, UK) were used for this approach. Proteins were separated in mini one-dimensional sodium dodecyl sulphate polyacrylamide gels (SDS-PAGE) containing 0.1% (*w*/*v*), with a separating gel prepared in 12% (w/v) and a stacker gel prepared in 4% (w/v) according to the methodology described by Laemmli [29]. Then, the proteins in SDS-PAGE were transferred to nitrocellulose membranes (Bio-Rad Laboratories Inc., Hercules, CA, USA). The same rabbit polyclonal antibody against human sAA used in the TR-IFMA (1:8000 dilution) was employed as primary antibody, while anti-rabbit IgG horseradish peroxidase (HRP)-conjugated goat polyclonal antibody (ab 6721, Abcam, Cambrigde, UK) (1:12000) was used as secondary antibody, and signal was detected using Pierce ECL2 kit (Pierce, Thermo Fisher Scientific, USA) and ImageQuant™ scanner (GE Healthcare, Uppsala, Sweden). The average intensity of each band, defined as the volume of the band feature divided by its area, was analyzed by using ImageQuant™ TL 8.1 (GE Healthcare, Uppsala, Sweden).

Cortisol measurement

Salivary cortisol was evaluated also for comparative purposes [30] with an automated chemiluminescent immunoassay (Immulite 1000 cortisol, Siemens Medical Solutions Diagnostics) validated for pigs' saliva [8]. The intra- and inter-assay CV was lower than 16%, and a limit of detection of 0.015 µg/dL.

Statistical methods

Arithmetic means, standard deviations (SD), CV and linear regression analyses were calculated using routine descriptive statistical procedures by spreadsheet (Excel 2000, Microsoft Corporation, Redmond, Washington, USA). To determine if sAA and salivary cortisol values obtained at different times in the stressful situation were statistically different, a Friedman test and a Dunn's multiple comparisons test were used. A Spearman correlation test was performed to compare sAA activity, sAA concentration and salivary cortisol results. The inter-individual variability of the sAA values (activity and concentration) and salivary cortisol in each time were expressed as the CV value, calculated as the SD divided by the mean of the values of the different individuals and then multiplied by 100. These statistical analyses were calculated using Graph Pad Prism 6 (GraphPad Software, San Diego, CA, USA).

Results

Activity and concentration of alpha-amylase in saliva

sAA activity (Fig. 1a) showed a significant change between the times ($\chi^2 = 12.76$, df = 5, $P = 0.026$), but the multiple comparisons test did not show any significant increase at any time ($P > 0.08$ for all times compared). sAA concentration (Fig. 1b) did not show significant changes along the times ($\chi^2 = 7.33$, df = 5, $P = 0.197$). Salivary cortisol significantly changed between the times ($\chi^2 = 13.71$, df = 5, $P = 0.033$), with an increase ($P = 0.045$) at T + 0B compared to TB (Fig. 1c). There was a significant correlation between sAA concentration and salivary cortisol ($n = 36$, $r = 0.48$, 95% confidence interval [CI] 0.18–0.71, $P = 0.003$). However, no correlation was observed between sAA activity and sAA concentration ($n = 36$, $r = 0.16$, 95% CI −0.18-0.47, $P = 0.338$), and between sAA activity and salivary cortisol ($n = 36$, $r = 0.14$, 95% CI −0.21-0.45, $P = 0.418$). Recurrent high-pitched vocalizations were observed in the six pigs during the restraint period.

When sAA activity values were individually evaluated (Fig. 2a), the differences of sAA activity between the times had an average value higher than 1000 U/L in pigs 1 (4166.4 U/L) and 6 (1225.5 U/L); higher than 500 U/L in pigs 2 (743.6 U/L), 3 (826.2 U/L) and 4 (548.1 U/L); and lower than 100 U/L in pig 5 (71.1 U/L). Peaks of activity were observed in pig 1 at T + 0A, in pig 2 at T + 0C and in pigs 3 and 6 at T + 0B. In pig 4, the peak was observed at T-5.

When sAA concentration was individually evaluated between times (Fig. 2b), a decrease was observed at T + 0C

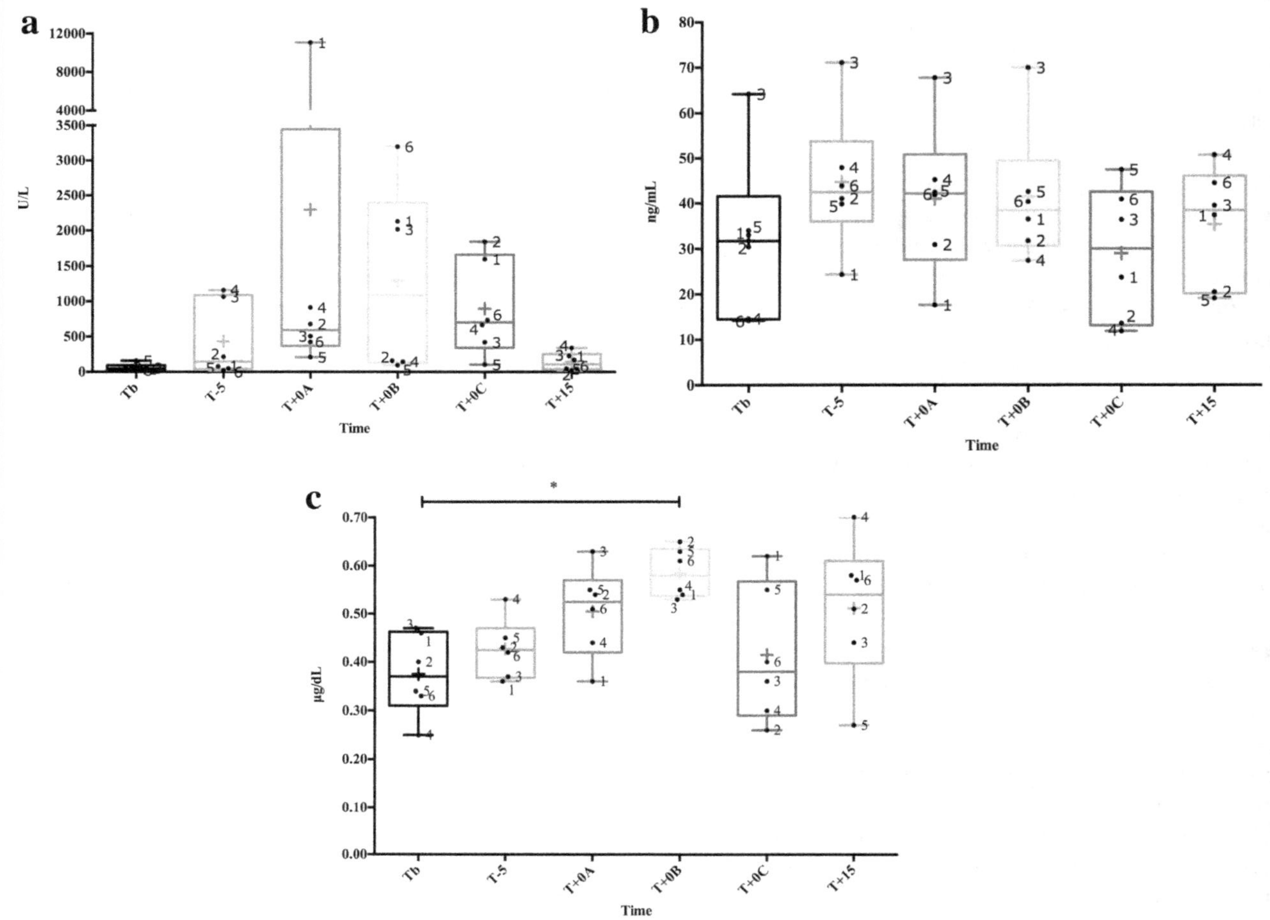

Fig. 1 Salivary alpha-amylase (sAA) activity (**a**), concentration (**b**) and salivary cortisol (**c**) during a nasal snare immobilization for 1 min from six pigs. The times were the day before at basal time (Tb), 5 min before (T-5), the firsts 30 s while the nasal snare immobilization was being performed (T + 0A), the seconds 30 s while the nasal snare immobilization was being performed (T + 0B), just after the immobilization (T + 0C) and 15 (T + 15) minutes later. The plots show medians (line within box), mean (cross inside the box), 25th and 75th percentiles (boxes), min and max values (whiskers) and individual values (points). The numbers mean the name of the pigs. Asterisks indicate significant post-hoc difference (Dunn's multiple comparisons test): * $P < 0.05$

in all pigs, with the exception of the pig 5 and 6. The inter-individual mean variability (Table 1) of the sAA activity (109.2% ± 42.2) was higher (2.5-fold and 5.1-fold, respectively) than in sAA concentration (42.7% ± 9.5) and salivary cortisol (21.2% ± 9.3).

Changes in isoforms patterns

WB results are presented in Fig. 3. Pigs saliva showed a band of 59–60 kDa in all times. On the other hand, pig 5 showed a band with 154–160 kDa along the different times. Additionally, a band at 65–66 kDa was observed in pigs 1 and 3 in the stress times only when sAA activity values were higher than 1000 U/L. The bands with 59–60 kDa and 154–160 kDa were also marked in the commercial human purified sAA (Additional file 1).

Discussion

In this paper, changes in sAA activity, concentration and its possible isoforms were evaluated after an experimental induced stress in pigs. The increase of salivary cortisol, considered as a biomarker of stress [7], that appeared in all pigs used in our study after the restraint would indicate that our experimental procedure was able to generate a stress in the animals. In addition, the high-pitched vocalizations emitted by the six pigs during the restrain period could indicate a negative emotional state [5]. sAA activity showed peaks of increase in four of the six pigs after the stressor at different times and with different intensity, however sAA concentration decreased in many animals after the stimulus. A reason for this different behavior could be the fact that activity and concentration are associated to different possible isoforms of sAA.

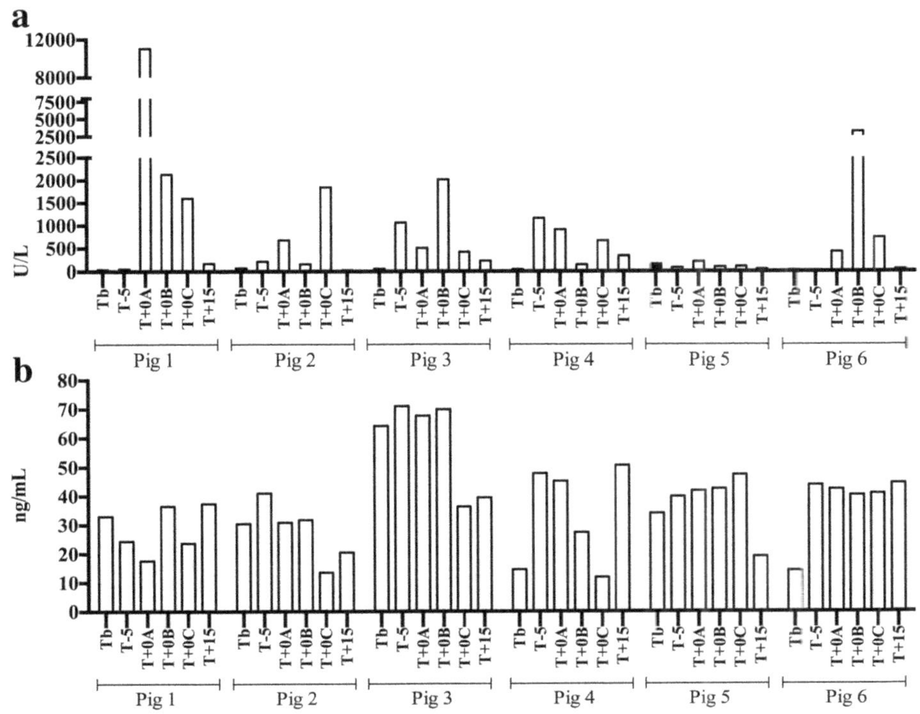

Fig. 2 Individual levels of salivary alpha-amylase (sAA) activity (**a**) and concentration (**b**) obtained from six pigs before and after nasal snare immobilization for 1 min. The times were the day before at basal time (Tb), 5 min before (T-5), the firsts 30 s while the nasal snare immobilization was being performed (T + 0A), the seconds 30 s while the nasal snare immobilization was being performed (T + 0B), just after the immobilization (T + 0C) and 15 (T + 15) minutes later. Bars show the total value from each individual at each time

For the analysis of sAA isoforms, serial samples from in-lividuals representing different sAA response (one with a najor sAA response, one with a moderate sAA response .nd one with a minor response) were analysed. According o the WB's results, different sAA isoforms appeared de-pending of the intensity of the sAA response. In humans t has been demonstrated that these sAA isoforms can change after sAA stimulation [22] and changes observed in these isoforms could influence the concentration and activity of the enzyme. However, as well as occurs with activity, there was a high inter-individual variability in the response of the different isoforms. The bands with 59–60 kDa and 154–160 kDa observed in the WB from porcine saliva had the same molecular weight than bands marked in the commercial purified sAA from humans (Additional file 1). In addition, the band with 59–60 kDa could correspond to the glycosylated isoform described in humans [21]. So it could be postulated that the changes observed in the bands in the WB study could be due to different amylase isoforms. This could open a new line for the evaluation of possible selected isoforms of sAA as potential biomarkers of stress, since for example the isoform with a molecular weight of 65–66 kDa could be related with major response in sAA activity after an stress, since appeared in pigs showing the higher sAA activity response to a stressful stimulus, whereas the isoform of 154–160 kDa could be related with minor response in sAA activity after a stress condition.

able 1 Inter-individual variability (%) of salivary alpha-amylase sAA) measured by enzymatic activity (U/L) and concentration ng/mL), and of salivary cortisol concentration (μg/dL) after the xperimental nasal snare immobilization for 1 min in 6 pigs

AA interindividual variability (%)			
	sAA		salivary cortisol
	U/L	ng/mL	μg/dL
b	75.3	57.51	22.5
-5	123.6	34.09	14.42
+ 0A	187.0	40.64	18.61
+ 0B	103.5	36.33	8.77
+ 0C	76.2	51.16	34.2
+ 15	89.4	36.43	28.6
lean	109.2	42.7	21.2
D[a]	42.2	9.5	9.3

SD standard deviation

A lack of correlation between sAA activity and concentration was observed in our study. Divergences between activity and concentration values have been described for other enzymes such as Paraoxonase-1 (PON1) in human

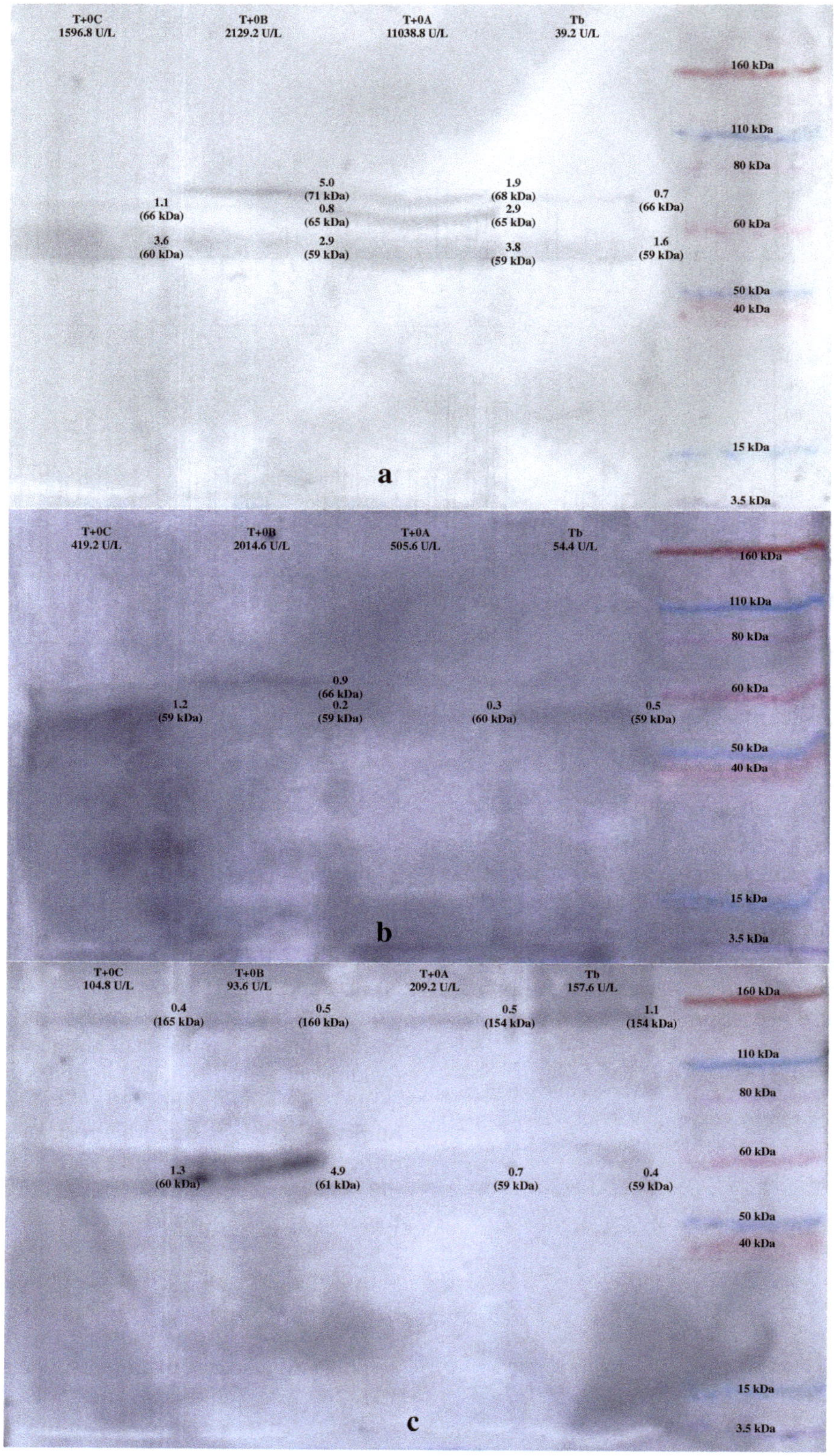

Fig. 3 (See legend on next page.)

(See figure on previous page.)
Fig. 3 Western blot from pig saliva in an experimental nasal snare immobilization. Saliva samples from Pig 1 (**a**), Pig 3 (**b**) and Pig 5 (**c**) with one ng per well of salivary alpha-amylase (sAA) at the day before at basal time (Tb), the firsts 30 s while the nasal snare immobilization was being performed (T + 0A), the seconds 30 s while the nasal snare immobilization was being performed (T + 0B) and just after the immobilization (T + 0C). Molecular weight markers (Novex Sharp Pre-Stained, Invitrogen, Carlsbad, California). Arrows mark positive bands in pig's saliva, and numbers above indicate the average intensity (× 10^3)

erum [31]. In the sAA case, it could be postulated that post-translational changes [21] could modify the enzyme's activity, although the concentration release does not show significant changes. In addition, we found no correlation between sAA activity and salivary cortisol. This is in line with previous reports previously described [15, 32] and could be due to the possible activation of the different related stress axis [33, 34] having a different time of reponse, with the sAA release being faster than the cortisol. Finally, the positive correlation between sAA concentration and salivary cortisol detected in our study should be taken with caution since r values below 0.50 are considered as weak [35], and both did not show a similar tendency along the times.

In this study, sAA activity showed a high inter-individual variability as it has been previously reported in pigs subjected to an acute stress model [15]. This high inter-individual variability was also observed in sAA concentration and it could be the cause for not obtaining significant differences in both sAA activity and concentration after the stress model. Biomarkers assessing of stress usually show inter-individual variability [8, 13, 36], probably due to the complexity of stress reaction [37] and because the stress response varies according to idiosyncrasy of the individual [38]. However, this inter-individual variability was higher in sAA activity, being in agreement with previous reports [10, 13, 20]. The higher inter-individual variability in sAA activity could be due to the fast-reacting biological response of the enzyme, and there is a large array of factors with potential to stimulate or inhibit amylase activity [13], that could be a potential limitation for its application as a stress biomarker.

It is important to point out that this is an exploratory study and the results observed should be taken as preliminary ones due to the low sample size. Further studies should be performed in large populations and with other different stress conditions in order to corroborate our findings. In addition, it would be of interest the development of studies to clarify the high inter-individual variability in sAA behavior after a stress induction that we found in our experimental conditions.

Conclusion

This study reveals that sAA activity and concentration behave in a different way in pigs after an experimental acute stress stimulus, showing a high inter-individual variation in their response. In addition, it reports the presence of sAA isoforms in pig saliva that show a different response after a stress. Although these results should be taken as preliminary ones due to the pilot nature of this study with a low sample size, it could open a new line for the evaluation of possible selected isoforms of sAA as potential biomarkers of stress.

Abbreviations

CI: Confidence interval; CP: Crude protein; CV: Coefficient of variation; HPA: Hypothalamic-pituitary-adrenocortical; HRP: Horseradish peroxidase; ME: Metabolizable energy; PON1: Paraoxonase-1; sAA: Salivary apha-amylase; SD: Standard deviation; SDS-PAGE: One-dimensional sodium dodecyl sulphate polyacrylamide gel electrophoresis; SNS: Sympathetic nervous system; TR-IFMA: Time-resolved immunofluorometric assay; WB: Western blot

Acknowledgements

This work was supported by the Seneca foundation of Murcia Regional Government, Spain (grant number 19894/GERM/15). D. Escribano was granted by the postdoctoral program 'Juan de la Cierva' of the 'Ministerio de Economía y Competitividad', Spain. M. Contreras-Aguilar was granted by the predoctoral contract 'FPU' of University of Murcia (R- 605/2016), Spain.

Funding

Seneca Foundation of Murcia Region (grant number: 19894/GERM/15).

Authors' contributions

MDCA and JJC conceived and designed the study. MDCA and DE collected the data. MDCA were involved in the chemical analysis. MDCA, DE, SMS, SMM, JJC and FT were involved in the data interpretation. MDCA drafted the manuscript and DE, SMS, SMM, JJC and FT critically read and edited the manuscript.

Consent for publication

Not applicable.

Competing interests

None of the authors has any financial or personal relationships that could inappropriately influence or bias the content of the paper.

Author details

[1]Interdisciplinary Laboratory of Clinical Analysis (Interlab-UMU), Veterinary School, Campus of Excellence Mare Nostrum, University of Murcia, 30100, Espinardo, Murcia, Spain. [2]Department of Food and Animal Science, School of Veterinary Medicine, Universitat Autònoma de Barcelona, 08193, Bellaterra, Barcelona, Spain. [3]Department of Animal Production, Veterinary school, Campus of Excellence Mare Nostrum, Murcia, Spain.

References

1. Prunier A, Heinonen M, Quesnel H. High physiological demands in intensively raised pigs : impact on health and welfare. Animal. 2010;4:886–98.
2. Smulders D, Verbeke G, Mormède P, Geers R. Validation of a behavioral observation tool to assess pig welfare. Physiol Behav. 2006;89:438–47.
3. Morton D, Griffiths P. Guidelines on the recognition of pain, distress and discomfort in experimental animals and an hypothesis for assessment. Vet Rec. 1985;116:431–6.
4. O'Driscoll K, Teixeira DL, O'Gorman D, Taylor S, Boyle LA. The influence of a magnesium rich marine supplement on behaviour, salivary cortisol levels, and skin lesions in growing pigs exposed to acute stressors. Appl Anim Behav Sci. 2013;145:92–101.
5. Dokmanović M, Velarde A, Tomović V, Glamočlija N, Marković R, Janjić J, et al. The effects of lairage time and handling procedure prior to slaughter on stress and meat quality parameters in pigs. Meat Sci. 2014;98:220–6.
6. Marx G, Horn T, Thielebein J, Knubel B, Von BE. Analysis of pain-related vocalization in young pigs. J Sound Vib. 2003;266:687–98.
7. Martínez-Miró S, Tecles F, Ramón M, Escribano D, Hernández F, Madrid J, et al. Causes , consequences and biomarkers of stress in swine : an update. BMC Vet Res. 2016;12:1–9.
8. Escribano D, Fuentes-Rubio M, Ceron JJ. Validation of an automated chemiluminescent immunoassay for salivary cortisol measurements in pigs. J Vet Diagn Investig. 2012;24:918–23.
9. Escribano D, Gutiérrez AM, Tecles F, Cerón JJ. Changes in saliva biomarkers of stress and immunity in domestic pigs exposed to a psychosocial stressor. Research in veterinary science. Elsevier BV. 2015;102:38–44.
10. Fuentes-Rubio M, Fuentes F, Otal J, Quiles A, Tecles F, Cerón JJ, et al. Measurements of salivary alpha-amylase in horse: comparison of 2 different assays. J Vet Behav: Clin Appl Res. 2015;10:122–7.
11. Lensen CMM, Moons CPH, Diederich C. Saliva sampling in dogs: how to select the most appropriate procedure for your study. J Vet Behav: Clin Appl Res Elsevier Inc. 2015;10:504–12.
12. Tsuchiya K, Saidin MY, Bin, Inoue T, Kajiwara K, Kimura M. Qualitative measurement of pain by analysing the salivary alpha amylase. Precision Eng Elsevier Inc. 2014;38:257–60.
13. Rohleder N, Nater UM. Determinants of salivary α-amylase in humans and methodological considerations. Psychoneuroendocrinology. 2009;34:469–85.
14. Petrakova L, Doering BK, Vits S, Engler H, Rief W, Schedlowski M, et al. Psychosocial stress increases salivary alpha-amylase activity independently from plasma noradrenaline levels. PLoS One. 2015;10:1–9.
15. Fuentes M, Tecles F, Gutierrez A, Otal J, Martinez-Subiela S, Ceron JJ. Validation of an automated method for salivary alpha-amylase measurements in pigs (Sus scrofa domesticus) and its application as a stress biomarker. J Vet Diagn Investig. 2011;23:282–7.
16. Kudielka BM, Schommer NC, Hellhammer DH, Kirschbaum C. Acute HPA axis responses, heart rate, and mood changes to psychosocial stress (TSST) in humans at different times of day. Psychoneuroendocrinology. 2004;29:983–92.
17. Behringer V, Deschner T, Möstl E, Selzer D, Hohmann G. Stress affects salivary alpha-amylase activity in bonobos. Physiol Behav. 2012;105:476–82.
18. Fuentes-Rubio M, Fuentes F, Otal J, Quiles A, Luisa HM. Validation of an assay for quantification of alpha-amylase in saliva of sheep. Can J Vet Res. 2016;80:197–202.
19. Contreras-Aguilar MD, Tecles F, Martínez-Subiela S, Escribano D, Bernal LJ, Cerón JJ. Detection and measurement of alpha- amylase in canine saliva and changes after an experimentally induced sympathetic activation. BMC Vet Res. 2017;13:1–6.
20. Contreras-Aguilar MD, Escribano D, Martínez-Subiela S, Martínez-Miró S, Rubio M, Tvarijonaviciute A, et al. Influence of the way of reporting alpha-amylase values in saliva in different naturalistic situations : a pilot study. PLoS One. 2017;12:1–13.
21. Hirtz C, Chevalier F, Centeno D, Rofidal V, Egea JC, Rossignol M, et al. MS characterization of multiple forms of alpha-amylase in human saliva. Proteomics. 2005;5:4597–607.
22. Yang Z, Chen L, Zhang M, Lin J, Zhang J, Chen W. Age differences of salivary alpha-amylase levels of basal and acute responses to citric acid stimulation between Chinese children and adults. Front Physiol. 2015;6:1–11.
23. Escribano D, Soler L, Gutiérrez AM, Martínez-Subiela S, Cerón JJ. Measurement of chromogranin a in porcine saliva: validation of a time-resolved immunofluorometric assay and evaluation of its application as a marker of acute stress. Animal. 2013;7:640–7.
24. O'Donnell K, Kammerer M, O'Reilly R, Taylor A, Glover V. Salivary alpha-amylase stability, diurnal profile and lack of response to the cold hand test in young women. Stress. 2009;12:549–54.
25. Nater UM, Rohleder N, Schlotz W, Ehlert U, Kirschbaum C. Determinants of the diurnal course of salivary alpha-amylase. Psychoneuroendocrinology. 2007;32:392–401.
26. van der Heiden C, Bais R, Gerhardt W, Lorentz K, Rosalki S. IFCC methods fo measurement of catalytic concentration of enzymes - part 9. IFCC method for alpha-amylase {[]1,4-alpha-D-glucan 4-glucanohydrolase, EC 3.2.1.1]. Clin Chim Acta. 1999;281:S5–39.
27. University of California B. Guidelines for the production of antibodies in laboratory animals. In: Animal care and use committee; 2014.
28. Peng Y, Chen X, Sato T, Rankin SA, Tsuji RF, Purification GY. High-resolution top-down mass spectrometric characterization of human salivary alpha-amylase. Anal Chem. 2012;84:3339–46.
29. Laemmli UK. Cleavage of structural proteins during assembly of head of bacteriophage-T4. Nature. 1970;227:680.
30. Cook NJ, Schaefer AL, Lepage P, Jones SDM. Radioimmunoassay for cortisol in pig saliva and serum. J Agric Food Chem. 1997;45:395–9.
31. Parra S, Alonso-Villaverde C, Coll B, Ferré N, Marsillach J, Aragonès G, et al. Serum paraoxonase-1 activity and concentration are influenced by human immunodeficiency virus infection. Atherosclerosis. 2006;194:175–81.
32. Contreras-Aguilar MD, Escribano D, Martín-cuervo M, Tecles F, Cerón JJ. Salivary alpha-amylase activity and cortisol in horses with acute abdominal disease : a pilot study. BMC Vet Res. 2018;14:1–7.
33. Engert V, Efanov SI, Duchesne A, Vogel S, Corbo V, Pruessner JC. Differentiating anticipatory from reactive cortisol responses to psychosocial stress. Psychoneuroendocrinology. 2013;38:1328–37.
34. Sumter SR, Bokhorst CL, Miers AC, Van Pelt J, Westenberg PM. Age and puberty differences in stress responses during a public speaking task: do adolescents grow more sensitive to social evaluation? Psychoneuroendocrinology. 2010;35:1510–6.
35. Milton JS. Statistical Methods in The biological and health sciences. 3th editio. Journal of chemical information and modeling. Radford, VA, USA: McGraw-HILL; 2013.
36. Lennartsson A. Effects of Psychosocial Stress on DHEA and DHEA-S levels. Acute and long-term effects. University of Gothenburg; 2013.
37. Fazio E, Ferlazzo A. Evaluation of stress during transport. Vet Res Commun. 2003;27:519–24.
38. Rushen J. Using aversion learning techniques to assess the mental state, suffering, and welfare of farm animals. J Anim Sci. 1996;74:1990–5.

22

Investigating porcine parvoviruses genogroup 2 infection using in situ polymerase chain reaction

Dinko Novosel[1,2*], Daniel Cadar[3,4], Tamás Tuboly[4], Andreja Jungic[5], Tomasz Stadejek[6], Tahar Ait-Ali[7] and Attila Cságola[4]

Abstract

Background: Porcine parvovirus 2 (PPV2) was detected in swine serum without showing any relationship with disease. The emergence of the virus seemed to be a unique event until other genetically highly similar parvoviruses were identified in China and, later in 2012, the presence of the virus was also described in Europe. PPV2 is widely distributed in pig populations where it is suspected to be involved in respiratory conditions, based on its frequent detection in lung samples. In order to investigate the potential pathogenic involvement of PPV2, 60 dead pigs were examined from two farms. They were necropsied and tested for PPV2 and PCV2 (Porcine circovirus type 2) by PCR; by Brown and Brenn (B&B) staining for bacteria; by immunohistochemistry (IHC) to detect CD3, Swine leukocyte antigen class II DQ (SLAIIDQ), lysozyme, porcine reproductive and respiratory syndrome virus (PRRSV), swine influenza (SIV), *Mycoplasma hyopneumoniae (Mhyo)*; and by in situ hybridization (ISH) to detect ssDNA and dsDNA of PCV2. PPV2 positive samples were subjected to in situ polymerase chain reaction (IS-PCR) including double staining method to detect PPV2 and host cell markers. To calculate statistical difference we used GENMOD or LOGISTIC procedures in Statistical Analysis System (SAS®).

Results: We found that the PPV2 was localized mostly in lymphocytes in lungs, lymph nodes and liver. Neither CD3 antigen nor lysozyme was expressed by these infected cells. In contrast, low levels of SLAIIDQ were expressed by infected cells, suggesting that PPV2 may have a specific tropism for immature B lymphocytes and/or NK lymphocytes though possibly not T lymphocytes.

Conclusion: The overall conclusion of this study indicates that PPV2 may contribute to the pathogenesis of pneumonia.

Keywords: In situ PCR, PPV2, Lungs, Lymphocytes

Background

Parvoviruses are small, non-enveloped icosahedral viruses that are ubiquitous in animal species. The *Parvoviridae* family is composed of two subfamilies: *Parvovirinae*, which infect vertebrates, and *Densovirinae*. *Parvovirinae* can be further divided into eight genera [1]. A number of parvoviruses (PPV) that infect pigs have been identified and include the classical PPV type 1 (PPV1, recently grouped into the *Protoparvovirus* genus as Ungulate protoparvovirus 1), PPV2 belonging to the *Tetraparvovirus* genus (*Ungulate tetraparvovirus 3*) and PPV3 (also known as *Hokovirus*), belong to the *Tetraparvovirus* genus (*Ungulate tetraparvovirus* 2), whereas PPV4 is a representative of the *Copiparvovirus* genus (*Ungulate copiparvovirus 2*). Two additional PPVs, namely PPV5 [2] and PPV6 [3], are still unclassified *Protoparvovirus*). Porcine bocaviruses are also prevalent in pigs and are members of the *Bocaparvovirus* genus, *Parvovirinae* subfamily [4]. All of these viruses are genetically divergent from each other [5–12]. Genomes of PPVs are single-stranded DNA molecules, with a size of approximately 4–6.3 kilobases (kb), that carry terminal palindromic sequences [5]. In general, they possess two

Correspondence: dinko.novosel@gmail.com
[1]Department of Pathology, Croatian Veterinary Institute, Savska cesta 143, 10000 Zagreb, Croatia
[2]Department for Animal science, Faculty of Agriculture, University of Zagreb, Svetosimunska 25, 10000 Zagreb, Croatia
Full list of author information is available at the end of the article

major open reading frames (ORFs) at e 5′- and ‘-3 end which encode for non-structural and capsid protein(s), respectively. An additional ORF3 exists in the middle of the viral genome in members of the *Copiparvovirus*, *Tetraparvovirus Bocaparvovirus* genus [5, 13]. The first newly discovered PPV species was PPV2 in 2005, which was detected in serum of otherwise clinically normal pigs [12]. The emergence of the virus appeared to be a unique event until befor 2006/7, when other genetically similar parvoviruses were identified in China [14], where PPV2 sequences were detected in serum from pigs with marked pyrexia and PCV2-induced post-weaning multisystemic wasting syndrome (PMWS). Later, in 2012, PPV2 was also described in Europe [15]. Phylodynamic analysis indicated that PPV2 had likely been present in Europe since 1920 in domestic and sylvatic hosts, representing a possible source of the virus [16]. Nowdays PPV2 is considered worldwide distributed in pig populations [15, 17, 18] and according to the frequent detection of the virus in lung samples it is suspected to be involved in respiratory conditions of pigs [2, 6, 19]. Recent investigations have indicated that PPV2 infection was correlated with the outbreak of clinically overt respiratory disease in pigs [20]. The aim of this study was to detect PPV2 using IS-PCR in order to investigate its possible implication in pathology of the lung and evaluate its association with PCV2 infections. In addition, we also applied immunohistochemistry to determine expression of host immune markers in infected cells.

Results

Of the 47 lungs tested, 24 were positive for the presence of PPV2 by PCR in farm E. All samples were positive for PCV2 by PCR (Additional file 1). However, using ISH only, 3 and 6 samples were weak and negative for PCV2, respectively, while the rest ranged from moderately to strongly positive (Additional file 1). Using PCR, several other viruses were confirmed in lungs including PPV3, PPV4, TTSuV1, TTSuV2, PoBolV, PoBoV3. PRRSV and SIV, while lungs were negative for presence of PPV1, PoBo1, 2 and 4, ADV and 6 V/7 V. Only 6 and 5 samples out of 47 were positive for PRRSV and SIV by PCR, however they were negative by IHC, respectively (Additional file 1). Statistical significance of the contribution of each virus in outbreak of PMWS is shown in Fig. 1a (Additional file 2). All examined lungs from farm E had a wide range of histopathological lesions and different PCV2 loads (Additional files 3 and 4). The statistical significance of these data is provided in Fig. 1b-d (Additional files 5, 6 and 7). We observed that the presence of PPV2 infection in the lung was significantly associated with a wide range of lesions (Fig. 1b). Notably, PPV2 infection correlated with a reduction in the size of the alveolar spaces, as well as increased numbers of CD3 cells in lungs (Fig. 1d) and a statistically significant increase of PCV2 load in cells of alveolar walls associated with a reduced replication in same cells (Fig. 1c). The level, intensity and aggregation of T lymphocytes, B lymphocytes and macrophages in specific parts of lungs were evaluated and correlated with the presence of PPV2 using IHC (Additional file 8). PPV2 was associated with increased levels of T-lymphocytes in the alveolar spaces and peribronchial area (Fig. 1d). On the other hand PMWS strongly influenced the level of macrophages. PPV2 was detected in the lungs of 4 of 13 animals from farm T. Results are summarised in Additional files 9 and 10. Using IS-PCR a moderate to severe PPV2 infection was detected in three lung samples (T2, T3 and T7) (Fig. 2a-c). Extensive areas exhibited positive signals were mostly found in cells morphologically characteristic of lymphocytes and macrophages in alveolar spaces (Fig. 2d). The presence of PPV2 in lung tissue was associated with marked vascular engorgement, lymphocytic infiltration, reduction of alveolar spaces, necrosis of ciliary epithelial cells and bronchial lumens filled with mucus and inflammatory cells (Fig. 2d). There was a moderate to severe infiltrate of T lymphocytes around bronchi whereas limited B lymphocytes were present around blood vessels (Fig. 2e). Macrophages were found throughout the lung sections, mostly in alveolar walls and spaces. PPV2 infected cells did not express any of the host markers (Fig. 2a-c) apart from SLAIIDQ antigen, expressed at a low level (Fig. 2f). All cases were negative for PCV2 by PCR and ISH. In contrast, every tested lung was positive for *Mhyo*, where a small amount of the surface lipo-protein was identified in macrophages (data not shown).

Discussion

The aim of this research was to investigate the potential involvement of PPV2 in lung pathology and its contribution to the pathogenesis of PCV2 associated diseases using in situ methods. PPV2 infections were detected on farm E by PCR but IS-PCR failed to detect the virus in situ. In contrast, PPV2 was detected using IS-PCR in non-PMWS affected pigs from farm T. IS-PCR is rarely employed therefore the experimental conditions had to be optimized to reach optimal sensitivity and specificity. PCR cycling conditions were based upon a pre-optimized method previously used to detect PPV2 using classic PCR. As described in the Materials and Methods, reducing the formalin fixation, protease pre-treatments, PCR hot start and use of single primer controls help to substantially improve the sensitivity and specificity of IS-PCR by reducing nucleic acid fragmentation and mis-priming during PCR amplification [21–24]. It is likely that further improvements will be required to

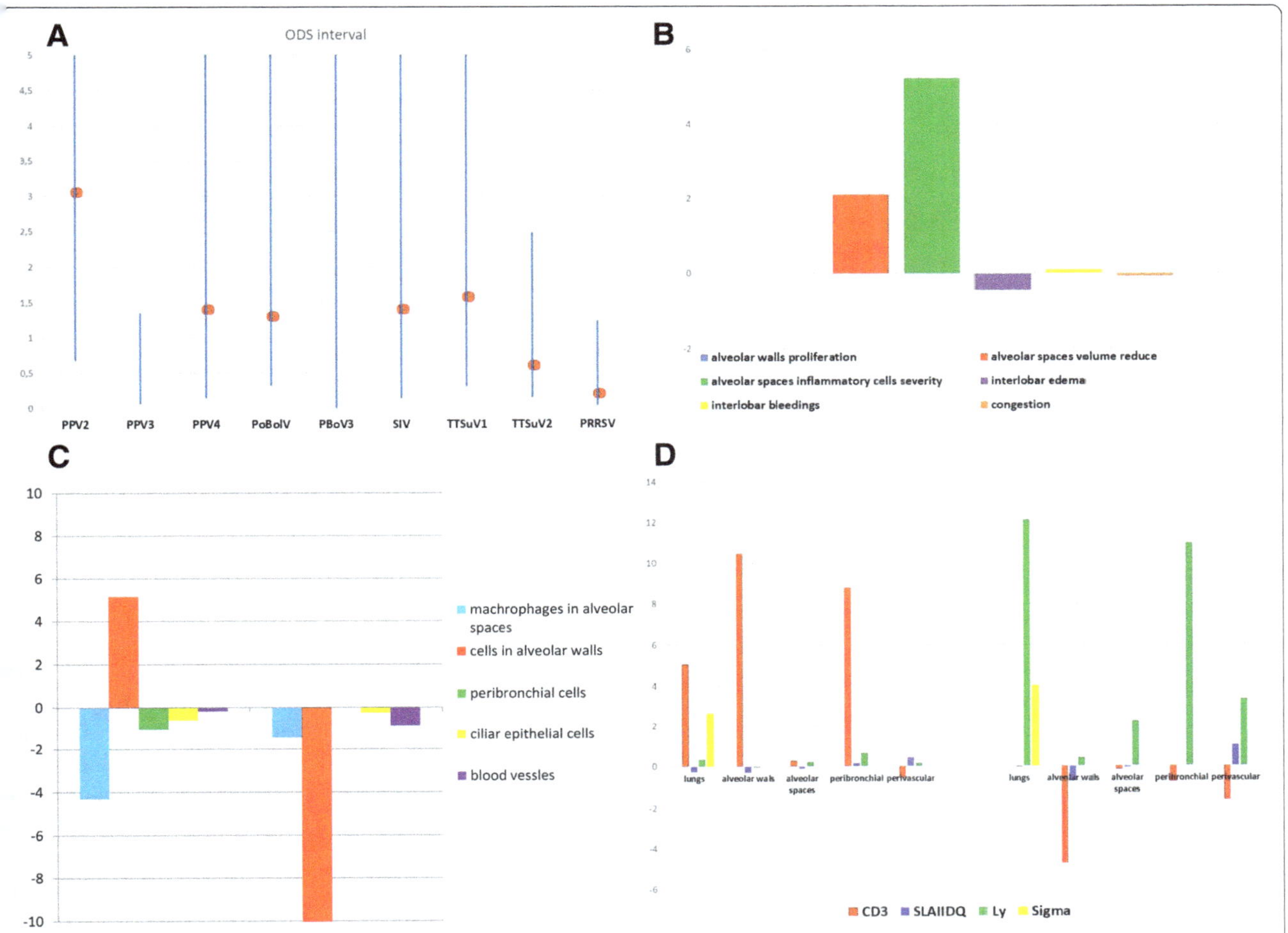

Fig. 1 ODDS ratio **a** for detected virus and PMWS; Wald Chi^2 test to evaluate the statistical significance of **b** specific lesions observed in lungs; **c** amount and level of replication PCV2 in PPV2 positive and PPV2 negative animals. **d** statistical significance in difference of presence of T lymphocytes, B lymphocytes and macrophages in alveolar walls; in alveolar spaces; in peribronchial area and in perivascular area in PPV2 positive and PPV2 negative. Positive Wald Chi2 values means that observed lesion was more frequently observed in PPV2 positive animals while negative Wald CHi2 value means that observed lesion was less frequently observed in PPV2 negative animals

ncrease further the sensitivity of the detection and lecrease background such as diffuse non-specific taining.

)eciphering PPV2 tropism

'ositive signals for PPV2 by IS-PCR were detected in ungs tissue in cells with morphology consistent with ymphocytes and macrophages. These results coincide vith the expected nature of parvoviruses in general, such s their requirement for rapid cellular division as it is ommonly seen during the S-phase of cell cycle [25, 26]. 'o further define the nature of the infected cells, double taining methods capable of simultaneously detecting either CD3, SLAIIDQ or lysozyme host markers and PV2 were optimized. In the lung tissue, PPV2 infected ells were associated with cells poorly expressing LAIIDQ antigen and, occasionally, CD3, but not lysoyme. Based on these observations it is tempting to suggest that PPV2 may have a tropism for SLAIIDQ-positive cells. It is noteworthy that, although CD3 antigen is exclusive to pro-thymocytes or mature T-cells, SLAIIDQ antigen can be expressed by B-cells, antigen presenting cells and subsets of resting and activated T-cells [27]. For example, porcine bone marrow progenitor cells have been shown to express low levels of SLA class II [28]. Furthermore, SLAIIDQ and CD3 antigens are not found on natural killer lymphocytes. Taken together, our investigations highlight a potential tropism of PPV2 for lymphocytes. However, because of the possibility that a virus may alter the regulation of SLAIIDQ or CD3 advocate the need for further investigations to ascertain the exact nature PPV2 infection.

Involvement of PPV2 infection in the pathology of lungs

The results from farm E suggest that PPV2 viruses may be associated with certain histopathological

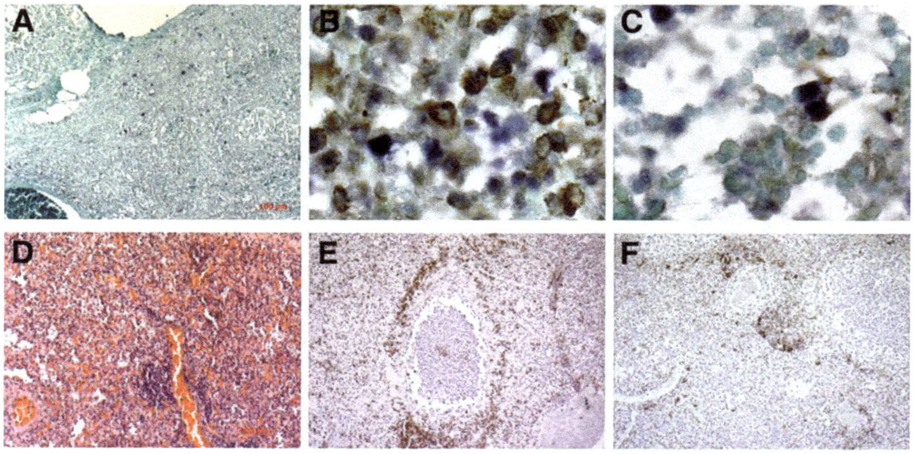

Fig. 2 Lungs T3. **a** Double staining IHC to detect CD3, DAB chromogen/IS PCR to detect PPV2, NBT chromogen 40X; **b** Double staining IHC to detect SLAIIDQ, DAB chromogen/IS PCR to detect PPV2, NBT chromogen 40X; **c** IS PCR to detect PPV2, NBT chromogen, 10X. **d** Severe pneumonia, H&E, 5X, **e** IHC to detect CD3, DAB chromogen, counterstained with Hematoxyline, 5X, **f** IHC to detect SLAIIDQ, DAB chromogen, counterstained with Hematoxyline 5X

lesions and host immune response alterations. All the samples on farm E were PCV2-positive and as a consequence may have been a confounding factor in this work. Nevertheless, our analysis indicates that PPV2 may have implication in the pathology of the lungs. Our statistical analysis indicates that the significance is higher if PMWS is observed. In lungs, irrespectively of the presence of PCV2, PPV2 was often associated with a severe reduction in size of alveolar spaces accompanied with an increase in the number of T lymphocytes in alveolar walls and peribronchial inflammatory reaction while significance is even higher when PMWS is observed. Whereas similar pathological conditions have often been attributed to infection by classical pathogens such as PCV2 [29], PRRSV [30] and SIV [31], in farm T none of the lung tissues tested positive for any of these classical viruses. Similarly, *Mycoplasma hyopneumonia* was not detected in areas where there was a strong peribronchial T-cell infiltrate [32]. Since none of these lesions could be directly attributed to any known pathogens and since there was a heavy PPV2 load in the lung parenchyma, associated with inflammatory lesions, we speculate that this virus may be a significant contributing factor in the development of those lesions. This conclusion is in agreement with the recent observation by Csagola and colleagues (2016) [20] which indicates that PPV2 infections are associated with respiratory health problems [20].

The results obtained in this study also indicate that IS PCR is a valuable diagnostic tool for the detection of PPV2.

Conclusions

We observed that PPV2 was localized mostly in lymphocytes in the lungs. Neither CD3 antigen nor lysozyme was expressed by these infected cells. In contrast, a low level of SLAIIDQ was expressed by infected cells suggesting that PPV2 may have a specific tropism for immature B lymphocytes and/or NK lymphocytes, rather than T lymphocytes. Furthermore, we conclude that PPV2 may contribute to the pathogenesis of pneumonia. Overall, these observations are consistent with the general nature of parvoviruses which enter into organism through the oropharyngeal route and replicate in lymphoid cells to ultimately alter the lymphoid system and the gastrointestinal tract. Similarly, canine minute virus (*Canine bocaparvovirus* 1) has been found to cause interstitial pneumonia and lymphoid necrosis in Peyer's patches [33]. Therefore, it is possible that all the lesions we have reported may be attributable, at least in part, to porcine parvovirus infection. To gather further evidence for this hypothesis, infections of SPF pigs will be required once in vitro PPV2 production in cell cultures is resolved.

Methods

Samples

Lungs were collected from 47 dead weaned pigs from a PMWS-positive farm (Farm E) and from 13 two to three-month-old dead pigs from a PMWS-negative farm (Farm T), both in Hungary. After post-mortem examination lungs were fixed in 10% neutral buffered formalin for 5–6 h, routinely processed, paraffin wax embedded, sectioned and stained for light microscopy as described above. To determine the presence of bacteria in tissue Brown and Brenn (B&B) staining method was used [34]. Parallel fresh lung samples were collected and stored at – 20 °C until processing. Lungs were tested for PPV2 and PCV2 by polymerase chain reaction (PCR). PPV2 complete genome sequence was revealed, designated as strain PPV2_Ted and deposited in Genbank, (access number: KX517759). Besides viruses of interest for this study all samples were checked for presence of Porcine parvovirus 1, 3 and 4, porcine Boca like virus (PBlV), Porcine boca virus 1, 2, 3 and 4 (PBoV), Torque teno sus virus 1 and 2 (TTSuV), Porcine cytomegalovirus (PCMV) (only in farm T), Aujezsky disease virus (ADV), Porcine reproductive and respiratory syndrome virus (PRRSV), Swine influence virus (H1N1/H3N2) (SIV) and Swine adenovirus (6 V/7 V). Paraffin wax embedded tissue was subjected to immunohistochemistry (IHC) to detect CD3, swine leukocyte antigen class II DQ (SLAIIDQ), lysozyme, PRRSV, swine influenza (SIV), *Mycoplasma hyopneumoniae (Mhyo)*, and ISH to detect ssDNA and dsDNA of PCV2. PPV2 positive samples were subjected to in situ PCR to detect the virus.

PCR test for PCV2,TTSuV, PPV1–4, PoBoV1–4, PoBolV, 6 V/7 V, PCMV, PRRSV, SIV and ADV

PCV2 was detected by real time qPCR according to previous protocols by Cadar et al. [35]; TTSuV1–2 by classical one step PCR according to previous protocols by Segales et al. [36]; PPV1 was checked using nested PCR according to Soares et al. [37]; PPV2–4, PoBoV1–4, PoBolV was detected by classical PCR according to previous protocols by Zhai et al., Csagola et al. and Ndze et al. [15, 38, 39]; PCMV was detected by classic PCR according to previous protocol by Hamel et al. [40]; 6 V/7 V by classical PCR according previous protocol by Kiss et al. [41]; ADV was detected by real-time PCR according to previous protocol by McKillen et al. [42]; PRRSV and SIV were detected by real time reverse nested RT PCR according to previous protocol by Biernacka et al. [43].

Immunohistochemistry to detect CD3, SLAIIDQ, lysozyme, PRRSV, SIV and *Mycoplasma hyopneumoniae*

Lung sections were dewaxed with xylene and rehydrated through graded alcohols to water. Endogenous peroxidase activity was blocked by incubation with 3% hydrogen peroxide in 0.1 M Tris-buffered saline (TBS, pH = 7.6) for 30 min. Immunohistochemistry was performed with seven primary antibodies: anti-human CD3, anti-SLAIIDQ, anti-lysozyme anti-PRRSV, anti-H1N1/H3N2 and anti-Mhyo with specific pretreatment and dilutions given in Additional file 11 as described previously [44–46]. For visualization of the positive reactions an anti-rabbit and anti-mouse labelled polymer HRP conjugated detection system (Envision, Dako) was used with a final incubation in diaminobenzidine (DAB)–hydrogen peroxide solution for 5 min (Dako, Denmark). Slides were counterstained in Mayer's haematoxylin, dehydrated, cover-slipped and microscopically examined. Lymph node from a slaughtered healthy pig served as positive control tissue. As negative controls, irrelevant primary antibodies at the same dilution were used as substitutes for the specific antibodies. The immune response observed in the lungs was graded as no immune cells or "0", weak infiltration or "1", moderate infiltration or "2" and severe infiltration or "3". For positive grading controls, lung sections positive for PRRSV, SIV or *Mhyo* were used. Negative controls were prepared by omitting the primary antibodies.

In situ hybridization to detect PCV2

To detect PCV2 DNA in tissues, ISH was carried out on paraffin-embedded samples as previously described [47]. The level of PCV2 ssDNA and/or dsDNA was estimated in different cell types.

In situ polymerase chain reaction (IS-PCR)

Direct IS-PCR was performed as previously described [23, 24, 48–50], with some modifications. Sections were dewaxed in xylene and rehydrated through different grades of ethanol to water. Dewaxed sections on DNase/RNase-free electrocharged slides were incubated with 40 μl Proteinase K (Dako) in 2 ml TBS (according to manufacturer's instructions) for 3 min at room temperature. Direct in situ PCR was performed using specific primers forward PPV2AF 5′-ACACGATGAGCGGTACGA-3′ and reverse PPV2AR 5′-TCCTCACGAGGTCTCTTCTG-3′ to amplify a 279 bp long ORF2 region sequence (GenBank access number NC_035180) as previously described [15]. After thorough washing of the slides with DEPC-treated water, 100% ethanol and air dry, 10 μl of PCR optimal solution (master mix) containing digoxigenin-11-(2′-deoxy-uridine-5′)-triphosphate (DIG-11-dUTP; Roche, USA) was added [23] on dried cut and the slides were covered. For amplification a Hot Start polymerase (Qiagen) was used. Cycling conditions and primers (Sigma-Aldrich) were used as described [15] and were further optimized for IS-PCR, such as increasing the denaturing and annealing temperatures by 1 °C and expanding to 15 s [24, 48–50]: activation step 95 °C/5 min; denaturation 95 °C/45 s, elongation 72 °C/1 min, annealing 57 °C/55 s and final elongation 72 °C/5 min during 30 cycles in in situ PCR thermal cycler (Perkin Elmer Geneamp In situ PCR System 1000 Thermal Cycler). Slides were stored overnight at 4 °C to immobilize in situ the amplicons. Sections were then washed 3X in 0.5 and 3X in 0.25 Saline-Sodium Citrate (SSC) buffer (Sigma-Aldrich) and finally 3X in Tris buffer pH 7.6. The detection was performed as described for ISH. To exclude primer independent amplification, positive samples were repeatedly tested with either the forward or reverse primer. As a negative control a paraffin block tissue from an animal that was PCR negative for PPV2 was used.

Double staining in situ PCR/IHC

Double staining to detect PPV2 and B and T lymphocytes and monocytes/macrophages was performed using a previously described protocol for in situ PCR to detect PPV2 and IHC to detect host markers CD3, SLAIIDQ and lysozyme. The forward order was detection of PPV2 nucleic acid first and then detection of host antigens (CD3, SLAIIDQ and lysozyme), while the reverse order started with the detection of the host antigens (CD3, SLAIIDQ and lysozyme) and then the viral nucleic acid.

IHC-is-PCR

Slides were processed with IS-PCR protocol until and incubated with NBT/BCIP to visualize positive signal for PPV2 presence without counterstaining. After incubation, the slides were placed in TBS and the appearance of blue chromogen was monitored under light microscope and were routinely subject to IHC protocol. Tissues were not pre-treated with *pronase* for CD3 and Lysozime detection but were incubated in citrate buffer pH 6 for 20 min at 96 °C for SLAIIDQ detection. Endogenous peroxidase activity was blocked by incubation with 3% hydrogen peroxide in TBS for 30 min. Tissue sections were rinsed in TBS and incubated with 20% normal goat serum solution in TBS for 1 h at room temperature.

Is-PCR-IHC

The slides were routinely subjected to IHC to detect CD3, SLAIIDQ and lysozyme followed by an incubation with DAB to visualize positive reaction. After incubation with DAB solution, without counterstaining, slides were placed in 100% ethanol and the appearance of brown chromogen was monitored under light microscope. Slides were then routinely processed to IS-PCR as previously described. Controls for IHC or in situ PCR were performed in single reaction.

Statistical analysis

Frequencies of pathological lesions and severity of immune cell infiltrations were assessed. The studied groups of samples were PCR positive and negative for the presence of PPV2; PMWS affected and non-affected (PCV2 positive) and PCV2-negative animals. All statistical analyses were performed using Statistical Analysis System (SAS®) for windows 6.14 (SAS Institute Inc., Cary, NC, USA). Depending on the parameterization (coding) of categorical explanatory variable we used GENMOD or LOGISTIC procedures and as our sample size was small we never used more than two explanatory variables in the model neither their interactions. Thus, the effects of age (defined in months, covariate in models) and/or other relevant dependent variables (see Additional files 5, 6 and 7) on the prevalence of PPV2 (categorized as 0 or 1) were analyzed by univariate generalized linear models (PROC GENMOD with normal distribution and link function identity). Furthermore, the effects of relevant dependent variables (see Additional file 2) on the prevalence of PMWS (categorized as 0 or 1) were analyzed by logistic regression (PROC LOGISTIC with link function logit and option ODDSRATIO).

Additional files

Additional file 1: Table presents results of PCR test for presence of following viruses: TTSuV, PPV1–4, PoBoV1–4, PoBolV, 6 V/7 V, PCMV, PRRSV, SIV and ADV in farm E.

Additional file 2: ODS results Farm E– PPV2 vs viruses.

Additional file 3: Table presents results of histopathological examination of lungs in farm E.

Additional file 4: Table presents results of presence of PCV2 in lungs tested by ISH in farm E.

Additional file 5: Wald Chi2-square Farm E: Histopathology.

Additional file 6: Wald Chi2-square Farm E: ISH PCV2.

Additional file 7: Wald Chi2-square Farm E: IHC immune cells.

Additional file 8: Results of IHC to detect specific immune cell markers in farm E.

Additional file 9: Presence of PPV2 by in situ PCR, histopathology findings and immune cell reaction in farm T.

Additional file 10: Presence of PPV2 by in situ PCR and other pathogens in farm T.

Additional file 11: Details of primary antibodies used for IHC.

Abbreviations

6 V/7 V: Porcine adenovirus; ADV: Aujezsky disease virus; B&B: Brown and Brenn; IHC: Immunohistochemistry; IS PCR: In situ polymerase chain reaction; *Mhyo*: *Mycoplasma hyopneumoniae*; ORFs: Open reading frames; PCMV: Porcine cytomegalovirus; PCV2: Porcine circovirus type 2; PMWS: post-weaning multi-systemic wasting syndrome; PoBolV: Porcine boca like virus; PoBoV: Porcine bocavirus; PPV: Porcine parvovirus; PRRSV: Porcine reproductive and respiratory syndrome virus; SIV: Swine influenza; SLAIIDQ: Swine leukocyte antigen class II DQ; TBS: Tris-buffered saline; TTSuV: Torque teno sus virus

Acknowledgements

We are grateful for support from the COST Action FA0902, KTIA_AIK_12-1-2012-0012, "MendTheGap" H2020-TWINN-2015 No 692249 and "MitoTAUROmics" HRZZ IP-11-2013-9070. We are grateful to Dr. sc. Petra Radulovic for assistance in immunohistochemistry. We are thankful for the comments and edits made by Dr. Sionagh H. Smith.We dedicate this work in memory of our friend and colleague Prof. Tuboly Tamás.

Funding

TA-A was support by BBSRC Institute Strategic Programme grants (BB/J004227/1, BB/P013740/1).

Authors' contributions

DN: drafted and wrote the manuscript, performed IHC and IS PCR; DC performed PCR; AJ review manuscript and analyze results; AC perform PCR, drafted and review manuscript and analyzed the data. TT, TA-A and TS: contributed to conception and design and wrote manuscript. All authors read and approved the final manuscript.

Competing interests

The authors declare that they have no competing interests.

Author details

Department of Pathology, Croatian Veterinary Institute, Savska cesta 143, 10000 Zagreb, Croatia. [2]Department for Animal science, Faculty of Agriculture, University of Zagreb, Svetosimunska 25, 10000 Zagreb, Croatia. WHO Collaborating Centre for Arbovirus and Haemorrhagic Fever Reference and Research, National Reference Centre for Tropical Infectious Diseases, Bernhard Nocht Institute for Tropical Medicine, Bernhard-Nocht-Strasse 74, 20359 Hamburg, Germany. [4]Department of Microbiology and Infectious Diseases, Faculty of Veterinary Science, Immunology, Szent István University, István u. 2, Budapest 1078, Hungary. [5]Department for Virology, Croatian Veterinary Institute, Savska cesta 143, 10000 Zagreb, Croatia. [6]Department of Pathology and Veterinary Diagnostic, Faculty of Veterinary Medicine, University of Life Science, Nowoursynowska 159C, 02-776 Warsaw, Poland. The Roslin Institute and Royal (Dick) School of Veterinary Studies, University of Edinburgh, Easter Bush, Edingburgh, United Kingdom.

References

1. International Committee on Taxonomy of Viruses. In. In. http://ictvonline.org/virusTaxonomy.asp. Accessed 3 Feb 2018.
2. Xiao CT, Gimenez-Lirola LG, Jiang YH, Halbur PG, Opriessnig T. Characterization of a novel porcine parvovirus tentatively designated PPV5. PLoS One. 2013;8(6):e65312.
3. Ni J, Qiao C, Han X, Han T, Kang W, Zi Z, Cao Z, Zhai X, Cai X. Identification and genomic characterization of a novel porcine parvovirus (PPV6) in China. Virol J. 2014;11:203.
4. NCBI. In. https://www.ncbi.nlm.nih.gov/taxonomy/?term=porcine+bocavirus. Accessed 3rd Feb 2018).
5. Tijssen P, Agbandje-McKenna M, Almendral JM, Bergoin M, Flegel TW, Hedman H, Kleinschmidt J, Li Y, Pintel DJ, Tattarsall P. Family Parvoviridae. In: AMQ K, Adams MJ, Carstens EB, Lefkowitz EJ, editors. Virus Taxonomy 9th report of the International Committee on Taxonomy of Viruses. London: Academic Press; 2011. p. 405–25.
6. Lau SK, Woo PC, Tse H, Fu CT, Au WK, Chen XC, Tsoi HW, Tsang TH, Chan JS, Tsang DN, et al. Identification of novel porcine and bovine parvoviruses closely related to human parvovirus 4. J Gen Virol. 2008;89(Pt 8):1840–8.
7. Cheung AK, Wu G, Wang D, Bayles DO, Lager KM, Vincent AL. Identification and molecular cloning of a novel porcine parvovirus. Arch Virol. 2010; 155(5):801–6.
8. Blomstrom AL, Belak S, Fossum C, McKillen J, Allan G, Wallgren P, Berg M. Detection of a novel porcine boca-like virus in the background of porcine circovirus type 2 induced postweaning multisystemic wasting syndrome. Virus Res. 2009;146(1–2):125–9.
9. Cheng WX, Li JS, Huang CP, Yao DP, Liu N, Cui SX, Jin Y, Duan ZJ. Identification and nearly full-length genome characterization of novel porcine bocaviruses. PLoS One. 5(10):e13583.
10. McKillen J, McNeilly F, Duffy C, McMenamy M, McNair I, Hjertner B, Millar A, McKay K, Lagan P, Adair B et al: Isolation in cell cultures and initial characterisation of two novel bocavirus species from swine in Northern Ireland. Vet Microbiol, 152(1–2):39–45.
11. Lau SK, Woo PC, Yip CC, Li KS, Fu CT, Huang Y, Chan KH, Yuen KY. Co-existence of multiple strains of two novel porcine bocaviruses in the same pig, a previously undescribed phenomenon in members of the family Parvoviridae, and evidence for inter- and intra-host genetic diversity and recombination. J Gen Virol. 92(Pt 9):2047–59.
12. Hijikata M, Abe K, Win KM, Shimizu YK, Keicho N, Yoshikura H. Identification of new parvovirus DNA sequence in swine sera from Myanmar. Jpn J Infect Dis. 2001;54(6):244 5.
13. Manteufel J, Truyen U. Animal bocaviruses: a brief review. Intervirology. 2008;51(5):328–34.
14. Wang F, Wei Y, Zhu C, Huang X, Xu Y, Yu L, Yu X. Novel parvovirus sublineage in the family of Parvoviridae. Virus Genes. 2010;41(2):305–8.
15. Csagola A, Lorincz M, Cadar D, Tombacz K, Biksi I, Tuboly T. Detection, prevalence and analysis of emerging porcine parvovirus infections. Arch Virol. 2012;157(6):1003–10.
16. Cadar D, Lorincz M, Kiss T, Novosel D, Podgorska K, Becskei Z, Tuboly T, Csagola A. Emerging novel porcine parvoviruses in Europe: origin, evolution, phylodynamics and phylogeography. J Gen Virol; 2013.
17. Opriessnig T, Xiao CT, Gerber PF, Halbur PG. Identification of recently described porcine parvoviruses in archived North American samples from 1996 and association with porcine circovirus associated disease. Vet Microbiol. 2014;173(1–2):9–16.
18. Sun J, Huang L, Wei Y, Wang Y, Chen D, Du W, Wu H, Liu C. Prevalence of emerging porcine parvoviruses and their co-infections with porcine circovirus type 2 in China. Arch Virol. 2015;
19. Saekhow P, Mawatari T, Ikeda H. Coexistence of multiple strains of porcine parvovirus 2 in pig farms. Microbiol Immunol. 2014;58(7):382–7.
20. Csagola A, Zadori Z, Meszaros I, Tuboly T. Detection of porcine parvovirus 2 (ungulate Tetraparvovirus 3) specific antibodies and examination of the serological profile of an infected swine herd. PLoS One. 2016;11(3): e0151036.
21. Mostegl MM, Richter B, Dinhopl N, Weissenbock H. Influence of prolonged formalin fixation of tissue samples on the sensitivity of chromogenic in situ hybridization. J Vet Diagn Investig. 2011;23(6):1212–6.
22. Ha Y, Chae C. Optimal probe size and fixation time for the detection of porcine circovirus-2 DNA by in situ hybridization in formalin-fixed, paraffin-embedded tissue. J Vet Diagn Investig. 2009;21(5):649–54.
23. Nuovo GJ. In situ PCR: protocols and applications. PCR Methods Appl. 1995; 4(4):S151–67.
24. Nuovo GJ. Co-labeling using in situ PCR: a review. J Histochem Cytochem. 2001;49(11):1329–39.
25. Cotmore SF, Tattersall P. The autonomously replicating parvoviruses of vertebrates. Adv Virus Res. 1987;33:91–174.
26. Kerr J, Cotmore S, Bloom ME, Linden RM, Parrish CR. Parvoviruses. London: Edward Arnold Ltd; 2006.
27. Lunney JK, Ho CS, Wysocki M, Smith DM. Molecular genetics of the swine major histocompatibility complex, the SLA complex. Dev Comp Immunol. 2009;33(3):362–74.
28. Perez C, Moreno S, Summerfield A, Domenech N, Alvarez B, Correa C, Alonso F, Ezquerra A, Dominguez J, Revilla C. Characterisation of porcine bone marrow progenitor cells identified by the anti-c-kit (CD117) monoclonal antibody 2B8/BM. J Immunol Methods. 2007;321(1–2):70–9.
29. Segales J, Rosell C, Domingo M. Pathological findings associated with naturally acquired porcine circovirus type 2 associated disease. Vet Microbiol. 2004;98(2):137–49.
30. Rossow KD, Collins JE, Goyal SM, Nelson EA, Christopher-Hennings J, Benfield DA. Pathogenesis of porcine reproductive and respiratory syndrome virus infection in gnotobiotic pigs. Vet Pathol. 1995;32(4):361–73.
31. Janke BH. Clinicopathological features of swine influenza. Curr Top Microbiol Immunol. 2013;370:69–83.
32. Whittlestone P. The role of mycoplasmas in the production of pneumonia in the pig. Amsterdam: Associated Scinetific Publishers; 1972.
33. Carmichael LE, Schlafer DH, Hashimoto A. Minute virus of canines (MVC, canine parvovirus type-1): pathogenicity for pups and seroprevalence estimate. J Vet Diagn Investig. 1994;6(2):165–74.
34. Luna L. Manual of histologic staining methods of AFIP. 3rd ed. New York: McGraw Hill Publications; 1968.
35. Cadar D, Csagola A, Spinu M, Dan A, Ursu K, Lorincz M, Tuboly T. Prevalence of porcine circoviruses in Transylvanian wild boars, detected by real-time PCR–short communication. Acta Vet Hung. 2010;58(4):475–81.
36. Segales J, Martinez-Guino L, Cortey M, Navarro N, Huerta E, Sibila M, Pujols J, Kekarainen T. Retrospective study on swine torque Teno virus genogroups 1 and 2 infection from 1985 to 2005 in Spain. Vet Microbiol. 2009;134(3–4): 199–207.
37. Soares RM, Durigon EL, Bersano JG, Richtzenhain LJ. Detection of porcine parvovirus DNA by the polymerase chain reaction assay using primers to the highly conserved nonstructural protein gene, NS-1. J Virol Methods. 1999;78(1–2):191–8.

38. Zhai S, Yue C, Wei Z, Long J, Ran D, Lin T, Deng Y, Huang L, Sun L, Zheng H, et al. High prevalence of a novel porcine bocavirus in weanling piglets with respiratory tract symptoms in China. Arch Virol. 2010;155(8):1313–7.
39. Ndze VN, Cadar D, Csagola A, Kisfali P, Kovacs E, Farkas S, Ngu AF, Esona MD, Dan A, Tuboly T, et al. Detection of novel porcine bocaviruses in fecal samples of asymptomatic pigs in Cameroon. Infect Genet Evol. 2013;17:277–82.
40. Hamel AL, Lin L, Sachvie C, Grudeski E, Nayar GP. PCR assay for detecting porcine cytomegalovirus. J Clin Microbiol. 1999;37(11):3767–8.
41. Kiss I, Matiz K, Allard A, Wadell G, Benko M. Detection of homologous DNA sequences in animal adenoviruses by polymerase chain reaction. Acta Vet Hung. 1996;44(2):243–51.
42. McKillen J, Hjertner B, Millar A, McNeilly F, Belak S, Adair B, Allan G. Molecular beacon real-time PCR detection of swine viruses. J Virol Methods. 2007;140(1–2):155–65.
43. Biernacka K, Karbowiak P, Wrobel P, Chareza T, Czopowicz M, Balka G, Goodell C, Rauh R, Stadejek T. Detection of porcine reproductive and respiratory syndrome virus (PRRSV) and influenza a virus (IAV) in oral fluid of pigs. Res Vet Sci. 2016;109:74–80.
44. Tanimoto T, Ohtsuki Y. Evaluation of antibodies reactive with porcine lymphocytes and lymphoma cells in formalin-fixed, paraffin-embedded, antigen-retrieved tissue sections. Am J Vet Res. 1996;57(6):853–9.
45. Evensen O. An immunohistochemical study on the cytogenetic origin of pulmonary multinucleate giant cells in porcine dermatosis vegetans. Vet Pathol. 1993;30(2):162–70.
46. Chianini F, Majo N, Segales J, Dominguez J, Domingo M. Immunohistological study of the immune system cells in paraffin-embedded tissues of conventional pigs. Vet Immunol Immunopathol. 2001; 82(3–4):245–55.
47. Rosell C, Segales J, Plana-Duran J, Balasch M, Rodriguez-Arrioja GM, Kennedy S, Allan GM, McNeilly F, Latimer KS, Domingo M. Pathological, immunohistochemical, and in-situ hybridization studies of natural cases of postweaning multisystemic wasting syndrome (PMWS) in pigs. J Comp Pathol. 1999;120(1):59–78.
48. Ocadiz-Delgado R, Castaneda-Saucedo E, Indra AK, Hernandez-Pando R, Flores-Guizar P, Cruz-Colin JL, Recillas-Targa F, Perez-Ishiwara G, Covarrubias L, Gariglio P. RXRalpha deletion and E6E7 oncogene expression are sufficient to induce cervical malignant lesions in vivo. Cancer Lett. 2012; 317(2):226–36.
49. Ocadiz-Delgado R, Castaneda-Saucedo E, Indra AK, Hernandez-Pando R, Gariglio P. Impaired cervical homeostasis upon selective ablation of RXRalpha in epithelial cells. Genesis. 2008;46(1):19–28.
50. Ocadiz-Delgado R, Marroquin-Chavira A, Hernandez-Mote R, Valencia C, Manjarrez-Zavala ME, Covarrubias L, Gariglio P. Induction of focal epithelial hyperplasia in tongue of young bk6-E6/E7 HPV16 transgenic mice. Transgenic Res. 2009;18(4):513–27.

23

Transmission parameters estimated for *Salmonella* typhimurium in swine using susceptible-infectious-resistant models and a Bayesian approach

Carla Correia-Gomes[1,7*], Theodoros Economou[2], Trevor Bailey[2], Pavel Brazdil[3,4], Lis Alban[5] and João Niza-Ribeiro[1,6]

Abstract

Background: Transmission models can aid understanding of disease dynamics and are useful in testing the efficiency of control measures. The aim of this study was to formulate an appropriate stochastic Susceptible-Infectious-Resistant/Carrier (SIR) model for *Salmonella* Typhimurium in pigs and thus estimate the transmission parameters between states.

Results: The transmission parameters were estimated using data from a longitudinal study of three Danish farrow-to-finish pig herds known to be infected. A Bayesian model framework was proposed, which comprised Binomial components for the transition from susceptible to infectious and from infectious to carrier; and a Poisson component for carrier to infectious. Cohort random effects were incorporated into these models to allow for unobserved cohort-specific variables as well as unobserved sources of transmission, thus enabling a more realistic estimation of the transmission parameters. In the case of the transition from susceptible to infectious, the cohort random effects were also time varying. The number of infectious pigs not detected by the parallel testing was treated as unknown, and the probability of non-detection was estimated using information about the sensitivity and specificity of the bacteriological and serological tests. The estimate of the transmission rate from susceptible to infectious was 0.33 [0.06, 1.52], from infectious to carrier was 0.18 [0.14, 0.23] and from carrier to infectious was 0.01 [0.0001, 0.04]. The estimate for the basic reproduction ration (R_0) was 1.91 [0.78, 5.24]. The probability of non-detection was estimated to be 0.18 [0.12, 0.25].

Conclusions: The proposed framework for stochastic SIR models was successfully implemented to estimate transmission rate parameters for *Salmonella* Typhimurium in swine field data. R_0 was 1.91, implying that there was dissemination of the infection within pigs of the same cohort. There was significant temporal-cohort variability, especially at the susceptible to infectious stage. The model adequately fitted the data, allowing for both observed and unobserved sources of uncertainty (cohort effects, diagnostic test sensitivity), so leading to more reliable estimates of transmission parameters.

Keywords: *Salmonella* typhimurium, Transmission parameters, Bayesian approach

Correspondence: carla.gomes@sruc.ac.uk
[1]ICBAS-UP - Department of Population Studies, Instituto de Ciências Biomédicas Abel Salazar – Universidade do Porto, Rua de Jorge Viterbo Ferreira, n°228, 4050-313 Porto, Portugal
[7]ERU-SRUC – Epidemiology Research Unit, Future Farming Systems, SRUC, Drummondhill, Inverness, IV2 4JZ, UK
Full list of author information is available at the end of the article

Background

Salmonella Typhimurium is one of the major food-borne pathogens currently causing disease in humans [1] and it is often related to consumption of pork products. Given its relevance to consumer food safety, *Salmonella spp.* control was considered necessary by the European food safety policy makers under the EC Regulation 2160/2003. In the near future, it is possible that a mandatory target reduction will be put in place in the European Union, regarding the *Salmonella* prevalence for pigs.

In practice, however, the control of this agent has proved to be difficult and expensive at the farm level [2]. Consequently, evaluating the efficiency of control strategies relating to this agent has become an important issue, as stated in recent reports [3]. Modelling the dynamics of *Salmonella* Typhimurium in pigs is important in evaluating alternative control strategies. The basic reproduction ratio (R_0) expresses the number of secondary cases to which a primary case gives rise during the infectious period and provides valuable information for simulation models. If R_0 is less than unity then the disease is receding, but when it is higher than unity the disease is spreading.

Susceptible – Infectious – Resistant (SIR) models are attractive tools that aid understanding of disease dynamics. The SIR model formulates the changes of individuals in the population between different disease states in terms of a system of ordinary differential equations (ODE), known as the Kermack-McKendrick ODE model [4]. The variables in the system are given by the three components groups: susceptible (S), infectious (I) and carriers (R). SIR models include a mathematical specification of the movement into and out of the three components. The key parameter in each of these mathematical specifications is the transition rate: from S to I (β), from I to R (α) and from R to I (ν). If such modelling is to be helpful in infectious disease control, it is critical to have the best possible estimates of these rates (β, α and ν), as all three are important for modelling the spread of infection. Transmission data, generated under controlled conditions (i.e. experimental studies or controlled field studies) are necessary to estimate the transition rates as accurately as possible.

In most cases *Salmonella* Typhimurium causes subclinical infection in swine with no apparent symptoms of disease. This makes it difficult to assess the infection status of individual pigs in an infected population without testing each animal several times. One of the difficulties in obtaining accurate estimates for β in *Salmonella* Typhimurium studies stems from the fact that the currently available bacteriological and serological tests used to assign the infection status are imperfect, introducing uncertainty when trying to classify each animal. Yet another source of uncertainty comes from the fact that pigs, once infected, shed the agent intermittently.

In the literature, it is conventional to use generalised linear models (GLMs) to describe the counts of animals moving between states (e.g. from S to I) using either Poisson [5-8] or Binomial distributions [4,9]. GLMs can be used to estimate all three transmission parameters although they lack flexibility, for example in capturing the effect of sensitivity and specificity of the diagnostic test used. GLMs also lack the flexibility to allow for unobserved effects of variables not recorded in the data but which influence the outcomes. The Bayesian framework proposed in this paper is flexible enough to incorporate such effects and also quantify the uncertainty due to imperfect diagnostic tests.

Following cohorts of animals in order to determine the dynamics of *S.* Typhimurium in susceptible populations is a very expensive procedure and only a few such studies exist. In this paper, we use data from a previous observational study designed and performed by Kranker *et al.* [10].

A Bayesian modelling framework was proposed and used to estimate transmission parameters (transition rate from S to I, transition rate from I to R and transition rate from R to I) for *Salmonella* Typhimurium in pig herds, using the longitudinal data from Kranker *et al.* [10]. The sensitivity and specificity of the tests used to classify the animals in the Kranker study were allowed for in the statistical model, which also incorporated random effects to allow for cohort heterogeneity.

Methods

Study herds, sampling, bacteriology and ELISA test

The data used have been previously described by Kranker *et al.* [10] and originate from three Danish pig herds known to be infected with *Salmonella* Typhimurium. The herds had moderate to high levels of *Salmonella* Typhimurium and therefore the within-herd prevalence was 40% or higher. These measures of prevalence were based on meat-juice samples collected over three months, evaluated by use of an optical density (OD) cut-off of 20%. Two of the farms, with 650 and 440 sows, respectively, were two-site operations; the remaining farm was a three-site operation with 300 sows. The three herds were self-supplying. In each herd, 10 litters were randomly selected, and in each litter, the ears of six randomly selected piglets were tagged. To account for variations in *Salmonella* shedding over time, litters from each herd were divided into two groups of five litters that were raised at approximately one-month intervals. Thus, on each farm there were two cohorts consisting of 30 pigs each, yielding a total of 180 piglets at the start of the study. All ear-tagged pigs from a given cohort were raised together for the entire observation period. The animals were followed longitudinally

10] and were first tested at the age of four weeks and hereafter at two to five week intervals until the age of laughter. Slaughter age varied between cohorts but was n average around 25 weeks. Cohorts were tested either ix to seven times in total. On each testing occasion, sera nd faeces from the animals were collected and tested for he presence of *Salmonella spp.*. At the age of four weeks nly faeces were collected, because maternal antibodies till present could give a false positive result. An animal vas considered serologically positive, wherever the sero-ogical test revealed a result of OD% >20, and bacterio-ogically positive if *Salmonella* was isolated from the aeces. The serological test used at this cut-off value is onsidered to have a sensitivity of 68% and to be 100% pecific [11]. The bacteriological test is considered to be 00% specific and the sensitivity is around 30 to 55% 12]. These test characteristics were incorporated in the tatistical model.

nfection status of the pigs

The testing time interval was different in each cohort, arying from two to five weeks. A homogenous dataset vas derived by inferring the infection status of each pig, very two weeks. The time step of two weeks was chosen ecause on average it takes two weeks for an animal to est positive to serology after being infected. It was herefore assumed that an animal was infectious in the wo weeks before being seropositive. The most likely nfection status of each pig was determined for each wo-week time step based on both faecal shedding and erology results from the sampling period closest to each ime step. Each animal was categorized as susceptible (S), nfectious (I) or carrier (R). An animal was considered usceptible if the agent was not present and the animal vas at the risk of infection. An animal was considered nfectious if it was shedding the agent and a potential ource of infection to other animals. An animal that was nfected with the agent but not shedding and therefore ot able to infect other animals was considered a car-ier. In the absence of reasonable sensitivity of the bac-eriological culture method, serology offered an alternative nd complementary way to assign the infection status of a ig and both methods were used in parallel to categorise he pigs' status.

Pigs were attributed status S when there was no pres-nce of bacteria in the faecal samples and the OD% was elow 20. Status I was assigned from the date when a ig was found to be bacteriologically positive until it was o longer positive by this testing method. Additionally, igs were assigned to status I based on seroconversion. The beginning of the infectious period was set to two veeks prior to the recorded date of seroconversion 13,14] and the duration was set to four weeks, assuming hat a pig would shed *Salmonella spp.* within an average of four weeks. This average period was based on experimental data regarding duration of the shedding period [13,15]. Thus, information was used from both tests in parallel for pig classification. Finally, status I was followed by status R and the pigs could return to status I if they were found to be culture positive later on during the study period. It was assumed that no pig would return to the susceptible status after being infected, because of the relative short life span of finisher pigs (after infection it takes around 112 days to clear the agent from the organs [14], and post-weaned pigs are generally slaughtered before this time). The following describes a particular example of how the classification was performed: if a pig was shedding at a specific testing time, it was considered infectious in the nearest bi-weekly time step, until it became bacteriologically negative, after which it was considered a carrier (in the nearest bi-weekly time step). If a pig was serologically positive, in the presence of a negative culture, it was considered infected and therefore classified as infectious for at least four weeks, from the nearest bi-weekly time step prior the testing time. If an animal was bacteriologically and serologically negative, it was considered susceptible. Given that testing of piglets was restricted to bacteriology (which has low sensitivity) at the beginning of the follow-up period, some piglets infected by the sow could have been erroneously classified as susceptible. For this reason, the analysis in each cohort started at the time infected animals were first detected (by either serology or bacteriology).

Estimation of the transmission parameters

Conventionally, transmission parameters of infectious disease, including *Salmonella spp.*, in swine herds [14,16-21] are estimated using regression models. These are often based on data describing the prevalence of that disease in the country or region to which the particular study refers. As suggested in some studies [5,22,23], we first applied a stochastic SIR models in the form of Generalised Linear Models (GLMs) in order to estimate the three transmission parameters. However, preliminary results (not reported here) suggested the presence of overdispersion in the GLMs, hinting towards unobserved sources of variation in the data such as cohort heterogeneity. Instead, we here report a framework for stochastic SIR models which i) extends the current GLM framework by including random effects, ii) is implemented using a Bayesian approach thus allowing incorporation of prior information (such as the sensitivity of *Salmonella* tests), iii) explicitly estimates the probability of not detecting infectious animals due to test sensitivity and iv) incorporates all sources of uncertainty/variation thus obtaining more realistic estimates of transmission parameters. As suggested by some authors [5], the inclusion of random effects automatically accounts for overdispersion by inflating the variance of the response variable while at the same time allowing for cohort heterogeneity.

Stochastic SIR models (and other variants such as SI or SIS models) are well-established in animal disease literature [4,19-21]. The benefit of using a stochastic SIR model is that transmission parameters can be estimated using statistical modelling; here the conventional stochastic SIR model was extended by explicitly allowing for cohort variation and unobserved temporal effects. The three components of the stochastic SIR model are described in detail below.

Transition from susceptible to infectious

It was assumed that pigs become infected by "infectious contacts" defined as: either contact with other infected animals, or contact with their environment (rodents, contaminated muck or feed). The rate at which a given animal has infectious contacts was assumed i) to be constant in time and ii) proportional to the density of infectious animals [19], with a constant of proportionality β, i.e. the transmission rate parameter. In other words, the infectious contacts per animal happen randomly in time so that their occurrence can be described by a Poisson process. More precisely, the number of infectious contacts per animal in a period Δt is Poisson distributed with mean $\lambda = \beta\ (I/N)\ \Delta t$, where I is the number of infectious animals and N is the total number of animals, at the beginning of Δt. As such, the probability of no infectious contacts per animal in Δt is $\exp(-\beta\ (I/N)\ \Delta t)$, implying that the probability of infection in Δt is $p = 1 - \exp(-\beta\ (I/N)\ \Delta t)$. This means that the number of new cases C at the end of Δt is Binomial with parameters S and p so that the mean of C is S*p.

Here, the current established methodology was extended to allow for the fact that i) λ may vary in time due to exogenous factors and ii) λ may vary across cohorts due to unobserved cohort effects. A random (scaling) effect $\exp(r_{jt})$ was included, for the jth cohort at time t, to get $\lambda_{jt} = \beta\ (I/N)\ \exp(r_{jt})\ \Delta t$ as the mean number of infectious contacts of a random animal, in herd j at time t. Note that Δt denotes the length of a time interval whereas t refers to actual time. On average, $\exp(r_{jt})$ was assumed to be equal to one, so that across all cohorts and time, the average transmission rate parameter is still β. By doing this, variation due to cohort or unknown temporal effects was explicitly modelled, which would otherwise contribute to the uncertainty in estimating β.

All time intervals in the data are equal to two weeks so for clarity, Δt = 1 was set so that one time step Δt corresponds to two weeks. This does not qualitatively affect the estimation of the transmission parameters. Because of the nature of the data, time t is now defined in discrete consecutive (bi-weekly) time steps.

The model may be formulated as follows:

$$\begin{aligned} C_{jt} &\sim \text{Binomial}\left(S_{jt}, p_{jt}\right) \\ p_{jt} &= 1 - \exp\{-\beta(I_{jt-1}/N_{jt-1})\exp(r_{1jt})\} \\ \text{cloglog}\left(p_{jt}\right) &= \log(\beta) + \log(I_{jt-1}) - \log(N_{jt-1}) + r_{1jt} \end{aligned} \quad (1$$

where:

- C_{jt} denotes the number of new infectious animals in cohort (j) at the end of the time step (t),.
- S_{jt-1} is the number of susceptible animals in cohort (j) at the end of the time step (t-1),
- p_{jt} is the probability of a susceptible animal in cohort (j) at the end of time step (t-1) becoming infectious by the end of time step (t),
- cloglog is the complementary log-log transformation,
- β is the transmission rate parameter for the transition from susceptible to infectious,
- I_{jt-1} is the number of infectious animals in cohort (j) at the end of the time step (t-1),
- N_{jt-1} is the total number of animals in cohort (j) at the end of the time step (t-1), and.
- r_{1jt} is a cohort time-dependent random effect (whic is zero on average).

Note that, at the beginning of the study, pigs wer considered to be either in the S or I status depending o the test results. When there was no infectious pi present at the end of the previous time step, i.e. $I_{jt-1} = 0$ the probability of becoming infectious was modelled as:

$\text{Cloglog}\ (p_{jt}) = \log\ (\beta) + r_{1jt}$. This is because even if ther are no infectious pigs present, animals can still be infecte (e.g., contaminated environment, feed, water, etc.). In thi formulation, β is seen as the underlying rate of transitio for a random pig in an average cohort with no infectiou animals, while r_{1jt} allows for unobserved cohort-time ef fects in the data e.g., anthropogenic influence, rodents etc Note that homogeneous mixing of the pigs in each cohor (i.e. all pigs could come into contact with each other) wa assumed, due to the small size of the cohorts.

In using the number of infectious pigs I_{jt}, in each co hort at the end of time step t, it was necessary to ac count for the sensitivity of both the serological an bacteriological test. Since the specificity in both tests i considered to be 100%, the parallel specificity is 1. Thi implies that $I_{jt} = Iobs_{jt} + Inob_{jt}$, where $Iobs_{jt}$ is the observe value and $Inob_{jt}$ is the number of infectious animals no detected (false negative pigs). In other words, $Iobs_{jt}$ is lower bound on the actual I_{jt}. The unobserved variabl $Inob_{jt}$ may be incorporated (and thus estimated) in th stochastic model and here it was assumed that it has a Bi nomial distribution with parameters N_{jt} and pND wher pND is the probability of not detecting infectious animals. This probability, pND, is of course dependent on the sensitivity probabilities of each test, which were assumed to be independent. $Inob_{jt}$ was modelled as follows:

$$\begin{aligned} I_{jt} &= Iobs_{jt} + Inob_{jt} \\ Inob_{jt} &\sim \text{Binomial}(N_{jt}, pND) \\ pND &= (1-SenC)*(1-SenE) \end{aligned} \tag{2}$$

where:

- *SenC* is the sensitivity probability of microbiological culture, and.
- *SenE* is the sensitivity probability of the ELISA test.

Treating $Inob_{jt}$ as an unobserved random variable allows formal quantification of the uncertainty in the data due to test sensitivity and constitutes one of the novelties of the proposed model. The Bayesian framework (see section 5 later on) used to estimate the stochastic SIR model can easily incorporate the estimation of $Inob_{jt}$ given prior information on SenC and SenE.

Transition from infectious (I) to resistant (R)

The rate α at which a random infectious animal in a given cohort becomes a carrier was assumed to be constant in time. As such, the length of time τ until an infectious animal becomes carrier can be modelled by an exponential distribution with rate parameter α. So, given that the animal is infectious at the start of time interval Δt, the probability pR of becoming carrier is $pR = Pr(\tau \leq \Delta t) = 1\text{-}\exp(-\alpha\Delta t)$ since τ is exponentially distributed (recall that $\Delta t = 1$ was set for conciseness). As before, a random cohort effect r_{2j} was added to allow for cohort heterogeneity in the data, to obtain $pR_j = 1\text{-}\exp(-\alpha \exp(r2_j))$. The number of new carrier animals $Rnew_{jt}$ at the end of time step t, is thus Binomial with parameters I_{jt} and pR_j. Note that a single parameter α was utilised, describing the rate at which a random infectious animal in an average cohort, becomes carrier, however, cohort variability (not all cohorts are average) was allowed for through r_{2j}, which in turn reduces uncertainty in estimating α. The I to R transition was modelled as follows:

$$\begin{aligned} Rnew_{jt} &\sim \text{Binomial}\left(I_{jt}, pR_j\right) \\ \text{cloglog}\left(pR_j\right) &= \log(\alpha) + r_{2j} \end{aligned} \tag{3}$$

Transition from resistant to infectious

For this compartment of the model, the rate of infectious contacts ν in a random carrier animal was assumed to be constant in time, where ν is the transmission rate parameter for the transition from carrier to infectious. With similar arguments as in the S to I compartment, the number of infectious contacts per animal in time period Δt is Poisson distributed with mean νΔt. Since this transition was actually a rare event (only happening three times in the entire study), the Poisson distribution can be used, as it approximates the Binomial when its probability parameter is close to zero. So if in cohort j, there are R_{jt-1} carrier animals at the end of the previous time step, the number of transitions from R to I in time step t may be modelled as a Poisson variable with mean $\mu_{jt} = \nu R_{jt-1}\exp(r_{3j})$. More explicitly:

$$\begin{aligned} Inew_{jt} &\sim \text{Poisson}\left(\mu_{jt}\right) \\ \log\left(\mu_{jt}\right) &= \log(\nu) + \log\left(R_{jt-1}\right) + r_{3j} \end{aligned} \tag{4}$$

where:

- $Inew_{jt}$ denotes the number of new infectious animals (that result from this transition) in cohort (j) at the end of the time step (t),
- μ_{jt} is the mean number of carrier animals that become infectious in the cohort ( ) during time step (t),
- ν is the transmission rate parameter for the transition from carrier to infectious state,
- R_{jt-1} is the number of carrier animals at the end of the time step (t-1) in cohort (j), and.
- r_{3j} is a cohort random effect that allows for cohort heterogeneity.

Note that $R_{jt-1} = 0$ is possible, in which case $\log(R_{jt-1}) = 0$ was set. The argument for doing this is that the transmission rate parameter ν may be defined as the limit of μ_{jt}/R_{jt-1} as R_{jt-1} goes to zero. As such, ignoring the random effect for a moment, μ_{jt}/R_{jt-1} should tend to a constant (i.e. ν) as R_{jt-1} goes to zero rather than infinity. Note that in our data, $R_{jt-1} = 0$ happened on 20% of occasions. In the hypothetical case that $R_{jt-1} = 0$ for the majority of time steps and cohorts, then this component of the model (i.e. the transition R to I) becomes redundant as there will ultimately be almost no information with which to estimate the transition parameter.

Cohort random effects

As indicated above, random cohort effects were incorporated into each transition step to allow for i) cohort heterogeneity/variability in the data, ii) unobserved cohort-specific factors, iii) unobserved temporal effects in the S to I compartment. These effects were different for each transition under the assumption that any unobserved cohort factors affect each transition in a different way. For the transitions S to I and R to I, these random effects also allow for factors which affect disease spread but which are not dependent on the animals themselves (such as contaminated environment, feed, water, etc.).

For the transition S to I, the cohort random effects were assumed to be time-varying and auto-correlated, and were modelled as:

$$r_{1j,t=1} \sim Normal(0, \sigma_1^2)$$
$$r_{1j,t} \sim Normal(r_{1j,t-1}, \sigma_1^2) \quad (5)$$

where the cohort random effect (r_{1jt}) for time step t depends on the previous cohort random effect at time (t-1). With this cohort time-dependent random effect any unobserved dynamic behaviour in the spreading of infection within cohorts was captured, such as that due to infected mice.

For the transition I to R and R to I, the random effects were modelled as:

$$r_{kj} \sim Normal(0, \sigma_k^2), k = 2, 3 \quad (6)$$

where:

- subscript *j* denotes cohorts and.
- σ_k^2 is the variance of the unobserved cohorts effects.

In a preliminary model building stage, a cohort time-dependent random effect, $r_{2jt,}$ was considered for the transition I to R; however the results showed no improvement to the model fit. Note that cohort time-dependent random effects were not considered for the Poisson model of the transition R to I. The transition only occurred three times in the entire study and it would be unreasonable to try to estimate unobserved temporal effects from this.

Model implementation

The overall SIR model described above was implemented in a Bayesian framework and fitted using Markov chain Monte Carlo (MCMC). In this framework, parameters are treated as random variables whose "prior" distribution expresses our uncertainty about their value before any data is observed. Prior distributions (priors) are combined with the observed data through Bayes theorem to produce the posterior distributions for each parameter (posteriors). The posteriors express the uncertainty about model parameters after data is observed and all statistical inference is based solely on the posteriors. MCMC is a numerical technique which produces samples of values that eventually converge (after a certain "burn-in" number) to samples of values from the posterior (distribution) of each parameter.

There was no historical information with which to inform the prior distributions of log (β), log (α) and log (ν), so Normal distributions with zero mean and a variance of 100 were used, reflecting prior ignorance while avoiding the use of improper prior distributions [24]. For the sensitivity probabilities of both serological and bacteriological tests, a Beta distribution was used as a prior. Previous information about the sensitivity of both tests [11,12] was used to inform those Beta distributions: a mean of 0.49 for faecal culture and a mean of 0.68 for Danish mix ELISA were assumed, so SenC ~ Beta (48.5, 50.5) and SenE ~ Beta (58.5, 27.5) were specified. These priors have means 0.49 and 0.68 respectively, and variances that match the range of possible values dictated by the findings of [11,12]. Specificity was assumed to be 100% in both tests. The precision (i.e. the inverse of the variance) of the Normal distribution for each random effect was given a Gamma (0.5, 0.005) prior distribution (large mean and very large variance to indicate prior ignorance).

The complete SIR model was implemented in the open-source statistical software WinBUGS [25]. Exactly 100,000 posterior samples were collected after a 5,000 sample burn-in to ensure convergence to the posterior distribution [26]. Two MCMC runs were performed, with different initial values, to ensure convergence and mixing. The samples were thinned by only collecting one in 10 consecutive samples to eliminate autocorrelation in posterior samples (the R package "coda" [27] was used) so that in total we ended up with 20,000 samples. Convergence was assessed by inspection of trace-plots but also more formally using the Raftery and Lewis diagnostic and the Gelman-Rubin R-hat diagnostic which should be sufficiently close to one if convergence has been achieved [28,29]. Mixing in the chains was assessed by comparing the Markov Chain (MC) error with the standard deviation for each parameter. Ideally the MC error for each parameter should be less than 5% of the standard deviation [30] for good mixing.

Posterior predictive simulation was used for model checking as described by Gilks *et al.* [24]. This technique is effectively testing whether the observed data are extreme in relation to the posterior predictive distribution of the observations (i.e., the fitted model). The deviance was the measure adopted for comparison. The technique involves the calculation of a "p-value" which should not be extreme (close to 0 or 1) for good model fit.

Calculations of the basic reproduction ratio (R_0)

Samples from the posterior distribution of R_0 were calculated from those of β and α using the following formula [5]:

$$R_0 = {}^{\beta}/_{\alpha} \quad (7)$$

where β is the transition rate from S to I, and α is the transition rate from I to R.

Results

Transmission parameters

Results, in terms of summary statistics from the posterior samples, are shown in Table 1. Note that the posterior

Table 1 Summary measures of the transmission parameters and random effects variances from the *Salmonella* transmission in pigs SIR model

Parameters	Mean	Standard deviation	Quartiles					Rhat
			2,5%	25%	50%	75%	97,5%	
β	0.44	0.49	0.06	0.20	0.33	0.52	1.52	1.0021
α	0.18	0.02	0.14	0.17	0.18	0.20	0.23	1.0009
v	0.02	0.03	0.0001	0.006	0.01	0.02	0.04	1.0009
σ_1^2	3.00	1.80	0.80	1.76	2.60	3.77	7.59	1.0011
σ_2^2	0.02	0.04	0.002	0.005	0.01	0.02	0.096	1.0009
σ_3^2	6.64	38.82	0.003	0.06	0.08	3.85	44.44	1.0010
pND	0.18	0.03	0.12	0.16	0.18	0.20	0.25	
R_0	2.20	1.25	0.78	1.46	1.91	2.56	5.24	

Legend: β – transition rate from susceptible to infectious, α – transition rate from infectious to carrier, v – transition rate from carrier to infectious, σ_1^2 – variance of the random effects for the transition from susceptible to infectious, σ_2^2 - variance of the random effects for the transition from infectious to carrier, σ_3^2 - variance of the random effects for the transition from carrier to infectious, *pND* – probability of non-detection of infectious animals, R_0 – basic reproduction ratio.

Samples are MCMC samples from the posterior distribution of each model parameter and inference is based on those samples. A point estimate, the standard error and the 95% credible interval for a parameter are, for example, calculated as the sample mean, the sample standard deviation and the sample 2.5% and 97.5% quantiles of the posterior samples for that parameter.

The MCMC convergence was considered acceptable since the R-hat for all parameters (including random effects) was never above 1.01. The results of the model did not significantly differ when the parameters of the priors for the sensitivity tests were varied (increasing and decreasing them by 10%).

The posterior distribution for transition rate α (I to R) was symmetric, but for the transition rate β (S to I) and v (R to I), the posterior distributions were asymmetric (Figures 1, 2 and 3). As such, the posterior median was chosen to best summarise the value of these parameters. The median for the transition rate β was 0.33, for α it was 0.18 while for v it was 0.01 (Table 1). The median of the variance of cohort random effects for the transitions I to R and R to I was close to zero, which implies that there was little significant variation between cohorts for these two transitions of the model. The median of the variance of the cohort-time dependent random effect for the transition S to I was 2.6 (95% credible interval [0.80; 7.59]), meaning that the cohort random effect is significant for this transition (Figure 4). The overall model fit was satisfactory with a "p-value" of 0.24 implying no significant difference between posterior predictive simulations (predictions from the model) and observed data.

Basic reproductive ratio (R_0)

Summary statistics of the posterior distribution of the R_0 parameter are shown in Table 1. The posterior median of R_0 was 1.91, with a 95% credible interval of 0.78 to 5.24. A density estimate of the posterior samples of R_0, which effectively describes the spread of *Salmonella spp.* in these three Danish pig herds known to be infected with *Salmonella*, is shown in Figure 5. For moderate to high within herd *Salmonella* prevalence, this R_0 distribution suggests that *Salmonella* Typhimurim can range from fading out scenarios to epidemic ones but most of the time the infection spread assumes an endemic form.

Diagnostic test sensitivity (pND)

Recall that this modelling framework includes the estimation of the probability of failing to detect infectious

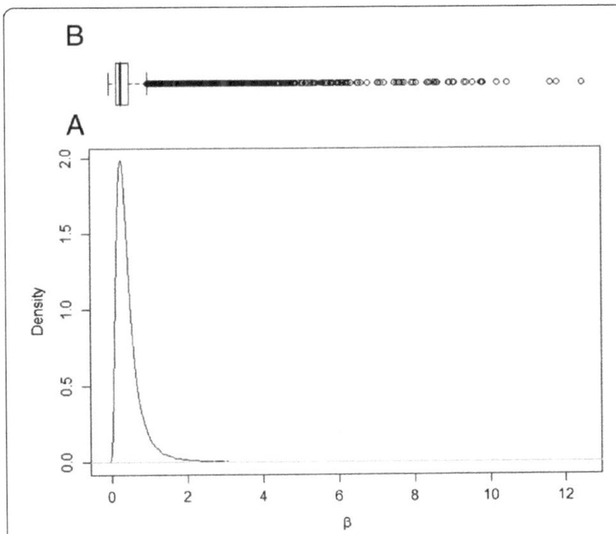

Figure 1 Posterior distribution of β. Legend: **A)** Plot of the posterior distribution for transmission parameter β, which describes the rate of spread of *Salmonella* Typhimurium from susceptible to infectious animals; **B)** Boxplot of the posterior samples used to produce the plot where the thick line in the box reflects the median.

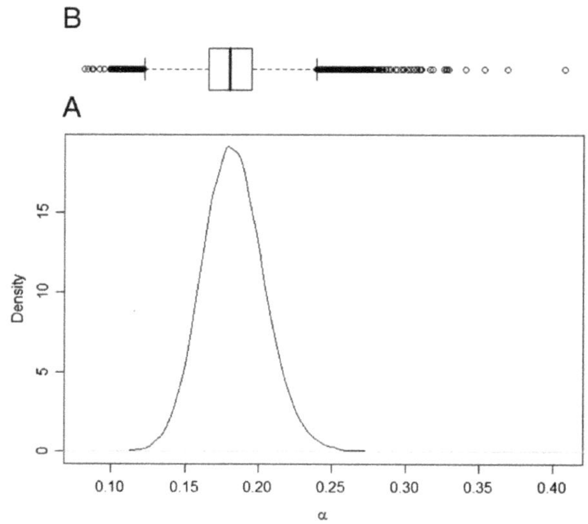

Figure 2 Posterior distribution of α. Legend: **A)** Plot of the posterior distribution for transmission parameter α, which describes the rate of spread of *Salmonella* Typhimurium from infectious to resistant animals; **B)** Boxplot of the posterior samples used to produce the plot where the thick line in the box reflects the median.

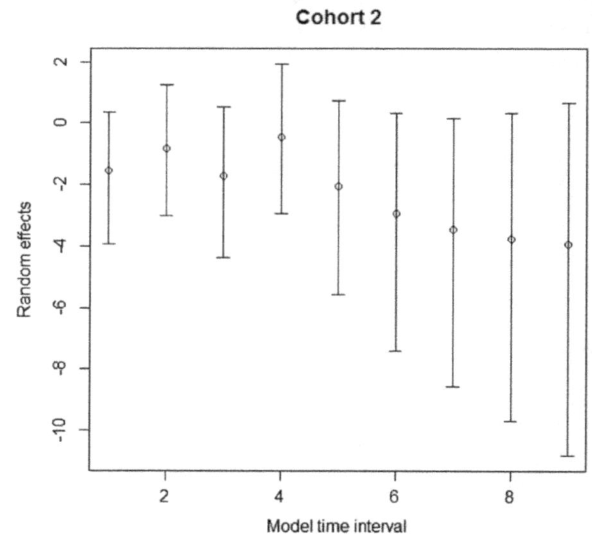

Figure 4 Posterior distribution of the β random effects for cohort two over time. Legend: Plot of the posterior distribution of the β random effects (time and cohort) for one cohort over time with the mean and 95% credible intervals.

animals, pND, using both the data but also prior information about the tests sensitivity [11,12]. Figure 6 shows a density estimate plot of the posterior distribution of pND.

Discussion

In this paper field data were used from a study conducted in three Danish pig herds which were known to be infected with *Salmonella* Typhimurium [10]. The data was considered sufficiently reliable to be used in estimating the transmission parameters of an SIR model describing the evolution of the disease and from that to infer R_0 for *Salmonella* Typhimurium in finisher pigs.

In comparing the parameters to those found in other studies (whether simulation- or observation-based studies

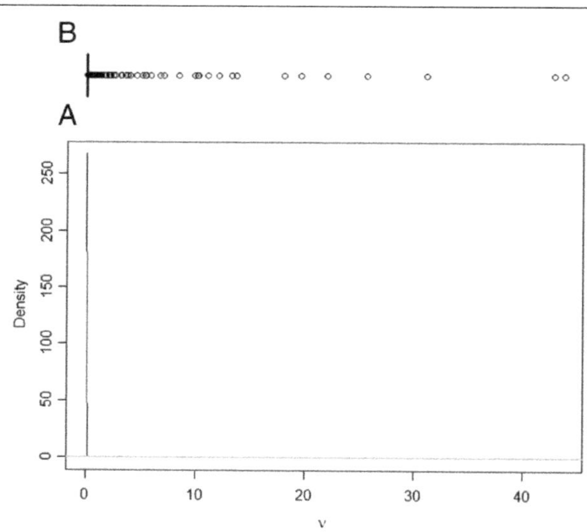

Figure 3 Posterior distribution of ν. Legend: **A)** Plot of the posterior distribution for transmission parameter ν, which describes the rate of spread of *Salmonella* Typhimurium from resistant to infectious animals; **B)** Boxplot of the posterior samples used to produce the plot where the thick line in the box reflects the median.

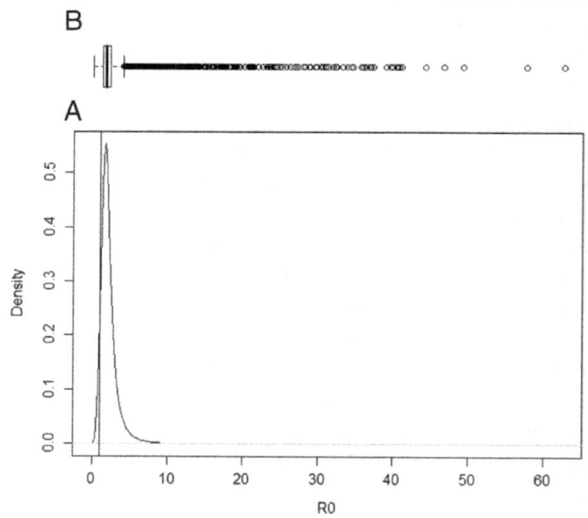

Figure 5 Posterior distribution of the basic reproduction ratio (R0). Legend: **A)** Plot of the posterior distribution for the basic reproduction ratio (R0). The vertical line shows the threshold value R0 = 1 where dissemination of the infection occurs; **B)** Boxplot of the posterior samples used to produce the plot where the thick line in the box reflects the median.

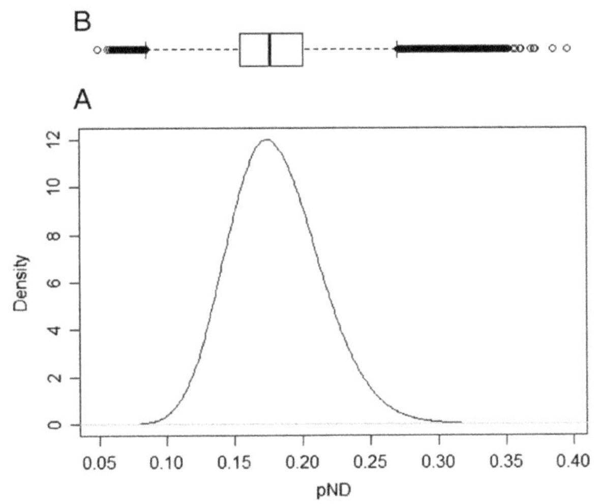

Figure 6 Posterior distribution of the probability of non-detection of infected animals (*pND*). Legend: **A)** Plot of the probability of non-detection of infected animals (*pND*) due to the test characteristics; **B)** Boxplot of the posterior samples used to produce the plot where the thick line in the box reflects the median.

It is important to take into consideration that the time interval used in this study was two weeks whereas in past simulation studies it varies from one day [14,17] to one week [18]. As the transmission parameters are rates, however, they can be easily transformed to relate to different time steps. Although the herds used in the Kranker study [10] had moderate to high levels of *Salmonella* Typhimurium prevalence, the median estimates of the transmission parameters from this study are lower than those found in previous simulation studies [16,18]. The transition rate β from S to I is slightly higher when compared to the Lurette *et al.* study [18] although the other rates (α, ν) are lower than the equivalent parameters in that same study. So the application of our proposed modelling framework to these Danish herds resulted in estimates comparable to similar studies (note that this approach could easily be used with data from other countries). Moreover, the prevalence of *Salmonella* in finishing pigs in Denmark is known to be close to the average prevalence in the EU [31].

To the best of our knowledge this is the first study of transmission rate parameters for *Salmonella* Typhimurium in swine that estimates the parameters using field data and a Bayesian probabilistic approach incorporating random effects.

Bias of the study

Correct classification of the infectious status of the individual pig is difficult for *Salmonella* Typhimurium infection, because the diagnostic tests currently used are imperfect [32-37]. Bacteriology lacks sensitivity given intermittent shedding of *Salmonella* by infected pigs, whereas using serology in individuals can be associated more with a past exposure to the agent than a current exposure; therefore it can lack specificity for detecting shedding animals. Positive serology also shows a delay between infection and expression, leading to some lack of sensitivity. When analysing the data, the lack of sensitivity was accounted for by: i) starting the analysis when at least one infected pig per cohort was observed and ii) using the probabilistic framework to predict the infectious animals that were not detected with these tests, from appropriately informed distributions based on the sensitivity of each test.

For optimal estimation of transmission parameters, the time step between each sampling should preferably be as short as the average generation interval, spanning the time when one animal becomes infectious to the time when a second animal becomes infectious because of the first animal. The time steps in this data (two weeks) are not ideal – preferably a few days or perhaps one week would be better [13]. However as previously discussed, the available data did not allow for such an option and it would be very costly to obtain new data. As data from a published study [10] were used, the time step was set to be an approximation of the different testing intervals within and between cohorts, given the limitations offered by the original set of data, and an approximation to the time of seroconversion [13,38]. This approximation could have affected the estimation of parameters due to the extended time interval between testing occasions. Nevertheless, comparison with the results published in other studies does not seem to support this hypothesis. Concerning the cohorts, it is clear from the Kranker study [10] that particular attention was paid to the selection of the herds, which were taken from a large population of Danish finishing herds with a well-known status for *Salmonella*. This gave us confidence regarding the generalization of our results, at least for herd infected with the same serotype (*S.* Typhimurium).

Transition parameters and R_0 values

Note that the stochastic SIR model presented here is only a discrete-time approximation to the real transmission dynamics, i.e. limited to bi-weekly intervals. In particular, when the number of susceptible animals is small and the infection intensity high, then the expected number of infectious animals will tend to be overestimated [5].

The estimate of the transition rate β (from S to I) is low compared with other infectious diseases (such as swine influenza) and reflects the fact that in most of the herds, *Salmonella* does not cause outbreaks but maintains a residual level of infection represented by infectious and carrier animals that enable the infection to persist in the herds. The credible interval for the transition parameter α (from I to R), matches the variability of shedding duration that is known from experimental and field studies [13,39]. The transition rate estimate ν (from R to I) is small and possibly dependent on stress events (the authors of the Kranker *et al.* study [10] report that two cohorts in which animals began shedding in a second round had a slurry overflow which can be considered a stressful event). The variance of the cohort time-dependent random effect was high and a possible explanation for that is the different management of cohorts which in turn induces high variability (between cohorts) in the transmission data. In future studies this should be taken into consideration as a way to minimize transmission of infection.

For spread to occur, R_0 should be above one. Looking at Figure 5 we can see that there is high probability that $R_0 > 1$, 94% specifically. The median R_0 value was 1.91 indicating that *Salmonella* Typhimurium was spreading in most of the cohorts. The value is not high (third quartile of R_0 is less than three) implying it would not spread rapidly through the susceptible populations under management systems similar to the ones used in these herds. With lower probability, R_0 is high enough to cause outbreaks, e.g. probability that $R_0 > 5$ is 2.5%.

The R_0 95% Credible Interval (CrI) ranges from 0.78 to 5.24. The higher values reflect that animals infected with a high infectious dose have a longer shedding period [13] than the ones infected with low infectious dose, and so the former can cause an outbreak. This makes sense because *Salmonella* Typhimurium is an agent that primarily spreads via the faecal-oral route.

Few studies are available to aid in defining infectious animals, but the experimental and field studies conducted by some authors [13,15] support the duration of infectiousness used in our study.

A next step in our investigation will be to include the estimated transmission parameters (β, α, ν) in a stochastic simulation model developed by the authors to simulate the spreading of *Salmonella* Typhimurium in swine herds and thus test the effectiveness of different control strategies.

Conclusions

A Bayesian framework was proposed, to estimate *Samonella* Typhimurium transmission parameters, and has been successfully implemented using data from Danish pig herds. The model extends the current established methodology of utilising GLMs to implement stochastic SIR models. Random effects were added to i) explicitly allow for cohort heterogeneity in the data (i.e. allow for the fact that pigs were grouped in cohorts), ii) capture possible unobserved cohort effects and iii) avoid the problem of overdispersion. Results in terms of posterior samples allow for direct probabilistic statements about model parameters which may be also used in other analyses such as simulation models for testing management strategies.

The issue of underestimating infectious pigs due to testing sensitivity was addressed by predicting the number of non-detected pigs, using i) prior information about test sensitivity and ii) the observed data. In doing that, the probability of non-detection was treated as an unknown parameter which was estimated at the same time as the transmission parameters.

All model unknowns (transmission parameters, cohort random effects, non-detected pigs, probability of non-detection) were estimated simultaneously, implying that all possible sources of uncertainty were modelled, in turn giving more confidence about the estimates of the transmission parameters.

Competing interests

The authors declare that they have no competing interests.

Authors' contributions

CCG and TE were involved in the design and performed the statistical modelling analysis and drafted the manuscript. TB was involved in the design of the statistical analysis and the revision of the manuscript for intellectual content. LA and PB were involved in the revision of the manuscript for intellectual content. JNR was involved in the drafting and revision of the manuscript for intellectual content. All authors approved the final manuscript.

Acknowledgements

We would like to thank the Danish Agriculture & Food Council and the authors of the study (Kranker et al., [10]) for allowing us to be using their data. This research was supported by FCT (PhD scholarship SFRH/BD/40932/2007 and pluriannual support of LIAAD-INESC Porto L.A). We are very grateful to Madeleine Henry for proof-reading this paper.

Author details

[1]ICBAS-UP - Department of Population Studies, Instituto de Ciências Biomédicas Abel Salazar – Universidade do Porto, Rua de Jorge Viterbo Ferreira, n°228, 4050-313 Porto, Portugal. [2]CEMPS, University of Exeter, Harrison Building, North Park Road, Exeter, EX4 4QF, UK. [3]LIAAD – INESC Porto L.A. Universidade do Porto, Rua de Ceuta, 118, 6, 4050-190 Porto, Portugal. [4]FEP-UP – Faculty of Economics - Universidade do Porto, Rua Dr. Roberto Frias, 4200-464 Porto, Portugal. [5]DMA - Danish Agriculture and Food Council, Axelborg, Axeltorv 3, DK-1609, Copenhagen, Denmark. [6]ISPUP – Institute of Public Health – Universidade do Porto, Rua das Taipas, 4099-003 Porto, Portugal. [7]ERU-SRUC – Epidemiology Research Unit, Future Farming Systems, SRUC, Drummondhill, Inverness, IV2 4JZ, UK.

References

1. EFSA: **The community summary report on trends and sources of Zoonoses and Zoonotic Agents and Food-Borne Outbreaks in the European Union 2008.** *EFSA J* 2010, **1496:**288.
2. Hurd HS, Enoe C, Sorensen L, Wachman H, Corns SM, Bryden KM, Grenier M: **Risk-based analysis of the Danish pork Salmonella program: past and future.** *Risk Anal* 2008, **28**(2):341–351.
3. FCC Consortium: **Analysis of the costs and benefits of setting a target for the reduction of *Salmonella* in slaughter pigs for European Commision Health and Consumers Directorate-General SANCO/2008/E2/036 Final Report.** 2010:1–198. http://ec.europa.eu/food/food/biosafety/salmonella/docs/fattening_pigs_analysis_costs.pdf.
4. Diekmann O, Heesterbeek JAP: *Mathematical Epidemiology of Infectious Diseases: Model Building, Analysis and Interpretation.* Chichester: John Wiley & Sons Ltd; 2000. Chapter 2.

5. Nielsen LR, van den Borne B, van Schaik G: **Salmonella Dublin infection in young dairy calves: transmission parameters estimated from field data and an SIR-model.** *Prev Vet Med* 2007, **79**(1):46–58.
6. Tsutsui T, Kobayashi S, Hayama Y, Nishiguchi A, Kameyama K, Konishi M, Murakami K: **Estimation of the within-herd transmission parameter of bovine leukemia virus.** *Prev Vet Med* 2010, **95**(1–2):158–162.
7. Bouma A, de Jong MCM, Kimman TG: **Transmission of pseudorabies virus within pig populations is independent of the size of the population.** *Prev Vet Med* 1995, **23**(3–4):163–172.
8. Yoshida N, Hara T: **Global stability of a delayed SIR epidemic model with density dependent birth and death rates.** *J Comput Appl Math* 2007, **201**(2):339–347.
9. Thomas E, Bouma A, Klinkenberg D: **A comparison of transmission characteristics of Salmonella enterica serovar Enteritidis between pair-housed and group-housed laying hens.** *Vet Res* 2011, **42**:40. http://www.veterinaryresearch.org/content/42/1/40.
10. Kranker S, Alban L, Boes J, Dahl J: **Longitudinal study of Salmonella enterica Serotype Typhimurium infection in three Danish farrow-to-finish swine herds.** *J Clin Microbiol* 2003, **41**(6):2282–2288.
11. Harris IT: **Serologic basis for assessment of subclinical Salmonella infection in swine: part 1.** *J Swine Health Prod* 2003, **11**(5):247–251.
12. Eriksson E, Aspan A: **Comparison of culture, ELISA and PCR techniques for salmonella detection in faecal samples for cattle, pig and poultry.** *BMC Vet Res* 2007, **3**:21.
13. Fravalo P, Cariolet R, Proux K, Salvat G: **Le portage asymptomatique de *Salmonella enterica* par les porcs: résultats issues de la constituition d'un modèle en conditions expérimentales.** In *35èmes Journées de la Recherche Porcine: 2003.* Paris, France: ITP, INRA; 2003:393–400.
14. Soumpasis I, Butler F: **Development and application of a stochastic epidemic model for the transmission of Salmonella Typhimurium at the farm level of the pork production chain.** *Risk Anal* 2009, **29**(11):1521–1533.
15. Nielsen B, Baggesen D, Bager F, Haugegaard J, Lind P: **The serological response to Salmonella serovars typhimurium and infantis in experimentally infected pigs. The time course followed with an indirect anti-LPS ELISA and bacteriological examinations.** *Vet Microbiol* 1995, **47**(3–4):205–218.
16. Hill AA, Snary EL, Arnold ME, Alban L, Cook AJ: **Dynamics of Salmonella transmission on a British pig grower-finisher farm: a stochastic model.** *Epidemiol Infect* 2008, **136**(3):320–333.
17. van der Gaag MA, Vos F, Saatkamp HW, van Boven M, van Beek P, Huirne RBM: **A state-transition simulation model for the spread of Salmonella in the pork supply chain.** *Eur J Oper Res* 2004, **156**(3):782–798.
18. Lurette A, Belloc C, Touzeau S, Hoch T, Ezanno P, Seegers H, Fourichon C: **Modelling Salmonella spread within a farrow-to-finish pig herd.** *Vet Res* 2008, **39**(5):49.
19. Velthuis AGJ, De Jong MCM, Kamp EM, Stockhofe N, Verheijden JHM: **Design and analysis of an *Actinobacillus pleuropneumoniae* transmission experiment.** *Prev Vet Med* 2003, **60**:53–58.
20. Broens EM, Espinosa-Gongora C, Graat EAM, Vendrig N, Van der Wolf PJ, Guardabassi L, Butaye P, Nielsen JP, De Jong MCM, Van De Giessen AW: **Longitudinal study on transmission of MRSA CC398 within pig herds.** *BMC Vet Res* 2012, **8**(58):10.
21. Romagosa A, Allerson M, Gramer M, Soo Joo H, Deen J, Detmer S, Torremorell M: **Vaccination of influenza a virus decreases transmission rates in pigs.** *BMC Vet Res* 2011, **42**(120):1–15.
22. Geenen PL, Dopfer D, Van der Meulen J, De Jong MC: **Transmission of F4+ E. coli in groups of early weaned piglets.** *Epidemiol Infect* 2005, **133**(3):459–468.
23. Eble P, de Koeijer A, Bouma A, Stegeman A, Dekker A: **Quantification of within- and between-pen transmission of foot-and-mouth disease virus in pigs.** *Vet Res* 2006, **37**(5):647–654.
24. Gilks WR, Richardson S, Spiegelhalter DJ: *Markov chain Monte Carlo in practice.* 1st edition. Boca Raton: Chapman & Hall/CRC; 1996.
25. Lunn DJ, Thomas A, Best N, Spiegelhalter D: **WinBUGS - a Bayesian modelling framework: concepts, structure, and extensibility.** *Stat Comput* 2000, **10**:325–337.
26. Spiegelhalter D, Thomas A, Best N, Lunn D: **WinBUGS Version 1.4.3 User Manual.** In *Medical Research Council Biostatistics Unit.* Cambridge: MRC; 2007.
27. Best NG, Cowles MK, Vines SK: *CODA Manual Version 0.30.* Cambridge, UK: MRC Biostatistics Unit; 1995.
28. Gelman A, Rubin DB: **Inference from iterative simulation using multiple sequences.** *Stat Sci* 1992, **7**:457–511.
29. Kostoulas P, Leontides L, Enøe C, Billinis C, Florou M, Sofia M: **Bayesian estimation of sensitivity and specificity of serum ELISA and faecal culture for diagnosis of paratuberculosis in Greek dairy sheep and goats.** *Prev Vet Med* 2006, **76**(1–2):56–73.
30. Congdon PD: *Applied Bayesian Hierarchical Methods.* London: Chapman and Hall/ CRC; 2010.
31. EFSA: **Report of the task force on Zoonoses data collection on the analysis of the baseline survey on the prevalence of *Salmonella* in slaughter pigs, PartA.** *EFSA J* 2008, **135**:111.
32. van Winsen RL, van Nes A, Keuzenkamp D, Urlings HAP, Lipman LJA, Biesterveld S, Snijders JMA, Verheijden JHM, van Knapen F: **Monitoring of transmission of Salmonella enterica serovars in pigs using bacteriological and serological detection methods.** *Vet Microbiol* 2001, **80**(3):267–274.
33. Nollet N, Maes D, Duchateau L, Hautekiet V, Houf K, Van Hoof J, De Zuttera L, De Kruif A, Geers R: **Discrepancies between the isolation of Salmonella from mesenteric lymph nodes and the results of serological screening in slaughter pigs.** *Vet Res* 2005, **36**(4):545–555.
34. Christensen J, Baggesen DL, Soerensen V, Svensmark B: **Salmonella level of Danish swine herds based on serological examination of meat-juice samples and Salmonella occurrence measured by bacteriological follow-up.** *Prev Vet Med* 1999, **40**(3–4):277–292.
35. Farzan A, Friendship RM, Dewey CE: **Evaluation of enzyme-linked immunosorbent assay (ELISA) tests and culture for determining Salmonella status of a pig herd.** *Epidemiol Infect* 2007, **135**(2):238–244.
36. Proux K, Houdayer C, Humbert F, Cariolet R, Rose V, Eveno E, Madec F: **Development of a complete ELISA using Salmonella lipopolysaccharides of various serogroups allowing to detect all infected pigs.** *Vet Res* 2000, **31**(5):481–490.
37. Szabo I, Scherer K, Roesler U, Appel B, Nockler K, Hensel A: **Comparative examination and validation of ELISA test systems for Salmonella typhimurium diagnosis of slaughtering pigs.** *Int J Food Microbiol* 2008, **124**(1):65–69.
38. Beloeil PA, Chauvin C, Proux K, Rose N, Queguiner S, Eveno E, Houdayer C, Rose V, Fravalo P, Madec F: **Longitudinal serological responses to Salmonella enterica of growing pigs in a subclinically infected herd.** *Prev Vet Med* 2003, **60**(3):207–226.
39. Nicholson FA, Groves SJ, Chambers BJ: **Pathogen survival during livestock manure storage and following land application.** *Bioresour Technol* 2005, **96**(2):135–143.

Actinobacillus pleuropneumoniae challenge in swine: diagnostic of lung alterations by infrared thermography

Anne Menzel[1*], Martin Beyerbach[2], Carsten Siewert[3], Melanie Gundlach[1], Doris Hoeltig[1], Robert Graage[4], Hermann Seifert[3], Karl-Heinz Waldmann[1], Jutta Verspohl[5] and Isabel Hennig-Pauka[4]

Abstract

Background: *Actinobacillus pleuropneumoniae (A.pp.)* is the causative agent of porcine pleuropneumonia leading to high economic losses in the pig industry. Infrared thermography (IRT) of the thorax might offer a new method to select swine with lung alterations for further diagnostics.
In this study 50 german landrace pigs were infected with *A.pp.* in an established model for respiratory tract disease, while 10 healthy pigs served as control animals. To avoid drift errors during IR measurements absolute skin temperatures and temperature differences between a thoracal and an abdominal region were assessed for its diagnostic validity.

Results: IRT findings during the course of experimental *A.pp.*-infection were verified by computed tomography (CT) before and on days 4 and 21 after infection. Significant correlations were found between clinical scores, CT score and lung lesion score. Ambient temperature, body temperature and abdominal surface temperature were factors influencing the skin surface temperature of the thorax. On day 4 but not on day 21 after infection the right thoracal temperature was significantly higher and the difference between a thoracal region in the height of the left 10th vertebra and an abdominal region was significantly lower in infected pigs than in control pigs. At a cut off of 28°C of right thoracal temperature the specificity of the method was 100% (CI 95%: 69-100%) and the sensitivity 66% (CI 95%: 51-79%).
At a cut off of 2°C temperature difference between thoracal and abdominal region on the left body site the specificity of the method was 100% (CI 95%: 69-100%) and the sensitivity 32% (CI 95%: 19-47%) with all control pigs detected negative.
Orientation for lung biopsy by IRT resulted in 100% specificity and sensitivity (CI 95%: 69-100%) of bacteriological examination of tissue samples during the acute stage of infection.

Conclusion: IRT might be a valuable tool for the detection of inflammatory lung alterations in pigs, especially during the acute stage of infection and if ambient temperatures are constant during individual measurements. External and internal factors interfere with this method, so that its application in the field might be restricted to a selection of pigs for further diagnostic with adequate specificity.

Keywords: Infrared thermography, Imaging techniques, Computed tomography, Aerosol challenge, Diagnostic method, Skin surface temperature, Regional temperature differences, Respiratory tract disease

* Correspondence: anne.menzel@tiho-hannover.de
[1]Clinic for Swine and Small Ruminants, Forensic Medicine and Ambulatory Services, University of Veterinary Medicine Hannover, Bischofsholer Damm 15Aff105, D-30173 Hannover, Germany
Full list of author information is available at the end of the article

Background

Porcine respiratory tract diseases lead to high economic losses in the swine industry worldwide. Clinical signs of disease can be reduced by vaccination against porcine respiratory tract pathogens, but under field conditions the protective effect is often limited in the case of multifactorial disease with several pathogens involved. In general, all vaccines available failed to prevent infection and transmission of pathogens [1,2]. In general, after the onset of acute respiratory disease on a farm, selected pigs are euthanized and necropsied to initiate bacteriological and virological examination of lung tissue. In addition, serological tests are performed in living pigs, which give information about contact with specific pathogens in the past, but not if lung tissue is affected or not [3].

Subclinically and chronically diseased animals do not show any clinical symptoms [4]; consequently, they cannot be selected efficiently for further diagnostic procedures or sorted out prior to slaughter. Therefore one clinical research aim in the field of diagnostic of respiratory diseases in pigs is to identify pigs with lung alterations which do not show clinical signs, to select them for further diagnostic procedures and by this increase the chance of a successful diagnosis as a basis for solving the herd problem.

The practicability of imaging techniques of the lung like digital radiography and computed tomography (CT) is restricted by high personal and investigation costs [5,6]. Ultrasonography was found to be more convenient but was of lower sensitivity, because lung lesions covered by aerated lung tissue were undetectable [7-9].

Infrared thermography (IRT) as an imaging method for the detection of elevated body temperature, circulatory disorders or circumscribed organ inflammation would be of high advantage in swine medicine because of its fast, cheap and non-invasive applicability.

One approach to overcome measurement inaccuracies due to a time-dependent drift error of the IR camera is the calculation of a difference temperature between two defined body localizations as an allocation base [10]. In the current study, temperature differences between regions of interest (ROI) were used to overcome IRT device errors and variations between different IRT images. Selected anatomical localizations could be reproducibly found in the IRT image. As depicted in the manufacturer's instruction of the used IR camera measurement accuracy was ± 1.5°C which is comparable to other IR cameras used in medicine diagnostics [11].

Dependence on ambient temperature is one major cause for the limited practical use of IRT in medicine up to now. In several studies in veterinary medicine IRT was tested as a diagnostic tool, e.g. to detect a pneumothorax in rats [12] or spine diseases and neuromuscular disorders in horses [13,14]. In calves, the skin temperature around the eyes was found to be a sensitive marker to detect changes in thermoregulation due to respiratory disease [15].

In pigs, IRT failed as a diagnostic tool for arthritis, because thick subcutaneous fatty tissue layers prevented the detection of a local inflammatory temperature increase [16].

In swine no reference values for thoracal skin temperatures in pigs with inflammatory lung alterations exist up to now. In the following study, a systematic approach was chosen to evaluate IRT as a diagnostic tool for the detection of changes in the surface temperature pattern of the thorax after infection with the lung pathogen *Actinobacillus pleuropneumoniae* (*A.pp.*).

The aim of this study was to examine the applicability of passive infrared thermography for the diagnostic of lung tissue alterations in pigs at different stages of infection. Clinical examination and CT were used to assess the lung health status during the experiment as an allocation base for IRT. Comparison between both imaging techniques resulted in the determination of specific regions of interest (ROI) for temperature measurements. At the end of the study, IRT findings were compared to findings from gross pathology and histological examinations.

Results

Animal model: clinical and post-mortem scores

Prior to infection all animals were tested negative for *A. pp.* in an Apx-II-Enzyme-linked immunosorbant assays (ELISA) and were defined as healthy according to a clinical score (CLS) and a CT score (CTS). After infection, challenged pigs developed respiratory disease of varying severity reflected by increased CLS, CTS, lung lesion scores (LLS) and scores according to S.P.E.S. (Table 1). A significant correlation was found between the S.P.E.S. score and the LLS ($r_{sp} = 0.72$, $p < 0.01$).

Several animals showed typical signs of acute pleuropneumonia, as elevated body temperature up to 41.8°C, dyspnoea, coughing, apathy and vomiting.

Twelve pigs had to be euthanized before the end of the experiment, because they suffered from generalized systemic disease with severe dyspnoea. They underwent CT and infrared thermographical examination prior to gross pathological examination.

The acute stage of infection was characterized by disseminated lung tissue alterations recorded by CT.

On day 21 after infection significant correlations were found between CLS, CTS and LLS (CLS-LLS: $r_p = 0.45$, $p = 0.01$; CTS-LLS: $r_p = 0.81$, $p < 0.01$ CLS - CTS: $r_p = 0.68$, $p < 0.01$). Gross pathological findings ranged from normal lung tissue to severe pleuropneumoniae.

Pigs of the control group stayed healthy until the end of the experiment.

Table 1 Clinical, computed tomographic and post-mortem scores in infected and control pigs

	Prior to infection (n = 50)	Day 4 (n = 47, CT score n = 46)	Day 21 (n = 40, CT score n = 39)
Clinical score			
Mean ± σ	**0.00** ± 0.02	**4.68** ± 3.86	**25.16** ± 33.13
Median	0.00	3.82	8.22
Range	0.00 – 0.13	1.16 – 17.63	4.52 – 92.63
CT score			
Mean ± σ	**0.03** ± 0.09	**5.39** ± 1.50	**2.11** ± 1.80
Median	0.00	5.25	1.63
Range	0.00 – 0.47	0.79 – 7.71	0.00 - 7.31
Lung lesion score [30] of infected pigs (n = 50)			
Mean ± σ			**12.45** ± 7.656
Median			11.7
Range			1.58 – 33.68
S.P.E.S. score [32] of infected pigs (n = 42)			
Median			4
75th percentil			4
Range			1-4
Lung lesion score [30] of control pigs (n = 10)			
Mean ± σ			**0.11** ± 0.33
Median			0
Range			0 – 1.05
S.P.E.S. score [32] of control pigs (n = 10)			
Median			0
75th percentil			0
Range			0-1

Surface skin temperatures measured by infrared thermography (IRT) during experimental infection and influencing factors

Data of ten control pigs and of all infected pigs were analyzed for surface skin temperature changes during the course of infection.

Multiple regression analysis revealed a variety of external and internal factors influencing the diagnostic command variables absolute surface temperatures of the thorax as well as skin surface temperature differences between thoracal and abdominal region (Tables 2 and 3). Most important influencing variables were ambient temperature, body core temperature and abdominal skin temperature.

Because individual pigs were examined subsequently by IRT imaging in a cooled chamber on fixed examination days, ambient temperature increased in parallel to the duration of examination due to the presence of the warm, living pigs and the examiner. The high impact also of a relatively cold ambient temperature (6-15°C) onto sensitivity and specificity of the method is reflected in the results of IRT measurements in this trial.

Student´s *t*-test for independent samples as well as t-tests for paired observations for the comparison of different stages of infection were performed with those pigs, which have been examined within an ambient temperature range of 7-14°C on all examination days (Figures 1 and 2). A significant difference between infected pigs and control pigs was found for the left skin surface difference temperature between lung ROI and abdominal ROI.

Differences in absolute skin surface temperatures between control pigs and infected pigs were significant already prior to infection (Figure 1), which might be due to the described order of examination. Control pigs were examined always at first in a relatively cool environment to avoid infection. A significant correlation was found between ambient temperature and thoracal skin surface temperatures ($p < 0.01$).

This obvious influence of ambient temperature onto the thoracal skin surface temperature was statistically corrected in an analysis of covariance. The corrected data revealed diagnostic significance for the skin surface temperature difference between abdominal and thoracal region on the left body site in the height of the 10th thoracic vertebrae ($p < 0.01$) during the acute stage of infection

As a result of this study, potential cut-offs were suggested which might allow a practical application of IRT by a specific preselection of pigs for further diagnostics although the method is influenced by ambient temperature and other internal factors.

During the acute stage of infection a cut off of 28°C of absolute right thoracal temperature resulted in a specificity of the method of 100% (95% confidence interval 69-100%) and a sensitivity of 66% (95% confidence interval 51-79%) as shown in Figure 3a. A cut off of 2°C temperature difference between thoracal and abdominal region on the left body site resulted in a specificity of 100% (95% confidence interval 69-100%) and a sensitivity of 32% (95% confidence interval 19-47%) (Figure 3b).

Maximal abdominal temperatures continuously increased with the days of examination in parallel to an increase in the body weight.

At the chronic stage of infection the lung lesion score was negatively correlated to body weight ($r_p = -0.5$, $p < 0.01$) and positively correlated to the clinical ($r_p = 0.5$, $p < 0.01$) and the CT score ($r_p = 0.8$, $p < 0.01$). No correlations were found between lung lesion and CT scores and the temperature parameters measured by IRT.

Validity of lung biopsy

A.pp. could be reisolated from lung biopsies in twelve out of 50 infected pigs. While the overall *A.pp.* detection rate using this method in comparison to positive lung tissue samples was 19-51% (CI 95%), all ten pigs with severe

Table 2 Correlations between dependent and independent variables on day 4 after infection

Influencing variables	Dependent variables							
	Pearsson's correlation coefficient, p- (probability) value, number of pigs							
	Temperature difference between thoracal and abdominal region on the left body site		Temperature difference between thoracal and abdominal region on the right body site		Left thoracal temperature		Right thoracal temperature	
	Infected	Control	Infected	Control	Infected	Control	Infected	Control
Age (living days)	0.07	0.42	−0.04	*0.72*	−0.08	−0.38	−0.03	−0.33
	0.63	0.23	0.78	*0.02*	0.53	0.28	0.85	0.36
	47	10	47	10	47	10	47	10
Body weight (kg)	−0.01	0.52	0.01	0.50	*0.33*	−0.18	*0.35*	0.05
	0.96	0.12	0.93	0.14	*0.02*	0.62	*0.01*	0.89
	47	10	47	10	47	10	47	10
Clinical score	0.06	0.28	−0.18	0.43	*−0.54*	−0.26	*−0.51*	0.06
	0.67	0.43	0.22	0.22	*<0.01*	0.46	*<0.01*	0.87
	47	10	47	10	47	10	47	10
Computed tomography score	−0.13	0.41	*−0.30*	0.47	−0.12	0.18	−0.12	−0.23
	0.40	0.23	*0.04*	0.17	0.43	0.62	0.42	0.53
	46	10	46	10	46	10	46	10
Breathing frequency (per minute)	−0.11	−0.08	−0.05	−0.20	0.29	0.44	0.27	0.14
	0.45	0.82	0.76	0.58	0.05	0.21	0.07	0.70
	46	10	46	10	46	10	46	10
Heart rate (per minute)	0.09	0.32	−0.03	0.09	0.07	*−0.65*	0.08	−0.45
	0.54	0.36	0.86	0.81	0.64	*0.04*	0.60	0.19
	46	10	46	10	46	10	46	10
Body temperature (rectal)	*0.34*	−0.35	*0.38*	−0.37	*0.30*	*0.83*	0.18	*0.82*
	0.02	0.33	*<0.01*	0.29	*0.05*	*<0.01*	0.22	*<0.01*
	46	10	46	10	46	10	46	10
Ambient temperature (°C)	0.03	−0.53	−0.00	−0.21	*0.75*	0.31	*0.78*	*0.64*
	0.89	0.11	0.98	0.56	*<0.01*	0.38	*<0.01*	*0.04*
	46	10	46	10	46	10	46	10
Abdominal temperature (left,°C)	−0.01	−0.21	*0.31*	−0.23	*0.96*	*0.75*	*0.94*	*0.89*
	0.93	0.56	*0.04*	0.44	*<0.01*	*0.01*	*<0.01*	*<0.01*
	47	10	47	10	47	10	47	10
Abdominal temperature (right,°C)	−0.10	−0.20	*0.31*	−0.04	*0.93*	0.58	*0.94*	*0.94*
	0.52	0.58	*0.04*	0.92	*<0.01*	0.08	*<0.01*	*<0.01*
	47	10	47	10	47	10	47	10
Lung lesion score	−0.21	−0.43	*−0.31*	−0.45	−0.11	0.51	−0.11	0.38
	0.15	0.22	*0.04*	0.19	0.48	0.13	0.48	0.27

Surface skin temperatures as well as temperature differences between thoracal and abdominal regions on the left and right body sites were influenced by several internal and external factors. Pearsson's Correlation Coefficients (upper lines) between dependent and influencing variables, their levels of significance (middle lines) and the number of evaluated pigs (lower line) are shown. From 50 infected pigs three pigs had died prior to day 4 after infection.

clinical symptoms, which had been sampled until day 4 after infection, had positive findings for *A. pp.* in bioptates (69-100%, CI 95%).

Only two animals belonging to the four pigs with the highest clinical score and showing also high lung lesion scores were *A.pp.*-positive in lung biopsy samples on day 21 after infection. Lung tissue samples of the respective pigs were also highly positive. Lung tissue samples of twenty-seven pigs were highly positive for *A.pp.*, while in five pigs only moderate and in four

Table 3 Correlations between dependent and independent variables on day 21 after infection

Influencing variables	Dependent variables							
	Pearsson´s correlation coefficient, p- (probability) value, number of pigs							
	Temperature difference between thoracal and abdominal region on the left body site		Temperature difference between thoracal and abdominal region on the right body site		Left thoracal temperature		Right thoracal temperature	
	Infected	Control	Infected	Control	Infected	Control	Infected	Contro
Age (living days)	−0.085	0.13	0.07	−0.03	0.13	0.36	0.18	0.44
	0.60	0.72	0.67	0.93	0.44	0.31	0.29	0.20
	40	10	40	10	40	10	40	10
Body weight (kg)	−0.04	−0.29	0.15	−0.33	*0.36*	*0.73*	*0.36*	*0.72*
	0.83	0.41	0.36	0.35	*0.02*	*0.02*	*0.02*	*0.02*
	40	10	40	10	40	10	40	10
Clinical score	−0.07	−0.30	−0.04	−0.18	−0.09	0.40	0.02	0.31
	0.68	0.34	0.82	0.63	0.58	0.25	0.91	0.38
	40	10	40	10	40	10	40	10
Computed tomography score	−0.17	0.17	−0.11	0.14	−0.07	0.13	−0.04	0.12
	0.30	0.65	0.50	0.69	0.68	0.72	0.81	0.74
	39	10	39	10	39	10	39	10
Breathing frequency (per minute)	0.09	0.28	0.04	0.56	0.23	−0.13	0.16	−0.22
	0.59	0.43	0.83	0.09	0.16	0.72	0.33	0.53
	40	10	40	10	40	10	40	10
Heart rate (per minute)	−0.02	0.18	0.00	0.41	*0.36*	−0.25	*0.44*	−0.30
	0.91	0.62	0.99	0.24	*0.02*	0.49	*<0.01*	0.40
	40	10	40	10	40	10	40	10
Body temperature (rectal)	0.28	0.15	*0.43*	−0.01	*0.64*	*0.67*	*0.72*	*0.73*
	0.08	0.68	*<0.01*	0.98	*<0.01*	*0.04*	*<0.01*	*0.02*
	40	10	40	10	40	10	40	10
Ambient temperature (°C)	−0.24	0.02	0.13	0.07	*0.72*	0.07	*0.59*	0.09
	0.14	0.96	0.43	0.86	*<0.01*	0.85	*<0.01*	0.80
	40	10	40	10	40	10	40	10
Abdominal temperature (left,°C)	0.08	0.42	*0.38*	0.33	*0.95*	*0.642*	*0.87*	*0.69*
	0.61	0.23	*0.02*	0.35	*<0.01*	*0.04*	*<0.01*	*0.03*
	40	10	40	10	40	10	40	10
Abdominal temperature (right,°C)	0.05	−0.03	*0.47*	0.02	*0.88*	*0.91*	*0.92*	*0.92*
	0.74	0.93	*<0.01*	0.97	*<0.01*	*<0.01*	*<0.01*	*<0.01*
	40	10	40	10	40	10	40	10
Lung lesion score	−0.20	−0.50	−0.09	−0.14	0.05	−0.12	0.10	−0.20
	0.21	0.14	0.57	0.70	0.76	0.75	0.54	0.57
	40	10	40	10	40	10	40	10

Surface skin temperatures as well as temperature differences between thoracal and abdominal regions on the left and right body sites were influenced by severa internal and external factors. Pearsson´s Correlation Coefficients (upper lines) between dependent and influencing variables, their levels of significance (middle lines) and the number of evaluated pigs (lower line) are shown.

pigs only low *A.pp.*-isolation rates were found (Figure 4). *A.pp.* was not reisolated from lung tissue of 14 pigs. A histological examination of lung tissue confirmed pneumonia and pleuritis in 44 out of 50 infected pigs (88%).

Discussion

The aim of this study was to evaluate IRT as an imagin technique for the diagnostic of respiratory disease in swine During the trial in living pigs the diagnostic potential o IRT was controlled by CT examination.

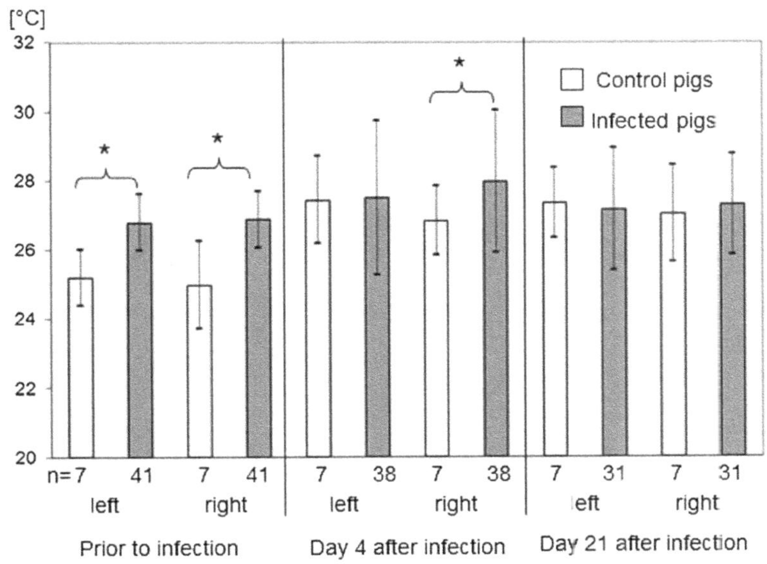

Figure 1 Absolute skin surface temperatures of the left and right thorax at different stages of infection. Asterics indicated significant differences between groups (p ≤ 0.05). Data of those pigs were evaluated which were measured in an ambient temperature range between 7-14°C.

Planning of the study was directed by preliminary findings supporting the hypothesis, that gross pathological lung lesions can be successfully detected in pigs by IRT and that the difference temperature between lung region and abdominal region is smaller in pigs with lung alterations due to an inflammatory increase in lung temperature [17]. Optimal ROIs for IRT on the pig thorax had been previously specified by measurement of tissue layer thicknesses in various anatomical positions (data not shown).

In general, IRT is a simple and non-invasive method to assess the surface temperature distribution of the body [18]. An increase in temperature is a basic physical reaction towards a harmful stimulus and is one sign of inflammation besides swelling, pain and redness.

Also under physiological conditions skin temperature - as the outer contact organ of the body with the environment - is influenced by many external and internal factors, e.g. sweat evaporation, vascular perfusion, local tissue metabolism and ambient temperature [19,20]. Anyhow, infrared

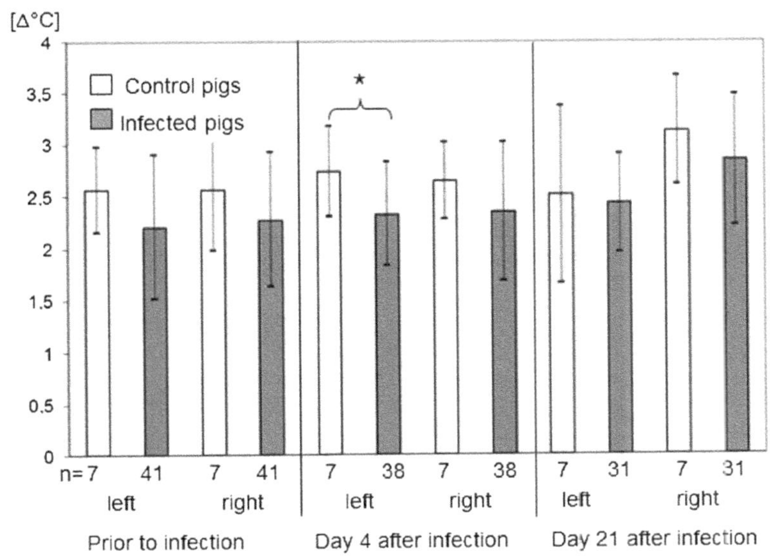

Figure 2 Temperature differences between thoracal and abdominal ROIs at different stages of infection. Asterics indicated significant differences between groups (p ≤ 0.05). Data of those pigs were evaluated which were measured in an ambient temperature range between 7-14°C.

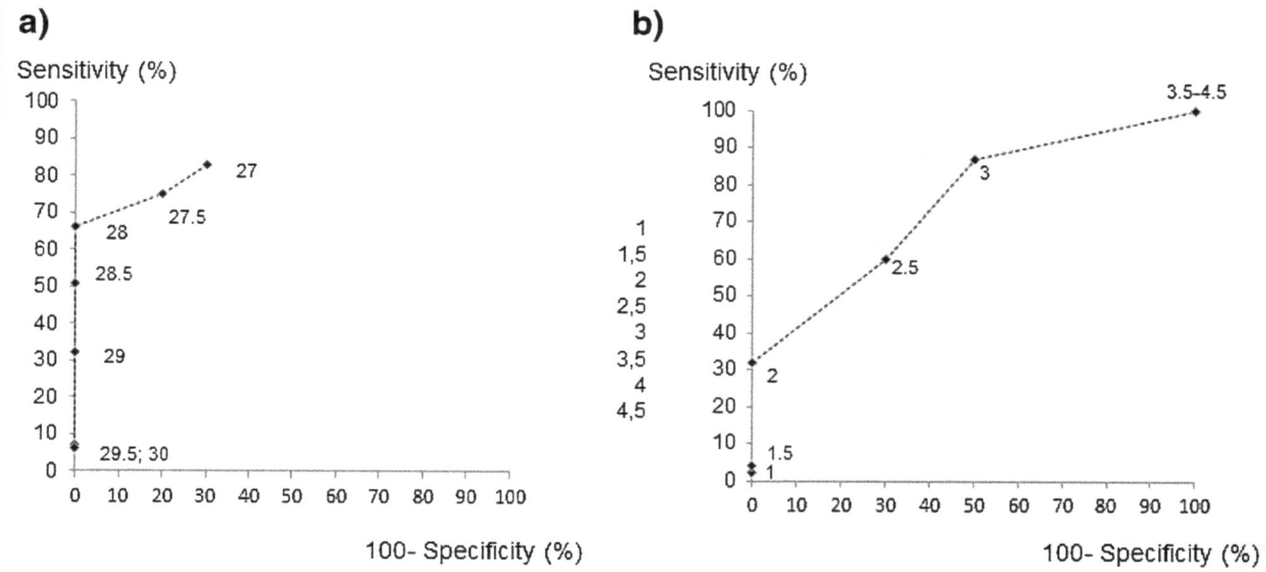

Figure 3 a, b: Receiver Operating Characteristics (ROC) –curves in the acute stage of infection. (a) absolute skin surface temperature of a thoracal region in the height of the 7th thoracic vertebrae on the right body site (cut-off values in °C). **(b)** the difference between abdominal and thoracal skin temperatures on the left body site (cut-off values in Δ°C). For every cut-off value the 100-specificity on the x-axe and the sensitivity on the y-axe is shown.

thermographical images captured under controlled conditions might be interpretable to diagnose specific pathological conditions and might be a helpful tool to monitor specific body reactions towards stress, especially thermal stress [21]. A satisfying reproducibility of IRT in a temperature-controlled environment has been shown previously [21,22].

As hypothezised, mean absolute surface temperatures of the thorax were rising after aerosol challenge during the acute stage of infection (day 4), when highest values were recorded. This temperature increase reflects inflammatory mechanisms in the lung (influx of exsudates, immune cell migration into tissue) as well as systemic reactions (increased body temperature, heart rate, changed respiratory rate). In contrast to that, prior to infection absolute surface temperatures were lower. Surface temperatures during the chronic stage of infection were slightly higher than those measured prior to infection but lower than in the acute stage of infection. The chronic stage of *A.pp.*-infection is characterized by sequestrated necrotic lung tissue, which is surrounded by a fibrotic capsule. In these altered lung areas neither tissue ventilation, nor blood circulation occur. Obviously these chronic inflammatory processes led not to an increased tissue blood perfusion accompanied by an increase in temperature which can be detected from the outside by IRT. Loca

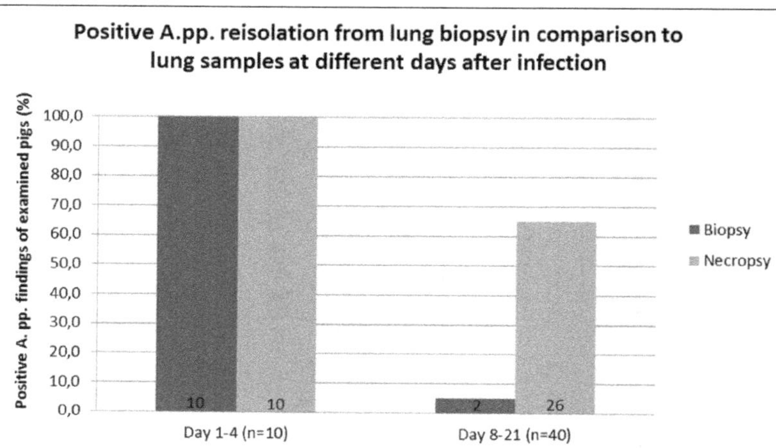

Figure 4 Comparison of *A.pp.* reisolation from lung tissue bioptates and lung samples from necropsied pigs.

temperatures in lung tissue sequesters might be lower than in non-affected lung areas.

Using difference temperatures ($\Delta\vartheta$) between the lung ROI and the abdominal ROI as an allocation base for the detection of inflammatory lung disorders, sensitivity and specificity of the method should be further improved for routine measurements under practical conditions. The hypothesis was that $\Delta\vartheta$ was highest prior to infection, due to physiological ventilation of lung tissue with cool air. During the acute stage of infection, when lung tissue was heated due to inflammation, $\Delta\vartheta$ was supposed to decrease. In contrast to that, in patient animals $\Delta\vartheta$ was not significantly different between the examination prior to infection and after infection. A significant difference was found between day 4 and 21 after infection with a higher difference temperature in the chronic stage of infection.

The high significant difference between lower absolute right lung ROI temperatures prior to infection in comparison to higher temperatures on day 21 after infection was found in all group constellations of patients. In parallel a higher difference temperature between lung and abdominal ROI was observed on day 21 after infection, which was contradictory to the hypothesis. This might be due to a steeper temperature increase of the abdominal ROIs on both body sites, which was obviously not proportional to a temperature increase of the lung ROIs.

The statistical comparison of patient animals with control animals showed, that infected pigs have disease-dependent thoracal surface temperature changes during the acute stage of infection, while no difference was found between both groups on day 21 after infection.

In the chronic stage of infection, three weeks later, abdominal ROI temperature significantly increased from day 4 to day 21 after infection in control pigs and to a much lesser extent in the patient pigs. Briefly, in healthy pigs a higher growth-dependent increase in abdominal than in lung temperature can be assumed. Additionally, differences in abdominal temperatures might be also due to differences in digestive activities. Feed depriviation before examination was at least 12 hours in all animals. Nevertheless, severity of disease affected the appetite of the pigs, so that individual differences in feed consumption occurred during the trial. Some animals still had intestinal contents during examination. The localization of intestine and liver tissue might also be an influencing factor onto thoracal temperatures. The left lung ROI was located at the height of the 10th vertebra where liver tissue was underlying. Filling of the stomach can dislocate the liver in a more cranial position close to the lung. Liver tissue is known to be approximately 1-2°C warmer than the body core temperature [23].

The chronological order of the examination of piglets is assumed to be also a factor influencing the thoracal surface. To avoid contamination of the healthy control pigs with *A.pp.*, they were always examined at first. For this reason the cooled chamber was warmer when patients were examined (ambient temperature during examination of control pigs: 8.47 ± 1.57°C and of infected pigs: 11.97 ± 1.23°C). As previously published, ambient temperature strongly affects the results of IRT measurements, although optimal ambient temperatures for IRT have been reported to be <18°C, which was realized in this study [24].

Not only the effect of ambient temperature on IRT measurement results might limit the application of this method on farms, but also the relative long time until an adequate IRT picture can be produced (approximately 30 seconds in anaesthetized pigs). Anatomical landmarks should be visible in the picture, so that the correct ROIs can be positioned for later temperature evaluation. Non-anaesthetized pigs are moving continuously, which will impair the quality of pictures. For this reason further technical improvement of IRT cameras will be necessary to pave the way for this technique for practical usage.

For the use of IRT adequate facilities and a profound knowledge of the anatomy and physiology of the examined species and the pathophysiology of the disease which should be examined might be important to avoid misdiagnosis. Because mostly several different bacterial and viral pathogens are involved in porcine respiratory diseases, also lung alterations will be a combination of different gross pathological findings. A detection of these inconsistent inflammatory findings might be even more difficult than those findings reported after experimental mono-infection in this study. Also under standardized external conditions, IRT is error-prone due to several influencing endogenous factors whose impact cannot adequately be corrected. IRT is not sensitive enough to assess the prevalence of pigs with lung alterations in a herd. But, using a cut off with a high specificity as suggested in this study, IRT might be a promising tool to detect pigs without clinical symptoms but with lung alterations. Using this 2-step diagnostic approach would enable a more targeted and cost-effective diagnostic of respiratory disease.

Bacteriological examination of lung tissue bioptates of infected pigs resulted in *A.pp.* reisolation in 24% of all animals. All animals with severe clinical symptoms, which were euthanized during the first days after infection, had positive findings for *A. pp.* in bioptates. Only 5% of pigs were detected positive by lung bioptates on day 21 after infection. For this reason, lung biopsy can be assessed to be a diagnostic option for *A. pp.* detection only during the acute stage of infection. Biopsy of the lung is highly invasive and can cause further problems as bleeding and sudden death.

It can be concluded, that the assessment of IRT for the diagnostic of lung alterations requires a comparison of infected and non-infected pigs of the same age and under same ambient temperature conditions. The interpretation of findings is complicated by a non-proportional, partly growth-dependent change in surface temperature of different body regions.

In this study, most appropriate surface temperature parameters for the diagnostic of the lung health status of pigs are the absolute temperature of the right thoracal region in the height of the 7th thoracic vertebra as well as the temperature difference between thoracal and abdominal region on the left body site on the height of the 10th thoracic vertebra.

With a next generation of IRT cameras both localizations should be further evaluated for their diagnostic significance in non-anaesthetized piglets with and without lung diseases and under moderate ambient temperature conditions.

Conclusion

Using IRT lung alternations are better detectable in the acute stage of infection 4 days after infection than in the chronic stage of infection 21 days after infection. The method is interfering with external and internal factors which have to be regarded during the examination and analysis. Especially the effect of ambient temperature on skin surface temperatures visualized in IR-images always has to be considered. The assessment of IRT requires a comparison of infected and non-infected pigs of the same age and under same ambient temperature conditions. The application of this tool in the field might be restricted to a selection of pigs for further diagnostic with adequate specificity.

Methods

Animals

A total of 60 clinically healthy male castrated pigs (German Landrace) in the age of four weeks were used in this study. All pigs were bred and raised in a closed breeding herd of high health status that is routinely tested negative for *A. pp.*, Porcine Reproductive and Respiratory Syndrome Virus (PRRSV), toxigenic *Pasteurella multocida*, endo- and ectoparasites.

To guarantee the health status of the pigs, all pigs used in this study were checked for antibodies against *A. pp.* using an Apx-II-Enzyme-linked immunosorbant assay (ELISA) after arrival [25]. Animals were housed and cared under standardized conditions according to the Directive of the European Convention for the Protection of Vertebrae Animals Used for Experimental and Other Scientific Purposes (European Treaty Series, nos. 123 [http://conventions.coe.int/treaty/EN/treaties/html/123.htm] and 170 [http://conventions.coe.int/treaty/EN/treaties/html/170.htm]) at the Institute for Microbiology, University of Veterinary Medicine Hannover, Germany. The study was approved from the local permitting authorities in the Lower Saxony State Office for Consumer Protection and Food Safety and in accordance with the requirements of the national animal welfare law (approval number: 33.9-42502-12/0835). Precautions aimed at avoiding unnecessary suffering were taken at all stages of the experiment.

Animals were randomised in two control groups of five and five challenge groups of ten.

Twice a day (8 am and 5 pm) a commercial weaner pig diet (Deuka Primo, Deutsche Tiernahrung Cremer GmbH & Co. KG, Bremen, Germany) was fed with exception of the examination days and the day of infection, when pigs were fed in the evening after the manipulations, to lower the risk of a circuit failure under anaesthesia and to minimize the effect of digestion onto the body surface temperature. Water was given ad libitum.

Experimental setup

Because of the high number of animals, which could not be examined within one trial due to logistic reasons, two sequential trials following the same protocol during the examination period of 28 days were performed. In the first trial 30 animals and in the second trial 20 animals were challenged with *A. pp.*, while 5 pigs served as a mock-infected control group during each trial. In total in this study data of 50 pigs challenged with *A.pp.* and 10 control pigs were evaluated. A clinical examination of all pigs with special emphasis onto gastrointestinal and respiratory signs, locomotory disorders, skin alterations and behaviour was performed daily in all pigs resulting in daily clinical scores. The first CT and IRT examination as well as blood sampling were performed in the first week when all pigs had been assessed as healthy.

As soon as deep anaesthesia was achieved by 15 mg ketamine (Ursotamin®, Serumwerk-Bernburg AG, Bernburg, Germany)/kg body weight (bw) intramuscularly (i.m.) and 2 mg azaperon (Stresnil®, Janssen-Cilag GmbH, Baar, Switzerland) /kg bw i.m., pigs were at first examined by computed tomography followed by a cooling down of 15 minutes in a cooling chamber (6-15°C) and then IRT examination of the thorax. Subsequently pigs were brought back to their stables and monitored until they awoke. A few days after the first examinations, aerosol challenge was performed on day 0 of the infection experiment.

The second examination was performed according to the same protocol on the fourth day after aerosol challenge during the acute stage of infection and the third examination on day 21 after infection during the chronic stage of infection. After the last examination, lung biopsies were sampled under deep anaesthesia and pigs were then euthanized (60 mg pentobarbital (Euthadorm®, CP-Pharma, Burgdorf, Germany)/ kg bw intravenously) and necropsied to assess gross pathological lung alterations and to take further diagnostic samples.

Aerosol challenge

Aerosol challenge was performed as previously described [26,27] using an *A.pp.* bioptype 1 serotype 2 strain for infection, which has been isolated from a naturally infected pig in Germany (lab identification number C3656/0271/11, Institute of Microbiology, University of Veterinary Medicine, Hannover, Germany).

Briefly, groups of five pigs were infected simultaneously in an aerosol chamber. Within 2 minutes at a pressure of 2 bar 13 ml of the diluted culture (containing $3 \times 10^7 - 8 \times 10^9$ bacteria) were nebulized in the chamber resulting in approximately 1×10^2 colony forming units (cfu) of *A.pp.* per litre aerosol. Subsequently pigs were exposed for 10 minutes to the aerosol in the closed chamber. Challenge doses were confirmed retrospectively by overnight culture of several dilutions of the bacterial inoculum and determination of the cfu.

For the mock challenge of control pigs 13 ml of a 154 mM sterile NaCl solution was nebulized in the aerosol chamber.

Clinical examination

Clinical scoring and the classification of disease severity were performed according to Hoeltig et al. [28] with the exception of pulse oxymetry. Animals were monitored daily for clinical signs of disease assessing the following parameters: breathing noise, type of respiration, breathing rate, coughing, skin colour, posture, behaviour, feed intake, body temperature, and symptoms of gastrointestinal disorders as vomiting or diarrhoea. Cumulative clinical scores were calculated for each pig as a sum of daily clinical scores from day of arrival to infection (day 0), from day 0 to 4 and from day 0 to 21. Disease classifications by clinical scores on day 0 and 4 were: not affected (0–0.70), slightly affected (0.71-7.13), moderately affected (7.14-13.56) and severely affected (>13.56). Disease classifications by clinical scores on day 21 were: not affected (0–2.00), slightly affected (2.01-34.7), moderately affected (34.71-67.3) and severely affected (>67.3).

CT examination

CT examination of the pig thorax has been described in detail by Brauer et al. [6]. Briefly, anaesthezised pigs were positioned symmetrically in sternal recumbency. From the cranial thoracic aperture to the caudal end of the lung the thorax was scanned by a third generation single-slice CT scanner (Philips Tomoscan M, Philips Medical Systems, Germany) with defined settings for scanogram and volume scan (tube voltage 120 kV, current 40 mA, slice thickness 7 mm, reconstruction interval 5 mm, pitch 1.5). CT scores (CTS) for each animal were calculated as previously described by Brauer et al. [6] taking morphological alterations and their distribution pattern, as well as absorption densities into account. Disease classification by CTS was: not affected (0–0.23), slightly affected (0.24-1.70), moderately affected (1.71-2.22) and severely affected (>2.23).

Infrared thermographical examination

Anaesthetized pigs were positioned in sternal recumbency on a plastic tray and metal markers were fixed at the 5th, 7th, 10th and 13th thoracic vertebrae left and right beside the spine to serve as anatomical landmarks. Pigs were left for acclimatization in a cooling chamber (average ambient temperature of 11.27 ± 2.29°C) for 15 minutes. Prior to and after this acclimatisation period heart frequency, respiratory rate, and body temperature were recorded. IRT images were made from the left and right side of the body in a constant distance, right-angled to the thorax with an IR camera (VarioCAM hr Inspec, Infratec, Dresden, Germany) after the acclimatization period. Presetting of the camera was a premium mode with a camera-internal repeated calibration prior to IRT imaging [11]. Thus, a continuous balancing of inhomogeneities in the microbolometer array was possible. An emissivity of 0.96, which is a good assumption for skin with little hair, was presetted [29]. Picture matrix was 384 x 288 pixels and the thermical resolution was 50 mK. Additionally, a reference body with constant room temperature placed next to the pig was recorded on each image as an internal standard. Room temperature was recorded prior to every single examination. For analysis of IR images a standard Windows PC and an image analysis software package (Irbis3, InfraTec GmbH, Dresden, Germany) were used.

Two certain ROIs, one on the right side of the thorax in the height of the 7th thoracic vertebra (R7vLr) and one on the left side of the thorax in the height of the 10th thoracic vertebra (R10vLl) were chosen as measurement localizations, because outer tissue layers (skin, fat, muscle) were thin at these anatomical positions (data not shown). These two ROIs were selected to evaluate thoracal surface temperatures in each pig at three examination days: prior to infection, when pigs were healthy, on day 4 after infection during the acute stage of disease and on day 21 after infection during the chronic stage of infection, when pigs did not show respiratory clinical signs any longer.

To transform real anatomical positions into two dimensional IR images, visible markers were positioned onto the pig. These metal markers served as anatomical landmarks and specific orientation points (OP) to reconstruct the exact positions of the 5th, 7th, 10th or 13th thoracic vertebra (TV) in the IR images

Two additional ROIs were positioned in the abdominal region in order to cover as much as possible of the abdominal area (Abd_1, Abd_2). Abd_1 touched tangentially the dorsal and ventral bodyline as well as the orientation point in the height of the 13th thoracic vertebra (OP13). Abd_2

was positioned adjacent to Abd_1 tangentially to the dorsal and ventral bodyline covering the remaining caudal part of the abdomen (Figure 5). Maximal abdominal surface temperatures (ϑ_{Max}) and standard deviations were recorded. The ROI of the reference body (Ref) with a radius of 18 pixels was representative for the ambient temperature measured onto the surface of a black reference body.

Mean (ϑ_M) temperature of the lung ROIs and the ROI of the reference body were documented.

Difference temperatures between mean lung ROI temperature and maximal abdominal ROI temperatures (Abd_1 or Abd_2) were calculated according to the following equation.

$$\Delta\vartheta Rx = \vartheta_{maxAbd1,\ Abd2} - \vartheta_{meanRx}$$

Measured absolute skin surface temperatures were corrected by the measurement error determined using the reference body as an allocation base.

Pathological, bacteriological and histological examination

Prior to euthanasia, those areas on the thoracal surface, which were obviously warmer than the surrounding tissue, were detected immediately by IRT imaging and directed lung biopsy was performed. If no warm areas could be detected by eye, lung biopsy was performed on the right side of the thorax between the fifth and the seventh rib. Lung tissue bioptates were divided and provided for histological and microbiological examinations.

After lung biopsy, control pigs and infected pigs were euthanized and necropsied. Macroscopic lung alterations were quantified according to the Lung Lesion Score (LLS) proposed by Hannan et al. [30] and specified in the European Pharmacopoeia for vaccine development [31] Briefly, lung tissue alterations assessed by visual inspection and palpation were recorded in a schematic map of the porcine lung consisting of 74 triangles (7 triangles for cardial and apical lobes each, 8 triangles for the accessory lobe, 19 triangles for each of the diaphragmatic lobes). The quotient of altered triangles and whole triangles of each lobe was multiplied by 5, so that each lobe could reach a maximum score of five and the whole lung a maximum lung lesion score of 35. The classification of the score was: not affected (0), slightly affected (0.1-5.0), moderately affected (5.1-10.0) and severely affected (>10.0). In addition, a score according to the Slaughterhouse Pleurisy Evaluation System (S.P.E.S.) was used, which allows a rapid and efficient quantification of pleuritis [32].

Altered lung tissue as well as lung bioptates were cultivated on selective meat and blood agar to reisolate *A.pp* or to confirm, that control pigs stayed *A.pp.*-negative until the end of the study [33]. Bacterial species diagnostic was confirmed by PCR for the ApxIIA gene and by urease activity [34,35].

Statistical analysis

Statistical analyses of data were performed using SAS® software, Version 9.3 (SAS Institute Inc., Cary, NC, USA). Right and left thoracal temperatures as well as the difference temperatures between thoracal and abdominal regions on the right and left body site were compared using student`s *t*-test for independent samples (2-sample-*t*-test) for group comparisons and *t*-test for dependent samples (1-sample-*t*-test for differences) for paired samples during the course of infection. Data were normally distributed

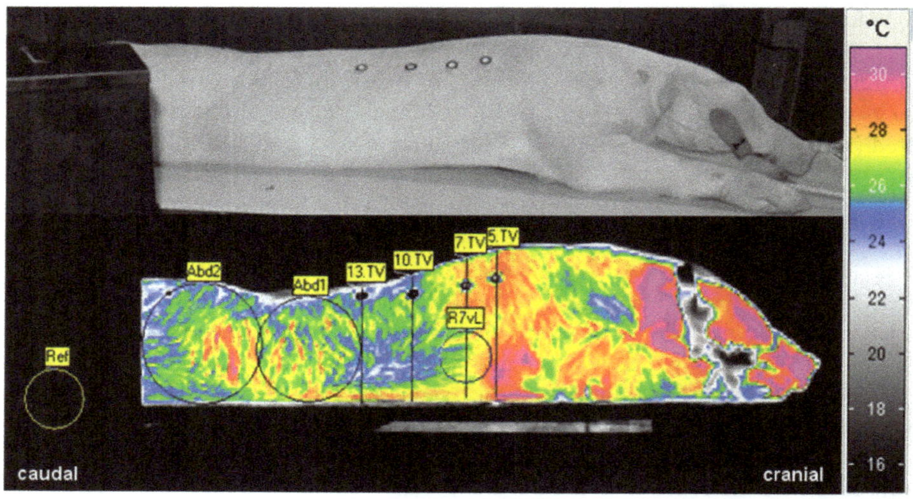

Figure 5 IR image of a highly infected pig in sternal recumbency with ROIs and reference lines. Day 4 after infection, right view. T_A = 13.6°C, colour range: SW-VarioCam, temperature range = 23–34°C, picture matrix: 384 x 288 pixel, emissivity of 0.96. 5.TV = vertical line of the 5th thoracic vertebra (TV), 7.TV = vertical line of the 7.TV,10.TV = vertical line of the 10.TV, 13.TV = vertical line of the 13.TV, Ref = ROI of the reference body, Abd1 and Abd2 = abdominal ROIs, R7vL = lung ROI of the 7.TV.

The Pearson´s correlation coefficients were calculated between these four dependent variables and various parameters as shown in Tables 2 and 3. The Spearman´s correlation coefficient was calculated for the S.P.E.S. and LLS scores. Multiple regression analysis was performed for the four diagnostic parameters, absolute left and right thoracal surface temperatures and left and right difference temperatures between thoracal and abdominal surfaces with various influencing variables as body weight, ambient temperature, body core temperature, right and left abdominal temperature, heart rate and breathing frequency (Tables 2 and 3). An analysis of covariance was performed to correct for the influence of ambient temperature onto the targeted variables.

Abbreviations

A.pp.: *Actinobacillus pleuropneumoniae*; IRT: Infrared thermography; CT: Computed tomography; ROI: Region of interest; ELISA: Enzyme-linked immunosorbant assays; CLS: Clinical score; CTS: Computed tomography score; LLS: Lung lesion score; CI: Confidence interval; PRRSV: Porcine Reproductive and Respiratory Syndrome Virus; bw: Body weight; i.m.: Intramuscularly; OP: Orientation point; TV: Thoracic vertebra; Abd_1, Abd_2: Abdominal ROIs; R10vLl: ROI of the 10.TV on the left side of the thorax; R7vLr: ROI of the 7.TV on the right side of the thorax; S.P.E.S.: Slaughterhouse Pleurisy Evaluation System.

Competing interests

The authors declare that they have no competing interests.

Authors' contributions

AM carried out the clinical examinations, performed statistical data analysis, elaborated the IRT protocol and drafted the manuscript. MB performed the statistical evaluation of data. CS was involved in IRT data analysis and statistical evaluation. MG performed computed tomography of the pigs. DH participated in the infection experiments and necropsy of the animals. RG was involved in clinical and computed tomography examinations. HS participated in the design of the studies. KHW participated in the design of the studies and in the development of the computed tomography protocol. V performed all bacteriological examinations and produced correct inoculation doses. IHP designed the study, performed the aerosol challenge, participated in necropsies, statistical evaluations and helped to draft the manuscript. All authors red and approved the final manuscript.

Acknowledgements

This research was supported by the German Research Community (DFG, HE 6419/1-1).

The authors wish to thank Prof. Mathias Ritzmann, Clinic for Swine, Ludwig-Maximilians-University, Munich, Germany, for providing biopsy equipment and giving scientific advice, Prof. Marion Hewicker-Trautwein, Institute of Pathology, University of Veterinary Medicine Hannover, Germany, for preparation and staining of histology sections and Prof. Martin Ganter and the staff of the laboratory, Clinic for Swine and Small Ruminants, Forensic Medicine and Ambulatory Services, University of Veterinary Medicine Hannover, Germany, for their support with the analysis of blood samples.

Author details

[1]Clinic for Swine and Small Ruminants, Forensic Medicine and Ambulatory Services, University of Veterinary Medicine Hannover, Bischofsholer Damm 15Aff105, D-30173 Hannover, Germany. [2]Institute for Biometry, Epidemiology and Information Processing, University of Veterinary Medicine, Hannover, Germany. [3]Institute for General Radiology and Medical Physics, University of Veterinary Medicine, Hannover, Germany. [4]Clinic for Swine, University of Veterinary Medicine, Vienna, Austria. [5]Institute for Microbiology, University of Veterinary Medicine, Hannover, Germany.

References

1. Opriessnig T, Giménez-Lirola LG, Halbur PG: **Polymicrobial respiratory disease in pigs.** *Anim Health Res Rev* 2011, **12**:133–148.
2. Hansen MS, Pors SE, Jensen HE, Bille-Hansen V, Bisgaard M, Flachs EM, Nielsen OL: **An Investigation of the pathology and pathogens associated with porcine respiratory disease complex in Denmark.** *J Comp Pathol* 2010, **143**:120–131.
3. Hensel A, Ganter M, Kipper S, Krehon S, Wittenbrink MM, Petzoldt K: **Prevalence of aerobic bacteria in bronchoalveolar lavage fluids from healthy pigs.** *Am J Vet Res* 1994, **55**:1697–1702.
4. Sorensen V, Jorsal SE, Mousing J: **Diseases of the respiratory system.** In *Diseases of Swine.* 9th edition. Edited by Straw BE, Zimmerman JJ, Allaire SD, Taylor DJ. Washington: Blackwell Publishing; 2006:149–177.
5. Brauer C, Hoeltig D, Hennig-Pauka I, Beyerbach M, Gasse H, Hewicker-Trautwein M, Gerlach GF, Waldmann KH: **Computed tomography of the pig lung: an innovative approach to the definition of the pulmonary health status.** *Tierärztl Prax G* 2011, **39**:205–214.
6. Brauer C, Hennig-Pauka I, Hoeltig D, Buettner FF, Beyerbach M, Gasse H, Gerlach GF, Waldmann KH: **Experimental *Actinobacillus pleuropneumoniae* challenge in swine: Comparison of computed tomographic and radiographic findings during disease.** *BMC Vet Res* 2012, **8**. online publication: doi:10.1186/1746-6148-8-47.
7. Heinritzi K, Beisl J: **Untersuchungen zur Verwendbarkeit der Sonographie beim Schwein.** *Dtsch tierärztl Wschr* 1995, **102**:4–15.
8. Hoeltig D, Hennig-Pauka I, Beyerbach M, Thies K, Rehm T, Gerlach GF, Waldmann KH, FUGATO-consortium IRAS: **Comparison of the diagnostic significance of clinical, radiographic and ultrasonographic results after an experimental aerosol infection of pigs with *Actinobacillus pleuropneumoniae*.** *Berl Munch Tierarztl Wochenschr* 2008, **121**:422–431.
9. Reinhold P, Rabeling B, Guenther H, Schimmel D: **Comparative evaluation of ultrasonography and lung function testing with the clinical sings and pathology of calves inoculated experimentally with *Pasteurella multocida*.** *Vet Rec* 2002, **150**:109–114.
10. Siewert C, Dänicke S, Kersten S, Brosig B, Rohweder D, Beyerbach M, Seifert H: **Difference method for analysing infrared images in pigs with elevated body temperatures.** *Z Med Phys* 2014, **24**:1.
11. Infratec GmbH: *Benutzerhandbuch VarioCAM high resolution, Stand.* ; 2009.
12. Rich PB, Dulabon GR, Douillet CD, Listwa TM, Robinson WP, Zarzaur BL, Pearlstein R, Katz LM: **Infrared thermography: a rapid, portable, and accurate technique to detect experimental pneumothorax.** *J Surg Res* 2004, **120**:163–170.
13. Schweinitz D: **Thermographic diagnostics in equine back pain.** *Vet Clin North Am Equine Pract* 1999, **15**:161–177.
14. Tunley BV, Henson FM: **Reliability and repeatability of thermographic examination and the normal thermographic image of the thoracolumbar region in the horse.** *Equine Vet J* 2004, **36**:306–312.
15. Schaefer AL, Cook NJ, Church JS, Basarab J, Perry B, Miller C, Tong AK: **The use of infrared thermography as an early indicator of bovine respiratory disease complex in calves.** *Res Vet Sci* 2007, **83**:376–384.
16. Savary P, Hauser R, Osse P, Jungbluth T, Gygax L, Wechsler B: **Eignung der Thermographie zur Erfassung von Entzündungen an den Gliedmaßen von Mastschweinen.** *Dtsch tierärztlWschr* 2008, **115**:324–329.
17. Siewert C, Hoeltig D, Brauer C, Seifert H, Hennig-Pauka I: **Medical infrared imaging of the porcine thorax for diagnosis of lung pathologies.** In *Proceedings of the 21th International Pig Veterinary Society Congress 2010 Vancouver.* Edited by D'Allaire S, Friendship R. Vancoiuver: 663. Volume II.
18. Fikackova H, Ekberg E: **Can infrared thermography be a diagnostic tool for arthralgia of the temporomandibular joint?** *Oral Surg Oral Med Oral Pathol Oral Radiol Endod* 2004, **98**:643–650.
19. So YT, Aminoff MJ, Olney RK: **The role of thermography in the evaluation of lumbosacral radiculopathy.** *Neurology* 1989, **39**:1154–1158.
20. Kateb B, Yamamoto V, Yu C, Grundfest W, Gruen JP: **Infrared thermal imaging: a review of the literature and case report.** *Neuroimage* 2009, **47**:T154–T126.
21. Zaproudina N, Varmavuo V, Airaksinen O, Naerhi M: **Reproducibility of infrared thermography measurements in healthy individuals.** *Physiol Meas* 2008, **29**:515–524.
22. Huygen FJ, Niehof S, Klein J, Zijlstra FJ: **Computer-assisted skin videothermography is a highly sensitive quality tool in the diagnosis and monitoring of complex regional pain syndrome type I.** *Eur J Appl Physiol* 2004, **91**:516–524.

23. Henssge C, Madea B, Benecke M, Berg S, Geyh MA, Karger B, Krause D, Lignitz E, Rothschild MA: **Leichenerscheinungen und Todeszeitbestimmung.** In *Handbuch gerichtliche Medizin.* Edited by Brinkmann B, Madea B. Berlin: Springer; 2004:102.
24. Roehlinger P: **Zur Anwendung der Infrarottechnik in der Veterinärmedizin.** *Arch Exper Vet med* 1979, **33:**851.
25. Leiner G, Franz B, Strutzberg K, Gerlach GF: **A novel enzyme-linked immunosorbent assay using the recombinant *Actinobacillus pleuropneumoniae* ApxII antigen for diagnosis of pleuropneumonia in pig herds.** *Clin Diagn Lab Immunol* 1999, **6:**630–632.
26. Jacobsen M, Nielsen J, Nielsen R: **Comparison of virulence of different *Actinobacillus pleuropneumoniae* serotypes and biotypes using an aerosol infection model.** *Vet Microbiol* 1996, **49:**159–168.
27. Maas A, Jacobsen ID, Meens J, Gerlach GF: **Use of an *Actinobacillus pleuropneumoniae* multiple mutant as a vaccine that allows differentiation of vaccinated and infected animals.** *Infect Immun* 2006, **74:**4124–4132.
28. Hoeltig D, Hennig-Pauka I, Thies K, Rehm T, Beyerbach M, Strutzberg-Minder K, Gerlach GF, Waldmann KH, FUGATO-consortium IRAS: **A novel Respiratory Health Score (RHS) supports a role of acute lung damage and pig breed in the course of an *Actinobacillus pleuropneumoniae* infection.** *BMC Vet Res* 2009, **5:**14.
29. Diakides NA, Bronzino JD: *Medical Infrared Imaging.* Boca Raton: CRC Press; 2008.
30. Hannan PC, Bhogal BS, Fish JP: **Tylosin tartrate and tiamutilin effects on experimental piglet pneumonia induced with pneumonic pig lung homogenate containing mycoplasmas, bacteria and viruses.** *Res Vet Sci* 1982, **33:**76–88.
31. European Pharmacopoeia (Ph. Eur.): **Porcine actinobacillosis vaccine (inactivated).** In *European Pharmacopoeia 7th edition.* 2008:926–927. Section: Vaccines.
32. Dottori M, Nigrelli AD, Bonilauri P, Merialdi G, Gozio S, Cominotti F: **Proposta per un nuovo sistema di punteggiatura delle pleuriti suine in sede di macellazione: La griglia SPES (Slaughterhouse Pleurisy Evaluation System).** *Large Anim Rev* 2007, **13:**161–165.
33. Jacobsen MJ, Nielsen JP: **Developement and evaluation of a selective and indicative medium for isolation of *Actinobacillus pleuropneumoniae*.** *Vet Microbiol* 1995, **47:**191–197.
34. Buettner FFR, Bendallah IM, Bosse JT, Dreckmann K, Nash JHE, Langford PR, Gerlach GF: **Analysis of the *Actinobacillus pleuropneumoniae* ArcA regulon identifies fumarate reductase as a determinant of virulence.** *Infect Immun* 2008, **76:**2284–2295.
35. Maas A, Meens J, Baltes N, Hennig-Pauka I, Gerlach GF: **Development of a DIVA subunit vaccine against *Actinobacillus pleuropneumoniae* infection.** *Vaccine* 2006, **24:**7226–7237.

PERMISSIONS

All chapters in this book were first published in VR, by BioMed Central; hereby published with permission under the Creative Commons Attribution License or equivalent. Every chapter published in this book has been scrutinized by our experts. Their significance has been extensively debated. The topics covered herein carry significant findings which will fuel the growth of the discipline. They may even be implemented as practical applications or may be referred to as a beginning point for another development.

The contributors of this book come from diverse backgrounds, making this book a truly international effort. This book will bring forth new frontiers with its revolutionizing research information and detailed analysis of the nascent developments around the world.

We would like to thank all the contributing authors for lending their expertise to make the book truly unique. They have played a crucial role in the development of this book. Without their invaluable contributions this book wouldn't have been possible. They have made vital efforts to compile up to date information on the varied aspects of this subject to make this book a valuable addition to the collection of many professionals and students.

This book was conceptualized with the vision of imparting up-to-date information and advanced data in this field. To ensure the same, a matchless editorial board was set up. Every individual on the board went through rigorous rounds of assessment to prove their worth. After which they invested a large part of their time researching and compiling the most relevant data for our readers.

The editorial board has been involved in producing this book since its inception. They have spent rigorous hours researching and exploring the diverse topics which have resulted in the successful publishing of this book. They have passed on their knowledge of decades through this book. To expedite this challenging task, the publisher supported the team at every step. A small team of assistant editors was also appointed to further simplify the editing procedure and attain best results for the readers.

Apart from the editorial board, the designing team has also invested a significant amount of their time in understanding the subject and creating the most relevant covers. They scrutinized every image to scout for the most suitable representation of the subject and create an appropriate cover for the book.

The publishing team has been an ardent support to the editorial, designing and production team. Their endless efforts to recruit the best for this project, has resulted in the accomplishment of this book. They are a veteran in the field of academics and their pool of knowledge is as vast as their experience in printing. Their expertise and guidance has proved useful at every step. Their uncompromising quality standards have made this book an exceptional effort. Their encouragement from time to time has been an inspiration for everyone.

The publisher and the editorial board hope that this book will prove to be a valuable piece of knowledge for researchers, students, practitioners and scholars across the globe.

LIST OF CONTRIBUTORS

Jana Pietschmann, Sandra Blome and Martin Beer
Institute of Diagnostic Virology, Friedrich-Loeffler-Institut, Suedufer 10, 17493 Greifswald—Insel Riems, Germany

José Manuel Sánchez-Vizcaíno and Lina Mur
VISAVET Center and Animal Health Department, Veterinary School, Universidad Complutense de Madrid, Avenida Puerta de Hierro s/n, 28040 Madrid, Spain

Ricardo Pérez-Sánchez and Ana Oleaga
Parasitología, IRNASA (CSIC), Cordel de Merinas, 40-52, 37008 Salamanca, Spain

Fernando Rodríguez
IRTA, Centre de Recerca en Sanitat Animal (CReSA, IRTA-UAB), Campus de la Universitat Autònoma de Barcelona, 08193 Bellaterra, Spain

Oscar Cabezón
IRTA, Centre de Recerca en Sanitat Animal (CReSA, IRTA-UAB), Campus de la Universitat Autònoma de Barcelona, 08193 Bellaterra, Spain
Servei d'Ecopatologia de Fauna Salvatge, Departament de Medicina i Cirurgia Animals, Universitat Autònoma de Barcelona, 08193 Bellaterra, Spain

Sara Muñoz-González, Marta Pérez-Simó and Llilianne Ganges
IRTA, Centre de Recerca en Sanitat Animal (CReSA, IRTA-UAB), Campus de la Universitat Autònoma de Barcelona, 08193 Bellaterra, Spain
OIE Reference Laboratory for Classical Swine Fever, IRTA-CReSA, Campus de la Universitat Autònoma de Barcelona, 08193 Barcelona, Spain

Rosa Rosell
IRTA, Centre de Recerca en Sanitat Animal (CReSA, IRTA-UAB), Campus de la Universitat Autònoma de Barcelona, 08193 Bellaterra, Spain
OIE Reference Laboratory for Classical Swine Fever, IRTA-CReSA, Campus de la Universitat Autònoma de Barcelona, 08193 Barcelona, Spain
Departament d'Agricultura, Ramaderia, Pesca i Alimentació (DARP), Centre de Recerca en Sanitat Animal (CReSA, IRTA-UAB), Campus de la Universitat Autònoma de Barcelona, 08193 Bellaterra, Spain

Andreu Colom-Cadena, Santiago Lavín and Ignasi Marco
Servei d'Ecopatologia de Fauna Salvatge, Departament de Medicina i Cirurgia Animals, Universitat Autònoma de Barcelona, 08193 Bellaterra, Spain

Lorenzo Fraile
Departament de Producció Animal, ETSEA, Universidad de Lleida, 25198 Lleida, Spain

Paloma Martínez de la Riva and Javier Domínguez
Departamento de Biotecnología, Instituto Nacional de Investigación y Tecnología Agraria y Alimentaria (INIA), 28040 Madrid, Spain

Amy L. Greer, Kelsey Spence and Emma Gardner
Department of Population Medicine, Ontario Veterinary College, University of Guelph, Guelph, ON N1G 2W1, Canada

Anna Borgström, Simone Scherrer, Constanze Kirchgässner, Sarah Schmitt, Daniel Frei and Max M. Wittenbrink
Institute of Veterinary Bacteriology, Vetsuisse Faculty, University of Zurich, Winterthurerstrasse 270, CH 8057 Zurich, Switzerland

A. G. Arruda and Z. Poljak
Department of Population Medicine, Ontario Veterinary College, University of Guelph, 50 Stone Rd East, Guelph, ON N1G 2W1, Canada

D. Knowles and A. McLean
Department of Computer Science, Computational Epidemiology and Public Health Informatics Lab, University of Saskatchewan, 176 Thorvaldson Bldg, 110 Science Place, Saskatoon, SK S7N 5C9, Canada

Katja Schulz, Christoph Staubach and Franz J. Conraths
Friedrich-Loeffler-Institut, Federal Research Institute for Animal Health, Institute of Epidemiology, Südufer 10, 17493 Greifswald, Insel Riems, Germany

Clémentine Calba and Marisa Peyre
Centre de Coopération Internationale en Recherche Agronomique Pour le Développement (CIRAD), Département ES, UPR AGIRs, TA C22/E, Campus International de Baillarguet, 34398 Montpellier Cedex 5, France

Nguyen Van Diep, Masuo Sueyoshi, Junzo Norimine, Takuya Hirai, Ohnmar Myint, Angeline Ping Ping Teh, Uda Zahli Izzati, Naoyuki Fuke and Ryoji Yamaguchi
Department of Veterinary Medicine, Faculty of Agriculture, University of Miyazaki, Gakuen-kibanadai-nishi-1-1, Miyazaki 889-2192, Japan

Longxian Zhang, Qinge Ren, Fuchang Yu and Yurong Yang
College of Animal Science and Veterinary Medicine, Henan Agricultural University, Zhengzhou 450002, Henan, People's Republic of China

Haiyan Wang
College of Animal Science and Veterinary Medicine, Henan Agricultural University, Zhengzhou 450002, Henan, People's Republic of China
Department of Animal Science, Henan Vocational College of Agriculture, Zhongmu, 451450 Henan, People's Republic of China

Nobuhiro Takemae, Ryota Tsunekuni and Yuko Uchida
Division of Transboundary Animal Disease, National Institute of Animal Health, NARO, 3-1-5 Kannondai, Tsukuba, Ibaraki 305-0856, Japan

Takehiko Saito
Division of Transboundary Animal Disease, National Institute of Animal Health, NARO, 3-1-5 Kannondai, Tsukuba, Ibaraki 305-0856, Japan
Thailand- Japan Zoonotic Diseases Collaboration Center, Kasetklang, Chatuchak, Bangkok 10900, Thailand
United Graduate School of Veterinary Sciences, Gifu University, 1-1, Yanagito, Gifu, Gifu 501-1112, Japan

Toshihiro Ito
The Avian Zoonosis Research Center, Faculty of Agriculture, Tottori University, 4-101 Koyama-cho Minami, Tottori, Tottori 680-8550, Japan

Fang Xie, Gang Li, Long Zhou, Yanhe Zhang, Ning Cui, Siguo Liu and Chunlai Wang
State Key Laboratory of Veterinary Biotechnology, Division of Bacterial Diseases, Harbin Veterinary Research Institute, Chinese Academy of Agricultural Sciences, Harbin, Heilongjiang, People's Republic of China

Scott Dee, Casey Neill and Gordon Spronk
Pipestone Applied Research, Pipestone Veterinary Services, 1300 Hwy 75 S, Pipestone, MN 56164, USA

Aaron Singrey, Travis Clement, Jane Christopher-Hennings and Eric Nelson
Animal Disease Research and Diagnostic Laboratory, South Dakota State University, Brookings, SD, USA

Roger Cochrane and Cassandra Jones
Department of Grain Science, Kansas State University, Manhattan, KS, USA

Gilbert Patterson
Center for Animal Health and Food Safety, University of Minnesota, St. Paul, MN, USA

Xiaohui Liu, Ting Ouyang, Teng Ma, Hongsheng Ouyang, Daxin Pang and Linzhu Ren
Jilin Provincial Key Laboratory of Animal Embryo Engineering, College of Animal Sciences, Jilin University, Changchun, Jilin 130062, China

Klaas Dietze, Anna Tucakov, Tatjana Engel, Sabine Wirtz, Klaus Depner, Anja Globig, Robert Kammerer and Susan Mouchantat
Friedrich-Loeffler-Institut, Federal Research Institute for Animal Health, Südufer 10, 17493 Greifswald Insel Riems, Germany

Lian F. Thomas, William A. de Glanville and E. Anne J. Cook
Centre for Infection Immunity and Evolution, Institute for Immunology and Infection Research, School of Biological Sciences, University of Edinburgh, Ashworth Labs, West Mains Rd, Edinburgh EH9 3JT, UK
International Livestock Research Institute, Nairobi 00100, Kenya

Richard P. Bishop and Cynthia Onzere
International Livestock Research Institute, Nairobi 00100, Kenya

Eric M. Fèvre
International Livestock Research Institute, Nairobi 00100, Kenya
Institute for Infection and Global Health, University of Liverpool, Leahurst Campus, Chester High Road, Neston CH64 7TE, UK

Michael T. Mcintosh and Karissa A. Lemire
United States Department of Agriculture, Foreign Animal Disease Diagnostic Laboratory, National Veterinary Services Laboratories, Animal and Plant Health Inspection Services, Greenport, NY 1944, USA

Kinga Urbaniak, Krzysztof Kwit, Małgorzata Pomorska-Mól, Barbara Frącek and Zygmunt Pejsak
Department of Swine Diseases, National Veterinary Research Institute, 57 Partyzantów Avenue, 24-100 Puławy, Poland

Iwona Markowska-Daniel
Department of Swine Diseases, National Veterinary Research Institute, 57 Partyzantów Avenue, 24-100 Puławy, Poland
Laboratory of Veterinary Epidemiology and Economics, Faculty of Veterinary Medicine, Warsaw University of Life Sciences, 159c Nowoursynowska Street, 02-776 Warsaw, Poland

Andrzej Kowalczyk
Department of Swine Diseases, National Veterinary Research Institute, 57 Partyzantów Avenue, 24-100 Puławy, Poland
Wrocław Research Centre EIT+, 147 Stabłowicka Street, 54-066 Wrocław, Poland

P. Sastre, A. Monedero, T. Ruiz, A. Sanz and P. Rueda
Inmunología y Genética Aplicada S. A. (INGENASA), Madrid, Spain

C. Gallardo and M. Arias
European Union Reference Laboratory for ASF (EURL), Centro de Investigación en Sanidad Animal, INIA, Madrid, Spain

Ji Eun Yu, Ji-Eun Shin, Jienny Lee, In-Soo Cho and Se-Eun Choe
Viral Disease Division, Animal and Plant Quarantine Agency, Gimcheon 39660, Republic of Korea

Hyeonjeong Kang
Viral Disease Division, Animal and Plant Quarantine Agency, Gimcheon 39660, Republic of Korea
Animal Virology Laboratory, School of Life Sciences, Kyungpook National University, Daegu 41566, Republic of Korea

Sang-Ho Cha
Viral Disease Division, Animal and Plant Quarantine Agency, Gimcheon 39660, Republic of Korea
PRRS research Laboratory, Viral Diseases Division, Animal and Plant Quarantine Agency, Gimcheon 39660, Republic of Korea

Changhee Lee
Animal Virology Laboratory, School of Life Sciences, Kyungpook National University, Daegu 41566, Republic of Korea

Areum Kang and Won-Il Kim
College of Veterinary Medicine, Jeonbuk National University, Iksan 54596Republic of Korea

Feng-shan Gao, Lei Feng, Ping Jiang, Hua Gao, Xiao-xin Zhai, Zong-hui Zhang and Xiao Hu
Department of Bioengineering, |College of Life Science and Technology, Dalian University, Xuefu street 10, Dalian, Liaoning 116622, People's Republic of China

Zi-bin Li
Department of Microbiology and Immunology, College of Veterinary Medicine, China Agricultural University, Beijing 100094, People's Republic of China

Slawomir Gonkowski, Krystyna Makowska and Jaroslaw Calka
Department of Clinical Physiology, Faculty of Veterinary Medicine, University of Warmia and Mazury, Oczapowski Str, 13 Olsztyn, Poland

Hongliang Zhang, Zhijun Tian, Chunxiao Liu, Jiazeng Chen, Yun Bai, Zhen Li, Lirun Xiang, Qian Wang, Jinmei Peng, Tongqing An and Xuehui Cai
State Key Laboratory of Veterinary Biotechnology, Harbin Veterinary Research Institute, Chinese Academy of Agricultural Sciences, Harbin 150001, China

Chaoliang Leng, Hongyue Zhai, Yunchao Kan and Lunguang Yao
Henan Key Laboratory of Insect Biology in Funiu Mountain, Henan Provincial Engineering Laboratory of Insects Bio-reactor, China-UK-NYNU-RRes Joint Laboratory of Insect Biology, Nanyang NormalUniversity, Nanyang 473061, China

Guangzhi Tong
Shanghai Veterinary Research Institute, Chinese Academy of Agricultural Sciences, No. 518, Ziyue Road, Minhang District, Shanghai 200241, China

Xufu Yang
North Guangdong Collaborative Innovation and Development Center of Pig Farming and Disease Control, Shaoguan University, Shaoguan 512005, China

María Dolores Contreras-Aguilar, Silvia Martínez-Subiela, Jose Joaquín Cerón and Fernando Tecles
Interdisciplinary Laboratory of Clinical Analysis (Interlab-UMU), Veterinary School, Campus of Excellence Mare Nostrum, University of Murcia, 30100, Espinardo, Murcia, Spain

Damián Escribano
Department of Food and Animal Science, School of Veterinary Medicine, Universitat Autònoma de Barcelona, 08193, Bellaterra, Barcelona, Spain

Silvia Martínez-Miró
Department of Animal Production, Veterinary school, Campus of Excellence Mare Nostrum, Murcia, Spain

Dinko Novosel
Department of Pathology, Croatian Veterinary Institute, Savska cesta 143, 10000 Zagreb, Croatia
Department for Animal science, Faculty of Agriculture, University of Zagreb, Svetosimunska 25, 10000 Zagreb, Croatia

Daniel Cadar
WHO Collaborating Centre for Arbovirus and Haemorrhagic Fever Reference and Research, National Reference Centre for Tropical Infectious Diseases, Bernhard Nocht Institute for Tropical Medicine, Bernhard-Nocht-Strasse 74, 20359 Hamburg, Germany
Department of Microbiology and Infectious Diseases, Faculty of Veterinary Science, Immunology, Szent István University, István u. 2, Budapest 1078, Hungary

Tamás Tuboly and Attila Cságola
Department of Microbiology and Infectious Diseases, Faculty of Veterinary Science, Immunology, Szent István University, István u. 2, Budapest 1078, Hungary

Andreja Jungic
Department for Virology, Croatian Veterinary Institute, Savska cesta 143, 10000 Zagreb, Croatia

Tomasz Stadejek
Department of Pathology and Veterinary Diagnostic, Faculty of Veterinary Medicine, University of Life Science, Nowoursynowska 159C, 02-776 Warsaw, Poland

Tahar Ait-Ali
The Roslin Institute and Royal (Dick) School of Veterinary Studies, University of Edinburgh, Easter Bush, Edingburgh, United Kingdom

Index

www.ingramcontent.com/pod-product-compliance
Lightning Source LLC
LaVergne TN
LVHW080725210926
848485LV00003B/518
* 9 7 8 1 6 3 9 8 7 1 6 7 4 *